Neuroendocrine Tumors: Review of Pathology, Molecular and Therapeutic Advances

Aejaz Nasir • Domenico Coppola
Editors

Neuroendocrine Tumors: Review of Pathology, Molecular and Therapeutic Advances

Springer

Editors
Aejaz Nasir
Diagnostic & Experimental Pathology
Lilly Research Laboratories,
Eli Lilly & Co.
Indianapolis
Indiana
USA

Domenico Coppola
University of South Florida
H. Lee Moffitt Cancer Ctr & Res
Tampa
Florida
USA

ISBN 978-1-4939-8047-5 ISBN 978-1-4939-3426-3 (eBook)
DOI 10.1007/978-1-4939-3426-3

Softcover reprint of the hardcover 1st edition 2016

Printed on acid-free paper

This Springer imprint is published by Springer Nature
The registered company is Springer Science+Business Media LLC New York

This book is dedicated

With love to:
My dear mother, *Bilqis Jehan*, and late father, *Muhammad Anwar*, for nurturing and supporting me to become a healer

With honor and gratitude to:
Prof. A. H. Nagi and *Prof. Hans E. Kaiser,* my role models, who profoundly influenced my career
Prof. Julia M. Polak and *Prof. Larry Kvols,* who inspired me to learn and practice Neuroendocrine Tumor Pathology for patients
Aejaz Nasir, MD, MPhil, FCAP

With love to:
My wife *Beverly* and to my family – *Stefano, David, Jennifer, Marc, and Christina* for their continuous support
Domenico Coppola, MD, FCAP

Preface

Neuroendocrine neoplasms involve many different organs in the human body and are characterized by diverse biology, unusual clinicopathologic and molecular profiles, and a number of unique challenges in their clinical management. With the exception of specialized centers, most institutions do not deal with these in sufficient frequency. Until recently, there has been lack of uniformly agreed diagnostic schemes and treatment guidelines for managing these patients. When dealing with these unusual neoplasms, some of the major challenges faced by the practicing pathologists include reference to internationally agreed, diagnostically reproducible, and clinically relevant classification schemes; unique patterns of tumor histology; and differentiation and patient outcomes. In recent years, there has been an unprecedented progress in diagnosis, prognostication, and treatment of these neoplasms both in the United States and Europe. In addition to efforts at standardization of histopathologic classification and grading schemes, recent advances in molecular pathology, diagnostic methodologies, and targeted therapeutics have also contributed a great deal to the recent progress in this field.

At the H. Lee Moffitt Cancer Center and Research Institute (Tampa, FL, USA), neuroendocrine tumor pathology has been practiced for many years by dedicated subspecialty pathologists, who serve a critical role not only in providing the highest standards in pathologic evaluation and diagnosis but they have also been an integral part of a large multidisciplinary NET patient management team led by world-renowned neuroendocrine oncologists, Professor Larry Kvols, M.D., and Jonathan Strosberg, M.D. Collaborative team efforts by pathologists, oncologists, surgeons, radiologists, and advanced researchers have led to a model of service excellence, which has made tremendous contribution to improve the quality of diagnostic service and patient care at this global center of excellence. Members of the clinical and subspecialty pathology team have also made major contributions to the recent development of comprehensive diagnostic and clinical guidelines by the North American Neuroendocrine Tumor Society (NANETS), the European Neuroendocrine Tumor Society (ENETS), and the World Health Organization (WHO).

In order to address some of the variations in the earlier NET classification schemes, the WHO has published revised histologic classifications of neuroendocrine neoplasms of the gastrointestinal tract and lung, including clinical, histopathologic, and molecular genetic features of these neoplasms. Furthermore, to help modern pathologists play an active role in the diagnosis, prognostication, and management of NET patients, a multidisciplinary team of experts in NETs proposed a consensus statement (Klimstra et al. 2010) on minimal data to be included in the NET pathology reports to ensure consistent patient management and reproducibility of data from clinical trials. It was heartening that agreement was reached among the members of the expert panel about the importance of tumor grading, staging landmarks, prognostic factors assessable by routine histology, the potential for tumors to metastasize, and the current status of advanced immunohistochemical and molecular testing for treatment-related biomarkers. This consensus statement could serve as an important resource for pathologists in their NET pathology practice. Another important advance in recent years is the addition of NET staging to the seventh edition of the *AJCC Cancer Staging Handbook*. The TNM staging for NETs of the GI tract and pancreas was proposed in line with the adenocarcinomas of these sites.

With the current progress in the practice of NET pathology, neuroendocrine markers, tissue-specific transcription factors (TTF1, CDX2), and other emerging immunohistochemical and molecular markers will need to be used more effectively by incorporating their use in the overall patient management plan. This will provide pathologists with more effective approaches to identify neuroendocrine differentiation in human cancer tissues, to workup metastatic neuroendocrine carcinomas (NECs) with unknown primaries, and to validate and assess newer molecular biomarkers of prognostic or therapeutic relevance. By implementation of these approaches, pathologists will make substantial contributions to advance the field of personalized oncology for NET patients.

Because of the differences in biology and clinical course of pancreatic, thoracic, and gastrointestinal NETs, advanced imaging and molecular diagnostic approaches will play an important role in the pathologic classification of NETs in the future. Although it is conventional to classify NETs based on embryologic origin (foregut, midgut, hindgut), anatomic location (lung, pancreas, GI tract), and their secreted products (insulin, glucagon, gastrin, others), the anatomic site of origin (pancreatic vs. nonpancreatic) is now being recognized as a key determinant decision regarding patient management because of important differences in NET biology and clinical course at these sites. Some NETs actively secrete hormones resulting in well-recognized clinical syndromes (functional NETs like insulinomas, VIPomas, etc.). In order to provide clinical teams with comprehensive surgical pathology reports for patient management, pathologists need to workup NET cases to be able to render both histopathologic and clinical classification in a given case of NET.

With improved understanding of the diverse biology and clinical course of NE malignancies, it is also becoming evident that NETs need to be separated into pancreatic and nonpancreatic NETs both for enrollment in clinical trials and treatment in the clinic. Until recently, there were only a few therapeutic options for patients with low- and intermediate-grade NETs. Promising clinical advances are being made to delay NET growth and improve patient survival. Recognition of PI3K/Akt/mTOR pathway, angiogenesis, and other biologic pathways as important "druggable" therapeutic targets offers further hope for NET patients in the future. A number of targeted therapies are under investigation and will offer additional therapeutic choices for NET patients in the future. In order to personalize therapies for individual NET patients, robust methodologies for predictive and prognostic biomarkers will need to be validated and implemented, so that newer targeted therapies may be tailored for specific subsets of NET patients. Emerging data suggest clinical relevance to assess methylguanine-methyltransferase (MGMT), PTEN, and TSC2 and other emerging biomarkers – findings that need to be validated in future studies.

In recent years, we offered a subspecialty training course in NET pathology for practicing pathologists and pathology residents and fellows titled "Diagnosis and Prognostication of Gastro-entero-pancreatic Neuroendocrine Neoplasms: A Multidisciplinary Approach" at the Joint American Society for Clinical Pathology (ASCP) Annual Meeting/World Association of Societies of Pathology and Laboratory Medicine (WASPaLM) XXVI World Congress in Las Vegas (NV, USA) (2011) and at the 2012 ASCP Annual Meeting in Boston (MA, USA). With the outstanding reviews and feedback from the audience, we felt the need for a more comprehensive reference book with a well-integrated subspecialty diagnostic pathology content, including a balanced review of recent advances in molecular aspects and targeted therapies for NET patients. In this regard, we are highly appreciative of the Anatomic Pathology faculty at Moffitt Cancer Center and at other institutions for sharing their advanced expertise in NET pathology. By providing a fully updated state of the science in NET pathology, this book is aimed to empower the practicing pathologists involved in NET diagnosis in their service work and the pathology residents, fellows, oncologists, radiologists, and NET researchers with the latest advances in the field.

Recent developments will serve as a landmark in the future progress in neuroendocrine tumor pathology and oncology and will set higher standards and uniformity both in the diagnostic services and patient care. In the near future, the field is also going to move closer to its twenty-first century goal of implementation of personalized oncology in order to maximize benefit to these patients. Some of the key areas of advancement for pathologists, who are actively engaged in the multidisciplinary management of NET patients, include more unified pathologic classification, histologic grading, reporting schemes, and molecular characterization, especially for development of promising biomarkers and diagnostics to predict response or resistance of NETs to more effective and safer targeted therapeutics.

We are confident that this comprehensive reference book with state of the science in cutting-edge advances in NET pathology will enable our fellow pathologists to take on a proactive role in application of recent NET pathologic typing, grading, and staging guidelines and integrate these with molecular and targeted therapeutic advances as part of a multidisciplinary model of NET oncology in the clinic. We envision that by doing so, pathologists can become major contributors to the forthcoming advancements not only in the diagnosis of NETs but also in the clinical management of neuroendocrine tumor patients in the twenty-first century.

Indianapolis, IN, USA — Aejaz Nasir
Tampa, FL, USA — Domenico Coppola

Contents

Part I General Topics in Neuroendocrine Tumor Pathology

Neuroendocrine Tumor Classification Systems: Grading 3
Shabnam Seydafkan and Domenico Coppola

Neuroendocrine Tumor Classification Systems: Staging 21
Shabnam Seydafkan and Domenico Coppola

Differential Diagnosis of Neuroendocrine Tumors 31
Kun Jiang and Domenico Coppola

Role of Immunohistochemistry and Molecular Genetics in Neuroendocrine Tumors 43
Kun Jiang, Ujalla Sheikh, Aejaz Nasir, and Domenico Coppola

Gastroenteropancreatic: Poorly Differentiated Neuroendocrine Carcinoma 57
Mulazim H. Bukhari, Ujalla Sheikh, Jalil Muhammad, Domenico Coppola, and Aejaz Nasir

Part II Systemic Aspects of Neuroendocrine Tumor Pathology

Neuroendocrine Neoplasms of the Brain 83
Yuan Frank Shan, Fulin Wang, Changshu Ke, and Meng Yan

Medullary Thyroid Carcinoma 117
Pablo Valderrabano, Stacey Simons, Jaime Montilla-Soler, Tuya Pal, Victor Zota, Kristen Otto, Bryan McIver, Domenico Coppola, and Marino E. Leon

Neuroendocrine Tumors (NETs) of the Mediastinum and Thymus 141
Sameer Al Diffalha and Farah Khalil

Neuroendocrine Tumors of the Lung 153
Farah Khalil

Breast Carcinomas with Neuroendocrine Features (Neuroendocrine Carcinomas of the Breast) 179
Marilin Rosa, Ujalla Sheikh, and Aejaz Nasir

Neuroendocrine Tumors of the Esophagus 203
Shabnam Seydafkan and Domenico Coppola

Neuroendocrine Neoplasms of the Stomach 217
Evita Henderson-Jackson, Ujalla Sheikh, Jalil Muhammad, Domenico Coppola, and Aejaz Nasir

Neuroendocrine Neoplasms of the Pancreas 245
Michael Markow and Barbara Ann Centeno

Neuroendocrine Neoplasms of the Small Intestine 273
Shabnam Seydafkan and Domenico Coppola

Neuroendocrine Neoplasms of the Appendix 289
Ujalla Sheikh, Evita Henderson-Jackson, Jalil Muhammad, Domenico Coppola, and Aejaz Nasir

Neuroendocrine Neoplasms of the Colon and Rectum 309
Masoumeh Ghayouri, Shabnam Seydafkan, Aejaz Nasir, and Domenico Coppola

Adrenal Neuroendocrine Tumors: Pheochromocytoma and Neuroblastic Tumors 323
Carmen M. Perrino and Debra L. Zynger

Neuroendocrine Tumors of the Urinary Bladder and Molecular Features 359
Jasreman Dhillon

Neuroendocrine Tumors of the Prostate and Molecular Features 369
Jasreman Dhillon

Neuroendocrine Tumors of the Female Genital Tract 379
Ozlen Saglam and Ardeshir Hakam

Pathology of Merkel Cell Carcinoma (Primary Neuroendocrine Carcinoma of the Skin) 393
Carlos N. Prieto-Granada and Jane L. Messina

Extraskeletal Ewing Sarcoma/Primitive Neuroectodermal Tumor 425
Rania Shamekh, Vicky Pham, and Marilyn M. Bui

Part III Molecular & Therapeutic Advances in Neuroendocrine Tumor Pathology

Molecular Pathology of Neuroendocrine Tumor: The Era of Targeted Therapeutics . . . 437
Anthony M. Magliocco

Somatostatin Receptors in Human Neuroendocrine Tumors . . . 445
Aejaz Nasir, Ujalla Sheikh, Jalil Muhammad, and Domenico Coppola

Pathologic Angiogenesis in Neuroendocrine Tumors . . . 457
Aejaz Nasir, Ujalla Sheikh, Jalil Muhammad, and Domenico Coppola

Molecular Targets in Human Neuroendocrine Tumors . . . 471
Ujalla Sheikh, Jalil Muhammad, Domenico Coppola, and Aejaz Nasir

Recent Advances in Molecular Pathology of Neuroendocrine Neoplasms . . . 487
Aejaz Nasir, Ujalla Sheikh, Kevin G Neill, Kun Jiang, Jalil Muhammad, and Domenico Coppola

Targeted Therapies for Neuroendocrine Neoplasms . . . 505
Heloisa Prado Soares and Jonathan Strosberg

Future Prospects in Neuroendocrine Tumor Pathology . . . 517
Aejaz Nasir and Domenico Coppola

Index . . . 525

Part I
General Topics in Neuroendocrine Tumor Pathology

Neuroendocrine Tumor Classification Systems: Grading

Shabnam Seydafkan and Domenico Coppola

General

Neuroendocrine tumors (NETs) are a diverse group of tumors that arise from neuroendocrine cells throughout the body and have similar features. NETs are classified according to their anatomical site; tumor differentiation; a marker of cell proliferation, for example, Ki-67; tumor grade and stage; and hormones or amines produced (Fig. 1).

In some instances, the term carcinoma has been applied to NET tumors. For example, versions 2001 and 2004 of the WHO classifications of digestive and pancreatic NETs used the term carcinoma when neoplasm had obvious evidence of malignant behavior, such as vascular invasion, gross local invasion, or metastases. However, the term neuroendocrine tumor has no prognostic or therapeutic meaning, and it should not be used in a pathology report without specifying the tumor grade and/or differentiation. The term carcinoid tumor was used in the past for tumors with or without the carcinoid syndrome (WHO 1980).

The presence of clinical symptoms and syndromes due to excessive hormone secretion, also referred as tumor functionality, has been applied to the tumor nomenclature for those NETs producing active biological products. An example of these is the pancreatic well-differentiated tumors producing insulin, glucagon, and gastrin. Although functionality has a role in determining prognosis in some subtypes (e.g., insulinomas are generally very indolent), it is the grade and stage of the tumor that determine the biological behavior of a functioning NET. Therefore, the pathological diagnosis of functional and nonfunctional NETs at the same anatomical site remains identical (Fig. 2).

S. Seydafkan, MD • D. Coppola, MD (✉)
Department of Anatomic Pathology, Moffitt Cancer Center, Tampa, FL, USA
e-mail: domenico.coppola@moffitt.org

A. Nasir, D. Coppola (eds.), *Neuroendocrine Tumors: Review of Pathology, Molecular and Therapeutic Advances*, DOI 10.1007/978-1-4939-3426-3_1

Table 3 General and tumour specific markers of GEP-NETs (27)
General markers
Chromogranins
Chromogranin A
Chromogranin B
Secretogranin II
Secretogranin III (1B1075)
Secretogranin IV (HISL-19)
Secretogranin V (7B2)
Secretogranin VI (NESP55)
Neuron Specific Enolase
Pancreatic polypeptide
Chorionic gonadotrophin
Tumor specific markers
Carcinoid tumors
24 h Urine 5-hydroxyindole acetic acid
24 h Urine 5-hydroxy-tryptophan
Plasma serotonin
Insulinoma
Fasting insulin
Fasting pro-insulin
Gastrinoma
Fasting/stimulated gastrin
Glucagonoma
Fasting glucagon
VIP-oma
Fasting vasoactive intestinal peptide
Somatostatinoma
Fasting somatostatin

Fig. 1 Summary of neuroendocrine tumor specific markers (Kizilgul et al. [1])

Table 2 Nomenclature, incidence, location and malignancy of pancreatic NETs

Name	Hormone	Cell type	Incidence (M)	Pancreas (%)	Duodenum (%)	Malignant (%)
Insulinoma	Insulin	β islet cells	1/1.25	>99		5-11
Gastrinoma	Gastrin	G cells	1/2.5	21-65	6-35	60
Glucagonoma	Glucagon	α cells	<1/5	>99		>70
VIPoma	VIP	δ cells	<1/5	85-90	10-15	50
Somatostatinoma	Somatostain	δ cells	<1/10	50	50	90
Nonfunctioning	Neuron-specific enolase, PP	F cells	1/5	>99		>50

Norton et al. Surgery: basic science and clinical evidence; 2000, 919-953. Reproduced with permission.

Fig. 2 Functional neuroendocrine tumors and their products (Kizilgul et al. [1])

Embryologic Classification of NENs [2]

An embryology-based classification of NENs categorizes it to three subtypes based on their original derivation site:

- Foregut NENs: (respiratory system, stomach, duodenum, proximal jejunum, and pancreas)
- Midgut NENs: (distal jejunum, ileum, appendix, and right-sided colon)
- Hindgut NENs: (transverse and left-sided colon and rectum)

Anatomic Distribution of NENs [3–5]

- *Pituitary gland*: Chromophobe anterior pituitary NETs
- *Thyroid gland*: Neuroendocrine thyroid tumors and thyroid medullary carcinoma (TMC)
- *Parathyroid tumors*
- *Gastroenteropancreatic neuroendocrine tumors (GEP-NET)*
  - *Foregut GEP-NET* (NETs of the stomach and proximal duodenum, pancreas, thymus, lung, and bronchus)
  - *Midgut GEP-NET* (From distal half of the 2nd part of the duodenum to the proximal two-thirds of the transverse colon, appendix)
  - *Hindgut GEP-NET (Distal colon and rectum)*
- *Liver and gallbladder*
- *Cervix*
- *Bladder*
- *Prostate*
- *Catecholamine-secreting tumors*
  - *Adrenal tumors and pheochromocytoma*
- *Merkel cell tumors*

Inherited Conditions

- Multiple endocrine neoplasia type 1 (MEN1)
- Multiple endocrine neoplasia type 2 (MEN2)
- Von Hippel-Lindau (VHL) disease
- Neurofibromatosis type 1
- Tuberous sclerosis

Differentiation [6–8]

Differentiation and grading express different concepts in tumor categorization, but they correlate intently. Differentiation represents the degree of tumor resemblance to its original nonneoplastic neuroendocrine cells equivalent.

Overall, neuroendocrine neoplasms are either well differentiated or poorly differentiated. Therapeutic approach is totally different between these two categories, and hence, it is very important to precisely separate well-differentiated from poorly differentiated NETs when performing tumor pathology assessment:

- *Well differentiated*: Nested, trabecular, or gyriform patterns of tumor cells, which are relatively uniform with abundant neurosecretory granules. Strong and diffuse immunoexpression of neuroendocrine markers: chromogranin A and synaptophysin.
- *Poorly differentiated NETs*: Less resemblance to nonneoplastic counterpart; sheetlike or diffuse architecture, irregular nuclei, and less cytoplasmic granularity. Immunoexpression of neuroendocrine markers is usually not prominent.

Grading

Grade reflects the tumor biological behavior, and it refers to the tumor proliferative activity. Grade of an NET determines its aggressiveness. Usually high-grade tumors have an aggressive behavior. Evidence of malignant and more aggressive behavior for an NET includes existence of vascular invasion, gross local invasion, and/or presence of metastases.

The first scientific pathologically and clinically based classification of GEP-NETs was proposed by the World Health Organization (WHO 2000) [9]. According to this classification, NETs were divided in three categories: benign, malignant, or of uncertain behavior. Although this system significantly influenced the common practice of medicine, it had limited practicality when classifying samples other than surgically resected cases [2].

Currently, there are three major systems to grade and stage NETs: NANET (North American NET Society), WHO (2010), and ENET (European Neuroendocrine Tumor Society).

The evolution of novel classification systems is worthy from the point of view that it took the clinicopathological, site-specific, differences into account and considered any NET as a potential malignant entity. Although, there is general consensus between the aforementioned classifications, however, there are slight differences between the NANETS and ENETS especially with regard to pancreatic and appendiceal NETs [2].

All systems use cell proliferation rate to separate tumor into three different categories of low, intermediate, and high grades. Low-grade NETs show indolent clinical course, whereas high-grade NETs are extremely aggressive. Intermediate-grade tumors usually have an uncertain clinical course and may have a moderately aggressive behavior.

The proliferative rate can be assessed by counting the number of mitoses per unit area of tumor (expressed as mitoses per 10 high-power microscopic fields (×40) each high-power field being 2 mm^2) or by assessing the percentage of Ki-67 immunopositivity of the neoplastic cells. Ki-67 is a proliferation marker marking all cells within the cell cycle. In addition the American Joint Committee on Cancer (AJCC) in the seventh edition of Cancer Staging Manual recommends expressing the Ki-67 proliferation index as % of 2000 cells counted in areas of highest nuclear labeling.

The well-differentiated category comprises low- and intermediate-grade tumors. The Ki-67 labeling rates are dramatically different between the well-differentiated and high-grade tumors.

Well differentiated: (NETs are either low or intermediate grade)

Low grade (ENETS G1)
Intermediate grade (ENETS G2)

Poorly differentiated: (are considered high grade in all cases)

High grade (ENETS G3)

Note: The well-differentiated intermediate-grade (G2) tumor variant could however biologically have a more aggressive behavior, but this concept is debated [10, 11].

The Ki-67 labeling index per se does not provide any additional or superior information over the mitotic count. However, when dealing with only a small amount of tumor tissue (usually small biopsies or cell blocks from cytologic preparations), 10 high-power microscopic fields may not be available for a proper mitotic count. In this context, evaluation with Ki-67 immunostain is recommended. In cases, where a sufficient amount of tissue is available, performing both methods is not recommended.

Due to the slight differences existent between classification systems, it is recommended to include the Ki-67 proliferation index in the pathology report when grading NETs. In the WHO classification system, the grading of pulmonary and thymic tumors is based only on the tumor mitotic rate, whereas in the ENETS classification system, the grading of gastroenteropancreatic and hindgut tumors uses either the mitotic rate or the Ki-67 labeling index. According to the WHO classification of pulmonary and thymic tumors, the presence and percent of necrosis distinguish intermediate-grade from low-grade tumors within the well-differentiated group.

WHO grading criteria for NET have undergone several modifications over the years. These changes have been shown very briefly in this review (Fig. 3). Terms "tumor" and "neuroendocrine" (instead of endocrine) have been favored by WHO 2010 as compared to previous versions.

Table 1 Definitions for GEP-NETs according to WHO classifications (22-24)

WHO 1980	WHO 2000	WHO 2010
Carcinoid	Well-differentiated endocrine tumor (WDET)	Neuroendocrine tumor G1 (carcinoid)
	Well-differentiated endocrine carcinoma (WDEC)	Neuroendocrine tumor G2
	Poorly differentiated endocrine carcinoma (PDEC)	Neuroendocrine carcinoma (large and small cell type)
Mucocarcinoid	Mixed exocrine-endocrine carcinoma (MEEC)	Mixed adenoneuroendocrine carcinoma (MANEC)
Mixed forms carcinoid adenocarcinoma		
Pseudoturmor lesions	Tumor-like lesions (TLL)	Hyperplastic and preneoplastic lesions

Fig. 3 WHO grading system evolution for neuroendocrine tumor classification (Kizilgul et al. [1])

WHO grading nomenclature for GEP-NENs (2010)		
Grade	Mitotic index	Ki-67
1. Grade 1 (G1)	Mitotic count <2 per 10 HPF	≤2
2. Grade 2 (G2)	Mitotic count 2–20 per 10 HPF	3–20 %
3. Grade 3 (G3) (Large cell or small cell)	Mitotic count >20 per 10 HPF	>20 %
4. Mixed adenoneuroendocrine carcinoma (MANEC)		
5. Hyperplastic and preneoplastic lesions		

The results of large series studies have supported the prognostic value of the WHO staging system in small intestine and pancreatic NETs [12]. A recent study assessing the WHO recommendations for grading GI-NETs supported the validity of this system [13].

Stomach [3, 14]

Less than 1 % of gastric neoplasms are neuroendocrine tumors (NETs). However, stomach is a common site for neuroendocrine neoplasms, and 10–30 % of all NENs are reported in the stomach.

In the classification systems proposed for gastroenteropancreatic NETs (GEP-NETs) by ENETS, NANETS, and WHO, neuroendocrine tumors of the stomach are classified histologically into 3 grades of low, intermediate, and high grade, using cell proliferation rate (using the mitotic rate or Ki-67 labeling index) and necrosis (Table 1).

Furthermore, NETs of the stomach are subclassified into three distinct groups based on the following criteria:

Type 1: In setting of chronic atrophic gastritis type A, the most common type
Type 2: In setting of ZES (Zollinger-Ellison syndrome), multiple endocrine neoplasia type I (MEN I)
Type 3: Sporadic

In previous classification systems, well-differentiated low- and intermediate-grade tumors were called typical and atypical carcinoid tumors:

- *Typical carcinoid tumor*: Well-differentiated, low-grade, neuroendocrine tumor grade 1

- *Atypical carcinoid tumor*: Well-differentiated, intermediate, neuroendocrine tumor grade 2

Pancreas

The pathological classification of pancreatic NETs (PNETs) is in general similar to that of NETs of the stomach and other GI-NETs (Table 1). However, the TNM staging system for PNETs differs depending on the site of origin of the tumor.

Table 1 Grading systems of nomenclature for NETs of the stomach and pancreas

Grade	GEP-NETs (ENETS)	GEP-NETs (WHO 2010)
Low grade	NET grade 1 (G1)	Neuroendocrine neoplasm grade 1
Intermediate grade	NET grade 2 (G2)	Neuroendocrine neoplasm grade 2
High grade	Neuroendocrine carcinoma grade 3 (G3), small cell carcinoma	Neuroendocrine carcinoma grade 3, small cell carcinoma
	Neuroendocrine carcinoma grade 3 (G3), large-cell neuroendocrine carcinoma	Neuroendocrine carcinoma grade 3, large cell neuroendocrine

For PNETs functionality also plays a role in classifying the tumor grade. A functional tumor refers to a tumor, which causes clinical symptoms due to excess hormone secretion.

Well-differentiated PNETs are divided into two groups:

- *Functional PNETs [FPNETs]*: Has a clinical syndrome
- *Nonfunctional PNETs [NFPNETs]*: Does not have a clinical syndrome

FPNETs are further divided and termed based on their clinical syndromes into insulinoma, glucagonoma, gastrinoma, VIPoma, and somatostatinoma subtypes. All PNETs are malignant except insulinoma.

The pathological diagnosis of functional NETs is identical to the nonfunctional NETs counterpart at the same anatomical site. Functionality status and the presence or absence of the clinical syndrome should be mentioned and attached to the diagnosis in the pathology report (Figs. 4 and 5).

Insulinoma Insulinomas are single tumors (except in MEN I cases) and generally small, intrapancreatic, and benign in more than 85–95 % of the cases. The diagnosis of insulinoma is by determining plasma proinsulin, insulin, C peptide, and glucose levels during a 72-h fast test.

Glucagonoma Glucagonomas present as a single, large (mean size 6 cm) intrapancreatic mass. Liver metastases are present at the time of diagnosis in more than 60 % of cases. Glucagonomas may be associated with glucose intolerance without significant hyperglycemia, in most of the cases.

Table 1 Cellular classifications of pancreatic neuroendocrine tumors (islet cell turnors)

	Secreted peptide hormone(s)	Pancreatic NET	Clinical manifestation/syndrome
Islet Cell			
Alpha (α)	Glucagon	Glucagonoma	Diabetes, dermatitis, NME
Beta (β)	Insulin	Insulinoma	Fasting hypoglycemia, neuroglycopenia
Delta (δ)	Somatostatin	Somatostatinoma	Steatorrhea, cholelithiasis, mild diabetes
A→D	VIP, other 5-HT ACTH MSH		WDHA Carcinoid Cushing Syndrome Hyperpigmentation
Interacinar cell			
F	Pencreatic polypeptide (PP)	PPoma	Non-functional or various syndromes
EC	5-HT	Carcinoid	Carcinoid syndrome (facial flushing. secretory diarrhea, wheezing right-sided heart vaive abnormalities)

VIP, Vasoactive intestinal peptide; 5-HT, serotonin; ACH, andrenocarticotropin; MSH, melanocyte stimulation hormone; WDHA, watery diarrhea, hypokalemia, achlorhydria; EC, enterochromaffin; Modified from: national cancer institute at the national institutes of health, pancreatic neuroendocrine tumors (islet cell tumors) Treatment (PDQ®); Health professional version, last modified: 06/29/2012, http://www.cancer.gov/cancertopics/pdq/treatment/isletcell/HealthProfessional.

Fig. 4 Functional NETs and their related clinical syndromes [15]

Table 2 Nomenclature, incidence, location and malignancy of pancreatic NETs

Name	Hormone	Cell type	Incidence (M)	Pancreas (%)	Duodenum (%)	Malignant (%)
Insulinoma	Insulin	β islet cells	1/1.25	>99		5-11
Gastrinoma	Gastrin	G cells	1/2.5	21-65	6-35	60
Glucagonoma	Glucagon	α cells	<1/5	>99		>70
VIPoma	VIP	δ cells	<1/5	85-90	10-15	50
Somatostatinoma	Somatostatin	δ cells	<1/10	50	50	90
Nonfunctioning	Neuron-specific enolase, PP	F cells	1/5	>99		>50

Norton et al. Surgery: basic science and clinical evidence; 2000, 919-953. Reproduced with permission.

Fig. 5 Functional NETs products, corresponding cells and the incidence by location [15]

VIPoma, Verner-Morrison Syndrome, and WDHA Syndrome (Watery Diarrhea, Hypokalemia, Achlorhydria) Usually presents as a single tumor secreting the vasoactive intestinal peptide (VIP), a neuropeptide member of the glucagon/secretin superfamily. VIP lowers arterial blood pressure and increases vasodilation and induces contraction of the heart. VIP is also upregulating glycogenolysis. These tumors are found to have metastases at the time of diagnosis in 70–80 % of cases. In adults, VIPomas are intrapancreatic. Childhood VIPomas are neural, adrenal, or periganglionic.

Gastrinoma, ZES Gastrinomas ectopically secrete gastrin and cause hypergastrinemia, which stimulates gastric acid oversecretion and results in Zollinger-Ellison syndrome (ZES). Gastrinomas are found in the duodenum in more than 60 % of patients with sporadic ZES, and they are usually single. The cases associated with MEN I/ZES are invariably multiple. Gastrinomas are malignant in 60–90 % of cases. Pancreatic tumors are more aggressive than duodenal tumors and more likely to metastasize to the liver and/or bone.

Somatostatinoma Somatostatinomas are usually single tumors found as a mass that can be found in the pancreas, in the duodenum, or in the small intestine. The overall malignancy rate for these tumors is around 50–60 %. Malignant potential and metastatic rate is higher in pancreatic somatostatinomas than in duodenal ones. About 10 % of duodenal somatostatinomas can be found in association with genetic syndromes (von Recklinghausen disease – NF-1). A PNET with clinical symptoms of somatostatin excess, in a setting of elevated plasma somatostatin level, is sufficient to diagnose somatostatinoma. Somatostatinomas are more commonly diagnosed by detection of somatostatin by immunohistochemistry and the presence of somatostatinoma syndrome, as the presenting symptom is rare.

Nonfunctional Nonfunctional PNETs are large intrapancreatic masses, which in 60–85 % of cases have liver metastasis at the time of diagnosis. These tumors do not secrete any hormonal product and are not associated with any clinical syndrome. NF-PNET is usually diagnosed as a pancreatic mass in a patient without hormonal symptoms but with elevated serum PP (pancreatic polypeptide) or CgA (chromogranin A) level or a positive OctreoScan (SRS) (biological active peptide products of tumor). However, elevated levels of PP or CgA are not specific for NF-PNETs [6, 9, 16–21].

Jejunum, Ileum, Appendix, and Cecum (Midgut NETs)

The term midgut NETs includes NETs arising in the jejunum, ileum, appendix, and cecum. These NETs have a common embryologic origin. Proliferative rate determines the low-, intermediate-, or high-grade midgut NETs. Both mitotic rate and Ki-67 labeling index are required to estimate cell proliferation rate. This grading system is shown in Table 2. It is recommended to specify the actual proliferative rate in the pathology report.

- Well-differentiated NETs of the midgut
- Well-differentiated NETs of the midgut may present with the classic carcinoid syndrome and therefore were previously described as midgut carcinoids.

Table 2 Grading systems of nomenclature for NETs jejunum, ileum, appendix, and cecum (midgut)

Grade	Traditional
Low grade, NET, grade 1 (G1)	<2 mitoses per 10 high-power fields AND <3 % Ki-67 index
Intermediate grade, NET grade 2 (G2)	2–20 mitoses per 10 high-power fields OR 3–20 % Ki-67 index
High grade	>20 Mitoses per 10 high-power fields OR >20 % Ki-67 index
	Neuroendocrine carcinoma, grade 3 (G3), small cell carcinoma
	Neuroendocrine carcinoma, grade 3 (G3), large-cell neuroendocrine carcinoma

- Mixed differentiation in NETs of the midgut
- Non-neuroendocrine components are relatively common in poorly differentiated (high-grade) neuroendocrine carcinomas throughout the gastrointestinal tract.
- Well-differentiated NETs of the appendix with glandular features
  In the appendix, it is common to observe mixed histology tumors having neuroendocrine and glandular features:

  1. *Tubular carcinoid tumors*
     Simple tubular arrangements of cells with uniform nuclei, with low proliferative rate, and with diffuse immunoexpression of neuroendocrine markers. Mimics classic NET.
     The prognosis of appendiceal tubular carcinoid tumors is the same as for classic tumor.
  2. *Goblet cell carcinoid tumors*
     Nests of cells with uniform nuclei, abundant cytoplasmic mucin, and low proliferative rate. The immunoexpression of neuroendocrine markers is usually limited to a subset of the neoplastic cells. These tumors have recently been divided in three groups: (1) typical goblet cell carcinoid; (2) adenocarcinoma ex goblet cell carcinoid, signet ring cell type; and (3) adenocarcinoma ex goblet cell carcinoid, poorly differentiated. Groups 2 and 3 show more aggressive behavior compared to typical goblet cell carcinoid. According to one study, the mean survival time for tumors in group 1 is approximately 119 months, while that of groups 2 and 3 is 43 and 31 months, respectively [22].
     There is high probability of transformation to adenocarcinoma with more aggressive behavior and worse prognosis, and they are treated and managed as primary adenocarcinomas of the appendix [23–25].

Distal Colon and Rectum (Hindgut)

NETs of the distal colon and rectum are known as hindgut carcinoids. Colorectal NETs are generally not associated with a hormonal syndrome such as flushing or diarrhea. The incidence of rectal NETs in African Americans and Asians is substantially higher than in Caucasians. As in other organ systems, hindgut NETs are divided into well- and poorly differentiated and include a combined (mixed) category.

Poorly differentiated hindgut NETs are called high-grade neuroendocrine carcinomas (neuroendocrine carcinoma, grade 3) and are further divided to small cell carcinoma and large-cell neuroendocrine carcinoma.

Combined tumors have elements of non-neuroendocrine tumors, mostly adenocarcinoma (mixed adenoneuroendocrine carcinoma or MANEC).

Well-differentiated (low- and intermediate-grade) tumors have been variably termed carcinoid tumor, neuroendocrine tumor (grade 1 and grade 2, respectively), or neuroendocrine carcinoma (low grade and intermediate grade, respectively).

At the moment the nomenclature for the grading of NETs of hindgut parallels that of midgut counterparts (shown in Table 2).

Rectal NETs are usually small, submucosal, and associated with a very low malignant potential. Tumors larger than 2 cm or those invading the muscularis propria are associated with a significantly higher risk of metastatic spread. Colonic NETs proximal to the rectum are less common and tend to behave more aggressively [26, 27].

Lung and Thymus (Thorax, Foregut) [28]

NETs of the thorax, including bronchial and thymic neuroendocrine NETs, are often referred to as NETs of the foregut, and the classification is uniform for these tumors.

The grading system recently proposed for all thoracic NETs by the WHO and the International Association for the Study of Lung Cancer (IASLC) uses either mitotic rate (expressed as mitoses per 10 HPF or 2 mm^2) or the presence and extent of necrosis. This grading system is shown in Table 3. As in other organ systems, it is recommended to include, in addition to the grade, the actual cell proliferation rate in the pathology report.

WHO System for Lung and Thymus

- *Well-differentiated NETs*: Carcinoid tumors, low and intermediate grade.
- *Poorly differentiated NETs*: High-grade neuroendocrine carcinomas, high grade: Small cell carcinoma and large-cell neuroendocrine carcinoma (cell size and nuclear morphology distinguish small cell carcinoma from large-cell neuroendocrine carcinoma)

Combined (mixed) form NET includes elements of both high-grade neuroendocrine carcinoma and non-neuroendocrine carcinoma (usually adenocarcinoma).

Bronchial Tumorlets Are solid nests or small monomorphic cells associated with bronchial epithelium. They are less than 0.5 cm in size and express neuroendocrine markers. They have very low risk of malignancy.

Table 3 Grading systems of nomenclature for NETs of the thorax (lung and thymus) (foregut)

Grade	WHO, IASLC
Low	<2 mitoses/10 HPF AND no necrosis, carcinoid tumor
Intermediate	2–10 mitoses/10 HPF, OF foci of necrosis, atypical carcinoid tumor
High	>10 mitoses/10 HPF
	Small cell carcinoma
	Large-cell neuroendocrine carcinoma

Pheochromocytoma, Paraganglioma, and Medullary Thyroid Cancer [24, 29]

Pheochromocytomas, intra-adrenal paraganglioma, and extra-adrenal sympathetic and parasympathetic paragangliomas are neuroendocrine tumors derived from adrenal chromaffin cells or similar cells in extra-adrenal sympathetic and parasympathetic paraganglia, respectively. Pheochromocytomas and paragangliomas exhibit similar basic histopathological characteristics. Familial subtypes show slight differences.

According to the 2004 World Health Organization criteria, malignancy is defined by the presence of metastases, not local invasion (significant invasion is considered by some pathologists as the sign of malignancy). There is currently no consensus for the adoption of a formal scoring system for these tumors. However, a system for the assessment of malignancy in pheochromocytomas exists (Pheochromocytoma of the Adrenal Gland Scaled Score [PASS]) [30].

Pheochromocytomas

Pheochromocytomas may occur sporadically or as part of hereditary syndromes. Up to approximately 24 % of tumors may be hereditary and are associated with multiple endocrine neoplasia type 2 (MEN2A or MEN2B), neurofibromatosis type 1 (NF-1), von Hippel-Lindau (VHL) syndrome, and familial paragangliomas and pheochromocytomas [due to germline mutations of genes encoding succinate dehydrogenase subunits B, C, and D (SDHB, SDHC, SDHD)]. In general, the traits are inherited in an autosomal dominant pattern.

Medullary Thyroid Cancer (MTC)

MTC is a malignancy of the thyroid C cells of the thyroid. Thyroid C cells secrete a number of peptides and hormones including calcitonin, carcinoembryonic antigen, and chromogranin A. These markers are elevated in circulation in patients with MTC and can be used to confirm the diagnosis or for early detection of tumor recurrence.

On gross examination, MTC lesions are whitish gray in color and firm to palpation. MTC is characterized by nests of uniform cells surrounded by a stroma rich in amyloid. Medullary thyroid cancer course has a wide range from extremely indolent tumors, which remain stable for many years, to aggressive tumors having a high mortality rate.

MTC can be sporadic or familial. Sporadic MTC is usually unifocal, while hereditary MCT is frequently multifocal and bilateral. Familial MTC is inherited in an autosomal dominant pattern, with variable expressivity and penetrance, and can be identified by the detection of RET mutations. In such cases, prophylactic thyroidectomy is recommended.

C Cell Hyperplasia

C cell hyperplasia is defined as more than 6 C cells per follicle or more than 50 C cells per low-power field. C cell hyperplasia is considered a tumor precursor lesion.

Anterior Pituitary

Pituitary adenomas are benign epithelial tumors derived from intrinsic cells of the adenohypophysis. The clinical manifestation may be the result of local mass effect with neurologic consequences, or it may be due to the excess of hormones produced. The majority of pituitary adenomas are composed of a proliferation of monomorphic cells with uniform round nuclei, delicate stippled chromatin, inconspicuous nucleoli, and a moderate amount of cytoplasm. Mitotic figures are uncommon in most adenomas, and Ki-67 antigen labeling indices are usually less than 3 %. Morphologic feature including invasive growth or elevated mitotic index (Ki-67 labeling index more than 3 %) and extensive nuclear immunostain for p53 can suggest aggressive behavior. The neoplastic progression of pituitary adenomas is related to oncogenes and defective tumor suppressor gene.

The classification of pituitary neoplasms has undergone a variety of modifications. Once, they were separated based on the light microscopy characteristics of cell cytoplasm and without considering the cell derivation and were included three categories of acidophilic, which assumed to produce excess amount of growth hormone, basophilic that was secreting adenocorticotrophic hormone (ACTH), and chromophobic tumors which were regarded as hormonally inactive. However, this system is not considered accurate and is not in use in clinical practice.

Currently adenomas are classified based upon their hormonal products:

1. Growth hormone-producing adenoma (GH producing)
2. Prolactin-producing adenoma (PRL producing)
3. Thyrotropin-producing adenoma (TSH producing)
4. ACTH-producing adenoma
5. Gonadotropin-producing adenoma (follicle-stimulating hormone (FSH), luteinizing hormone (LH), and or α-subunit)

Pituitary adenomas from endocrinological standpoint are considered to be *active* or *inactive* based on the amount of the hormone that they secrete. This is considered as a type of *Functional Classification* in which active adenomas are the ones that secrete amount of hormone that exceeds normal levels in the blood and causes overt clinical symptoms. Inactive adenomas although are composed of secretory and cellular components for hormone production, but they are not associated with clinical syndromes. This can be either due to undetectable amount of hormones secreted by these tumors or secretion of an abnormal hormone, which is not being detected with regular antibodies in radioimmunoassays, or simply due to a genetic defect that bans hormone secretion.

Functional Classification of Pituitary Adenomas

1. *Endocrine hyperfunction*
    - Elevated serum GH/IGF (insulin-like growth factor 1) levels: Causes acromegaly and gigantism
    - Hyperprolactinemia
    - Elevated ACTH and consequent cortisol level: Causes Cushing disease
    - Inappropriate TSH secretion and consequent hyperthyroidism
    - Significantly elevated FSH/LH and/or α-subunit levels
    - Multiple hormone overproduction from multihormonal tumors or double adenomas
2. *Clinically nonfunctioning*
    - No known hormone produced or released
    - Hormones or hormone fragments produced which may not cause clinical manifestation – FSH, LH, and or α-subunit
    - Hormones normally cause clinical sign and symptoms, but at times they are produced without clinical manifestation – silent ACTH or GH-producing adenomas.
    - Biological inactive hormone fragment or hormone product.
3. *Functional status undetermined*

WHO Classification of Pituitary Tumors

Pituitary adenoma

Typical adenoma
Atypical adenoma

Pituitary carcinoma

Radiologic Classification of Pituitary Tumors

Microadenoma: Small tumor <= 10 mm
Macroadenoma: Tumor >10 mm

Giant adenoma: Tumor >4 cm

References [31, 32]

Abbreviations

NEN	Neuroendocrine neoplasm
GI-NENs	Gastrointestinal neuroendocrine neoplasms
NET	Neuroendocrine tumor
NEC	Neuroendocrine carcinoma
GEP-NETs	Gastroenteropancreatic neuroendocrine tumors
PNET	Pancreatic neuroendocrine tumor
MANEC	Mixed adenoneuroendocrine carcinoma
SCNEC	Small cell neuroendocrine carcinoma
WHO	World Health organization
NANET	North American Neuroendocrine Society
ENET	European Neuroendocrine Tumor Society
NSE	Neuron-specific enolase
CgA	Chromogranin
Syn	Synaptophysin
HPF	High-power field

References

1. Kizilgul M, Delibasi T. Gastroenteropancreatic neuroendocrine tumors (gep-nets). Transl Gastrointest Cancer. 2014;4:39–56.
2. Capelli P, Fassan M, Scarpa A. Pathology – grading and staging of gep-nets. Best Pract Res Clin Gastroenterol. 2012;26:705–17.
3. Strosberg JR, Coppola D, Klimstra DS, Phan AT, Kulke MH, Wiseman GA, Kvols LK, North American Neuroendocrine Tumor Society. The nanets consensus guidelines for the diagnosis and management of poorly differentiated (high-grade) extrapulmonary neuroendocrine carcinomas. Pancreas. 2010;39:799–800.
4. Park CH, Chung JW, Jang SJ, Chung MJ, Bang S, Park SW, Song SY, Chung JB, Park JY. Clinical features and outcomes of primary hepatic neuroendocrine carcinomas. J Gastroenterol Hepatol. 2012;27:1306–11.
5. Almeida MQ, Stratakis CA. Solid tumors associated with multiple endocrine neoplasias. Cancer Genet Cytogenet. 2010;203:30–6.
6. Klimstra DS, Modlin IR, Coppola D, Lloyd RV, Suster S. The pathologic classification of neuroendocrine tumors: a review of nomenclature, grading, and staging systems. Pancreas. 2010;39:707–12.
7. Vinik AI, Woltering EA, Warner RR, Caplin M, O'Dorisio TM, Wiseman GA, Coppola D, Go VL, North American Neuroendocrine Tumor Society. Nanets consensus guidelines for the diagnosis of neuroendocrine tumor. Pancreas. 2010;39:713–34.
8. Niederle MB, Hackl M, Kaserer K, Niederle B. Gastroenteropancreatic neuroendocrine tumours: the current incidence and staging based on the who and european neuroendocrine tumour society classification: an analysis based on prospectively collected parameters. Endocr Relat Cancer. 2010;17:909–18.

9. Nilsson O, Van Cutsem E, Delle Fave G, Yao JC, Pavel ME, McNicol AM, Sevilla Garcia MI, Knapp WH, Kelestimur F, Sauvanet A, Pauwels S, Kwekkeboom DJ, Caplin M, Frascati Consensus C, European Neuroendocrine Tumor Society. Poorly differentiated carcinomas of the foregut (gastric, duodenal and pancreatic). Neuroendocrinology. 2006;84:212–5.
10. Strosberg JR, Weber JM, Feldman M, Coppola D, Meredith K, Kvols LK. Prognostic validity of the American Joint Committee on cancer staging classification for midgut neuroendocrine tumors. J Clin Oncol (Official Journal of the American Society of Clinical Oncology). 2013;31:420–5.
11. Sorbye H, Strosberg J, Baudin E, Klimstra DS, Yao JC. Gastroenteropancreatic high-grade neuroendocrine carcinoma. Cancer. 2014;120:2814–23.
12. Rindi G, Falconi M, Klersy C, Albarello L, Boninsegna L, Buchler MW, Capella C, Caplin M, Couvelard A, Doglioni C, Delle Fave G, Fischer L, Fusai G, de Herder WW, Jann H, Komminoth P, de Krijger RR, La Rosa S, Luong TV, Pape U, Perren A, Ruszniewski P, Scarpa A, Schmitt A, Solcia E, Wiedenmann B. Tnm staging of neoplasms of the endocrine pancreas: results from a large international cohort study. J Natl Cancer Inst. 2012;104:764–77.
13. Yamaguchi T, Fujimori T, Tomita S, Ichikawa K, Mitomi H, Ohno K, Shida Y, Kato H. Clinical validation of the gastrointestinal net grading system: Ki67 index criteria of the who 2010 classification is appropriate to predict metastasis or recurrence. Diagn Pathol. 2013;8:65.
14. Delle Fave G, Kwekkeboom DJ, Van Cutsem E, Rindi G, Kos-Kudla B, Knigge U, Sasano H, Tomassetti P, Salazar R, Ruszniewski P, Barcelona Consensus Conference participants. Enets consensus guidelines for the management of patients with gastroduodenal neoplasms. Neuroendocrinology. 2012;95:74–87.
15. Lairmore TC, Quinn CE, Martinez MJ. Neuroendocrine tumors of the pancreas: molecular pathogenesis and current surgical management. Transl Gastrointest Cancer. 2013;3:29–43.
16. Falconi M, Plockinger U, Kwekkeboom DJ, Manfredi R, Korner M, Kvols L, Pape UF, Ricke J, Goretzki PE, Wildi S, Steinmuller T, Oberg K, Scoazec JY, Frascati Consensus C, European Neuroendocrine Tumor Society. Well-differentiated pancreatic nonfunctioning tumors/carcinoma. Neuroendocrinology. 2006;84:196–211.
17. Falconi M, Bartsch DK, Eriksson B, Kloppel G, Lopes JM, O'Connor JM, Salazar R, Taal BG, Vullierme MP, O'Toole D, Barcelona Consensus Conference participants. Enets consensus guidelines for the management of patients with digestive neuroendocrine neoplasms of the digestive system: well-differentiated pancreatic non-functioning tumors. Neuroendocrinology. 2012;95:120–34.
18. Ahlman H, Nilsson O, McNicol AM, Ruszniewski P, Niederle B, Ricke J, Jensen R, Kos-Kudla B, Oberg K, O'Connor JM, Pavel ME, Vullierme MP, Frascati Consensus Conference participants. Poorly-differentiated endocrine carcinomas of midgut and hindgut origin. Neuroendocrinology. 2008;87:40–6.
19. Schott M, Kloppel G, Raffel A, Saleh A, Knoefel WT, Scherbaum WA. Neuroendocrine neoplasms of the gastrointestinal tract. Dtsch Arztebl Int. 2011;108:305–12.
20. Kulke MH, Anthony LB, Bushnell DL, de Herder WW, Goldsmith SJ, Klimstra DS, Marx SJ, Pasieka JL, Pommier RF, Yao JC, Jensen RT, North American Neuroendocrine Tumor Society. Nanets treatment guidelines: well-differentiated neuroendocrine tumors of the stomach and pancreas. Pancreas. 2010;39:735–52.
21. Jensen RT, Cadiot G, Brandi ML, de Herder WW, Kaltsas G, Komminoth P, Scoazec JY, Salazar R, Sauvanet A, Kianmanesh R, Barcelona Consensus Conference participants. Enets consensus guidelines for the management of patients with digestive neuroendocrine neoplasms: functional pancreatic endocrine tumor syndromes. Neuroendocrinology. 2012;95:98–119.
22. Tang LH, Shia J, Soslow RA, Dhall D, Wong WD, O'Reilly E, Qin J, Paty P, Weiser MR, Guillem J, Temple L, Sobin LH, Klimstra DS. Pathologic classification and clinical behavior of the spectrum of goblet cell carcinoid tumors of the appendix. Am J Surg Pathol. 2008;32:1429–43.

23. Pape UF, Perren A, Niederle B, Gross D, Gress T, Costa F, Arnold R, Denecke T, Plockinger U, Salazar R, Grossman A, Barcelona Consensus Conference participants. Enets consensus guidelines for the management of patients with neuroendocrine neoplasms from the jejuno-ileum and the appendix including goblet cell carcinomas. Neuroendocrinology. 2012;95:135–56.
24. Baloch ZW, LiVolsi VA. Neuroendocrine tumors of the thyroid gland. Am J Clin Pathol. 2001;115(Suppl):S56–67.
25. Boudreaux JP, Klimstra DS, Hassan MM, Woltering EA, Jensen RT, Goldsmith SJ, Nutting C, Bushnell DL, Caplin ME, Yao JC, North American Neuroendocrine Tumor Society. The nanets consensus guideline for the diagnosis and management of neuroendocrine tumors: well-differentiated neuroendocrine tumors of the jejunum, ileum, appendix, and cecum. Pancreas. 2010;39:753–66.
26. Fenoglio-Preiser CM. Gastrointestinal neuroendocrine/neuroectodermal tumors. Am J Clin Pathol. 2001;115(Suppl):S79–93.
27. Anthony LB, Strosberg JR, Klimstra DS, Maples WJ, O'Dorisio TM, Warner RR, Wiseman GA, Benson AB, Benson 3rd AB, Pommier RF, North American Neuroendocrine Tumor Society. The nanets consensus guidelines for the diagnosis and management of gastrointestinal neuroendocrine tumors (nets): well-differentiated nets of the distal colon and rectum. Pancreas. 2010;39:767–74.
28. Phan AT, Oberg K, Choi J, Harrison Jr LH, Hassan MM, Strosberg JR, Krenning EP, Kocha W, Woltering EA, Maples WJ, North American Neuroendocrine Tumor Society. Nanets consensus guideline for the diagnosis and management of neuroendocrine tumors: well-differentiated neuroendocrine tumors of the thorax (includes lung and thymus). Pancreas. 2010;39:784–98.
29. Chen H, Sippel RS, O'Dorisio MS, Vinik AI, Lloyd RV, Pacak K, North American Neuroendocrine Tumor Society. The North American neuroendocrine tumor society consensus guideline for the diagnosis and management of neuroendocrine tumors: pheochromocytoma, paraganglioma, and medullary thyroid cancer. Pancreas. 2010;39:775–83.
30. Thompson LD. Pheochromocytoma of the adrenal gland scaled score (pass) to separate benign from malignant neoplasms: a clinicopathologic and immunophenotypic study of 100 cases. Am J Surg Pathol. 2002;26:551–66.
31. Barakat MT, Meeran K, Bloom SR. Neuroendocrine tumours. Endocr Relat Cancer. 2004;11:1–18.
32. Wick MR. Neuroendocrine neoplasia. Current concepts. Am J Clin Pathol. 2000;113:331–5.

Neuroendocrine Tumor Classification Systems: Staging

Shabnam Seydafkan and Domenico Coppola

General [1, 2]

Staging of the NETs classifies patients into prognostic groups.

WHO has proposed a more scientific and clinically related tumor based classification in 2000. The most recent WHO classification suggests that neuroendocrine neoplasms are potentially malignant and consequently should be staged according to a site-specific staging system (TNM) (Fig. 1) (TNM classification of NETs).

WHO 2000 classification system used the generic name of neuroendocrine tumor and classified the lesions based on their size, cell proliferation rate, localization, differentiation, and hormone production. Before formal TNM-based staging systems being used for NETs, data submitted to the Surveillance, Epidemiology, and End Results (SEER) program of the National Cancer Institute classified these tumors into localized, regional, and distant stages based on the absence or presence of lymph node or distant metastases without taking into consideration the extent of the primary tumor. For NETs, metastasis represents the most important prognostic determinant after grading.

Initial WHO classifications (NETs of the gastrointestinal tract 2000 and pancreatic NETs 2004) incorporated both staging information (size and extent of tumor) and grading information (number of mitoses/Ki-67 proliferative index) into a single prognostic predictive system, with a different name being applied to the tumors in each prognostic group.

Other widely used and accepted TNM staging systems for NETs are the one proposed by the American Joint Committee on Cancer (AJCC) and the one proposed

S. Seydafkan, MD • D. Coppola, MD (✉)
Department of Anatomic Pathology, Moffitt Cancer Center, Tampa, FL, USA
e-mail: domenico.coppola@moffitt.org

A. Nasir, D. Coppola (eds.), *Neuroendocrine Tumors: Review of Pathology, Molecular and Therapeutic Advances*, DOI 10.1007/978-1-4939-3426-3_2

Fig. 1 General approach TNM classification of NETs [3]

GI tract:
– Carcinoid: separate staging by site
– Small cell/large cell: stage as carcinoma
Pancreas: stage as carcinoma
Lung: stage as carcinoma
Skin: separate classification for Merkel cell carcinoma

Adapted from Sobin L, Gospodarowicz M, Wittekind C (eds) (2010) TNM classification of malignant tumours, 7th edn, Wiley-Blackwell, Oxford

by the European Neuroendocrine Tumor Society (ENETS). Both systems are site specific. The system proposed by AJCC includes NETs of all anatomic sites whereas ENETS recommendations are limited to the TNM staging of gastroenteropancreatic NETs. These systems do not optimally distinguish survival outcomes among patients with early-stage tumors.

Similarly to other broadly accepted classification systems, the most recent WHO classification separate provided grading and staging of the tumors. The most recent WHO classification applies to all gastroenteropancreatic NETs arising throughout the body based on the organ of origin (including thyroid, adrenal gland, and endocrine pancreas). The small bowel, in general, is the most common site for NET and within the small bowel; the terminal ileum is the NET's most common location. Pituitary tumors are rare and usually benign and there is no staging system for them (American Cancer Society).

NETs spread equally via blood or lymphatic system. The most common metastatic site for GEP-NETs is the lymph nodes, followed by the liver, lung, peritoneum, and pancreas. Local spread to neighboring organs is usually associated with extensive fibrosis. The North American Neuroendocrine Tumor Society (NANETS) Consensus Guidelines for the Diagnosis of Neuroendocrine Tumor proposes that the goals for the initial staging of NET include: "identification of primary tumor, assessment of extent of disease, treatment planning and recommendations for imaging studies to be performed for initial staging." Imaging studies recommended by NANETS for initial staging include plain film of the chest, cross-sectional imaging (CT or MRI) of the abdomen and pelvis, and [111In-DTPA0] octreotide scintigraphy. It is suggested to perform small-bowel series or multiphasic CT of the abdomen and pelvis with thin section in suspected but not yet confirmed cases of midgut primary NET (e.g., a mesenteric mass in the ileal mesentery).

At this time, no sufficient data is available to validate any of the staging systems. Therefore, it is recommended to provide in the pathology report the extent of tumor involvement at the primary site and at the metastatic site, to allow validation and modifications to the staging systems in the future, if required. It is also recommended to reference in the pathology report the TNM system used for the staging [4].

ENETS System for Classification of NETs [1, 2]

ENETS has published recommendations for TNM staging of gastroenteropancreatic (GEP) NETs based on the clinical, surgical, and imaging data. ENETS staging system applies to all grades of NETs.

Information on the presence or absence of metastasis has to be available as a minimum requirement for ENETS staging [1]. ENET system applies to GI-NETs of foregut, midgut, and hindgut. Foregut NETs are further divided into three groups: (1) gastric NETs; (2) duodenum, ampulla, and proximal jejunum NETs; and (3) pancreatic NETs. Midgut and hindgut NET category includes lower jejunum/ileum, appendix, and colon/rectum.

ENETS staging criteria use stage 0 only for the stomach because this is the only anatomic site where Tis is defined. Stage I includes the T1 NETs with limited growth. Stage II applies to the tumors larger in size or more invasive, either T2 or T3, but always in the absence of metastasis. Stage III includes tumors with invasion into surrounding structures but without lymph node metastasis (stage IIIA) and tumors of any AJCC T stages (T1, T2, T3, and T4) in the presence of regional node metastasis (stage IIIB). Stage IV includes tumors of any AJCC T stage and of any AJCC N stage (N0 or N1) with the presence of distal metastasis (M1) at the time of initial diagnosis.

UICC/AJCC System for Classification of NETs [5]

The seventh edition of the UICC/AJCC staging system recommends for GI-NETs to have a specific staging depending on the site of origin, whereas GI neuroendocrine carcinomas (large-cell and small-cell carcinoma) and all pancreatic NENs to be staged like conventional carcinomas [5].

AJCC System for Classification of NETs

Clinical staging based on AJCC recommendations depends on the anatomic extent and the pathologic staging that can be obtained using endoscopic biopsies, percutaneous biopsies, fine needle aspirations, surgical explorations, and examination of primary surgically resected tumors, lymph nodes, and distant metastasis. Capsule endoscopy and enteroscopy are useful to identify small-bowel lesions. MRI and computed tomography are effective in the initial localization of NETS or other metastases. Somatostatin receptor scintigraphy (SRS) and positron emission tomography (PET) are useful in localizing GI-NETs. The combination of SRS or PET with CT or MRI is highly sensitive in NET detection.

By AJCC/UICC convention, the "T" stands for primary tumor that is not yet treated. "P" is used to indicate pathologic classification and it is based on gross and microscopic examinations (in contrast to clinical staging which is usually performed by the referring physician). pT signifies an adequate resected primary tumor or biopsy specimen pathologically evaluated. pN represents adequate LN removal to assess LN metastases. pM indicates adequate microscopic examination of distant lesions.

Pathologic staging does not necessarily need the primary tumor to be completely removed, and as long as the highest category of T and N and M can be conformed microscopically, the criteria for pathology staging are achieved without the need for total removal of the tumor.

Despite considerable similarity, differences in staging of primary tumors between ENETS and UICC staging systems still exist and should be considered when managing patient care.

In the case of pancreatic NENs, a discrepancy in the T stage (primary tumor stage) between ENETS and UICC staging systems has been noticed (Cienfuegos et al. (Fig. 2)) [6–9]. In the case of GI-NENs, the definitions of T stage for appendiceal and gastric NENs differ between the two staging systems [4, 10] (Figs. 3 and 4).

However, the main classification criteria used for both systems include the size and the extent of invasion to landmarks similar to that used for non-neuroendocrine tumors of the same site. It is recommended that the pathologic features, such as tumor size, extent of involvement, and invasion of these structures, be particularly indicated in the pathology reports in addition to providing a TNM stage and it is critical to clarify which classification system is being used to allow for the interpretation of T stage between ENETS and UICC classification [6] (Tables 1 and 2).

AJCC Staging Classification		ENETS Staging Classification	
T1	Tumor limited to the pancreas, <2 cm	T1	Tumor limited to the pancreas, <2 cm
T2	Tumor limited to the pancreas, >2 cm	T2	Tumor limited to the pancreas, 2-4 cm
T3	Tumor extends beyond the pancreas, but not Involving the celiac axis or SMA	T3	Tumor limited to the pancreas, >4 cm, or invading duodenum or CBD
T4	Tumor involves the celiac axis or SMA	T4	Tumor invades adjacent structures
N0	No regional LN metastasis	N0	No regional LN metastasis
N1	Regional LN metastasis	N1	Regional LN metastasis
M0	No distant metastasis	M0	No distant metastasis
M1	Distant metastasis	M1	Distant metastasis

Stage	T	N	M	Stage	T	N	M
IA	T1	N0	M0	I	T1	N0	M0
IB	T2	N0	M0	IIA	T2	N0	M0
IIA	T3	N0	M0	IIB	T3	N0	M0
IIB	T1-3	N1	M0	IIIA	T4	N0	M0
III	T4	N0-1	M0	IIIB	Any T	N1	M0
IV	Any T	Any N	M1	IV	Any T	Any N	M1

	ENETS I	ENETS II	ENETS III	ENETS IV
AJCC I	25	59	0	0
AJCC II	0	4	37	0
AJCC III	0	0	18	0
AJCC IV	0	0	0	282

CBD = common bile duct; LN = lymph node; SMA = superior mesenteric artery.

Fig. 2 Comparison of TNM classification of pancreatic NENs according to ENETS versus UICC/AJCC (TNM classification) [6, 7]

ENETS	UICC
Tis In situ tum or / dysplasia (<0.5 mm)	Mucosa 0.5 mm
T1 Tumor invades lamina propria or submucosa and ≤ 1	Mucosa 0.5 –1 cm or submucosa ≤ 1 cm
T2 Tumor invades muscularis propria or submucosa or >	Muscularis propria or > 1 cm
T2 Tumor penetrates serosa	Subserosa
T2 Tumor invades adjacent structures	Perforates serosa; adjacent structures

Fig. 3 Comparison of TNM classification of gastric NENs according to ENETS versus UICC/AJCC (TNM classification) [4]

E NETS stage:			
stage 0:	Tis	N0	M0
stage I:	T1	N0	M0
stage IIa:	T2	N0	M0
stage IIb:	T3	N0	M0
stage IIIa:	T4	N0	M0
stage IIIb:	any T	N1	M0
stage IVb:	any T	any N	M1
UICC/AJCC stage:	T1		
stage I:	T1	N0	M0
stage II:	T2–3	N0	M0
stage III:	T4	N0	M0
	any T	N1	M0
stage IV:	any T	any N	M1

Fig. 4 Comparison of TNM classification of appendiceal NEN according to ENETS versus UICC/AJCC (TNM classification) [10]

Table 1 Anatomic stage/prognostic group (TNM classification, AJCC recommendations)

Stage 0	Tis (applies only for stomach)	N0	M0
Stage I	T1	N0	M0
Stage IIA	T2	N0	M0
Stage IIB	T3	N0	M0
Stage IIIA	T4	N0	M0
Stage IIIB	Any T	N1	M0
Stage IV	Any T	Any N	M1

Table 2 Neuroendocrine tumor staging form

NEUROENDOCRINE TUMOR STAGING FORM		
CLINICAL *Extent of disease before any treatment*	**STAGE CATEGORY DEFINITIONS**	**PATHOLOGIC** *Extent of disease through completion of definitive surgery*
❑ y clinical– staging completed after neoadjuvant therapy but before subsequent surgery	TUMOR SIZE: ____________	❑ y pathologic – staging completed after neoadjuvant therapy AND subsequent surgery
	PRIMARY TUMOR (T)	
	Stomach	
❑ TX	Primary tumor cannot be assessed	❑ TX
❑ T0	No evidence of primary tumor	❑ T0
❑ Tis	Carcinoma *in situ*/dysplasia (tumor size <0.5mm), confined to mucosa	❑ Tis
❑ T1	Tumor invades lamina propria or submucosa and ≤1cm in size	❑ T1
❑ T2	Tumor invades muscularis propria or >1cm in size	❑ T2
❑ T3	Tumor penetrates subserosa	❑ T3
❑ T4	Tumor invades visceral peritoneum (serosa) or other organs or adjacent structures	❑ T4
	For any T, add (m) for multiple tumors	
	Duodenum/Ampulla/Jejunum/Ileum	
❑ TX	Primary tumor cannot be assessed	❑ TX
❑ T0	No evidence of primary tumor	❑ T0
❑ T1	Tumor invades lamina propria or submucosa and size ≤1 cm* (small intestinal tumors); tumor ≤1 cm (ampullary tumors)	❑ T1
❑ T2	Tumor invades muscularis propria or size >1 cm (small intestinal tumors); tumor >1 cm (ampullary tumors)	❑ T2
❑ T3	Tumor invades through the muscularis propria into subserosal tissue without penetration of overlying serosa (jejunal or ileal tumors) or invades pancreas or retroperitoneum (ampullary or duodenal tumors) or into non-peritonealized tissues.	❑ T3
❑ T4	Tumor invades visceral peritoneum (serosa) or invades other organs	❑ T4
	For any T, add (m) for multiple tumors *Tumor limited to ampulla of Vater for ampullary gangliocytic paraganglioma	
	Colon or Rectum	
❑ TX	Primary tumor cannot be assessed	❑ TX
❑ T0	No evidence of primary tumor	❑ T0
❑ T1	Tumor invades lamina propria or submucosa and size ≤2 cm	❑ T1
❑ T1a	Tumor size <1 cm in greatest dimension	❑ T1a
❑ T1b	Tumor size 1 to 2 cm in greatest dimension	❑ T1b
❑ T2	Tumor invades muscularis propria or size >2 cm with invasion of lamina propria or submucosa	❑ T2
❑ T3	Tumor invades through the muscularis propria into the subserosa, or into non-peritonealized pericolic or perirectal tissues	❑ T3
❑ T4	Tumor invades peritoneum or other organs	❑ T4
	For any T, add (m) for multiple tumors	
	REGIONAL LYMPH NODES (N)	
	Stomach	
❑ NX	Regional lymph nodes cannot be assessed	❑ NX
❑ N0	No regional lymph node metastasis	❑ N0
❑ N1	Regional lymph node metastasis	❑ N1

HOSPITAL NAME/ADDRESS	PATIENT NAME/INFORMATION

(continued)

Table 2 (continued)

NEUROENDOCRINE TUMOR STAGING FORM

Clinical		Pathologic
❑ NX ❑ N0 ❑ N1	***Duodenum/Ampulla/Jejunum/Ileum*** Regional lymph nodes cannot be assessed No regional lymph node metastasis Regional lymph node metastasis	❑ NX ❑ N0 ❑ N1
❑ NX ❑ N0 ❑ N1	***Colon or Rectum*** Regional lymph nodes cannot be assessed No regional lymph node metastasis Regional lymph node metastasis	❑ NX ❑ N0 ❑ N1
	DISTANT METASTASIS (M)	
❑ M0 ❑ M1	***Stomach*** No distant metastasis (no pathologic M0; use clinical M to complete stage group) Distant metastasis	❑ M1
❑ M0 ❑ M1	***Duodenum/Ampulla/Jejunum/Ileum*** No distant metastasis (no pathologic M0; use clinical M to complete stage group) Distant metastasis	❑ M1
❑ M0 ❑ M1	***Colon or Rectum*** No distant metastasis (no pathologic M0; use clinical M to complete stage group) Distant metastasis	❑ M1

ANATOMIC STAGE • PROGNOSTIC GROUPS

CLINICAL				PATHOLOGIC			
GROUP	T	N	M	GROUP	T	N	M
❑ 0	Tis*	N0	M0	❑ 0	Tis*	N0	M0
❑ I	T1	N0	M0	❑ I	T1	N0	M0
❑ IIA	T2	N0	M0	❑ IIA	T2	N0	M0
❑ IIB	T3	N0	M0	❑ IIB	T3	N0	M0
❑ IIIA	T4	N0	M0	❑ IIIA	T4	N0	M0
❑ IIIB	Any T	N1	M0	❑ IIIB	Any T	N1	M0
❑ IV	Any T	Any N	M1	❑ IV	Any T	Any N	M1
❑ Stage unknown				❑ Stage unknown			
**Note*: Tis applies only to stomach.				**Note*: Tis applies only to stomach.			

PROGNOSTIC FACTORS (SITE-SPECIFIC FACTORS)

REQUIRED FOR STAGING: None

CLINICALLY SIGNIFICANT:

Pre-operative plasma chromogranin A level (CgA) ____________

Urinary 5-hydroxyindolacetic acid (5-HIAA) level ____________

Mitotic count ____________

Histologic Grade (G) *(also known as overall grade)*

Grading system	***Grade***
❑ 2 grade system	❑ Grade I or 1
❑ 3 grade system	❑ Grade II or 2
❑ No 2 or 3 grade system is available	❑ Grade III or 3

General Notes:

For identification of special cases of TNM or pTNM classifications, the "m" suffix and "y," "r," and "a" prefixes are used. Although they do not affect the stage grouping, they indicate cases needing separate analysis.

m suffix indicates the presence of multiple primary tumors in a single site and is recorded in parentheses: pT(m)NM.

y prefix indicates those cases in which classification is performed during or following initial multimodality therapy. The cTNM or pTNM category is identified by a "y" prefix.

HOSPITAL NAME/ADDRESS	PATIENT NAME/INFORMATION

Table 2 (continued)

NEUROENDOCRINE TUMOR STAGING FORM

ADDITIONAL DESCRIPTORS

Lymphatic Vessel Invasion (L) and Venous Invasion (V) have been combined into Lymph-Vascular Invasion (LVI) for collection by cancer registrars. The College of American Pathologists' (CAP) Checklist should be used as the primary source. Other sources may be used in the absence of a Checklist. Priority is given to positive results.

- ❑ Lymph-Vascular Invasion Not Present (absent)/Not Identified
- ❑ Lymph-Vascular Invasion Present/Identified
- ❑ Not Applicable
- ❑ Unknown/Indeterminate

Residual Tumor (R)

The absence or presence of residual tumor after treatment. In some cases treated with surgery and/or with neoadjuvant therapy there will be residual tumor at the primary site after treatment because of incomplete resection or local and regional disease that extends beyond the limit of ability of resection.

- ❑ RX Presence of residual tumor cannot be assessed
- ❑ R0 No residual tumor
- ❑ R1 Microscopic residual tumor
- ❑ R2 Macroscopic residual tumor

General Notes (continued):

The ycTNM or ypTNM categorizes the extent of tumor actually present at the time of that examination. The "y" categorization is not an estimate of tumor prior to multimodality therapy.

r prefix indicates a recurrent tumor when staged after a disease-free interval, and is identified by the "r" prefix: rTNM.

a prefix designates the stage determined at autopsy: aTNM.

surgical margins is data field recorded by registrars describing the surgical margins of the resected primary site specimen as determined only by the pathology report.

neoadjuvant treatment is radiation therapy or systemic therapy (consisting of chemotherapy, hormone therapy, or immunotherapy) administered prior to a definitive surgical procedure. If the surgical procedure is not performed, the administered therapy no longer meets the definition of neoadjuvant therapy.

❑ Clinical stage was used in treatment planning (describe): ____________________

❑ National guidelines were used in treatment planning ❑ NCCN ❑ Other (describe): ____________________

____

Physician signature Date/Time

HOSPITAL NAME/ADDRESS	PATIENT NAME/INFORMATION

Abbreviations

NEN	Neuroendocrine neoplasm
GI-NENs	Gastrointestinal neuroendocrine neoplasms
NET	Neuroendocrine tumor
NEC	Neuroendocrine carcinoma
GEP-NETs	Gastroenteropancreatic neuroendocrine tumors
PNET	Pancreatic neuroendocrine tumor
MANEC	Mixed adenoneuroendocrine carcinoma
SCNEC	Small cell neuroendocrine carcinoma
WHO	World Health Organization
NANET	North American Neuroendocrine Tumor Society
ENET	European Neuroendocrine Tumor Society
UICC	Union for International Cancer Control

References

1. Rindi G, Kloppel G, Alhman H, Caplin M, Couvelard A, de Herder WW, Erikssson B, Falchetti A, Falconi M, Komminoth P, Korner M, Lopes JM, McNicol AM, Nilsson O, Perren A, Scarpa A, Scoazec JY, Wiedenmann B, all other Frascati Consensus Conference Participants, European Neuroendocrine Tumor Society. TNM staging of foregut (neuro)endocrine tumors: a consensus proposal including a grading system. Virch Arch (Int J Pathol). 2006;449:395–401.
2. Rindi G, Kloppel G, Couvelard A, Komminoth P, Korner M, Lopes JM, McNicol AM, Nilsson O, Perren A, Scarpa A, Scoazec JY, Wiedenmann B. Tnm staging of midgut and hindgut (neuro) endocrine tumors: a consensus proposal including a grading system. Virch Arch (Int J Pathol). 2007;451:757–62.
3. Diez M, Teule A, Salazar R. Gastroenteropancreatic neuroendocrine tumors: diagnosis and treatment. Ann Gastroenterol. 2013;26:29–36.
4. Hirabayashi K, Zamboni G, Nishi T, Tanaka A, Kajiwara H, Nakamura N. Histopathology of gastrointestinal neuroendocrine neoplasms. Front Oncol. 2013;3:2.
5. Sobin LH, Compton CC. Tnm seventh edition: what's new, what's changed: communication from the international union against cancer and the american joint committee on cancer. Cancer. 2010;116:5336–9.
6. Kloppel G, Rindi G, Perren A, Komminoth P, Klimstra DS. The Enets and ajcc/uicc tnm classifications of the neuroendocrine tumors of the gastrointestinal tract and the pancreas: a statement. Virch Arch (Int J Pathol). 2010;456:595–7.
7. Oberg K. Diagnostic work-up of gastroenteropancreatic neuroendocrine tumors. Clinics. 2012;67 Suppl 1:109–12.
8. Liszka L, Pajak J, Mrowiec S, Zielinska-Pajak E, Golka D, Lampe P. Precursor lesions of early onset pancreatic cancer. Virch Arch (Int J Pathol). 2011;458:439–51.
9. Discrepancies between two staging systems (European-ENETS versus. American-AJCC) of neuroendocrine neoplasms of the pancreas: A study of 77 cases. J Clin Oncol. 2015;33(suppl 3; abstr 318). 2015 Gastrointestinal Cancers Symposium. http://hwmaint.meeting.ascopubs.org/cgi/content/abstract/33/3_suppl/318
10. Pape UF, Perren A, Niederle B, Gross D, Gress T, Costa F, Arnold R, Denecke T, Plockinger U, Salazar R, Grossman A, Barcelona Consensus Conference Participants. Enets consensus guidelines for the management of patients with neuroendocrine neoplasms from the jejuno-ileum and the appendix including goblet cell carcinomas. Neuroendocrinology. 2012;95:135–56.

Differential Diagnosis of Neuroendocrine Tumors

Kun Jiang and Domenico Coppola

Introduction

Well-differentiated NETs are generally composed of a uniform population of oval, round, to polygonal cells with medium to moderate granular cytoplasm, "salt-to-pepper" chromatin pattern, and inconspicuous nucleoli. NET cells are usually growing in nodular, nested, organoid, trabecular, tubular, rosette, and pseudoglandular patterns. Microscopic foci of degenerative atypia can be seen. Degenerative nuclear atypia and pleomorphism could be seen occasionally and focally in any given tumor, even within grade 1 well-differentiated NETs. Attention should be made not to interpret these features to distinguish tumor grades or predicting prognosis [1–5]. These "pseudo-dysplastic foci" include enlarged nuclei and cell bodies, nuclear hyperchromasia, and smudgy chromatin texture. These seemingly alarming phenomena should not be interpreted as true dysplasia or features associated with higher-grade NETs. Focal whirling and spindling of tumor cells usually exists; however, none of the abovementioned histology has been proven clinically significant for disease progression and prognosis.

In NETs, the intervening and surrounding stroma is generally rich in vasculature and shows focal or diffuse hyalinization, which has been attributed to the deposition of hormonal secretion by these cells (see Fig. 1 in the chapter "Immunophenotypical

K. Jiang, MD, PHD (✉)
Anatomic Pathology, H. Lee Moffitt Cancer Center, Tampa, FL 33612, USA

Department of Oncologic Science, University of South Florida, Tampa, FL 33612, USA
e-mail: kun.jiang@moffitt.org

D. Coppola, MD
Department of Anatomic Pathology, Moffitt Cancer Center, Tampa, FL, USA
e-mail: domenico.coppola@moffitt.org

A. Nasir, D. Coppola (eds.), *Neuroendocrine Tumors: Review of Pathology, Molecular and Therapeutic Advances*, DOI 10.1007/978-1-4939-3426-3_3

Profile and Molecular Genetics of Neuroendocrine Tumors"). A special stain with Congo red could highlight the amyloid deposition. Dense fibrosis and abundant collagen deposition are also not infrequent. Occasional cases have been reported to contain foci of microcalcification (psammomatous calcification) and cartilaginous or osseous metaplasia. It should be noted that the presence of metaplastic tissue does not impact NET grades or prognosis.

One of the most import prognostic factors in NETs is the grade, which can be determined using the tumor proliferation index and presence/absence of necrosis. The tumor proliferation index can be assessed using the tumor nuclear labeling with Ki-67 or MIB-1. MIB-1 is a monoclonal antibody directed against a different epitope of the same proliferation-related antigen recognized by Ki-67 antibody [1, 3, 6, 7]. In pathology practice, counting tumor cell mitoses in 10 high-power fields cannot always be accomplished on biopsy material, when the tumor tissue is scant or contains only a few tumor cells. In these situations, Ki-67 proliferation index becomes an essential tool for determining neuroendocrine tumors grade. Ki-67 immunostain will decorate the nuclei of all cells present in the cell cycle between G1 and M phases [1, 3, 6, 7]. According to the current criteria, NETs are well differentiated and grade 1 if Ki-67 index is equal to or less than 2 % and grade 2 if the Ki-67 index is between 2 and 20 % (AJCC, seventh edition). One potential technical challenge and diagnostic pitfall is the presence of intratumoral and peritumoral lymphocytic infiltrates, which may determine a falsely high Ki-67 labeling rate. The nuclei of lymphocytic are Ki-67 positive and if they are counted in error as tumor cells will inevitably and falsely increase the Ki-67 proliferation index in a given tumor. One method to avoid this issue is the adoption of a double staining technique (we use the Ki-67/keratin cocktail where the Ki-67 antibody is labeled with a brown chromogen (peroxidase) and the cytokeratin antibody is labeled with a red chromogen (alkaline phosphatase)). This method will effectively eliminate the erroneous counting of interspersed lymphocytes within the NETs (the lymphocytes will be labeled with nuclear Ki-67 only and not with the cytoplasmic keratin signal). Optimal interpretation of the double immunostain requires the tissue to be well preserved and well processed. Significant crushing artifact may pose a great challenge when dealing with a mixture of dark brown-red signal coloring the smeared cells.

In high-grade (grade 3) neuroendocrine carcinoma (NEC), the malignant morphological features will include increased tumor proliferation rate (20 or more mitoses per 10 high-power fields, or a Ki-67 nuclear labeling index equal or more than 20 %), usually accompanied by frequent single cell apoptosis and/or confluent "geographic" necrosis, and an infiltrative growth pattern [1, 3, 6, 7]. Fragile, smudgy nuclei with molding and/or overlapping, irregularly bizarre nuclear shape and giant cells, as well as intermediate cell morphology are also identified frequently; the three latter features have been frequently observed in small cell carcinoma (SCC) among NECs [1, 3, 6–8]. Importantly, in our daily pathology practice, we have seen tumors that were morphologically well-differentiated neuroendocrine neoplasms, but demonstrated a higher than 20 % Ki-67 proliferation index and demonstrated an aggressive clinical course, while the mitotic count was well under 10 %. These peculiar tumors were seen especially in MEN 1 patients. Therefore, we suggest that mitotic rate alone may not

Table 1 Differentiating neuroendocrine tumor from various adenocarcinomas

NET (grades 1 and 2)	Adenocarcinoma
Bland cytology, maybe degenerative atypia	Dysplastic cytology
Chromogranin, synaptophysin, or CD56 positivity	Chromogranin and synaptophysin negative; focal weak signal can be seen in poorly differentiated tumors
Hyalinization, amyloid, and psammomatous calcification; no desmoplastic response	Desmoplastic response frequently present; invading adjacent stroma
0–20 mitotic counts per 10 high-power fields	Mitotic figures frequent; atypical mitosis present
Nodules, cohesive nests, and strands; pushing boarders	Infiltrative, invasive, Indian files, destructive growth
Ki-67 usually between 0 and 20 %	Significantly higher Ki-67, usually well above 50 %
Mucicarmine and PAS-D both negative	Mucicarmine and PAS-D highlight intra- and extra-cytoplasmic mucin

be an accurate measure of neuroendocrine tumor grade without determination of the Ki-67 proliferative index. One frequent challenge in GI pathology is to differentiate GI NETs from other morphologically similar entities. This chapter aims to cover the major differential diagnoses to consider when dealing with a possible GI NET. However, we cannot describe all of the possible scenarios that can be encountered in a daily pathology practice. Please refer to Table 1 for a summary of these entities.

Neuroendocrine Tumor Versus Adenocarcinoma

When facing gastrointestinal NETs, we should be sure to eliminate the possibility of mimickers, which include both primary and secondary adenocarcinomas, and a spectrum of other entities. Histologically, NETs may grow in tubular, nodular, or pseudoglandular configurations that may mimic adenocarcinoma, either primary or metastatic [1, 3, 4, 7]. When differentiating an NET from a poorly differentiated adenocarcinoma, attention must be paid to the peculiar morphological, histochemical, and immunoprofile details. Making the correct diagnosis is of the outmost importance as it will impact therapy and the clinical management of the patient [3, 9].

Histochemically, adenocarcinomas produce mucin which is positive with a periodic acid–Schiff–diastase (PAS-D) special stain, and it will appear as either intracellular or extracellular bright red vacuoles. NETs are negative by PAS-D staining due to the lack of mucin production. Similarly, mucicarmine stain can also be used to highlight mucin in adenocarcinomas, and it will be negative in NETs. However, although specific, PAS-D and mucicarmine are not sensitive histochemical markers, and false-negative results are not infrequent, especially when dealing with a poorly differentiated adenocarcinoma. When assessing PAS-D and mucicarmine in these cases, it is important to examine the entire tumor because both stains can be positive only in focal areas or in rare tumor cells. Hence, histochemical stains alone may not be sufficient to detect a poorly differentiated adenocarcinoma. Histological and immunohistochemical studies and detailed evaluation of the clinical history, radiological findings, and laboratory (i.e., 5-hydroxyindoleacetic acid or 5-HIAA levels in urine) and serological tests (i.e., serum chromogranin A levels) are all essential in reaching the correct diagnosis.

Immunohistochemically, adenocarcinomas and NETs are both positive for multiple cytokeratin markers (if not all of them), including pan-cytokeratin, GI, or pancreatobiliary-related markers, such as CK20, CK7, CK17, CK19, CK8/CK18, and MOC-31. Therefore, cytokeratin staining alone is not a suitable marker for neuroendocrine differentiation. It is important that at least one neuroendocrine marker be unequivocally positive in NET cells. Usually multiple positive markers are positive in low-grade NETs. The most frequently used are synaptophysin and chromogranin. CD56 and neuron-specific enolase (NSE) are also used frequently [1, 3, 4, 10, 11]. In addition, Ki-67 proliferation index is essential when grading NETs, but it can also aid in differentiating a low-grade NETs from adenocarcinoma [10–13]. Ki-67 positivity is within 20 % in low-grade NETs but always significantly higher in adenocarcinomas (usually between 50 and 90 %). A higher than 20 % proliferative index is also seen in neuroendocrine carcinomas, including both small cell carcinoma and large-cell NEC; but these two entities show distinct histological differences from adenocarcinoma. Other immunohistochemical markers such as gastrin, somatostatin, glucagon, insulin, histamine, and bradykinin are less frequently utilized [10–13]. Serological and laboratory markers, such as urine 5-HIAA, have mostly clinical significance It should also be kept in mind that occasionally, poorly differentiated adenocarcinomas can be focally and weakly positive for a neuroendocrine marker such as synaptophysin or chromogranin. This positivity, however, should be viewed as reflection of the poorly differentiated nature of the tumors, instead of an indication of neuroendocrine differentiation. Rarely, mixed adenocarcinoma and neuroendocrine carcinoma (MANEC) has been reported in the literature and encountered in practice; detailed inspection of the histological sections, PAS-D, and/or mucicarmine special staining, immunohistochemical staining for neuroendocrine markers, Ki-67 proliferation index, and clinical information can all aid in reaching the correct diagnosis [11, 14, 15]. Importantly, for a tumor to be classified as MANEC, each of the two components must represent at least 30 % of the total tumor. Clinically, MANEC behaves aggressively, and the consensus is to manage this malignancy as neuroendocrine carcinoma [15].

Neuroendocrine Tumors Versus Primary Tumors Originated in the Liver

One frequently encountered clinical scenario is that of a patient presenting with liver nodule(s) and clinical suspicion of a primary neoplasm(s) of the liver (HCC, cholangiocarcinoma, or other hepatic types of tumor) which needs to be differentiated from a metastatic NET involving the liver. A large proportion of these lesions represent hepatocellular neoplasms including benign and dysplastic hepatocellular lesions as well as hepatocellular carcinoma (HCC). One common feature of these primary hepatocellular lesions is that most of them are immunohistochemically positive for hepatocellular specific antigen (HepPar-1) and arginase, represented by a diffuse granular cytoplasmic labeling [16]. In the case of HCC, ancillary staining with alpha fetoprotein (AFP) (cytoplasmic labeling), glypican-3 (cytoplasmic and membranous labeling), polyclonal CEA (canalicular pattern), CD34 (sinusoidal pattern), and CD-10 (canalicular pattern) can all be used to differentiate HCC from NET. Clinically, HCC patients frequently show an elevated serum AFP levels; however, this is not always the case especially when dealing with a fibrolamellar type of HCC. On the other hand, hepatocellular adenoma and focal nodular hyperplasia are also positive for HepPar-1 and arginase, and a reticulin stain will highlight benign 1–2 cell thick hepatic plates in adenoma and focal nodular hyperplasia as compared to thick hepatocyte cords seen in HCC. Imaging study often can detect scar-like central areas in focal nodular hyperplasia, but this is not always the case. All these hepatocellular lesions are negative for neuroendocrine markers. Moreover, metastatic NETs to the liver usually express markers related to the site of origin, for example, NETs of colonic origin will stain for CDX-2 and CK20, those of pulmonary origin will be TTF-1 positive, and those deriving from a pancreatic primary will be PAX8 positive [17–19]. It should be noted that all high-grade neuroendocrine carcinoma may express TTF-1 regardless of the site of origin [8].

Neuroendocrine Tumors Versus Other Neoplasms

Primary liver endothelial neoplasms including hemangioma, epithelioid hemangioendothelioma, and angiosarcoma can all be distinguished from NETs by morphological evaluation and essential immunostains for endothelial, epithelial, and neuroendocrine markers. Intrahepatic cholangiocarcinoma and most secondary adenocarcinomas involving the liver, such as metastatic pancreatobiliary, lung, and upper and lower GI tract adenocarcinomas, can be differentiated by histological evaluation, mucicarmine and PAS-D special stains, and immunostains for neuroendocrine markers, as mentioned above. In addition, comparison with previous biopsy or resection material, radiological findings, and related clinical history may clarify the diagnosis. Detailed review of clinical information and image findings will aid in forming a differential list, and additional confirmatory workup can help narrow down the differential.

Neuroendocrine Tumors Versus Solid Pseudopapillary Neoplasm (SPN) of the Pancreas

SPN is a relatively rare entity which has been predominantly diagnosed in female patients [20], usually of young to middle age. Morphological distinction of NET and SPN, either grossly or microscopically, can be challenging. The typical histological features of NET (i.e., organoid and pseudoglandular patterns) and of SPN (pseudopapillary fibrovascular core wrapped by bland-appearing neoplastic cells) may not be well preserved on the H&E-stained sections, due to sampling issue, tissue degeneration, or surgical-related change. Therefore, immunohistochemical workup becomes essential in discriminating one from the other. SPN expresses epithelial markers such as AEI/AE3 and CAM 5.2, although usually focally and weakly; SPN cells are usually immunohistochemically positive for CD56 and synaptophysin (patchy stain) but negative for chromogranin. Importantly, SPN shows abnormal beta-catenin expression (nuclear and cytoplasmic stain), a reflection of a mutation in CTNNB1 gene (cyclin-D1) which is invariably present in SPN [21]. SPN tumor cells express progesterone receptors, but not androgen receptors [20, 21], and galectin-3, which will help in differentiating SPN from pancreatic NET [22]. Of notice, both NET and SPN demonstrate low Ki-67 proliferative index, usually lower than 5 %, indicating a low growth potential for SPN.

Neuroendocrine Tumors Versus Paragangliomas

NET cells are generally arranged in a nodular, nested, and trabecular pattern of growth, intermingled by subtle fibrovascular stroma. Cytologically NET cells display mild to moderately eosinophilic, clear, or finely granular cytoplasm and nuclei with a “salt-to-pepper” chromatin distribution pattern [3, 4, 23]. Paragangliomas (so-called extra-adrenal pheochromocytomas) are originated in the ganglia of the sympathetic nervous system in the body, known for their “zellballen” pattern of growth [24, 25]. Architecturally paragangliomas can mimic NETs in terms of nodular and nested growth pattern and rich vasculatures embedded within fibrovascular septa [24, 25]. In the presence of a metastatic tumor, it can be difficult to differentiate one entity from the other, and both NET and malignant paraganglioma are capable of metastasis. Immunohistochemistry may be helpful in this differential: paraganglioma contains sustentacular cells which are highlighted by S-100 stain, and paraganglioma is not labeled by cytokeratin.

Neuroendocrine Tumors Versus Nonepithelial Neoplasms

Differentiating lymphomas, small blue cell tumors such as Ewing sarcoma, and desmoplastic small round cell tumor and malignant melanoma from NET may occasionally be difficult. Careful histological analysis, essential immunohistochemical study, and related molecular and genetic test(s) can aid in reaching the correct diagnosis. Noticeably, S-100 protein is frequently expressed by both NETs and NECs, and it should not be used in this differential. It is wise to test separate melanoma markers such as tyrosinase, Mitf, melan-A, and HMB-45. Desmoplastic small round cell tumor, a soft tissue sarcoma that usually occurs as masses in young adults and teenagers involving multiple organ sites, displays densely fibrotic stroma, mimicking fibrovascular septa within NETs [26]. However, the clinical presentation, the clinical history, and both immunohistochemical and molecular studies are essential to identify this malignant and aggressive tumor which is typically positive for cytokeratins, desmin, epithelial membrane antigen, and vimentin [26]. Metastatic thyroid medullary carcinoma is immunohistochemically positive for neuroendocrine markers, but also for TTF-1, calcitonin, and CEA. These markers, in the presence or absence of a clinical history of primary medullary carcinoma, will help in reaching the correct diagnosis [27].

Determination of Origin for Metastatic NET

One frequently encountered clinical scenario is a patient presenting with a diagnosis of metastatic NET, without a known primary site. Recent publications have indicated that while most NETs from small intestine (especially those from the terminal ileum) and appendix are positive for CDX-2, less than 20 % of NETs from the upper GI tract, including the stomach and duodenum, display CDX-2 labeling [18]. Rectal NETs show a CDX-2 labeling rate which is in between the two listed above. On the other hand, while a similar low percentage of pancreatic NETs are positive for CDX-2, around two-thirds of pancreatic NETs are positive for PAX-8 [17]. Interestingly, NETs from the duodenum show a similar rate of PAX-8 positivity. A metastatic low-grade NET from the lung is usually TTF-1 positive [19]. Of course, clinical history, imaging findings, and laboratory results are all required to generate a complete differential list and to reach a corrected diagnosis.

Neuroendocrine Tumors Versus Prostate Cancer

Prostate cancer, especially when metastatic or when involving the rectum, can be misinterpreted as NET on small biopsies and on frozen section. The small prostatic acini, especially when confluent (tumors with high-grade Gleason score), may mimic an NET with nested growth pattern. To compound this problem is the fact that rectal NETs may express prostatic acid phosphatase (PAP). Also on a frozen section sample, the prominent nucleoli of prostatic carcinoma cells may be less prominent. The suspicion of prostate cancer in a male patient should prompt the pathologist to perform PSA immunostain when dealing with a tumor believed to be a NET.

Figure 1 and Tables 1 and 2 summarize features and tests that can help in differentiating an NET from its mimickers.

In summary, diagnosing an epithelial neoplasm as an NET, NEC, or other types of tumors (i.e., adenocarcinoma) is a frequently encountered event during a daily pathology practice. Please refer to Fig. 1 for the H&E images of the most relevant mimickers of NET and NEC. In addition, the attached Table 1 summarizes the major criteria that could be adopted when differentiating any given neuroendocrine neoplasm from its mimickers.

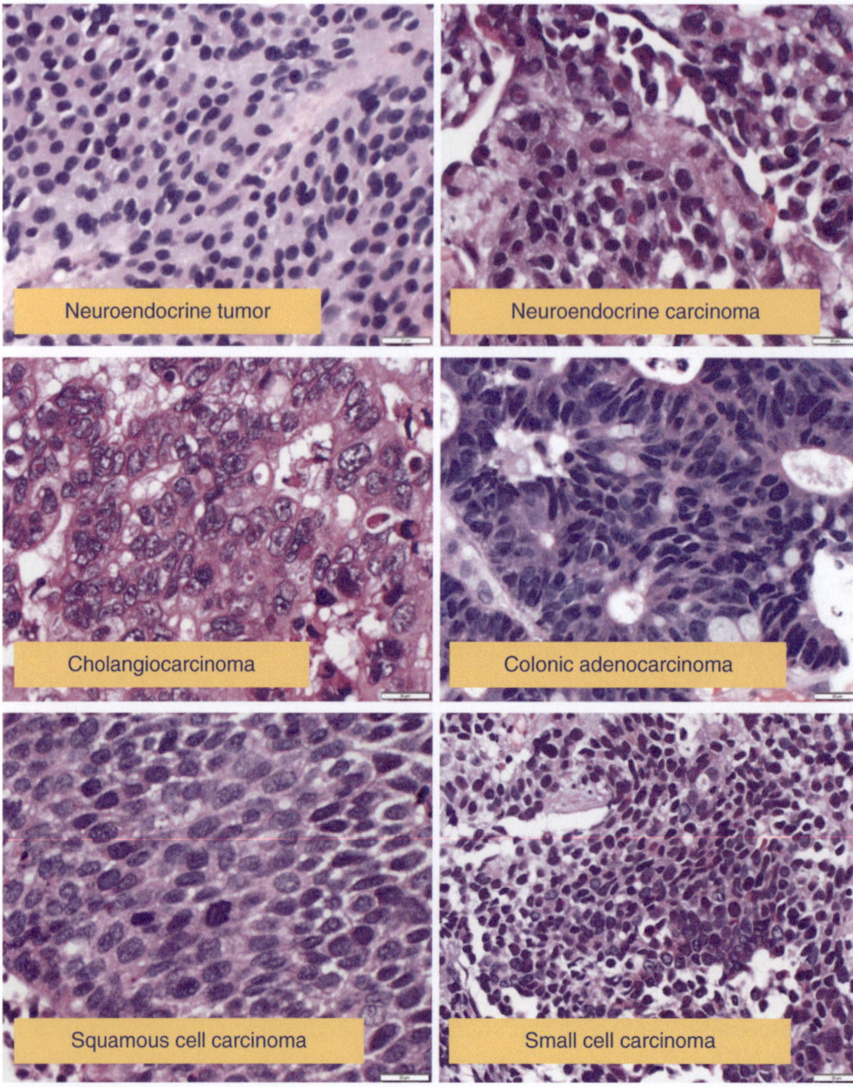

Fig. 1 Neuroendocrine neoplasms and the most relevant mimickers (H&E sections, 40×)

Table 2 Differentiating neuroendocrine neoplasms from various malignancies

Neuroendocrine neoplasms	Frequent mimickers of neuroendocrine neoplasms
Neuroendocrine tumor Neuroendocrine carcinoma	Bland cytology (NET grades 1 and 2); frank cytological atypia or infiltrative growth (NEC); positive neuroendocrine markers
Adenocarcinoma from a spectrum of origins (GI and pancreatobiliary tract, lung, GYN, GU, and skin adnexal appendages)	A wide spectrum of cytological and architectural dysplasia; frequent mitoses and potentially necrosis; positive mucicarmine and PAS-D; negative neuroendocrine markers
Pancreatic acinar cell carcinoma (usually in senior patients, large tumor size, aggressive behavior with frequent mitoses)	Focal weak synaptophysin labeling; negative chromogranin; positive trypsin, chymotrypsin and Bcl-10, invading adjacent stroma with nuclear signal for beta-catenin
Pancreatic solid pseudopapillary neoplasm (SPN, mostly in middle-age female patients, located in pancreatic tail)	Positive CD10 and nuclear beta-catenin; focal synaptophysin; negative or focally label by cytokeratin; PAS-D (+) intracytoplasmic globules; positive alpha-1 antitrypsin
Malignant melanoma (usually with but occasionally without a clinical history of melanoma)	Markedly dysplastic morphology (monster cells), destructive growth; positive S-100, melan-A, Mitf, and tyrosinase; negative cytokeratin by IHC
Lymphoma (clinical history or frankly de novo diagnosis; a history or clinical evidence of lymphoma could give a way)	Discohesive clusters, nests, or sheets of atypical monomorphic lymphoid proliferation; positive for CD45 and lymphoma markers by IHC and flow cytometry; negative for cytokeratin and neuroendocrine markers
Ki-67 usually between 0 and 20 % for NET; >20 % for NEC	Significantly higher Ki-67 in various malignancies, usually at least 50 % (adenocarcinoma, acinar cell carcinoma, melanoma, and lymphoma); only 1–4 % for SPN

Abbreviations

NET	Neuroendocrine tumor
NEC	Neuroendocrine carcinoma
NSE	Neuron-specific enolase
GI	Gastrointestinal
SCC	Small cell carcinoma
LCNEC	Large-cell neuroendocrine carcinoma
MANEC	Mixed adenoneuroendocrine carcinoma
SPN	Solid pseudopapillary neoplasm

References

1. Rindi G, Petrone G, Inzani F. 25 Years of neuroendocrine neoplasms of the gastrointestinal tract. Endocr Pathol. 2014;25:59–64.
2. Hirabayashi K, Zamboni G, Nishi T, Tanaka A, Kajiwara H, Nakamura N, et al. Histopathology of gastrointestinal neuroendocrine neoplasms. Front Oncol. 2013;3:2.

3. Anthony LB, Strosberg JR, Klimstra DS, Maples WJ, O'Dorisio TM, Warner RR, et al. The NANETS consensus guidelines for the diagnosis and management of gastrointestinal neuroendocrine tumors (nets): well-differentiated nets of the distal colon and rectum. Pancreas. 2010;39:767–74.
4. Kloppel G, Rindi G, Perren A, Komminoth P, Klimstra DS. The ENETS and UICC TNM classification of neuroendocrine tumors of the gastrointestinal tract and the pancreas: comment. Pathologe. 2010;31:353–4.
5. Leja J, Essaghir A, Essand M, Wester K, Oberg K, Totterman TH, et al. Novel markers for enterochromaffin cells and gastrointestinal neuroendocrine carcinomas. Mod Pathol. 2009;22:261–72.
6. Castano JP, Sundin A, Maecke HR, Villabona C, Vazquez-Albertino R, Navarro E, et al. Gastrointestinal neuroendocrine tumors (NETs): new diagnostic and therapeutic challenges. Cancer Metastasis Rev. 2014;33:353–9.
7. Fottner C, Weber MM. Neuroendocrine neoplasms of the gastrointestinal tract. Classification, clinical presentation and diagnosis. Internist (Berl). 2012;53:131–44.
8. Verset L, Arvanitakis M, Loi P, Closset J, Delhaye M, Remmelink M, et al. TTF-1 positive small cell cancers: don't think they're always primary pulmonary! World J Gastrointest Oncol. 2011;3:144–7.
9. Schott M, Kloppel G, Raffel A, Saleh A, Knoefel WT, Scherbaum WA, et al. Neuroendocrine neoplasms of the gastrointestinal tract. Dtsch Arztebl Int. 2011;108:305–12.
10. Rorstad O. Prognostic indicators for carcinoid neuroendocrine tumors of the gastrointestinal tract. J Surg Oncol. 2005;89:151–60.
11. Grabowski P, Scherubl H. Expression of neuroendocrine markers in undifferentiated carcinomas of the gastrointestinal tract. J Clin Oncol. 2005;23:4795–6; author reply 4796–7.
12. Oberg K. Neuroendocrine tumors of the gastrointestinal tract: recent advances in molecular genetics, diagnosis, and treatment. Curr Opin Oncol. 2005;17:386–91.
13. Norton JA. Endocrine tumours of the gastrointestinal tract. Surgical treatment of neuroendocrine metastases. Best Pract Res Clin Gastroenterol. 2005;19:577–83.
14. Nikou GC, Lygidakis NJ, Toubanakis C, Pavlatos S, Tseleni-Balafouta S, Giannatou E, et al. Current diagnosis and treatment of gastrointestinal carcinoids in a series of 101 patients: the significance of serum chromogranin-A, somatostatin receptor scintigraphy and somatostatin analogues. Hepatogastroenterology. 2005;52:731–41.
15. La Rosa S, Marando A, Sessa F, Capella C. Mixed adenoneuroendocrine carcinomas (MANECs) of the gastrointestinal tract: an update. Cancers (Basel). 2012;4:11–30.
16. Timek DT, Shi J, Liu H, Lin F. Arginase-1, HepPar-1, and Glypican-3 are the most effective panel of markers in distinguishing hepatocellular carcinoma from metastatic tumor on fine-needle aspiration specimens. Am J Clin Pathol. 2012;138:203–10.
17. Sangoi AR, Ohgami RS, Pai RK, Beck AH, McKenney JK. PAX8 expression reliably distinguishes pancreatic well-differentiated neuroendocrine tumors from ileal and pulmonary well-differentiated neuroendocrine tumors and pancreatic acinar cell carcinoma. Mod Pathol. 2011;24:412–24.
18. Erickson LA, Papouchado B, Dimashkieh H, Zhang S, Nakamura N, Lloyd RV, et al. Cdx2 as a marker for neuroendocrine tumors of unknown primary sites. Endocr Pathol. 2004;15:247–52.
19. Du EZ, Goldstraw P, Zacharias J, Tiffet O, Craig PJ, Nicholson AG, et al. TTF-1 expression is specific for lung primary in typical and atypical carcinoids: TTF-1-positive carcinoids are predominantly in peripheral location. Hum Pathol. 2004;35:825–31.
20. Vassos N, Agaimy A, Klein P, Hohenberger W, Croner RS. Solid-pseudopapillary neoplasm (SPN) of the pancreas: case series and literature review on an enigmatic entity. Int J Clin Exp Pathol. 2013;6:1051–9.
21. Chetty R, Serra S. Loss of expression of E-cadherin in solid pseudopapillary tumors of the pancreas. Pancreas. 2009;38:338; author reply 338–9.
22. Jiang K, Lawson D, Cohen C, Siddiqui MT. Galectin-3 and PTEN expression in pancreatic ductal adenocarcinoma, pancreatic neuroendocrine neoplasms and gastrointestinal tumors on fine-needle aspiration cytology. Acta Cytol. 2014;58:281–7.
23. Williams GT. Endocrine tumours of the gastrointestinal tract-selected topics. Histopathology. 2007;50:30–41.

24. McNicol AM. Histopathology and immunohistochemistry of adrenal medullary tumors and paragangliomas. Endocr Pathol. 2006;17:329–36.
25. He J, Wang X, Zheng W, Zhao Y. Retroperitoneal paraganglioma with metastasis to the abdominal vertebra: a case report. Diagn Pathol. 2013;8:52.
26. Hayes-Jordan A, Anderson PM. The diagnosis and management of desmoplastic small round cell tumor: a review. Curr Opin Oncol. 2011;23:385–9.
27. Fischer S, Asa SL. Application of immunohistochemistry to thyroid neoplasms. Arch Pathol Lab Med. 2008;132:359–72.

Role of Immunohistochemistry and Molecular Genetics in Neuroendocrine Tumors

Kun Jiang, Ujalla Sheikh, Aejaz Nasir, and Domenico Coppola

Introduction

Neuroendocrine tumors (NETs) are a family of neoplasms that arises from nervous (neuro-) system and hormonal (endocrine) cells. These tumors may originate from a variety of organs [1]. In the gastrointestinal (GI) tract, NET has been identified in each organ and site, mostly in the small intestine and appendix, followed by the stomach and colon. The esophagus and anal region are less involved than the rest of the GI tract [1]. Neuroendocrine cells in the GI tract may be viewed as the largest endocrine organ in the human body. NET frequently occurs in the luminal parts of the GI tract but also in the pancreatobiliary system, where they often involve the pancreas. It has been well recognized that most NETs are low grade, while a minority of neuroendocrine neoplasms demonstrate an aggressive behavior and are classified as neuroendocrine carcinoma (NEC) [1].

Histologically, the cells of NET share common characteristics, typically associated with neuroendocrine differentiation: medium to abundant amount of slightly eosinophilic, finely granular cytoplasm, containing neurosecretory

K. Jiang, MD, PHD
Anatomic Pathology, H. Lee Moffitt Cancer Center, Tampa, FL, USA

Department of Oncologic Science, University of South Florida, Tampa, FL 33612, USA
e-mail: kun.jiang@moffitt.org

U. Sheikh, MD • D. Coppola, MD (✉)
Department of Anatomic Pathology, Moffitt Cancer Center, Tampa, FL, USA
e-mail: domenico.coppola@moffitt.org

A. Nasir, MD, MPhil, FCAP (✉)
Diagnostic & Experimental Pathology (Tailored Therapeutics), Lilly Research Laboratories, Eli Lilly & Co., Indianapolis, IN, USA
e-mail: nasirae@lilly.com

A. Nasir, D. Coppola (eds.), *Neuroendocrine Tumors: Review of Pathology, Molecular and Therapeutic Advances*, DOI 10.1007/978-1-4939-3426-3_4

granules (as it can be visualized by electron microscopy). The nuclei are oval to round and pericentrally or centrally located, which cytologically exhibit the "salt-pepper-like" chromatin pattern [1–4]. These morphological features are demonstrated in Fig. 1a, b, where a well-differentiated NET involving the terminal ileum is shown. Despite the absence of necrosis and the low mitotic rate (less than 2 mitoses per 10 high-power fields), the tumor infiltrated the nests and nodules of the perienteric adipose tissue. This tumor was classified as pathological stage T3. Perineural invasion and lymphovascular invasion were both present (photos not shown here). Immunohistochemically, NET cells in the GI tract produce common polypeptide hormones and multiple biogenic amines. These substances modulate the biological functions of the organs where these tumors arise [1, 2, 5–7]. Accordingly, the immunophenotypical profiles of these neoplasms are relatively specific: they are positive for markers of neuroendocrine differentiation and may produce various polypeptides and hormones unique to their subtypes [1, 2, 5–7]. NETs from a particular anatomical origin usually have similar behavior; occasionally, individual tumor within the same group may display distinct biological and biochemical characteristics [2]. There are also certain histochemical differences among various NETs, depending on their location and the grade of differentiation [4] [4]. Specifically, foregut and hindgut NETs are predominantly argentaffin negative, while midgut NETs are mostly argentaffin positive [2, 6, 8, 9]. However, for practical purposes, the workup of GI NETs does not routinely include argentaffin staining. Immunohistochemical examination of common neuroendocrine markers (usually synaptophysin, chromogranin, CD56, neuron-specific enolase) and of cell proliferation 0 markers (Ki-67 or MIB-1 labeling index) are regularly performed [2, 6, 8, 9].

Immunophenotypical Profiles of Neuroendocrine Tumors

Immunohistochemical Markers of Epithelial Differentiation and Neuroendocrine Tumors

When dealing with an unknown, newly identified epithelioid neoplasm exhibiting histological features reminiscent of neuroendocrine cells (more frequently NET instead of NEC), one essential step, prior to testing the neuroendocrine nature of the lesion, is to prove that the lesional cells are epithelial in nature, usually an immunostain for cytokeratin(s) (AE1/AE3 or CAM5.2). The utility of these two markers has been displayed in a terminal ileum NET shown in Fig. 1c, d. The neuroendocrine markers are generally tested immunohistochemically at the same time or right after the cytokeratin examination. Positive synaptophysin and chromogranin A immunostains are represented by moderately to darkly labeled cytoplasm where the fine neuroendocrine granules within the cytoplasm will be highlighted by one or both markers (Fig. 1e, f).

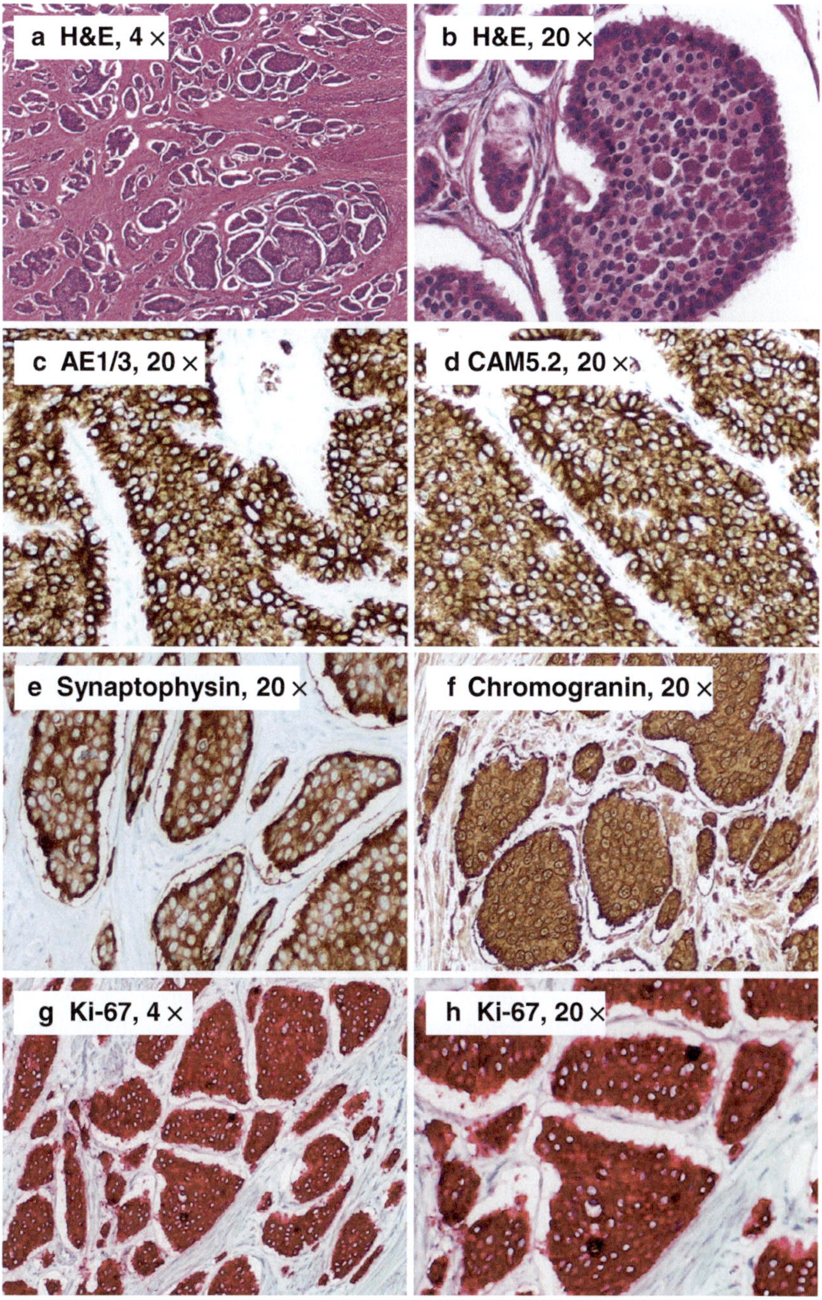

Fig. 1 Morphological futures and immunoprofile of a well-differentiated neuroendocrine tumor of the terminal ileum. (**a**, **b**) Hematoxylin and eosin-stained sections. (**c**–**f**) Cytokeratin AE1/3 and CAM5.2 and neuroendocrine (synaptophysin and chromogranin A) labeling in this grade 1 well-differentiated neuroendocrine tumor. (**g**, **h**) Ki-67 nuclear index illustrated by Ki-67 and cytokeratin (AE1/3) double staining method. *Ki-67* dark brown, *AE1/3* red. Less than 2 % Ki-67 index is seen by this double staining

Immunohistochemical Markers of Neuroendocrine Differentiation

Synaptophysin, a protein encoded by the *SYP* gene, also named the major synaptic vesicle protein p38, is a 313 amino acid synaptic vesicle glycoprotein with a molecular weight of 38 kDa [10]. Synaptophysin is extensively detected in a variety of neuroendocrine cells in the human body and was believed to play a key role in synaptic transmission. Still, the exact function of this protein remains incompletely understood. Recent research has implicated synaptophysin in the development of the nervous system and has suggested a potential modulator function of this protein in biological behavioral regulation [10, 11]. Nonetheless, due to its almost universal distribution in NETs, positive immunohistochemical staining of synaptophysin has been used as the standard for diagnosing these tumors. A diffuse unequivocal labeling for synaptophysin indicates neuroendocrine differentiation (see Fig. 1e which shows an example of synaptophysin expression in an NET of the terminal ileum. Both well-differentiated NETs and poorly differentiated NECs express synaptophysin; the latter includes small cell carcinoma and large cell neuroendocrine carcinoma [1, 5–7]. In addition, synaptophysin can be also detected in the neuroblastoma, pheochromocytoma, and medullary thyroid carcinoma, which should be included in the differential diagnosis of an NET.

Another most frequently used marker of NETs is chromogranin A. This protein is the product of *CHGA* gene, which is also called parathyroid secretory protein 1, being a member of the granin family of neuroendocrine proteins [12, 13]. Chromogranin A is located within the neurosecretory vesicles of neuroendocrine cells such as those of pancreatic islet beta cell and enterochromaffin-like (ECL) cells in the luminal GI mucosa. Chromogranin A seems to be involved in the modulation of the autocrine and paracrine function of neuroendocrine cells, and it has been recognized as the precursor of multiple functional peptides implicated in neuroendocrine functions [14, 15]. As a specific marker for NETs, chromogranin A can be detected in both low and malignant (high-grade) neuroendocrine neoplasms [1, 5–7]. Both synaptophysin and chromogranin A positivity are represented by a moderate to strong staining of the cytoplasm corresponding to the visualization of the neurosecretory granules (demonstrated in Fig. 1f).

In addition to immunoreactivity for the abovementioned neuroendocrine markers, GI NETs regularly secrete a spectrum of peptides and hormones that have been acknowledged as NET markers. For example, the majority of NETs show cellular immunoreactivity for several molecules involved in neuroendocrine functions, such as neuron-specific enolase (NSE), UCH-L1, and CD56; the latter two being regarded as relatively sensitive but less specific markers of neuroendocrine differentiation [6, 8, 16, 17]. Although historically these molecules had been holding their status as neuroendocrine markers, currently they are not routinely utilized for immunohistochemical examination.

Immunohistochemistry for Secretory Proteins and Receptors

A number of secretory molecules are important because of their site-specific expression and their involvement in the so-called carcinoid syndrome. Serotonin, for example, is mainly produced by serotonin-producing enterochromaffin cells in NETs. These NETs are most frequently identified in the small intestine (mostly in the terminal ileum and jejunum). These tumors grow in nested, insular, pseudoglandular, and rosette-like patterns [5, 6]. Approximately 90 % of small intestinal NETs express high levels of serotonin and substance P. They also occasionally express prostatic acid phosphatase. These tumors are always argentaffinic and argyrophilic. Frequently, these neuroendocrine tumors possess high levels of hormone receptors, especially somatostatin receptors, and uptake this hormone and its analogues strongly [5, 6, 18]. With the availability of newer somatostatin receptor analogues, it is becoming more relevant to evaluate the expression of various somatostatin receptors (SSTRs 1-5) in NE tumor tissues. Investigators from our institute have shown differential levels of expression of the five SSTRs in intestinal and pancreatic endocrine tumors [19]. Clinical validation and utility of such advanced immunohistochemical approaches can further contribute to the success of newer somatostatin analogues. Through their unique receptor profiles, the avidity of NETs for various hormones has been widely utilized in the studies and diagnostic workup of both primary and metastatic NETs and also in the clinical management of patients with advanced-stage GI NETs which have shown vulnerability to hormone receptor antagonists [6, 20].

Location of Neuroendocrine Neoplasms and Choice of Immunohistochemical Markers

It should be noted that sometimes the utilization of these NET markers could be restricted depending on the primary site of the neoplasm. In other words, NETs identified in the foregut (also including the pancreas, thymus, airway, and lung), midgut, and hindgut will show distinct immunoprofiles. For example, foregut NETs express serotonin and are argentaffin negative; they frequently produce histamine and are often associated with carcinoid syndrome. Hindgut NETs are also argentaffin negative, but they seldom secrete serotonin or any vasoactive peptides [1, 6, 20]. In contrast, midgut NETs are argentaffin positive; they often secrete high levels of serotonin, kinins, prostaglandins, substance P (SP), and vasoactive peptides [1, 6, 20]. Usually aware that these hormones and protein markers are not routinely examined when studying and diagnosing GI NETs. We must be aware that occasionally small intestinal NETs express only synaptophysin but not chromogranin A, and that rare cases have even shown positivity for chromogranin B but not chromogranin A.

Epithelial Versus Site-specific Immunohistochemical Markers

The majority of NETs stain with pan-cytokeratin AE1/AE3 and CAM5.2 and diffusely and strongly for neuroendocrine marker(s). In addition, depending on the site of origin, NETs may be positive for relatively specific "site of origin"-related markers. For example, NETs originating in the GI tract are usually positive for CDX-2 [21], although this is not always the case [20, 22]. NETs originating in the pancreas are usually immunohistochemically positive for nuclear PAX-8 [23]. Similarly, pulmonary NETs are often positive for nuclear TTF-1 [22]. However, be aware that, when dealing with a high-grade neuroendocrine carcinoma (NEC), a positive nuclear labeling of TTF-1 does NOT necessarily indicate a lung origin [24], and positivity for TTF-1 has been frequently seen in NECs from a wide spectrum of primary sites [25, 26].

Importantly, one must keep in mind that occasionally NETs may be cytokeratin negative. In the presence of such a case, one should consider to perform S-100 immunostaining to rule out a pheochromocytoma/paraganglioma. The latter is characterized by typical sustentacular cells which are highlighted by the S-100 stain. Careful histological examination will also identify the "zellballen" arrangement of the tumor cells and a rich fibrovascular background.

Immunohistochemistry and Grade of Neuroendocrine Neoplasms

Compared with grade 1 and grade 2 well-differentiated NETs, small cell carcinoma (SCC) and large cell neuroendocrine carcinoma (LCNEC) may show similar or weaker and focal staining for neuroendocrine markers. In some occasions, they may actually be negative or display only very focal areas of positivity for certain but not all neuroendocrine markers (Fig. 2). Hence, immunohistochemical negativity for the common neuroendocrine markers in a poorly differentiated tumor with histological features resembling a neuroendocrine carcinoma does not necessarily exclude such diagnosis. When possible, alternative marker(s) should be attempted to determine neuroendocrine differentiation. At the same time, one needs to pay attention to the histological features. In a large cell NEC, the abundant cytoplasm, the vesicular nuclei with coarse chromatin distribution and prominent nucleoli, and the high mitotic rates will be storytelling. In a small cell carcinoma, features such as scant cytoplasm, smaller cell size, extensive necrosis, frequent single cell apoptosis, fine chromatin distribution, characteristic nuclear molding, and a high Ki-67 proliferative index will direct to the correct diagnosis, even in the absence of ancillary stains.

Role of Immunohistochemistry in Differentiating Neuroendocrine from Other Malignancies

At times poorly differentiated adenocarcinoma may mimic neuroendocrine carcinoma both morphologically and immunophenotypically, causing a diagnostic dilemma. These rare tumors may occasionally form ill-formed glandular and tubular

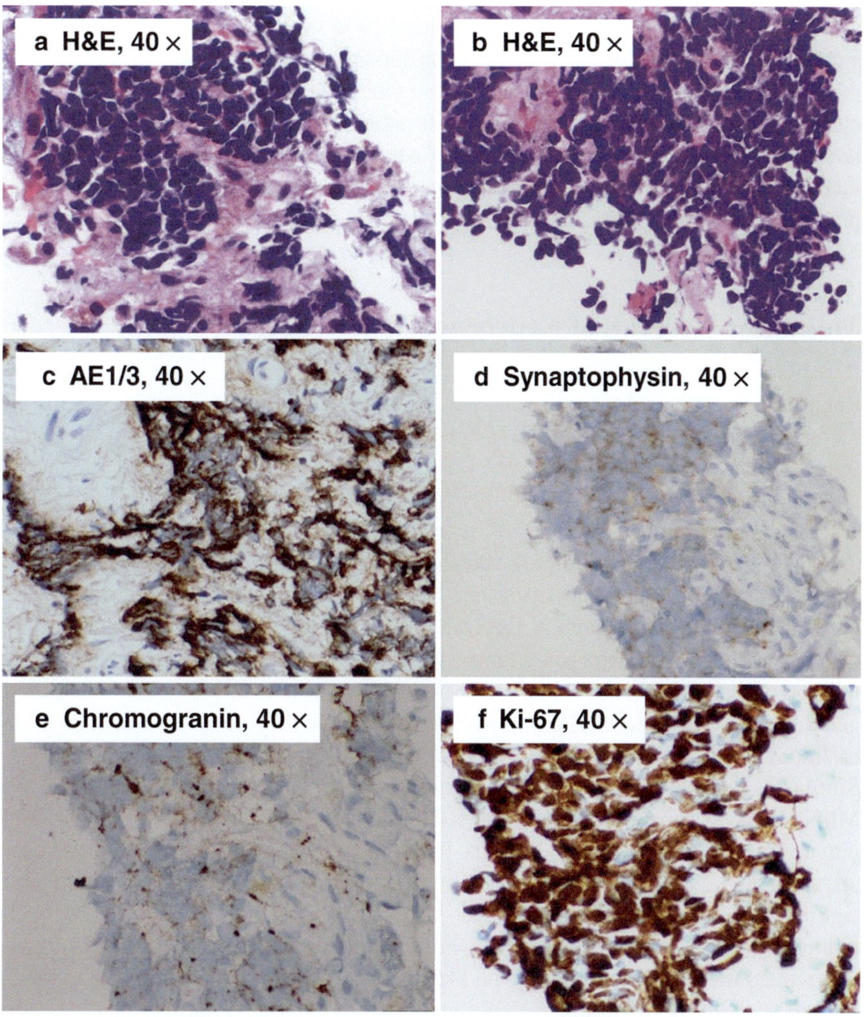

Fig. 2 Morphological features and immunoprofiles of a metastatic small cell carcinoma (SCC) involving the liver. (**a**, **b**) Hematoxylin and eosin-stained sections. (**c**) AE1/3 cytokeratin immunostain. (**d**, **e**) Relatively weak synaptophysin and chromogranin A labeling in this SCC. (**f**) Ki-67 nuclear index illustrated by Ki-67 immunostaining: more than 90 % SCC cells nuclei were labeled positive, reflecting its highly aggressive nature

structures, with subtle, intracytoplasmic, or extracellular mucinous vacuoles on H&E-stained sections. Sometimes the mucinous vacuoles are near invisible by H&E staining, but they can be highlighted by a PAS-diastase or mucicarmine special stains. Even when these tumors are positive for synaptophysin, chromogranin A, and/or CD56, the presence of positive PAS-D or mucicarmine stain should raise the suspicion of a poorly differentiated adenocarcinoma. These rare tumors are classified as either mixed adenoneuroendocrine carcinoma (MANEC) or poorly differentiated adenocarcinoma with neuroendocrine differentiation. The WHO guidelines have clear criteria on the classification of these tumors, and only when both neuroendocrine and adenocarcinoma components represent at least 30 % of the total tumor it can be classified as MANEC. In our era of precision medicine and personalized therapy, the molecular background of a tumor is becoming integral part of the data required by the clinicians for the proper management of a patient. With the recent progress in our understanding of the molecular genetics of neuroendocrine tumors, we will now provide a brief overview of these developments to the extent that they can impact the practice of diagnostic neuroendocrine pathology in the twenty-first century.

Molecular Genetics of Neuroendocrine Tumors

Regarding the molecular profile and genetic background of NETs, it has been well recognized that although most NETs are sporadic, certain patients present with multiple simultaneous NETs and/or carry a strong family history of NETs, indicating molecular and/or genetic susceptibility to NET.

One main group of disorders is represented by multiple endocrine neoplasia (MEN) types 1 and 2, which are rare hereditary cancer syndromes expressing a wide spectrum of neuroendocrine neoplasms. The current investigations on the molecular and clinical genetics associated with these entities demonstrate that the gene responsible for MEN1 is a tumor suppressor gene, which acts as a regulator of the nuclear transcriptional machinery in tumor cells [27–29]. The newly acquired genetic and diagnostic modalities will be able to identify neoplastic lesions at an earlier stage, potentially improving outcome and quality of life in those patients. Similarly, our knowledge on genotype-phenotype correlations is illustrated by MEN2, caused by a mutation in the RET oncogene [27, 30]. Novel genetic and diagnostic methods have enabled us to identify NETs lesions at much earlier stages. This advancement has led to improved outcome and quality of life in a significant number of patients [30, 31], which also facilitates more individualized treatment strategies for these patients. For example, MEN1 encodes a nuclear protein named menin, which binds to and modulates directly the transcriptional function of Jun-D. In particular, menin's tumor suppressor function involves the inhibition of Jun-D-activated transcription [31]. Predominant germline or somatic mutations in MEN1 gene are truncation or absence of the encoded product [29]; similarly, 11q13 loss of heterozygosity in tumors predicts inactivation of the other

MEN1 copy. MEN1 somatic mutation is prevalent in nonhereditary, MEN1-like tumor types [29].

Other hereditary disorders in which patients may be affected with an NET include the von Hippel-Lindau (VHL)-related syndrome, von Recklinghausen's disease or neurofibromatosis type 1 (NF-1), and tuberous sclerosis (so-called TSCs, including TSC1 and TSC2) [32]. In these patients, the genetic abnormalities play a significant role in the development of NETs, which are frequently multifocal. The pathological features of familial/hereditary NETs are generally similar to the sporadic form, with subtle differences [33]. For example, VHL disease has an incidence of one in near 36,000 births. There is over 90 % penetrance by the age of 65. Age at diagnosis ranges from as young as a few years to late 70s, with an average patient age at clinical diagnosis of 26 [34]. NF-1 or TSC1/2 mutations result in loss of function of the corresponding protein products neurofibromin and tuberin, respectively [35]. Specifically, the intact proteins of these NET-related genes suppress the function of a common target, namely, mammalian target of rapamycin (mTOR) [35], which is a key regulator of cell growth and integrates a wide variety of cellular inputs, such as growth factors, nutrients, energy status, and hypoxia-induced stress; thus, it is regarded as a potential therapeutic target for NETs in the pancreas [36, 37]. Recent investigation has indicated that everolimus significantly prolonged progression-free survival among patients with advanced stages of pancreatic neuroendocrine tumors and was associated with a low rate of severe adverse events [37].

In sporadic cases, GI NETs show predominantly genetic alterations concentrated on chromosome 18; and losses of the entire chromosome as well as smaller deletions have both been documented. The most frequently identified mutation in GI NETs is that of beta-catenin, with overexpression of cyclin D1 and c-Myc. Of notice, a set of genes including NAP1L1, MAGE-2D, and MTA1 has been correlated with prognosis [38]. In parallel, in sporadic pancreatic NETs, the newly updated WHO 2010 classification scheme adopts a proliferation-based grading system together with the classical histopathological diagnostic criteria for NETs [39]. Molecular genetics and comparative genomic hybridization (CGH) indicate that the chromosomal losses occur more frequently than the gains, whereas amplifications are uncommon. Especially, losses of chromosome 1 and 11q as well as gains of 9q appear to be early events in the development of pancreatic tumors [40, 41]. These findings demonstrate that chromosomal instability and alterations of tumor suppressor pathways are crucial mechanisms associated with NET progression and behavior. In addition, gains of chromosome 4 and losses of 6q have been found in about 50 % of functioning tumors, among which, the majority were confirmed to be insulinomas [42]. Recent genome-wide single nucleotide polymorphism (SNP) analysis observed that about up to one-third of pancreatic endocrine tumors had genetic imbalances and chromosomal aberrations [43]. Furthermore, homozygous deletion and hypermethylation of p16/MTS1 or a deletion of the p16INK4a tumor suppressor gene on chromosome 9p21 has also been demonstrated in sporadic gastrinomas, while both benign and malignant insulinomas possess high LOH rates for chromosome 22q [38]. Moreover, cyclin D1 overexpression was identified by both protein and nucleic acid analyses in 43 % of NETs [44]. Lastly, high-grade pancreatic NETs display a marked fraction of genetic abnormalities usually seen with conventional cancers, the most frequently observed abnormality being the cell cycle key regulatory TP53.

In pancreatic NETs, whole exome sequencing has shown nonsynonymous mutations that were far fewer in numbers than those in ductal pancreatic adenocarcinoma [45]. The genes commonly involved in pancreatic NETs include MEN1, DAXX, and ATRX, and genes coding for various members of the mammalian target of rapamycin (mTOR) pathway [46]. DAXX (death-domain-associated protein) and ATRX (α thalassemia/mental retardation syndrome, X-linked) are chromatin remodeling genes, and one of these genes is somatically mutated in 45 % of sporadic pancreatic NETs. Mutations in these genes are associated with the alternative lengthening of telomeres (ALT) phenotype, a telomerase-independent mechanism for telomere maintenance [47].

Pancreatic NETs with mutant MEN1, DAXX, and ATRX genes have better prognosis than wild-type tumors. As such, somatic mutations in DAXX and ATRX genes are late events in pancreatic NETs, evidenced by their absence in microadenomas [48]. Mutations in mTOR (mammalian target of rapamycin) pathway, including PIK3CA, PTEN, and TSC2 are present in 14 % of pancreatic NETs, and be targeted by mTOR pathway inhibitors [37, 45]. Similarly, the VHL/HIF pathway is also important in the genesis of pancreatic NETs [49], and pancreatic neuroendocrine microadenomas are present in about three-fourths of patients with vHL syndrome. Sporadic pancreatic NETs can rarely harbor somatic VHL gene mutation, but promoter hypermethylation and deletion of VHL occur in up to 25 % sporadic pancreatic NETs and are associated with adverse outcome [50].

Accumulating evidence suggests that a wide spectrum of molecular and genetic abnormalities could be involved in the initiation and progression of NETs. Therefore, it is conceivable that such new information may be used to predict tumor behavior and prognosis in a given case of NET. Recent work from our institution has identified several novel molecular markers of tumor progression, including RUNX1T1, palladin, and others, in localized pancreatic endocrine tumors [51, 52]. Molecular and immunohistochemical evaluation of these and other progression genes/proteins in otherwise low-grade NETs may identify subsets within otherwise indolent NETs that may benefit patients by more aggressive monitoring and evaluation of newer therapies. The epigenetic modifications and differential microRNA expression patterns examined in the aberrant signaling pathways of NETs are still being investigated; the relevant findings hopefully will shed light on predicting a given NET behavior and improving patient management. While NETs remain a group of intriguing diseases continuously posing diagnostic and management challenges [39], with the availability of higher quality immunohistochemical markers and molecular genetic approaches, we not only hope to improve diagnostic standards in the practice of neuroendocrine pathology, but we, as modern-age pathologists, will also contribute more actively to the management of NET patients by our clinical oncology colleagues.

In conclusion, immunohistochemistry plays an important role, not only in the diagnosis, differential diagnosis, and grading of neuroendocrine neoplasms, it is also relevant in the localization of various peptides secreted by the NET cells. More recently, the applications of immunohistochemistry are becoming even broader and will continue to serve the anatomic pathologists interested in cost-effective and reliable evaluation of newer protein targets, as we implement more personalized approaches to diagnose and classify NETs in the age of molecular advancement. Advances in the molecular genetics of NETs have already contributed a large body of useful knowledge regarding pathogenesis, clinical behavior, and response of NETs to the emerging targeted therapies. In future, with the advancements in genetic technologies and cost-effectiveness, it is hoped that anatomic and molecular pathologists will be able to contribute even more effectively to the management of patients with neuroendocrine malignancies.

Abbreviations

ATRX	α Thalassemia/mental retardation syndrome X-linked
DAXX	Death-domain-associated protein
NET	Neuroendocrine tumor
NSE	Neuron-specific enolase
GI	Gastrointestinal
SCC	Small cell carcinoma
LCNEC	Large cell neuroendocrine carcinoma
MANEC	Mixed adenoneuroendocrine carcinoma
VHL	Von Hippel-Lindau
MEN	Multiple endocrine neoplasms
SSTRs	Somatostatin receptors (1-5)
mTOR	Mammalian target of rapamycin

References

1. Rindi G, Petrone G, Inzani F. 25 Years of neuroendocrine neoplasms of the gastrointestinal tract. Endocr Pathol. 2014;25(1):59–64.
2. Hirabayashi K, Zamboni G, Nishi T, Tanaka A, Kajiwara H, Nakamura N. Histopathology of gastrointestinal neuroendocrine neoplasms. Front Oncol. 2013;3:2.
3. Maillard MH, Hiroz P, Wagner D, Prior J, Boubaker A, Pralong F, et al. Gastrointestinal neuroendocrine tumors: pleomorphic and often ignored. Rev Med Suisse. 2012; 8(352):1658–63.
4. Williams GT. Endocrine tumours of the gastrointestinal tract-selected topics. Histopathology. 2007;50(1):30–41.
5. Kloppel G, Rindi G, Perren A, Komminoth P, Klimstra DS. The ENETS and UICC TNM classification of neuroendocrine tumors of the gastrointestinal tract and the pancreas: comment. Pathologe. 2010;31(5):353–4.

6. Anthony LB, Strosberg JR, Klimstra DS, Maples WJ, O'Dorisio TM, Warner RR, et al. The NANETS consensus guidelines for the diagnosis and management of gastrointestinal neuroendocrine tumors (nets): well-differentiated nets of the distal colon and rectum. Pancreas. 2010;39(6):767–74.
7. Amarapurkar DN, Juneja MP, Patel ND, Amarapurkar AD, Amarapurkar PD. A retrospective clinico-pathological analysis of neuroendocrine tumors of the gastrointestinal tract. Trop Gastroenterol. 2010;31(2):101–4.
8. Oberg KE. Gastrointestinal neuroendocrine tumors. Ann Oncol. 2010;21 Suppl 7:vii72–80.
9. Leja J, Essaghir A, Essand M, Wester K, Oberg K, Totterman TH, et al. Novel markers for enterochromaffin cells and gastrointestinal neuroendocrine carcinomas. Mod Pathol. 2009;22(2):261–72.
10. Sudhof TC, Lottspeich F, Greengard P, Mehl E, Jahn R. The cDNA and derived amino acid sequences for rat and human synaptophysin. Nucleic Acids Res. 1987;15(22):9607.
11. Schmitt U, Tanimoto N, Seeliger M, Schaeffel F, Leube RE. Detection of behavioral alterations and learning deficits in mice lacking synaptophysin. Neuroscience. 2009;162(2):234–43.
12. Helman LJ, Ahn TG, Levine MA, Allison A, Cohen PS, Cooper MJ, et al. Molecular cloning and primary structure of human chromogranin A (secretory protein I) cDNA. J Biol Chem. 1988;263(23):11559–63.
13. Gazdar AF, Helman LJ, Israel MA, Russell EK, Linnoila RI, Mulshine JL, et al. Expression of neuroendocrine cell markers L-dopa decarboxylase, chromogranin A, and dense core granules in human tumors of endocrine and nonendocrine origin. Cancer Res. 1988;48(14): 4078–82.
14. Nikou GC, Lygidakis NJ, Toubanakis C, Pavlatos S, Tseleni-Balafouta S, Giannatou E, et al. Current diagnosis and treatment of gastrointestinal carcinoids in a series of 101 patients: the significance of serum chromogranin-A, somatostatin receptor scintigraphy and somatostatin analogues. Hepatogastroenterology. 2005;52(63):731–41.
15. Cetin Y, Aunis D, Bader MF, Galindo E, Jorns A, Bargsten G, et al. Chromostatin, a chromogranin A-derived bioactive peptide, is present in human pancreatic insulin (beta) cells. Proc Natl Acad Sci U S A. 1993;90(6):2360–4.
16. Schott M, Kloppel G, Raffel A, Saleh A, Knoefel WT, Scherbaum WA. Neuroendocrine neoplasms of the gastrointestinal tract. Dtsch Arztebl Int. 2011;108(18):305–12.
17. Modlin IM, Moss SF, Oberg K, Padbury R, Hicks RJ, Gustafsson BI, et al. Gastrointestinal neuroendocrine (carcinoid) tumours: current diagnosis and management. Med J Aust. 2010;193(1):46–52.
18. Burke AP, Thomas RM, Elsayed AM, Sobin LH. Carcinoids of the jejunum and ileum: an immunohistochemical and clinicopathologic study of 167 cases. Cancer. 1997;79(6):1086–93.
19. Nasir A, Stridsberg M, Strosberg J, Su PH, Livingston S, Malik HA, et al. Somatostatin receptor profiling in hepatic metastases from small intestinal and pancreatic neuroendocrine neoplasms: immunohistochemical approach with potential clinical utility. Cancer Control. 2006;13(1):52–60.
20. Rothenstein J, Cleary SP, Pond GR, Dale D, Gallinger S, Moore MJ, et al. Neuroendocrine tumors of the gastrointestinal tract: a decade of experience at the Princess Margaret Hospital. Am J Clin Oncol. 2008;31(1):64–70.
21. Erickson LA, Papouchado B, Dimashkieh H, Zhang S, Nakamura N, Lloyd RV. Cdx2 as a marker for neuroendocrine tumors of unknown primary sites. Endocr Pathol. 2004;15(3):247–52.
22. Srivastava A, Hornick JL. Immunohistochemical staining for CDX-2, PDX-1, NESP-55, and TTF-1 can help distinguish gastrointestinal carcinoid tumors from pancreatic endocrine and pulmonary carcinoid tumors. Am J Surg Pathol. 2009;33(4):626–32.
23. Sangoi AR, Ohgami RS, Pai RK, Beck AH, McKenney JK, Pai RK. PAX8 expression reliably distinguishes pancreatic well-differentiated neuroendocrine tumors from ileal and pulmonary well-differentiated neuroendocrine tumors and pancreatic acinar cell carcinoma. Mod Pathol. 2011;24(3):412–24.

24. Du EZ, Goldstraw P, Zacharias J, Tiffet O, Craig PJ, Nicholson AG, et al. TTF-1 expression is specific for lung primary in typical and atypical carcinoids: TTF-1-positive carcinoids are predominantly in peripheral location. Hum Pathol. 2004;35(7):825–31.
25. Verset L, Arvanitakis M, Loi P, Closset J, Delhaye M, Remmelink M, et al. TTF-1 positive small cell cancers: don't think they're always primary pulmonary! World J Gastrointest Oncol. 2011;3(10):144–7.
26. Agoff SN, Lamps LW, Philip AT, Amin MB, Schmidt RA, True LD, et al. Thyroid transcription factor-1 is expressed in extrapulmonary small cell carcinomas but not in other extrapulmonary neuroendocrine tumors. Mod Pathol. 2000;13(3):238–42.
27. Carling T. Multiple endocrine neoplasia syndrome: genetic basis for clinical management. Curr Opin Oncol. 2005;17(1):7–12.
28. Chandrasekharappa SC, Guru SC, Manickam P, Olufemi SE, Collins FS, Emmert-Buck MR, et al. Positional cloning of the gene for multiple endocrine neoplasia-type 1. Science. 1997;276(5311):404–7.
29. Agarwal SK, Lee Burns A, Sukhodolets KE, Kennedy PA, Obungu VH, Hickman AB, et al. Molecular pathology of the MEN1 gene. Ann N Y Acad Sci. 2004;1014:189–98.
30. Brandi ML, Gagel RF, Angeli A, Bilezikian JP, Beck-Peccoz P, Bordi C, et al. Guidelines for diagnosis and therapy of MEN type 1 and type 2. J Clin Endocrinol Metab. 2001;86(12):5658–71.
31. Agarwal SK, Guru SC, Heppner C, Erdos MR, Collins RM, Park SY, et al. Menin interacts with the AP1 transcription factor JunD and represses JunD-activated transcription. Cell. 1999;96(1):143–52.
32. Rindi G, Wiedenmann B. Neuroendocrine neoplasms of the gut and pancreas: new insights. Nat Rev Endocrinol. 2012;8(1):54–64.
33. Frankel WL. Update on pancreatic endocrine tumors. Arch Pathol Lab Med. 2006;130(7):963–6.
34. Kim JJ, Rini BI, Hansel DE. Von Hippel Lindau syndrome. Adv Exp Med Biol. 2010;685:228–49.
35. Ehehalt F, Saeger HD, Schmidt CM, Grutzmann R. Neuroendocrine tumors of the pancreas. Oncologist. 2009;14(5):456–67.
36. Wiedenmann B, Pavel M, Kos-Kudla B. From targets to treatments: a review of molecular targets in pancreatic neuroendocrine tumors. Neuroendocrinology. 2011;94(3):177–90.
37. Yao JC, Shah MH, Ito T, Bohas CL, Wolin EM, Van Cutsem E, et al. Everolimus for advanced pancreatic neuroendocrine tumors. N Engl J Med. 2011;364(6):514–23.
38. Oberg K. Genetics and molecular pathology of neuroendocrine gastrointestinal and pancreatic tumors (gastroenteropancreatic neuroendocrine tumors). Curr Opin Endocrinol Diabetes Obes. 2009;16(1):72–8.
39. Klimstra DS, Modlin IR, Coppola D, Lloyd RV, Suster S. The pathologic classification of neuroendocrine tumors: a review of nomenclature, grading, and staging systems. Pancreas. 2010;39(6):707–12.
40. Lubensky IA, Zhuang Z. Molecular genetic events in gastrointestinal and pancreatic neuroendocrine tumors. Endocr Pathol. 2007;18(3):156–62.
41. Bloomston M, Durkin A, Yang I, Rojiani M, Rosemurgy AS, Enkmann S, et al. Identification of molecular markers specific for pancreatic neuroendocrine tumors by genetic profiling of core biopsies. Ann Surg Oncol. 2004;11(4):413–9.
42. Arnold C. Neuroendocrine tumors of the gastrointestinal tract. Praxis (Bern 1994). 2007;96(1-2):19–28.
43. Kimdo H, Nagano Y, Choi IS, White JA, Yao JC, Rashid A. Allelic alterations in well-differentiated neuroendocrine tumors (carcinoid tumors) identified by genome-wide single nucleotide polymorphism analysis and comparison with pancreatic endocrine tumors. Genes Chromosomes Cancer. 2008;47(1):84–92.
44. Chung DC, Brown SB, Graeme-Cook F, Seto M, Warshaw AL, Jensen RT, et al. Overexpression of cyclin D1 occurs frequently in human pancreatic endocrine tumors. J Clin Endocrinol Metab. 2000;85(11):4373–8.

45. Jiao Y, Shi C, Edil BH, de Wilde RF, Klimstra DS, Maitra A, et al. DAXX/ATRX, MEN1, and mTOR pathway genes are frequently altered in pancreatic neuroendocrine tumors. Science. 2011;331(6021):1199–203.
46. Hessman O, Lindberg D, Einarsson A, Lillhager P, Carling T, Grimelius L, et al. Genetic alterations on 3p, 11q13, and 18q in nonfamilial and MEN 1-associated pancreatic endocrine tumors. Genes Chromosomes Cancer. 1999;26(3):258–64.
47. Heaphy CM, de Wilde RF, Jiao Y, Klein AP, Edil BH, Shi C, et al. Altered telomeres in tumors with ATRX and DAXX mutations. Science. 2011;333(6041):425.
48. de Wilde RF, Heaphy CM, Maitra A, Meeker AK, Edil BH, Wolfgang CL, et al. Loss of ATRX or DAXX expression and concomitant acquisition of the alternative lengthening of telomeres phenotype are late events in a small subset of MEN-1 syndrome pancreatic neuroendocrine tumors. Mod Pathol. 2012;25(7):1033–9.
49. Speisky D, Duces A, Bieche I, Rebours V, Hammel P, Sauvanet A, et al. Molecular profiling of pancreatic neuroendocrine tumors in sporadic and Von Hippel-Lindau patients. Clin Cancer Res. 2012;18(10):2838–49.
50. Schmitt AM, Schmid S, Rudolph T, Anlauf M, Prinz C, Kloppel G, et al. VHL inactivation is an important pathway for the development of malignant sporadic pancreatic endocrine tumors. Endocr Relat Cancer. 2009;16(4):1219–27.
51. Nasir A, Helm J, Turner L, Chen DT, Strosberg J, Hafez N, et al. RUNX1T1: a novel predictor of liver metastasis in primary pancreatic endocrine neoplasms. Pancreas. 2011;40(4):627–33.
52. Henderson-Jackson EB, Helm J, Strosberg J, Nasir NA, Yeatman TJ, Kvols LK, et al. Palladin is a marker of liver metastasis in primary pancreatic endocrine carcinomas. Anticancer Res. 2011;31(9):2957–62.

Gastroenteropancreatic: Poorly Differentiated Neuroendocrine Carcinoma

Mulazim H. Bukhari, Ujalla Sheikh, Jalil Muhammad, Domenico Coppola, and Aejaz Nasir

Introduction

Neuroendocrine carcinomas (NECs) are a rare and heterogeneous group of malignancies characterized by differences in embryologic, biologic, histopathologic, and molecular characteristics [1–5]. NECs are characterized by the expression of immunohistochemical markers of neuroendocrine differentiation and include two main histologic entities: small cell carcinoma (SCC) and large-cell NEC (LCNEC) [1]. LCNECs can be difficult to distinguish from poorly differentiated adenocarcinomas, supporting the need for synaptophysin and CgA IHC in the pathologic evaluation of such tumors. Up to 40 % of NECs contain elements of non-neuroendocrine histology, which varies depending on the primary location [6].

Neuroendocrine tumors (NETs) arise from the cells of the disseminated neuroendocrine system, which is widely distributed in the body, including the gastrointestinal tract, pancreas, lung, thyroid, adrenal gland and many other organs. In the entire

M.H. Bukhari, MBBS, DCP, MPhil, FCPS, PhD (✉)
Department of Anatomic Pathology, H. Lee Moffitt Cancer Center, Tampa, FL, USA

Department of Pathology, King Edward Medical University, Lahore, Pakistan
e-mail: mulazim.hussain@gmail.com

U. Sheikh, MD • D. Coppola, MD
Department of Anatomic Pathology, H. Lee Moffitt Cancer Center, Tampa, FL, USA

J. Muhammad
George Mason University, Fairfax, VA, USA

A. Nasir, MD, MPhil, FCAP (✉)
Diagnostic & Experimental Pathology (Tailored Therapeutics),
Lilly Research Laboratories,
Room 2391, Building 98C/2C, Eli Lilly & Co., 893 South Delaware St.,
Indianapolis, IN, USA
e-mail: nasirae@lilly.com

A. Nasir, D. Coppola (eds.), *Neuroendocrine Tumors: Review of Pathology, Molecular and Therapeutic Advances*, DOI 10.1007/978-1-4939-3426-3_5

human body, the gastrointestinal tract has the largest population of neuroendocrine (NE) cells. Despite this, NECs of the colon and rectum are rare.

Epidemiology

NECs are rare in the large intestine, but more common than elsewhere in the intestines [7]. NECs comprise 0.6 % of all carcinomas of the large intestine [4]. Also, PD-NECs account for as much as 10–20 % of malignant digestive NETs [8]. They are mainly located in the esophagus, pancreas, ampulla of Vater, and large bowel but very rarely in the ileum [9–13]. On the basis of the Surveillance, Epidemiology, and End Results (SEER) database, colorectal NEC has an incidence of 0.2 per 100,000 inhabitants, and 62 % of patients have distant disease at diagnosis [14]. In the pancreas, high-grade NECs account for <1 % of pancreatic carcinomas and no more than 2–3 % of all pancreatic NETs [14].

Molecular Pathology

The molecular pathogenesis of GEP-NEC is uncertain. It has been suggested that they either originate from multipotent stem cells, which may also be the origin of non-neuroendocrine adenocarcinomas, or arise from the dedifferentiation of well-differentiated neuroendocrine neoplasms (NENs) [15–20]. The latter possibility is less likely, because although not entirely impossible as shown in Fig. 4, it is rare to identify tumors that have separate components of well-differentiated NET and poorly differentiated NEC [21].

Colorectal NECs show higher frequency of allelic imbalances, especially involving the p53, CDKN2A/Rb pathway, FHIT (3p), DCC/SMAD4 (18q), and MEN1 [22, 23]. They may also share some molecular abnormalities with colorectal adenocarcinomas, suggesting a common origin [15, 17]. In contrast to CRCs, colorectal NECs (especially SCCs) often show Rb (protein) loss similar to pulmonary PD-NECs [24]. Most NECs have intact mismatch repair proteins [25].

Some genetic alterations are site specific, e.g., TMPRSS2-ERG gene rearrangement in PD-NECs arising in the prostate gland [26].

Histopathologic Classification Schemes

According to the earlier World Health Organization (WHO) classifications, the GEP-NETs were classified into well-differentiated NETs (WD-NETs, benign or uncertain malignant potential), well-differentiated neuroendocrine carcinomas

(WD-NECs, low-grade malignancy), and poorly differentiated NECs, "usually small-cell" neuroendocrine carcinomas (high-grade malignancy) [27, 28].

The 2010 WHO classification of digestive neoplasms [7] redefined the terminology to classify neuroendocrine neoplasms of the gastrointestinal tract and pancreas [29] to include three groups: G1 NET, G2 NET, and neuroendocrine carcinoma (NEC) that, by definition, are grade 3 (G3) neoplasms. This last category should correspond to the previously defined PD-NEC category. In general, both G1 and G2 NETs correspond to the previous well-differentiated NET (both benign and uncertain behavior categories) and well-differentiated neuroendocrine carcinoma categories [30]. However, there is no strict relationship between the G1 and G2 NETs under current WHO classification and the categories of the previous classification. Indeed, G1 NETs do not necessary correspond to WD-NETs of the previous classification just as G2 NETs do not strictly correspond to WD-NECs [30].

Histologic Subtypes of PDNEC

In 2010, WHO defined poorly differentiated neuroendocrine carcinomas to include both small cell carcinoma and large-cell neuroendocrine carcinoma [7]. The NECs are characterized by the expression of immunohistochemical markers of neuroendocrine differentiation and include two main histologic entities: small cell carcinoma and large-cell NEC [1].

Small Cell Carcinoma (SCC)

Morphologically, these are identical to SCCs arising from lungs with few differences, as mentioned in the section on esophageal SCC. The tumor cells are arranged in solid, organoid, trabecular, or pseudoglandular patterns and show high nuclear grade, minimal cytoplasm, indistinct nucleoli, and nuclear molding, increased mitotic activity, and necrosis (Fig. 1).

Large Cell Carcinoma (LCC)

These are composed of large cells arranged in organoid, nested, trabecular, rosette-like and palisading patterns that suggest neuroendocrine origin. In contrast to SCC, LCC cells exhibit more abundant cytoplasm and vesicular nuclei with prominent nucleoli (Fig. 2).

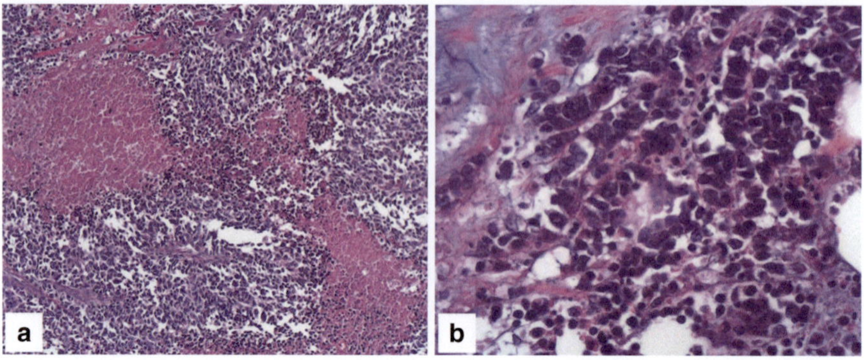

Fig. 1 Small cell neuroendocrine carcinoma of the colon characterized by sheets of neoplastic cells with abundant necrosis (**a**). Tumor cells are round to oval, small- to medium-sized (2–4 times of lymphocyte size) with scant cytoplasm and hyperchromatic nuclei and indistinct nucleoli (**b**) (Reproduced with permission from La Rosa et al. [30])

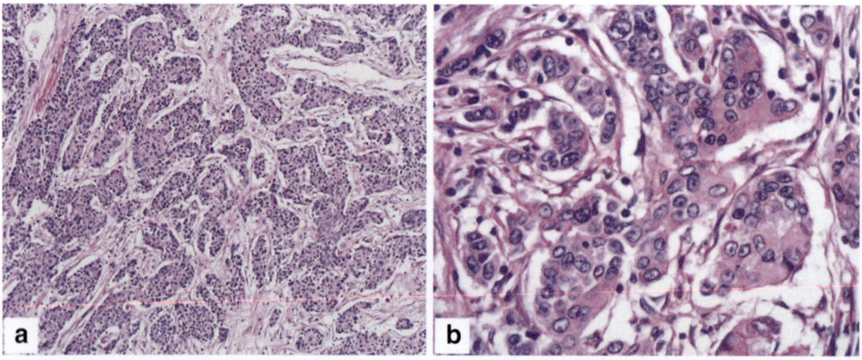

Fig. 2 Large cell neuroendocrine carcinoma showing trabecular architecture (**a**) is composed of large cells with vesicular nuclei showing prominent nucleoli and abundant eosinophilic cytoplasm (**b**) (Reproduced with permission from La Rosa et al. [30])

Mixed Adenoneuroendocrine Carcinoma (MANEC)

This has both exocrine and neuroendocrine components, with each component exceeding 30 % [7].

Site-Specific PD-NECs

Esophageal Poorly Differentiated NEC (PD-NEC)

Esophageal PDNECs are high-grade neuroendocrine carcinomas and are further divided into three categories, i.e., small cell carcinoma, mixed neuroendocrine carcinoma, and large-cell neuroendocrine carcinoma [6]. In a comprehensive histomorphologic analysis by Shia et al., most HGNECs arising in the squamous-lined GI tract (esophagus and anal canal) were small cell type (78 %), whereas most involving the glandular mucosa were large cell (53 %) or mixed (82 %) [6].

Gastric PD-NEC

Poorly differentiated neuroendocrine carcinoma of the stomach is comprised of small cell and large cell carcinoma. Large-cell neuroendocrine carcinoma (LCNEC) is the recently described member of this family, originally reported in the lung by Travis et al. Since then, LCNEC has been described in many extrapulmonary sites including the stomach, gall bladder, urinary bladder, uterine cervix, and kidney [31].

PD-NEC of the Colon and Rectum

Neuroendocrine carcinomas of the colon and rectum are uncommon, comprising less than 1 % of the colorectal cancers. These include small cell, large cell, and intermediate carcinoma [4, 32–35]. Usually found in the right colon, they have an associated adenoma or adenocarcinoma [6, 36]. In colorectum, 75 % of PD-NECs are LCC type, while in the anus, most are SCCs [6]. Primary colonic NECs without associated adenoma need to be differentiated from metastatic pulmonary SCC or cutaneous Merkel cell carcinoma [37, 38].

Histopathologic Findings

Small-cell NEC: These show diffuse or nested growth pattern and are composed of small-medium cells with minimal cytoplasm, fusiform nuclei with granular chromatin, and inconspicuous nucleoli [7]. Some larger cells or less than 25 % cells with nucleoli are acceptable [7]. Mitoses average 65/10HPFs; one-quarter of cases have a minor (<30 %) adenocarcinoma or, in case of anal canal, squamous cell carcinoma component [6].

Large-cell NEC: Tumor cells have more abundant cytoplasm and more vesicular nuclei, often with prominent nucleoli [6, 39], and are disposed in organoid, nested, trabecular, rosette-like or palisading patterns [7]. Sixty-one percent cases have a component of adenocarcinoma, which may exceed 30 % of the total tumor mass, justifying the diagnosis of MANEC [6].

MANECs: Most MANECs of the large intestine consist of adenocarcinoma (or squamous cell carcinoma in case of anal canal), mixed with high-grade NEC, which may be SCC or LCC [6, 40]. Up to 41 % of colorectal adenocarcinomas can have immunohistochemically detectable neuroendocrine cells [41–43].

Carcinoma: A malignant neoplasm with morphologically recognizable adenocarcinoma and NEC components is carcinoma, in which both components should be graded [7].

Based on the WHO criteria for pulmonary neuroendocrine tumors (Travis 2004) [44], Shia et al. [6] classified 87 high-grade GI tract tumors that initially carried a diagnosis of either poorly differentiated carcinoma with or without any neuroendocrine characteristics, SCC, or combined adenocarcinoma-neuroendocrine carcinoma into (1) *SCC* with features typical of pulmonary SCC (although cells had more round nuclear contours); (2) *LCNEC*, morphologically similar to its pulmonary counterpart and positive immunoreactivity for chromogranin (71 %) or synaptophysin (94 %) or both; (3) *mixed neuroendocrine carcinoma with intermediate histologic features* (e.g., cells with an increased nuclear/cytoplasmic ratio but with apparent nucleoli) and positive immunoreactivity for at least 1 neuroendocrine marker; and (4) *poorly differentiated adenocarcinoma* [6]. A few cases showed either non-small cell-type neuroendocrine morphology or immunoreactivity for NE markers, but not both. Most HGNECs arising in the squamous-lined GI tract (esophagus and anal canal) were small cell type (78 %), whereas most involving the glandular mucosa were large cell (53 %) or mixed (82 %) type; associated adenocarcinomas were more frequent in large cell (61 %) or mixed (36 %) type than in small cell type (26 %) [6].

Since LCNEC may not be as chemosensitive as SCC (even in the lung), the above analysis supported a dichotomous classification scheme (small cell vs. non-small cell) for HGNEC of the GI tract [6]. Separation of non-small cell type into large cell and mixed subtypes may not be necessary, as all these cancers are clinically aggressive. However, it will be important for pathologists to uniformly apply respective diagnostic criteria in classifying these malignancies, so that their pathobiologic characteristics and optimal management strategies can be determined in future studies.

Pancreatic PD-NEC

Mostly located in the head of the pancreas [45], poorly differentiated NEC of the pancreas is a highly aggressive neoplasm, with frequent metastases and poor survival, as most patients die within less than a year [37, 46]. In order to establish this diagnosis, it is necessary to demonstrate immunolabeling with general neuroendocrine markers (CgA, Syn) [7].

Histopathologic Findings Pancreatic PD-NECs are composed of tightly packed nests and diffuse irregular sheets of cells, often with extensive/geographic necrosis. NECs are classified as small-cell NECs or large-cell NECs depending on the size of the tumor cells, the prominence of the nucleoli, and the amount of cytoplasm, using criteria similar to those used for pulmonary NECs [44, 47, 48]. Mitoses are abundant (>20/10HPFs), frequently >40–50/10HPFs. In the pancreas large-cell NECs are more common than small-cell NECs [7]. The tumor cells may have variable amount of cytoplasm in intermediate and large cell variants [37]. In the pancreas, mixed adenoneuroendocrine carcinomas (MANECs) include the following subtypes: mixed acinar-neuroendocrine carcinoma, mixed ductal-neuroendocrine carcinoma, and mixed acinar-neuroendocrine-ductal carcinoma [7].

In a recent study, 107 pancreatic resections for PDNECs were critically reassessed using the 2010 WHO classification and grading (mitotic rate/index) criteria [7], including IHC markers of neuroendocrine (CgA, Syn) and acinar (trypsin, chymotrypsin) differentiation [46]. Sixty-three of 107 cases were reclassified, mostly as WD-NETs, or acinar cell carcinoma, and excluded. Of the remaining 44 definitive PDNECs, majority (61 %) were large-cell NECs, and some were combined NECs and adenocarcinoma (Fig. 3) or combined WD-NETs and PD-NEC (Fig. 4) [46]. This analysis underscored the value of careful application of diagnostic criteria and IHC markers to ensure accurate diagnosis of these unusual malignancies [46]. In the future it will be relevant to characterize the biology of these malignancies, since in addition to different morphologies, there may also be prognostic and/or therapeutic implications.

Neoplasms featuring organized pattern, uniform nuclei with salt-and-pepper chromatin, and >20 mitoses/10HPFs are currently classified as NECs, based solely

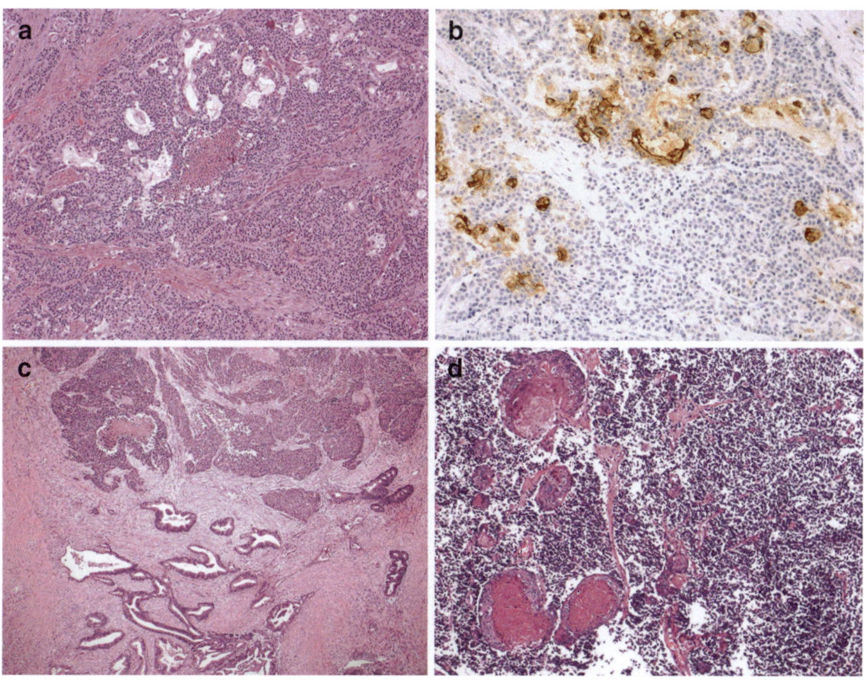

Fig. 3 Combined neuroendocrine carcinomas: Individual ductal adenocarcinoma glands are intimately admixed with nests of neuroendocrine tumor cells (**a**). The ductal adenocarcinoma glands express glycoprotein marker, CEA (**b**). Conventional ductal adenocarcinoma and neuroendocrine carcinoma components are sharply segregated (**c**). Small cell carcinoma exhibits widespread squamous differentiation (**d**) (Reproduced with permission from Basturk O et al. [46])

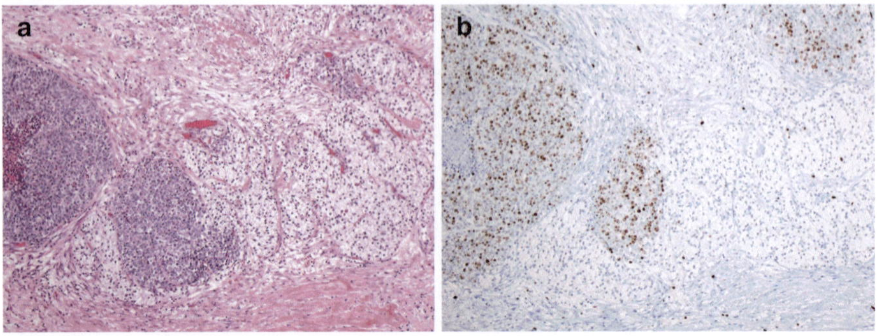

Fig. 4 Foci of poorly-differentiated NEC sharply segregated from well differentiated neuroendocrine tumor regions, composed of cells with clear cytoplasm and monotonous, round nuclei, exhibit a nested growth pattern (**a**). A Ki67 stain shows a labeling index of 1 % in this component (as opposed to 50 % in the poorly differentiated NEC component (**b**) (Reproduced with permission from Basturk O et al. [46])

on mitotic count [7]. Further studies will be important to determine the biology and clinical behavior of such neoplasms.

Clinical Features of PD-NEC

The presenting symptoms of the GEP PDNEC are nonspecific and depend to some extent on the anatomic location and spread. Symptoms may include abdominal pain, nausea, diarrhea, weight loss, and carcinoid syndrome (10 %) [49]. The most common site of metastases is regional lymph nodes. Distant metastatic sites include the liver (44 %), lung (14 %), peritoneum (14 %), and pancreas (7 %) [39].

Role of Immunohistochemistry in PD-NEC

The histologic diagnosis of SC-NEC (small cell type) is to be made based on cytomorphologic features (high N/C ratio, fine chromatin, little or invisible cytoplasm, crush artifact) on optimal quality H & E-stained sections as long as other diagnostic considerations are ruled out by appropriate workup [7]. The histologic diagnosis of LC-NEC (large cell type) needs to be supported by immunolabeling for general neuroendocrine markers (CgA, Syn, NSE, CD56) to avoid possible misdiagnoses either with the more frequent poorly differentiated adenocarcinomas and squamous cell carcinomas or with lymphomas and mesenchymal neoplasms [7, 30]. While classic SC-NEC may be negative for NE markers, usually a variable proportion of neoplastic cells stain for general NE markers in LC-NEC but less intensely than in WD-NETs [7, 50].

To some extent, IHC can also be used in the differential diagnosis of GEP PD-NEC with those arising from the lung, skin, cervix, bladder, liver, or elsewhere and to identify various diagnostic or prognostic markers by using appropriate IHC marker panels [51–53]. Once diagnosis of PD-NEC has been established, it is necessary to classify the tumor as a high-grade neuroendocrine carcinoma (small cell carcinoma or large cell type, based on morphology) and to differentiate it from low-grade NETs [54], which may also have Ki-67 index well above >20 %. All high-grade NECs are analyzed under the umbrella of PD-NECs, and it is important to determine their primary site of origin for further management.

Immunohistochemistry often plays a pivotal role in determining the cell lineage as well as the primary site of the malignancy [55, 56]. Routine measurement of urine 5-hydroxyindoleacetic acid is not useful, because GEP-NECs are rarely associated with serotonin secretion [10]. Usually, 18F-fluorodeoxyglucose positron emission tomography (FDG-PET) is strongly positive in NEC [42] and can be useful for staging, especially in patients with locoregional presentation. The relevance of somatostatin receptor imaging is uncertain [10, 57–60]. A positive imaging may indicate a relatively well-differentiated NET, despite high proliferative activity (>20 mitoses/10HPFs), although latest recommendation from WHO is to classify such tumors as PDNEC [7]. In contrast to patients with pulmonary NEC (SCLC), imaging of the brain is only indicated in patients with GEP-NEC who are symptomatic [21].

Neuroendocrine and Other IHC Markers

Synaptophysin (Syn)

Synaptophysin is an integral membrane glycoprotein found in presynaptic neuronal vesicles and in the small clear vesicles of normal and neoplastic neuroendocrine cells. It is expressed independently of other neuroendocrine markers in PD-NEC. It is used to identify and classify these tumors. Several studies have indicated the usefulness of synaptophysin [52, 61–70]. In our Neuroendocrine Tumor Pathology practice, we generally use both synaptophysin and chromogranin A because they balance specificity with sensitivity [30].

Chromogranin A (CgA)

Chromogranins are acidic glycoproteins located in neurosecretory granules. The most abundant is chromogranin A (molecular weight 68 kDa) [71, 72]. Chromogranins can be detected immunohistochemically in nearly all neuroendocrine tumors. Positivity depends on the number of dense core granules, but there may be a lack of immunoreactivity in small cell carcinoma and Merkel cell carcinoma, where secretory granules are sparse [73, 74]. Greater sensitivity in small cell carcinomas may be achieved with improved antigen retrieval methods [75, 76]. In one study, CgA was elevated in 66 % of 188 patients who had advanced GEP-NEC [10]. Care must be taken not to use CgA alone because it can be only focally positive and lead to underdiagnosis. To avoid diagnostic pitfalls, it should be used with synaptophysin, which is expressed intensely and diffusely in all PD-NECs [30].

Neuron-Specific Enolase (NSE)

NSE is a glycolytic enzyme composed of dimers of three subunits: alpha, beta, and gamma. The gamma-gamma dimers of enolase are found mainly in neurons and neuroendocrine cells and are referred to as neuron-specific enolase. However, gamma subunits have been found in other cells as well. NSE is a useful generic for neuroendocrine cells of the gastrointestinal tract and pancreas and PD-NECA arising from them. In our experience, 88 % of GEP PD-NECs were immunoreactive for NSE. Neuron-specific enolase has been tested as a marker primarily in patients with pulmonary NEC [77, 78].

CD56

Neural cell adhesion molecule (NCAM, also the cluster of differentiation CD56) is a homophilic binding glycoprotein expressed on the surface of the neurons, glia, skeletal muscle, and natural killer cells. In the future, specific detection of CD56 isoforms will help to elucidate their individual functions in the pathogenesis and progression of malignant neoplasms and may have a positive impact on the development of CD56-based immunotherapeutic strategies [79].

The sensitivity of synaptophysin IHC tends to be same for SCC, LCC, and moderately differentiated neuroendocrine carcinoma (MD-NEC), whereas CD56 and NSE immunoreactivity tend to be more intense in SCC as compared to LCC and MD-NEC. Furthermore, while NSE, PGP 9.5, and CD56 have good sensitivity, they are not highly specific as they can also be expressed in other types of non-neuroendocrine neoplasms [80, 81]

CAM 5.2

CAM 5.2 is a murine monoclonal antibody, raised against the colon carcinoma cell line HT29, which recognizes lower molecular weight intracellular cytokeratin proteins within secretory epithelia. Anti-cytokeratin (CAM 5.2) is composed of mouse IgG2a heavy chains and kappa light chains. It is usually used to study the human keratin proteins 7 and 8, which are low molecular weight proteins and are expressed on secretory epithelium and are negative in squamous epithelium [82–84]. CAM 5.2 also detects neuroendocrine carcinomas (including small cell carcinoma and Merkel cell carcinomas), germ cell tumors (with the exception of seminoma), and synovial and epithelioid sarcomas [85]. In a metastatic setting, it is important to document neuroendocrine differentiation by conventional neuroendocrine markers [86], like CgA, Syn, CD56, and NSE.

CDX2

CDX2 is a critical nuclear transcription factor for intestinal development and is expressed in neuroendocrine tumors arising from intestinal epithelium and adenocarcinomas. So far, the use of CDX2 positivity along with conventional neuroendocrine markers can differentiate intestinal adenocarcinoma and PD-NEC. In a PD-NEC, CDX2 positivity supports intestinal origin, while PD-NECs of the gall bladder and pancreas tend to be CDX2 negative. Therefore, CDX2 can be used in the workup of a case of metastatic PD-NEC with unknown primary in the right setting.

CEA

Carcinoembryonic antigen (CEA) is a glycoprotein involved in adhesion, but its production is decreased before birth. It is a prognostic and predictive factor for carcinoma of intestinal origin, especially from the colon. It can be used to differentiate primary site of PD-NECs for intestinal origin when used along other conventional neuroendocrine markers.

TTF-1

Thyroid transcription factor (TTF)-1 is a tissue-specific gene, with expression mediated largely by transcription factors. It is also a master regulatory gene and thus a potential marker of cellular lineage. This marker is useful for the diagnosis of neuroendocrine and adenocarcinoma arising from the lung [87]. Its expression in neuroendocrine tumors (NETs) has not been studied as widely as in non-NETs, with the exception of SCCs, in which TTF-1 is highly sensitive but not specific for lung primary, and is frequent in extrapulmonary SCCs. The expression of *TTF-1 in gastric or intestinal biopsy specimens may suggest the diagnosis of pulmonary or other extrapulmonary PD-NEC, because TTF1 immunoreactivity is practically absent in gastrointestinal or pancreatic NETs* [30].

ASH1

The expression of the transcription achaete-scute homolog 1 (ASH1) has also recently been investigated in a large series of lung and extrapulmonary PD-NECs with the aim of using it as a marker of lung origin since ASH1 is involved in the development of fetal lung neuroendocrine cells [88]. However, as it has been observed for other transcription factors, ASH1 expression was found in both lung and extrapulmonary PDNECs. In this study, ASH1 expression was almost exclusively restricted to PD-NECs and was negative in NETs, with the only exception of rare lung carcinoids showing a focal and faint immunoreactivity. For this reason, *ASH1 has been proposed as a marker of poor differentiation rather than a marker of lung origin* [88]. ASH1 immunohistochemistry may be useful in small biopsy specimens when morphology alone is not sufficient to make a diagnosis of PD-NEC [30].

P53

The expression of p53 can also help, because it can be frequently observed in GEP PD-NECs while it is rather rare in NETs [19, 89, 90].

Organ-Specific IHC Markers in the Workup of PD-NEC

Organ-specific IHC markers may be used to recognize clues about the possible primary source in the case of metastatic PD-NEC, unknown primary. In some cases, if further questions regarding identification remain, genetic and molecular analyses may be performed to confirm the proper diagnosis [91]. Some potential site-specific IHC markers include CK7/20, CDX2, TTF-1, trypsin, and chymotrypsin [92–98], although their specificity is not absolute and frequently needs clinical correlation.

Gastrointestinal PD-NECs

In colorectal PD-NECs, neuroendocrine differentiation is supported by reactivity for NSE, Syn, CgA, or CD56 [6, 99–104]. Some poorly differentiated LCCs may be negative for CgA.

Colorectal SCCs: 95 % colorectal SCCs express either CgA, Syn, or CD56 [6]. Ki-67 proliferative index is usually >50 % and may be almost 100 % {Bosman, 2010 #2006}. Keratin expression (AE1:AE3 or CAM 5.2) is often dot-like [105]. A proportion of colorectal SCCs may express CDX2, CK20, TTF1, CEA, CK-7, and mucin [106, 107, 108]. Since TTF-1 has been reported in a wide range of other extrapulmonary SCCs, its use to define the site of origin is limited [108].

Colorectal LCCs: At least two NE markers (Syn, CgA, or CD56) must be diffusely positive to establish this diagnosis [7]. Ki-67 proliferative index is usually 30–80 % [7]. Colorectal LCCs may be positive for CDX2, but are usually negative for TTF-1 [106], a tissue-specific transcription factor specific for the thyroid, lung, and brain tissues [4, 103]. Mucin is positive in few of the large-cell NECs [6, 106, 109].

Pancreatic PD-NECs

Immunoreactivity for NE markers (CgA, Syn) is essential to support the diagnosis of PD-NEC and to distinguish from poorly differentiated ductal adenocarcinomas of the pancreas [7]. Immunoreactivity for trypsin and chymotrypsin can help differentiate pancreatic acinar cell carcinomas from PD-NECs [7]. In the case of pancreatic PD-NECs, the possibility of metastasis from an extrapancreatic NEC must be considered and ruled out by clinical correlation and appropriate IHC workup. ISL1 [21], commonly considered as a marker of pancreatic origin, has recently been found in several extrapancreatic PD-NECs [110], including rectal NETs [111].

PD-NEC Unknown Primary

Results of IHC workup suggested that markers alone could not reliably distinguish neuroendocrine carcinomas of unknown primary in fine-needle aspiration or biopsy specimens because of low sensitivity and specificity. Therefore, use of a panel of antibodies may be helpful in identifying the site of origin of neuroendocrine carcinoma of unknown primary [112–114].

An important point about the application of IHC in the workup of PD-NEC is that any of the above markers should be used and interpreted with great caution in the right clinical setting with required clinical correlation and by considering their respective limitations.

Prognosis

Both pulmonary and extrapulmonary PDNECs appear to be highly aggressive malignancies with a propensity for early metastases and unfavorable outcomes, whether presenting as a pure histologic pattern or as component of a combined carcinoma [4, 6, 7, 9, 10, 14, 44, 60, 115–117]. HG-NECs of the pancreas are usually advanced and unresectable at diagnosis with 100 % mortality [7]. Patients with pancreatic HG-NECs survive 1 month to 1 year despite some initial favorable responses to chemotherapy [118, 119]. In a recent series of extrapulmonary PD-NECs, patients with GI primaries had more extensive disease and poorer prognoses than those with primary tumors at other locations. 70 % of patients with colorectal NECs have metastases at presentation; median survival is 10.2 months, and 5-year survival is 13 % [4, 6, 9, 105]. Prognosis of colorectal MANECs is uncertain.

Interestingly, 100 % of the patients with SCC of the uterine cervix had limited disease at the time of diagnosis and showed a favorable clinical course [115]. The survival of patients who have tumors that are well differentiated but high grade appears to be significantly longer than the survival of patients who have poorly differentiated high-grade tumors (40 months vs. 17months) [120].

Prognostic Markers

Although it is well known that GEP PDNECs are high-grade cancers associated with a poor prognosis [6], data from a few published studies [6, 89, 121] and from anecdotal experience seem to suggest that there is a fraction of patients with PD-NECs, who have a better survival rate than expected. However, it is difficult to identify this small group of patients. La Rosa et al. have recently demonstrated that the simultaneous presence of microsatellite instability (MSI) and widespread gene methylation is a predictor of better outcome in patients with colorectal PD-NECs [89]. Interestingly, this specific molecular category of PD-NECs was associated with large cell subtype, abundant peri-tumoral lymphoid infiltrate, and lack of both histologically documented vascular invasion and CD117 expression. The peri-tumoral lymphoid infiltration may represent host lymphoid response as part of biology of this type of PDNEC, as already demonstrated in patients with colorectal adenocarcinomas [122]. There is a good correlation of MSI with the immunohistochemical loss of MLH1 protein, suggesting that immunohistochemistry for the mismatch repair proteins (MLH1, MSH2, MSH6, and PMS2) should be included in the diagnostic panel to identify MSI-high PD-NECs potentially correlated with a better prognosis [30].

Response to Therapy in PD-NEC

Poorly differentiated neuroendocrine carcinomas, especially the small cell subtype (SCC), tend to have a favorable but short-lived response to platinum-based chemotherapy [4, 6, 7, 9, 10, 14, 44, 60, 115–117]. In a recent review [21] of several retrospective first-line chemotherapy studies in GEP PD-NEC, in which patients were treated with cisplatin-etoposide combinations or other chemotherapy regimens, median overall survival ranged from 10.6 to 19 months and the overall response rates ranged from 27 to 67 % [10, 21, 123–125]. It is quite obvious in these studies that span over last few decades that there is a need to improve clinical outcome in this deadly disease. This may be achieved by combining the available chemotherapy regimens with newer, more effective, and safer targeted therapies or other alternative approaches.

Diagnostic Challenges for Pathologists

Discrepancy Between Mitotic and Ki-67 Indices: Importance of Cytomorphology

Although the 2010 WHO classification of the Tumors of the GI Tract (Bosman 2010) has the great advantage of being easier to use than the previous WHO classification, especially for the diagnosis of low and intermediate malignant NET types, it still has some challenges with reference to the NECs. This is mainly due to the fact that NECs are neoplasms that, by definition, show a wide range of proliferation rates with a Ki-67 index ranging from 20 to 100 % and a mitotic index >20 mitoses × 10 HPF, independent of the morphologic picture. The observation that some tumors show a well to moderate (morphologic) differentiation together with a Ki-67 index higher than 20 % has led to some discussion as to how such cases be classified and managed. In the stomach, these tumors were defined as histologically moderately differentiated with high proliferation [126], while in the pancreas, they were defined as neuroendocrine neoplasms G3 and separated from other neuroendocrine carcinomas [110]. These studies only described the dichotomy between morphology and proliferation without studying, in detail, the clinical and therapeutic features of this intermediate category [30], which will be an area for future investigation.

Clinical Considerations for Pathologists

A number of recent studies have investigated some of the challenging areas that we think may be of interest to diagnostic pathologists with expertise in neuroendocrine tumor pathology. Basturk et al. [127] demonstrated that pancreatic neuroendocrine neoplasms showing a G2 mitotic count (2–20 mitoses × 10 HPF) but a G3 Ki-67 proliferative index (>20 %) were associated with a statistically ($p = 0.017$) better behavior than G3 tumors characterized by both >20 mitoses × 10 HPF and >20 % Ki-67 index. Similar results were found by Vélayoudom-Céphise et al. [120] who investigated a series of 28 cases of neuroendocrine neoplasms with a Ki-67 proliferative index >20 % in which 12 showed a well-differentiated morphology and 16 a poorly differentiated morphology resembling large-cell neuroendocrine carcinomas. These authors first classified tumors morphologically following the criteria proposed for the lung [128] and GEP neuroendocrine neoplasms [129]. They did not find a significant difference in the overall survival between the two categories ($p = 0.34$). However, they more rarely observed a short survival (<2 years) in G3 well-differentiated NETs (25 % of the cases) than in G3 large-cell neuroendocrine carcinomas (62.5 % of the cases, $p = 0.049$). An important finding of therapeutic relevance in this study was that patients with G3 well-differentiated NETs did not show a response to cisplatin-based chemotherapy in contrast to high-grade large-cell neuroendocrine carcinomas [120]. The different response to cisplatin-based chemotherapy was also found by Sorbye et al. who observed a statistical difference in survival and response to therapy when NECs were divided into two categories using a cutoff of 55 % for the Ki-67 index [10]. In particular, patients bearing gastrointestinal neuroendocrine neoplasms with less than 55 % had a significant longer survival ($p < 0.05$), even if it was only 4 months, than patients with highly proliferative neoplasms (Ki-67 > 55 %). More interestingly, these patients were also less responsive to chemotherapy resembling the patients with G3 well-differentiated NETs described by Vélayoudom-Céphise et al. [120].

Taken together, all these new findings suggest that high proliferative activity, as defined by G3 grading according to the ENETS and 2010 WHO proposals, should not be considered per se as synonymous of poorly differentiated NEC. This implies that proliferation alone is not sufficient for the classification of high-grade NECs, and we need to go back to morphology and add it to proliferative indices to correctly classify these neoplasms [30]. A new category of high-grade NENs defined by the combination of G3 proliferation grade and well- to moderately differentiated morphologic features should be created and separated from neoplasms showing the typical morphologic features of either small- or large-cell neuroendocrine carcinomas [30].

Although the prognostic significance of this distinction needs to be validated in large tumor series, data so far reported seem to suggest that this difference is mainly important for the choice of chemotherapy treatment [30]. The evaluation of the immunohistochemical pattern of CgA immunoreactivity has recently been proposed as an additional useful tool to help in the differential diagnosis between high-grade PD-NECs and NETs with high proliferation [130]. Indeed, chromogranin A is generally focal with a dot-like paranuclear expression in PD-NECs, while it is diffusely and strongly positive in the cytoplasm of most cells in NETs with high proliferation [30].

For these reasons, the 2010 WHO classification may be modified to introduce a new category between G2 NET and NEC that could be defined as G3 NET. In this new possible classification, the term NEC should be restricted to those neoplasms showing the typical morphologic features of either small- or large-cell neuroendocrine carcinomas as defined in the 2000 WHO classification which also show more than 55 % of Ki-67 index [30].

In conclusion, PD-NECs (grade 3, small cell or large cell) of all sites often demonstrate alterations in P53 and Rb, pursue an aggressive clinical course, and are treated with platinum-based chemotherapy. Further advances in our understanding of the molecular basis of PDNECs should lead to new diagnostic and therapeutic strategies and are an area of active investigation, as we further implement the newer model of precision oncology in the near future.

Abbreviations

ASH1	Achaete-scute homolog 1
CEA	Carcinoembryonic antigen
FDG-PET	18F-fluorodeoxyglucose positron emission tomography
IHC	Immunohistochemistry markers
ISL1	Islet 1
LCC	Large cell carcinoma
LCNEC	Large-cell neuroendocrine carcinoma
MEN1	Multiple endocrine neoplasia 1
MSI	Microsatellite instability
NCAM	Neural cell adhesion molecule
NEC	Neuroendocrine carcinoma
NENs	Neuroendocrine neoplasms

NET	Neuroendocrine tumor
NF-PET	Nonfunctioning pancreatic endocrine tumor
NSE	Neuron-specific enolase
PDNEC	Poorly differentiated neuroendocrine carcinoma
PET	Pancreatic endocrine tumor
PMH	Peptide histidine methionine
PNET	Pancreatic neuroendocrine tumor
SCC	Small cell carcinoma
SCLC	Small cell lung carcinoma
TTF-1	Thyroid transcription factor-1
WDNET	Well-differentiated neuroendocrine tumor
WHO	World Health Organization

References

1. Malhotra RK, Li W. Poorly differentiated gastroenteropancreatic neuroendocrine carcinoma associated with X-linked hyperimmunoglobulin M syndrome. Arch Pathol Lab Med. 2008;132(5):847–50.
2. Bajetta E, Catena L, Procopio G, Bichisao E, Ferrari L, Della Torre S, et al. Is the new WHO classification of neuroendocrine tumours useful for selecting an appropriate treatment? Ann Oncol. 2005;16(8):1374–80.
3. Pearse AG. The diffuse neuroendocrine system and the apud concept: related "endocrine" peptides in brain, intestine, pituitary, placenta, and anuran cutaneous glands. Med Biol. 1977;55(3):115–25.
4. Bernick PE, Klimstra DS, Shia J, Minsky B, Saltz L, Shi W, et al. Neuroendocrine carcinomas of the colon and rectum. Dis Colon Rectum. 2004;47(2):163–9.
5. Saclarides TJ, Szeluga D, Staren ED. Neuroendocrine cancers of the colon and rectum. Results of a ten-year experience. Dis Colon Rectum. 1994;37(7):635–42.
6. Shia J, Tang LH, Weiser MR, Brenner B, Adsay NV, Stelow EB, et al. Is nonsmall cell type high-grade neuroendocrine carcinoma of the tubular gastrointestinal tract a distinct disease entity? Am J Surg Pathol. 2008;32(5):719–31.
7. Bosman FT, Carneiro F, Hruban RH, Theise ND. World Health Organization (WHO) classification of tumours of the digestive system. Geneva: WHO Press; 2010.
8. Lepage C, Ciccolallo L, De Angelis R, Bouvier AM, Faivre J, Gatta G. European disparities in malignant digestive endocrine tumours survival. Int J Cancer. 2010;126(12):2928–34.
9. Brenner B, Tang LH, Klimstra DS, Kelsen DP. Small-cell carcinomas of the gastrointestinal tract: a review. J Clin Oncol. 2004;22(13):2730–9.
10. Sorbye H, Welin S, Langer SW, Vestermark LW, Holt N, Osterlund P, et al. Predictive and prognostic factors for treatment and survival in 305 patients with advanced gastrointestinal neuroendocrine carcinoma (WHO G3): the NORDIC NEC study. Ann Oncol. 2013;24(1):152–60.
11. Brenner B, Shah MA, Gonen M, Klimstra DS, Shia J, Kelsen DP. Small-cell carcinoma of the gastrointestinal tract: a retrospective study of 64 cases. Br J Cancer. 2004;90(9):1720–6.
12. Machida N, yamaguchi T, Kasuga A, et al. Multicenter retrospective analysis of systemic chemotherapy for advanced poorly differentiated neuroendocrine carcinoma of the digestive system [abstract]. J Clin Oncol. 2012;30(15S):Abstract 4046.
13. Walter T, Tougeron D, Manfredi S, et al. Clinical characteristics in 127 patients with advanced G3 gastrointestinal neuroendocrine carcinoma: the FFCD-GTE national cohort study

[abstract 2464]. Paper presented at: European Cancer Congress 2013; September 27 to October 1, 2013; Amsterdam, the Netherlands. Available at: http://2013.europeancancercongress.org/Scientific-Programme/Abstract-search.aspx#.
14. Kang H, O'Connell JB, Leonardi MJ, Maggard MA, McGory ML, Ko CY. Rare tumors of the colon and rectum: a national review. Int J Colorectal Dis. 2007;22(2):183–9.
15. Vortmeyer AO, Lubensky IA, Merino MJ, Wang CY, Pham T, Furth EE, et al. Concordance of genetic alterations in poorly differentiated colorectal neuroendocrine carcinomas and associated adenocarcinomas. J Natl Cancer Inst. 1997;89(19):1448–53.
16. Kim KM, Kim MJ, Cho BK, Choi SW, Rhyu MG. Genetic evidence for the multi-step progression of mixed glandular-neuroendocrine gastric carcinomas. Virchows Arch. 2002;440(1):85–93.
17. Ubiali A, Benetti A, Papotti M, Villanacci V, Rindi G. Genetic alterations in poorly differentiated endocrine colon carcinomas developing in tubulo-villous adenomas: a report of two cases. Virchows Arch. 2001;439(6):776–81.
18. Pizzi S, Azzoni C, Bassi D, Bottarelli L, Milione M, Bordi C. Genetic alterations in poorly differentiated endocrine carcinomas of the gastrointestinal tract. Cancer. 2003;98(6):1273–82.
19. Yachida S, Vakiani E, White CM, Zhong Y, Saunders T, Morgan R, et al. Small cell and large cell neuroendocrine carcinomas of the pancreas are genetically similar and distinct from well-differentiated pancreatic neuroendocrine tumors. Am J Surg Pathol. 2012;36(2):173–84.
20. Karkouche R, Bachet JB, Sandrini J, Mitry E, Penna C, Cote JF, et al. Colorectal neuroendocrine carcinomas and adenocarcinomas share oncogenic pathways. A clinico-pathologic study of 12 cases. Eur J Gastroenterol Hepatol. 2012;24(12):1430–7.
21. Sorbye H, Strosberg J, Baudin E, Klimstra DS, Yao JC. Gastroenteropancreatic high-grade neuroendocrine carcinoma. Cancer. 2014;120(18):2814–23.
22. Furlan D, Cerutti R, Genasetti A, Pelosi G, Uccella S, La Rosa S, et al. Microallelotyping defines the monoclonal or the polyclonal origin of mixed and collision endocrine-exocrine tumors of the gut. Lab Invest. 2003;83(7):963–71.
23. Platt CC, Haboubi NY, Schofield PF. Primary squamous cell carcinoma of the terminal ileum. J Clin Pathol. 1991;44(3):253–4.
24. Kitamura H, Yazawa T, Sato H, Okudela K, Shimoyamada H. Small cell lung cancer: significance of RB alterations and TTF-1 expression in its carcinogenesis, phenotype, and biology. Endocr Pathol. 2009;20(2):101–7.
25. Stelow EB, Moskaluk CA, Mills SE. The mismatch repair protein status of colorectal small cell neuroendocrine carcinomas. Am J Surg Pathol. 2006;30(11):1401–4.
26. Klimstra DS, Beltran H, Lilenbaum R, Bergsland E. The spectrum of neuroendocrine tumors: histologic classification, unique features and areas of overlap. Am Soc Clin Oncol Educ Book. 2015;35:92–103.
27. Solcia EKG, Sobin LH. WHO: histological typing of endocrine tumors. Berlin/New York: Springer; 2000.
28. Faggiano A, Mansueto G, Ferolla P, Milone F, del Basso de Caro ML, Lombardi G, et al. Diagnostic and prognostic implications of the World Health Organization classification of neuroendocrine tumors. J Endocrinol Invest. 2008;31(3):216–23.
29. Rindi G, Arnold R, Bosman FT, et al. Nomenclature and classification of neuroendocrine neoplasms of the digestive system. In: Bosman FT, Carneiro F, Hruban RH, Theise ND, editors. WHO classification of tumours of the digestive system. Lyon: IARC Press; 2010. p. 13–4.
30. La Rosa S, Sessa F. High-grade poorly differentiated neuroendocrine carcinomas of the gastroenteropancreatic system: from morphology to proliferation and back. Endocr Pathol. 2014;25(2):193–8.
31. Travis WDCT, Corrin B, Shimosato Y, Brambilla E. in collaboration with Sobin, LH and pathologists from 14 countries. World Health Organization International Classification of Tumors. Histological typing of lung and pleural tumors. 3rd ed. Berlin: Springer; 1999.
32. Sigel JE, Goldblum JR. Neuroendocrine neoplasms arising in inflammatory bowel disease: a report of 14 cases. Mod Pathol. 1998;11(6):537–42.

33. Spigel DR, Hainsworth JD, Greco FA. Neuroendocrine carcinoma of unknown primary site. Semin Oncol. 2009;36(1):52–9.
34. Staren ED, Gould VE, Jansson DS, Hyser M, Gooch GT, Economou SG. Neuroendocrine differentiation in "poorly differentiated" colon carcinomas. Am Surg. 1990;56(7):412–9.
35. Vilor M, Tsutsumi Y, Osamura RY, Tokunaga N, Soeda J, Ohta M, et al. Small cell neuroendocrine carcinoma of the rectum. Pathol Int. 1995;45(8):605–9.
36. Mills SE, Allen Jr MS, Cohen AR. Small-cell undifferentiated carcinoma of the colon. A clinicopathological study of five cases and their association with colonic adenomas. Am J Surg Pathol. 1983;7(7):643–51.
37. Huang WS, Lin PY, Lee IL, Chin CC, Wang JY, Yang WG. Metastatic Merkel cell carcinoma in the rectum: report of a case. Dis Colon Rectum. 2007;50(11):1992–5.
38. Lau CP, Leung WK. Caecal metastasis from a primary small-cell lung carcinoma. Hong Kong Med J. 2008;14(2):152–3.
39. Travis WD, Linnoila RI, Tsokos MG, Hitchcock CL, Cutler Jr GB, Nieman L, et al. Neuroendocrine tumors of the lung with proposed criteria for large-cell neuroendocrine carcinoma. An ultrastructural, immunohistochemical, and flow cytometric study of 35 cases. Am J Surg Pathol. 1991;15(6):529–53.
40. Makino A, Serra S, Chetty R. Composite adenocarcinoma and large cell neuroendocrine carcinoma of the rectum. Virchows Arch. 2006;448(5):644–7.
41. Indinnimeo M, Cicchini C, Memeo L, Stazi A, Provenza C, Ricci F, et al. Correlation between chromogranin-A expression and pathological variables in human colon carcinoma. Anticancer Res. 2002;22(1A):395–8.
42. Sun MH. Neuroendocrine differentiation in sporadic CRC and hereditary nonpolyosis colorectal cancer. Dis Markers. 2004;20(4–5):283–8.
43. Yao GY, Zhou JL, Lai MD, Chen XQ, Chen PH. Neuroendocrine markers in adenocarcinomas: an investigation of 356 cases. World J Gastroenterol. 2003;9(4):858–61.
44. Kleihues P, Sobin L, editors. Tumors of the lung, pleura, thymus and heart. Lyon: IARC Press; 2004.
45. McLoughlin JM, Kuhn JA, Lamont JT. Neuroendocrine tumors of the pancreas. Curr Treat Options Gastroenterol. 2004;7(5):355–64.
46. Basturk O, Tang L, Hruban RH, Adsay V, Yang Z, Krasinskas AM, et al. Poorly differentiated neuroendocrine carcinomas of the pancreas: a clinicopathologic analysis of 44 cases. Am J Surg Pathol. 2014;38(4):437–47.
47. Reyes CV, Wang T. Undifferentiated small cell carcinoma of the pancreas: a report of five cases. Cancer. 1981;47(10):2500–2.
48. Klimstra DS. Tumors of the Pancreas, Atlas of Tumor Pathology, Armed Forces Institute of Pathology. American Registry of Pathology (ARP), Washington DC, USA. Third Series, Fascicle 20, 1997.
49. Odze RGJ, Crawford J. Surgical pathology of GI tract, liver, biliary tract, and pancreas. Philadelphia: WB Saunders; 2004.
50. Hammond EH, Yowell RL, Flinner RL. Neuroendocrine carcinomas: role of immunocytochemistry and electron microscopy. Hum Pathol. 1998;29(12):1367–71.
51. Wenig BM. Undifferentiated malignant neoplasms of the sinonasal tract. Arch Pathol Lab Med. 2009;133(5):699–712.
52. Capelozzi VL. Role of immunohistochemistry in the diagnosis of lung cancer. J Bras Pneumol. 2009;35(4):375–82.
53. Kim HS, Yi SY, Jun HJ, Ahn JS, Ahn MJ, Lee J, et al. L1 cell adhesion molecule as a predictor for recurrence in pulmonary carcinoids and large-cell neuroendocrine tumors. APMIS. 2009;117(2):140–6.
54. Frankel WL. Update on pancreatic endocrine tumors. Arch Pathol Lab Med. 2006;130(7):963–6.
55. Dabbs D, Silverman J. Immunohistochemical workup of metastatic carcinoma of unknown primary. Pathol Case Rev. 2001;6(4):146–53.

56. Strosberg J, Nasir A, Coppola D, Wick M, Kvols L. Correlation between grade and prognosis in metastatic gastroenteropancreatic neuroendocrine tumors. Hum Pathol. 2009;40(9):1262–8.
57. Welin S, Sorbye H, Sebjornsen S, Knappskog S, Busch C, Oberg K. Clinical effect of temozolomide-based chemotherapy in poorly differentiated endocrine carcinoma after progression on first-line chemotherapy. Cancer. 2011;117(20):4617–22.
58. Hentic O, Hammel P, Couvelard A, Rebours V, Zappa M, Palazzo M, et al. FOLFIRI regimen: an effective second-line chemotherapy after failure of etoposide-platinum combination in patients with neuroendocrine carcinomas grade 3. Endocr Relat Cancer. 2012;19(6):751–7.
59. Binderup T, Knigge U, Loft A, Mortensen J, Pfeifer A, Federspiel B, et al. Functional imaging of neuroendocrine tumors: a head-to-head comparison of somatostatin receptor scintigraphy, 123I-MIBG scintigraphy, and 18F-FDG PET. J Nucl Med. 2010;51(5):704–12.
60. Faggiano A, Sabourin JC, Ducreux M, Lumbroso J, Duvillard P, Leboulleux S, et al. Pulmonary and extrapulmonary poorly differentiated large cell neuroendocrine carcinomas: diagnostic and prognostic features. Cancer. 2007;110(2):265–74.
61. Kulshrestha R, Vijayan VK. Immunohistochemical staining on fine needle aspiration biopsy-cell block specimens in the differential diagnosis of lung cancers. Indian J Chest Dis Allied Sci. 2009;51(1):21–5.
62. Bruder G, Wiedenmann B. Identification of a distinct 9S form of soluble clathrin in cultured cells and tissues. Exp Cell Res. 1986;164(2):449–62.
63. Gould VE, Lee I, Wiedenmann B, Moll R, Chejfec G, Franke WW. Synaptophysin: a novel marker for neurons, certain neuroendocrine cells, and their neoplasms. Hum Pathol. 1986;17(10):979–83.
64. Navone F, Jahn R, Di Gioia G, Stukenbrok H, Greengard P, De Camilli P. Protein p38: an integral membrane protein specific for small vesicles of neurons and neuroendocrine cells. J Cell Biol. 1986;103(6 Pt 1):2511–27.
65. Rehm H, Wiedenmann B, Betz H. Molecular characterization of synaptophysin, a major calcium-binding protein of the synaptic vesicle membrane. EMBO J. 1986;5(3):535–41.
66. Seemuller U, Arnhold M, Fritz H, Wiedenmann K, Machleidt W, Heinzel R, et al. The acid-stable proteinase inhibitor of human mucous secretions (HUSI-I, antileukoprotease). Complete amino acid sequence as revealed by protein and cDNA sequencing and structural homology to whey proteins and Red Sea turtle proteinase inhibitor. FEBS Lett. 1986;199(1):43–8.
67. Wiedenmann A, Langhammer W, Botzenhart K. Enterobacteria as quality criteria in unprocessed, drinking and swimming pool water. Comparative study of the occurrence of enterobacteria, Escherichia coli, coliforms, colony count, fecal streptococci and Pseudomonas aeruginosa. Zentralbl Bakteriol Mikrobiol Hyg B. 1988;187(2):91–106.
68. Wiedenmann B, Franke WW, Kuhn C, Moll R, Gould VE. Synaptophysin: a marker protein for neuroendocrine cells and neoplasms. Proc Natl Acad Sci U S A. 1986; 83(10):3500–4.
69. Wiedenmann B, Kuhn C, Schwechheimer K, Waldherr R, Raue F, Brandeis WE, et al. Synaptophysin identified in metastases of neuroendocrine tumors by immunocytochemistry and immunoblotting. Am J Clin Pathol. 1987;88(5):560–9.
70. Gould VE, Wiedenmann B, Lee I, Schwechheimer K, Dockhorn-Dworniczak B, Radosevich JA, et al. Synaptophysin expression in neuroendocrine neoplasms as determined by immunocytochemistry. Am J Pathol. 1987;126(2):243–57.
71. Kasprzak A, Zabel M, Biczysko W. Selected markers (chromogranin A, neuron-specific enolase, synaptophysin, protein gene product 9.5) in diagnosis and prognosis of neuroendocrine pulmonary tumours. Pol J Pathol. 2007;58(1):23–33.
72. Shy SW, Lee WH, Chou MC, Lai YS, Tu YC. Small cell lung carcinoma: clinicopathological, immunohistochemical, and ultrastructural study. J Surg Oncol. 1990;45(3):146–61.
73. Erickson LA, Lloyd RV. Practical markers used in the diagnosis of endocrine tumors. Adv Anat Pathol. 2004;11(4):175–89.

74. Kimura N, Pilichowska M, Okamoto H, Kimura I, Aunis D. Immunohistochemical expression of chromogranins A and B, prohormone convertases 2 and 3, and amidating enzyme in carcinoid tumors and pancreatic endocrine tumors. Mod Pathol. 2000;13(2):140–6.
75. Tony JC. The chromogranin-secretogranin family. N Engl J Med. 2003;348(25):2579–80; author reply –80.
76. Taupenot L, Harper KL, O'Connor DT. The chromogranin-secretogranin family. N Engl J Med. 2003;348(12):1134–49.
77. Korse CM, Taal BG, Vincent A, van Velthuysen ML, Baas P, Buning-Kager JC, et al. Choice of tumour markers in patients with neuroendocrine tumours is dependent on the histological grade. A marker study of Chromogranin A, Neuron specific enolase, Progastrin-releasing peptide and cytokeratin fragments. Eur J Cancer. 2012;48(5):662–71.
78. Baudin E, Gigliotti A, Ducreux M, Ropers J, Comoy E, Sabourin JC, et al. Neuron-specific enolase and chromogranin A as markers of neuroendocrine tumours. Br J Cancer. 1998;78(8):1102–7.
79. Gattenlohner S, Stuhmer T, Leich E, Reinhard M, Etschmann B, Volker HU, et al. Specific detection of CD56 (NCAM) isoforms for the identification of aggressive malignant neoplasms with progressive development. Am J Pathol. 2009;174(4):1160–71.
80. DeLellis RA, Shin SJ, Treaba DO. Immunohistology of endocrine tumors. In: Dabbs DJ, editor. Diagnostic immunohistochemistry: theranostic and genomic applications. Philadelphia: Saunders Elsevier; 2010. p. 291–339.
81. Wick MR. Immunohistology of neuroendocrine and neuroectodermal tumors. Semin Diagn Pathol. 2000;17(3):194–203.
82. Moll R, Franke WW, Schiller DL, Geiger B, Krepler R. The catalog of human cytokeratins: patterns of expression in normal epithelia, tumors and cultured cells. Cell. 1982;31(1):11–24.
83. Smedts F, Ramaekers F, Robben H, Pruszczynski M, van Muijen G, Lane B, et al. Changing patterns of keratin expression during progression of cervical intraepithelial neoplasia. Am J Pathol. 1990;136(3):657–68.
84. Makin CA, Bobrow LG, Bodmer WF. Monoclonal antibody to cytokeratin for use in routine histopathology. J Clin Pathol. 1984;37(9):975–83.
85. Leader M, Patel J, Makin C, Henry K. An analysis of the sensitivity and specificity of the cytokeratin marker CAM 5.2 for epithelial tumours. Results of a study of 203 sarcomas, 50 carcinomas and 28 malignant melanomas. Histopathology. 1986;10(12):1315–24.
86. Raymond WA, Leong AS. Immunoperoxidase staining in the detection of lymph node metastases in stage I breast cancer. Pathology. 1989;21(1):11–5.
87. Yatabe Y, Mitsudomi T, Takahashi T. TTF-1 expression in pulmonary adenocarcinomas. Am J Surg Pathol. 2002;26(6):767–73.
88. La Rosa S, Marando A, Gatti G, Rapa I, Volante M, Papotti M, et al. Achaete-scute homolog 1 as a marker of poorly differentiated neuroendocrine carcinomas of different sites: a validation study using immunohistochemistry and quantitative real-time polymerase chain reaction on 335 cases. Hum Pathol. 2013;44:1391–9.
89. La Rosa S, Marando A, Furlan D, Sahnane N, Capella C. Colorectal poorly differentiated neuroendocrine carcinomas and mixed adenoneuroendocrine carcinomas: insights into the diagnostic immunophenotype, assessment of methylation profile, and search for prognostic markers. Am J Surg Pathol. 2012;36(4):601–11.
90. La Rosa S, Sessa F, Capella C, Riva C, Leone BE, Klersy C, et al. Prognostic criteria in nonfunctioning pancreatic endocrine tumors. Virchows Arch. 1996;429:323–33.
91. Bishop AE, Power RF, Polak JM. Markers for neuroendocrine differentiation. Pathol Res Pract. 1988;183(2):119–28.
92. Shimizu T, Miwa W, Nakamori S, Ishikawa O, Konishi Y, Sekiya T. Absence of a mutation of the p21/WAF1 gene in human lung and pancreatic cancers. Jpn J Cancer Res. 1996;87(3):275–8.
93. Balta Z, Sauerbruch T, Hirner A, Buttner R, Fischer HP. Primary neuroendocrine carcinoma of the liver. From carcinoid tumor to small-cell hepatic carcinoma: case reports and review of the literature. Pathologe. 2008;29(1):53–60.

94. De Lott LB, Morrison C, Suster S, Cohn DE, Frankel WL. CDX2 is a useful marker of intestinal-type differentiation: a tissue microarray-based study of 629 tumors from various sites. Arch Pathol Lab Med. 2005;129(9):1100–5.
95. Schmitt AM, Riniker F, Anlauf M, Schmid S, Soltermann A, Moch H, et al. Islet 1 (Isl1) expression is a reliable marker for pancreatic endocrine tumors and their metastases. Am J Surg Pathol. 2008;32(3):420–5.
96. Winn B, Tavares R, Fanion J, Noble L, Gao J, Sabo E, et al. Differentiating the undifferentiated: immunohistochemical profile of medullary carcinoma of the colon with an emphasis on intestinal differentiation. Hum Pathol. 2009;40(3):398–404.
97. Yatabe Y, Koga T, Mitsudomi T, Takahashi T. CK20 expression, CDX2 expression, K-ras mutation, and goblet cell morphology in a subset of lung adenocarcinomas. J Pathol. 2004;203(2):645–52.
98. Ha Kim G, Am Song G, Youn Park D, Han Lee S, Hyun Lee D, Oh Kim T, et al. CDX2 expression is increased in gastric cancers with less invasiveness and intestinal mucin phenotype. Scand J Gastroenterol. 2006;41(8):880–6.
99. Hoda SA, Hajdu SI. Small cell carcinoma of the esophagus. Cytology and immunohistology in four cases. Acta Cytol. 1992;36(2):113–20.
100. Ikeda Y, Ozawa S, Ando N, Kitagawa Y, Ueda M, Kitajima M. Meanings of c-erbB and int-2 amplification in superficial esophageal squamous cell carcinomas. Ann Thorac Surg. 1996;62(3):835–8.
101. Mori M, Matsukuma A, Adachi Y, Miyagahara T, Matsuda H, Kuwano H, et al. Small cell carcinoma of the esophagus. Cancer. 1989;63(3):564–73.
102. Tsushima T, Tsuji Y, Abe S, Tamura F, Mizushima T, Nagashima H, et al. A case of metastatic gastric endocrine cell carcinoma which could be curably resected after chemotherapy with S-1/CDDP. Gan To Kagaku Ryoho. 2008;35(5):817–20.
103. Shpaner A, Yusuf TE. Primary gastric small-cell neuroendocrine carcinoma. Endoscopy. 2007;39 Suppl 1:E310–1.
104. Nugent SL, Cunningham SC, Alexiev BA, Bellavance E, Papadimitriou JC, Hanna N. Composite signet-ring cell/neuroendocrine carcinoma of the stomach with a metastatic neuroendocrine carcinoma component: a better prognosis entity. Diagn Pathol. 2007;2:43.
105. Gaffey MJ, Mills SE, Lack EE. Neuroendocrine carcinoma of the colon and rectum. A clinicopathologic, ultrastructural, and immunohistochemical study of 24 cases. Am J Surg Pathol. 1990;14(11):1010–23.
106. Kato T, Terashima T, Tomida S, Yamaguchi T, Kawamura H, Kimura N, et al. Cytokeratin 20-positive large cell neuroendocrine carcinoma of the colon. Pathol Int. 2005;55(8):524–9.
107. Erickson LA, Papouchado B, Dimashkieh H, Zhang S, Nakamura N, Lloyd RV. Cdx2 as a marker for neuroendocrine tumors of unknown primary sites. Endocr Pathol. 2004;15(3):247–52.
108. Cheuk W, Chan JK. Thyroid transcription factor-1 is of limited value in practical distinction between pulmonary and extrapulmonary small cell carcinomas. Am J Surg Pathol. 2001;25(4):545–6.
109. Kodama T, Shimosato Y, Koide T, Watanabe S, Teshima S. Large cell carcinoma of the lung–ultrastructural and immunohistochemical studies. Jpn J Clin Oncol. 1985;15(2):431–41.
110. Agaimy A, Erlenbach-Wunsch K, Konukiewitz B, Schmitt AM, Rieker RJ, Vieth M, et al. ISL1 expression is not restricted to pancreatic well-differentiated neuroendocrine neoplasms, but is also commonly found in well and poorly differentiated neuroendocrine neoplasms of extrapancreatic origin. Mod Pathol. 2013;26(7):995–1003.
111. Koo J, Zhou X, Moschiano E, De Peralta-Venturina M, Mertens RB, Dhall D. The immunohistochemical expression of islet 1 and PAX8 by rectal neuroendocrine tumors should be taken into account in the differential diagnosis of metastatic neuroendocrine tumors of unknown primary origin. Endocr Pathol. 2013;24(4):184–90.
112. Iacangelo AL, Eiden LE. Chromogranin A: current status as a precursor for bioactive peptides and a granulogenic/sorting factor in the regulated secretory pathway. Regul Pept. 1995;58(3):65–88.

113. Rindi G, Luinetti O, Cornaggia M, Capella C, Solcia E. Three subtypes of gastric argyrophil carcinoid and the gastric neuroendocrine carcinoma: a clinicopathologic study. Gastroenterology. 1993;104(4):994–1006.
114. Janson ET, Holmberg L, Stridsberg M, Eriksson B, Theodorsson E, Wilander E, et al. Carcinoid tumors: analysis of prognostic factors and survival in 301 patients from a referral center. Ann Oncol. 1997;8(7):685–90.
115. Lee SS, Lee JL, Ryu MH, Chang HM, Kim TW, Kim WK, et al. Extrapulmonary small cell carcinoma: single center experience with 61 patients. Acta Oncol. 2007;46(6):846–51.
116. Walenkamp AM, Sonke GS, Sleijfer DT. Clinical and therapeutic aspects of extrapulmonary small cell carcinoma. Cancer Treat Rev. 2009;35(3):228–36.
117. Garcia-Carbonero R, Capdevila J, Crespo-Herrero G, Diaz-Perez JA, Martinez Del Prado MP, Alonso Orduna V, et al. Incidence, patterns of care and prognostic factors for outcome of gastroenteropancreatic neuroendocrine tumors (GEP-NETs): results from the National Cancer Registry of Spain (RGETNE). Ann Oncol. 2010;21(9):1794–803.
118. O'Connor TP, Wade TP, Sunwoo YC, Reimers HJ, Palmer DC, Silverberg AB, et al. Small cell undifferentiated carcinoma of the pancreas. Report of a patient with tumor marker studies. Cancer. 1992;70(6):1514–9.
119. Morant R, Bruckner HW. Complete remission of refractory small cell carcinoma of the pancreas with cisplatin and etoposide. Cancer. 1989;64(10):2007–9.
120. Velayoudom-Cephise FL, Duvillard P, Foucan L, Hadoux J, Chougnet CN, Leboulleux S, et al. Are G3 ENETS neuroendocrine neoplasms heterogeneous? Endocr Relat Cancer. 2013;20(5):649–57.
121. Power DG, Asmis TR, Tang LH, Brown K, Kemeny NE. High-grade neuroendocrine carcinoma of the colon, long-term survival in advanced disease. Med Oncol. 2011;28 Suppl 1:S169–74.
122. Pages F, Galon J, Dieu-Nosjean MC, Tartour E, Sautes-Fridman C, Fridman WH. Immune infiltration in human tumors: a prognostic factor that should not be ignored. Oncogene. 2010;29(8):1093–102.
123. Moertel CG, Kvols LK, O'Connell MJ, Rubin J. Treatment of neuroendocrine carcinomas with combined etoposide and cisplatin. Evidence of major therapeutic activity in the anaplastic variants of these neoplasms. Cancer. 1991;68(2):227–32.
124. Mitry E, Baudin E, Ducreux M, Sabourin JC, Rufie P, Aparicio T, et al. Treatment of poorly differentiated neuroendocrine tumours with etoposide and cisplatin. Br J Cancer. 1999;81(8):1351–5.
125. Hainsworth JD, Spigel DR, Litchy S, Greco FA. Phase II trial of paclitaxel, carboplatin, and etoposide in advanced poorly differentiated neuroendocrine carcinoma: a Minnie Pearl Cancer Research Network Study. J Clin Oncol. 2006;24(22):3548–54.
126. La Rosa S, Inzani F, Vanoli A, Klersy C, Dainese L, Rindi G, et al. Histologic characterization and improved prognostic evaluation of 209 gastric neuroendocrine neoplasms. Hum Pathol. 2011;42:1373–84.
127. Basturk O, Yang Z, Tang LH, et al. Increased (>20 %) Ki67 proliferation index in morphologically well differentiated pancreatic neuroendocrine tumors (PanNETs) correlates with decreased overall survival. Mod Pathol. 2013;26 Suppl 2:423A.
128. Travis WD. Advances in neuroendocrine lung tumors. Ann Oncol. 2010;21 Suppl 7:vii65–71.
129. Kloppel G, Anlauf M. Epidemiology, tumour biology and histopathological classification of neuroendocrine tumours of the gastrointestinal tract. Best Pract Res Clin Gastroenterol. 2005;19(4):507–17.
130. Volante M, Birocco N, Gatti G, Duregon E, Lorizzo K, Fazio N, et al. Extrapulmonary neuroendocrine small and large cell carcinomas: a review of controversial diagnostic and therapeutic issues. Hum Pathol. 2014;45(4):665–73.

Part II
Systemic Aspects of Neuroendocrine Tumor Pathology

Neuroendocrine Neoplasms of the Brain

Yuan Frank Shan, Fulin Wang, Changshu Ke, and Meng Yan

Introduction

The central nervous system (CNS) harbors a few primary neuroendocrine neoplasms, the most common being pituitary adenomas, followed by central neurocytomas and pineal tumors, while the not very common would be metastatic neuroendocrine carcinomas from other body origins. These tumors mainly affect young adults and adult patients. As more and more clinical and research data about those tumors' histogenesis and oncogenes emerge, we understand deeper on those tumors' biology, and as this era of the personalized medicine is becoming a reality, this knowledge will help us to identify the small subsets of atypical tumors and develop more therapeutic agents for target treatment in the future.

Y.F. Shan, MD, PhD (✉)
Department of Pathology and Laboratory Medicine, University of South Florida at Tampa General Hospital, 1 Tampa General Circle, Tampa, FL 33606, USA
e-mail: yshan918@gmail.com

F. Wang, MD
Department of Pathology, China General Hospital of PLA, 28 Fuxing Road, Beijing 100853, China
e-mail: wfl301@yeah.net

C. Ke, MD, PhD • M. Yan, MD
Department of Pathology, Tongji Hospital, Tongji Medical College, Huazhong University of Sciences and Technology, 1095 Jie Fang Avenue, HanKou, Wuhan, Hubei 430030, China
e-mail: kecs@hust.edu.cn; Yanmeng529@163.com

A. Nasir, D. Coppola (eds.), *Neuroendocrine Tumors: Review of Pathology, Molecular and Therapeutic Advances*, DOI 10.1007/978-1-4939-3426-3_6

Pituitary Adenomas

Introduction

The anterior pituitary comprises several different cell types, responsible for the synthesis and secretion of a group of specific hormones, such as growth hormone (GH) and adrenocorticotropic hormone (ACTH). Each of these cell types may give rise to a discrete pituitary tumor subtype that is either hormonal active or inactive (nonfunctional). The serum test may be helpful for the diagnosis of those hormonal active pituitary tumors, such as prolactinomas (lactotroph adenomas). These tumors are the most frequent type of hyperfunctioning pituitary adenoma, and usually show increased serum prolactin level (prolactinemia). While the majority of pituitary tumors comprise nonmetastasizing slowly growing adenomas, approximately one third will become invasive and a very small proportion (about 0.1 %) will become malignant. Clinically, hormonal active tumors may give rise to syndromes like acromegaly or Cushing's disease, which in some cases are lethal. Equally, the more aggressive (fast-growing) tumors may show symptoms of intracranial mass with hypopituitarism and/or extracranial spread. The monoclonal nature of the majority of pituitary tumor subtypes was supported by data from loss of heterozygosity (LOH) analysis and by X-chromosomal inactivation analysis in female patients, which strongly suggest the view that pituitary adenomas result from a clonal expansion of a single mutated pituitary cell [1].

Although human pituitary adenomas represent one of the most common intracranial neoplasms in our practice, routine histopathological examination cannot identify which tumors are likely to progress toward an invasive phenotype or which are destined toward recurrence. Recent advances in the molecular pathology of these tumors hold significant promise for prediction of recurrence and the design of novel treatment strategies. Moreover, emerging data clearly indicate that different molecular mechanisms are involved in the pathogenesis of the various pituitary tumor subtypes. Until recently the *gsp* oncogene was the only oncogene significantly associated with pituitary tumors; however, emerging data have described a role for PTTG and cyclin D1 in pituitary tumorigenesis. For known and putative tumor suppressor gene (TSG) loci, allelic losses on the long arms of chromosomes 10, 11, and 13 are significantly associated with the transition from the noninvasive to the invasive and metastatic phenotypes, while losses on chromosome 9p occur early in pituitary tumorigenesis [1, 7].

Pituitary tumors are the result of a monoclonal outgrowth where the intrinsic genetic defects involve oncogenes, tumor suppressor genes (TSG), and most likely genes responsible for differentiation. In addition, hypothalamic- and intrapituitary-derived growth factors are imposed upon these aberrant cells, contributing to their growth characteristics. Furthermore, their genetics, as with most other tumor types, is a consequence of the combined contribution of genetic and epigenetic aberrations, targeting the genome and epigenome, respectively [1]. In these cases, "epigenetics" can be defined as "a process that heritably influences the expression of a gene without genetic change to the underlying DNA sequence itself" [3]. In these cases, heritability is principally mediated by postreplicative modifications that include methylation of cytosine bases in DNA, modification of histone proteins, and expression of microRNA (miRNA). Multiple reports show that for tumors of pituitary origin, epigenetic changes appear to be the major contributors to tumor genetics and outgrowth [3], in which frequent CpG island methylation and/or modification of histone tails is considered as the major player [3, 12, 13].

Pathology Diagnosis of Pituitary Adenoma

Routine diagnosis of pituitary adenomas is usually not challenging. One of the most characteristic features of pituitary adenoma is its monotonous histological feature, which can be easily appreciated by touch or smear preparation during intraoperative consultation/frozen section. This feature is probably due to its molecular pathogenesis of single mutated cell clonal proliferation.

In order to determine the disrupture of pituitary acini, the characteristic feature of pituitary adenoma, a reticulin stain is often requested to demonstrate the disrupture of pituitary acini. The reticulin stain can also be helpful in differential pituitary adenoma from pituitary hyperplasia, the later showing only expansion rather than disrupture of pituitary acini.

A minimal panel of immunostains is helpful to the diagnosis of pituitary adenomas, which includes synaptophysin and CAM 5.2. Pituitary adenomas are uniformly immunoreactive for synaptophysin and variably for chromogranin and CAM 5.2. In addition, synaptophysin immunohistochemically positive in a finely fibrillary pattern highlights small fragments of posterior pituitary gland that can also be included in the specimen, especially in specimens being assessed for Rathke cleft cyst.

In terms of specific anterior pituitary hormones necessary for subtyping pituitary adenomas, FSH, ACTH, GH, and PRL as a small group are recommended [132].

Oncogenes in Pituitary Adenomas

GSP

The G proteins comprise a family of heterotrimeric proteins that transduce signals from the cell surface, via ligand-receptor interactions, to downstream effectors. The alpha subunit of this complex (Gs, Gi, and Gq) in their active (GTP bound) form represents the proximal effector molecules in these signaling cascades. Heterozygous activating somatic point mutations in the alpha subunit of the stimulatory Gs protein were the earliest dominant activating mutations described in endocrine tumors [17]. Activation results when missense mutations replace residues 201 (Arg to either Cys or His) or 227 (Gln to Arg or Leu). The resultant oncogene, termed *gsp*, occurs predominantly in growth hormone (GH) secreting pituitary tumors and shows ethnic or geographic variability in its frequency in somatotropinomas. *Gsp* mutations are found in 30–40 % of Caucasians, 40 % of Koreans, and 10 % of Japanese [20] with acromegaly. However, they are infrequently detected in other pituitary adenoma subtypes [11].

The direct mechanism by which the ensuing elevated cAMP levels stimulate proliferation and GH hypersecretion is not known but may involve the phosphorylated form (activated) of the transcription factor CREB. A study of 15 somatotropinomas showed elevated levels of phosphorylated CREB in all tumors investigated, irrespective of the *gsp* status of the tumor [1].

ras

ras proto-oncogenes including H-ras, K-ras, and N-ras are all similar to the membrane-anchored G proteins. Mutations in H-ras have been detected in metastatic pituitary carcinomas and in one aggressive prolactinoma. The findings suggest that H-ras is a late event in human pituitary tumorigenesis [2, 21].

Pituitary Tumor-Transforming Gene (PTTG)

Melmed and colleagues isolated a cDNA encoding a novel pituitary tumor-transforming gene, termed PTTG. Initially isolated from a rat pituitary cell line, and later on isolated in the human homologue of the rat sequence [10], they showed that increasing levels of PTTG mRNA were found in all GH, 9 of 10 prolactinomas, 23 of 30 nonfunctional tumors, and in a single corticotropinoma [9, 10]. In addition, the human sequence was also shown to have transforming potential in vitro and in vivo similar to that of the rat sequence. The expression of PTTG in most pituitary tumors studied suggests this to be an early change in pituitary tumorigenesis.

Allelic Imbalance of the CCND1 Gene and Cyclin D1 Expression

The cyclin D1 gene (*CCND1*) located on chromosome 11q13, and is one of the most frequently amplified genes observed in human tumors, with amplification of *CCND1* usually leading to cyclin D1 protein overexpression [32]. Some reports have described this phenomenon by using allelic imbalance studies within the *CCND1* gene in which they exploited a common polymorphism in the gene coding cyclin D1 (CCND1). Hibberts et al. determined allelic imbalance of the *CCND1* gene utilizing a PCR-based analysis of microdissected tumor material [22, 23, 34]. The study showed that of 60 tumors that were informative at this locus, 25 % showed allelic imbalance, with imbalance occurring more frequently in invasive tumors than in their noninvasive counterparts ($p=0.02$). Further study showed immunohistochemical (IHC) expression of cyclin D1. Of 46/60 available for staining, 25/46 (54 %) showed positive staining, either nuclear or cytoplasmic expression of cyclin D1, while the surrounding normal cells and normal pituitaries failed to stain for this protein [4]. In tumors staining positive for cyclin D1, 9/46 (20 %) showed nuclear staining, and in 16/46 (35 %), it was exclusively confined in the cytoplasm [27]. The functional significance of cyclin D1 within the cytoplasmic compartment is unclear, but is a well-recognized event in several tumor types. Both nuclear and cytoplasmic stainings were found more frequently in nonfunctional tumor than in somatotropinomas. However, there was no correlation between cyclin D1 expression and tumor grade or between allelic imbalance and expression of this protein. The results would suggest that expression of cyclin D1 occurs early in pituitary tumorigenesis and more frequently in nonfunctional tumors. The lack of an association between allelic imbalance and expression would suggest that mechanisms in addition to amplification are responsible for deregulated expression and await further study [1].

Tumor Suppressor Genes (TSG)

Several suppressor genes have been associated with pituitary tumorigenesis in human and experimental animals [2].

MEN1

The cloning of the MEN1 gene has led to the discovery of germline mutations in many familial and some sporadic MEN1 patients. Interestingly, few patients with sporadic pituitary tumors have mutations or other alterations in MEN1 or menin gene, suggesting a limited role of the menin gene in pituitary tumorigenesis and progression [2].

Retinoblastoma Susceptibility Gene (Rb)

Mutations of the Rb gene are rare in human pituitary tumors, although mice with knockout of Rb gene frequently develop tumors of the pituitary intermediate lobe [24].

p53

Although the p53 is the most commonly altered gene in human cancers, genetic alteration in the p53 gene is uncommon in human pituitary tumors. Interestingly, overexpression of p53 protein, which usually suggests alterations in p53 synthesis or processing in the tumor cells, is common in pituitary carcinomas. In addition, please note that overexpression of p53 by immunohistochemical stain is usually helpful for the diagnosis of atypical pituitary adenomas (see below). Apparently, overexpression of p53 protein in a pituitary adenoma indicates a more aggressive clinical behavior of this tumor [14, 16].

nm23

This protein is a purine factor binding substrate present in a wide spectrum of metastatic human cancers. One report suggested that an isoform of the nm23 protein had reduced expression of the protein and mRNA in invasive pituitary tumors. Genetic mutations were not associated with this decreased expression. Further studies are needed to learn about the role of nm23 in pituitary tumor progression [18].

p16/CDKN2A

The cyclin-dependent kinase (CDK) inhibitor p16 is recognized as a tumor suppressor associated with numerous tumor types. As a cell cycle regulator, by binding or sequestration of CDK4, it prevents the phosphorylation of pRB and is responsible for inhibiting progress through the G1/S cell cycle checkpoint. Loss of p16/CDKN2A by several mechanisms results in pRB remaining in its hyperphosphorylated form, negating its ability to inhibit progress through this cell cycle checkpoint. The p16/CDKN2A gene is inactivated in numerous different human cancers, and the principal mechanisms appear to be either homozygous deletion or gene silencing through methylation of its associated CpG island [3, 19, 25, 27].

The p16 gene is located on chromosome 9p21, and its mutation in several tumors supports its role as a tumor suppressor gene (TSG). A few studies indicated that epigenetic changes of p16 gene in pituitary tumors were hypermethylated [27]. Further study showed that specific subtypes of pituitary tumors, namely, nonfunctional tumors, were hypermethylated, while growth hormone tumors were not [1]; among the nonfunctional tumors, it is usually null cell adenomas, and less frequently FSH/LH tumors, that are hypermethylated, confirming the specificity of this epigenetic change in subgroups of adenomas [2].

A study by immunohistochemical stain showed that p16 protein was expressed in normal pituitary tissue and unmethylated tumors (somatotropinomas), while the methylated nonfunctional tumors were stain negative for p16 [27]. Additional study of the subdivision of nonfunctional tumors into invasive and noninvasive types showed an approximately equal frequency of methylation, suggesting, as with chromosome 9p LOH, that this represents an early change in pituitary tumorigenesis [1, 24, 30].

p27/Kip1

Another family of CDKI includes Kip/Cip proteins which include p27/Kip1 (p27), P21/WAF1/CIP1 (p21), and p57/Kip2 (p57). These proteins inhibit kinase activities of pre-activated G1 cyclin E-CDK2, cyclin D-CDK4/6, and other cyclins [15]. Many studies in human cancers have shown that p27 is probably important in tumor development of pituitary and other tumors. In the human pituitary, p27 protein decreases from normal pituitary to adenomas and carcinomas, but mutations in the p27 gene are very uncommon [15]. A few studies reported that ACTH cells and tumors have the lowest level of p27 expression and there are significant differences in p27 expression in functional and nonfunctional tumors [2]. Most interestingly, animals with both p27 and p18 knockouts develop massive pituitary tumors as well as hyperplasia and tumors of other endocrine tissue [29].

Regions of Chromosomal Loss Associated with the Progression of Pituitary Tumors

Several groups of researchers identified regions of allelic loss in pituitary tumors at known or putative TSG loci. Allelic losses on chromosomes 10q26, 11q13, and 13q12-14 mark these regions as harboring putative TSG in pituitary tumors [7]. This study also showed that allelic deletion correlated with increasingly invasive behavior as well as a significantly higher frequency of loss (at one or more loci) in invasive pituitary adenomas (33 %) and pituitary carcinomas (73 %) compared to their noninvasive counterparts (9.5 %) [7]. Other studies of the 11q13 region, at what was then the presumed site of the *MEN1* gene, had also shown this to be a frequent region of loss in pituitary tumors [31]. For losses of 13q, the map position of the tumor suppressor *RB1*, another study found that, in their sample, all 13 highly invasive or malignant pituitary tumors and 4 of their metastases had sustained deletion of one *RB1* allele, but no losses were found in four benign adenomas [4, 24]. A large cohort study showed that a loss of one or more loci was more frequent in invasive nonfunctional tumors (54 %) than in their noninvasive counterparts (29 %) [4].

The Pituitary Tumor-Associated Methylome

The first study of the major pituitary adenoma subtypes, describing a comprehensive genome-wide investigation of the DNA methylome, was published in the late part of 2012 [8]. However, advances in microarray technologies, pioneered by Illumina, have made possible the determination of, on a genome-wide scale, the methylation status at more than 27,000 CpG dinucleotides sites that span approximately 14,000 genes. These technologies also made possible the interrogation of multiple samples in a single experiment. Bioinformatic analysis, on the basis of stringent criteria, identified hypermethylated genes in each of the major pituitary adenoma subtypes [3, 26–28]. In some cases, the genes identified as inappropriately methylated were restricted to a single adenoma type, whereas others were common to two or more subtypes.

The Pituitary Tumor-Associated Methylome: The Histone Connection

The epidermal growth factor (EGF) containing fibulin-like extracellular matrix protein 1 (EFEMP1) gene, also known as fibulin 3, was initially identified as inappropriately methylated by Duong et al. [3, 8]. Further study showed that expression of this multifunctional protein was found to be significantly reduced in the majority of pituitary adenomas and irrespective of their subtypes [3]. Another study revealed that histone modifications associated with condensed chromatin were apparent in all of the tumors in which EFEMP 1 expression was reduced.

MicroRNA: Multi-target Posttranscriptional Repressors

miRNAs play important roles in a range of essential, albeit diverse, cellular process that include differentiation, cell growth, and cell death [5, 6]. Reports of their inappropriate expression in disparate tumor types are persuasive with respect to their role in tumorigenesis, including those of pituitary origin. They comprise a class of endogenous, nonprotein-coding, single-stranded RNAs that range in size from 20 to 25 nucleotides, repressing posttranscriptional protein synthesis by pairing to the 3′-untranslated regions of target mRNAs [33]. The integrity of the pairing is dependent upon the complementarity between the miRNA and the target transcript, resulting in either perfect or imperfect pairing, wherein the former leads to mRNA degradation and the latter translational repression [5, 6].

Inappropriate miRNA Expression Patterns (and Its Functional Consequences) in Pituitary Adenomas

Many data in recent years showed inappropriate expression of miRNA in pituitary tumors as either an increase or decrease, as related to the normal gland. Several reports have addressed and determined the potential of miRNAs to elicit tumor suppressor activity. Another study on GH3 cells showed that miR-15, miR-16, miR-26a, miR-19a2, and let-7a inhibited cell proliferation, colony-forming activity (CFA), and led to a decrease in cell viability. Further study showed that a majority of these miRNAs showed significant reduced expression in growth hormone adenomas and also in most other pituitary adenoma subtypes [1, 3].

Diagnostic and Clinical Management on Pituitary Adenomas

Routine histological diagnoses of pituitary adenomas are usually not difficult, and confirming the diagnosis usually requests a reticulin stain to confirm the neoplastic nature of the pituitary adenoma by demonstrating the disrupture of the normal pituitary fiber network (acini). In addition, the reticulin stain may be helpful to identify the expanded, but not ruptured, pituitary acini structure as in pituitary hyperplasia rather than adenoma. Most laboratories routinely perform the immunohistochemical stains to identify the endocrine abnormality in pituitary adenomas. A subtype of pituitary adenomas should be mentioned here as “atypical pituitary adenomas” since it carries more recurrence. The diagnosis of an atypical pituitary adenoma should be considered when the tumor shows mitosis, and/or is positive for p53, and has more than 3 % proliferation index of Ki-67 (MIB-1) by immunohistochemistry, which indicates an unusually high recurrent rate in this type of tumor.

Clinically, more active management on those nonfunctional pituitary adenomas should be considered since accumulating data indicates that those nonfunctional pituitary adenomas usually are associated with more aggressive clinical behavior due to their underlying molecular abnormalities.

Conclusion

Recent research findings attest to the significant impact of aberrations that target the epigenomic landscape as contributors to the genetics and outgrowth of pituitary adenomas. These changes are found in each of the principle targets that influence chromatin remodeling, namely, CpG island methylation, histone tail modification, and inappropriate expression of miRNAs. Different from genetic changes, epigenetic changes are reversible and thereby offer the prospect of restoring gene expression. The ability of epidrugs to induce expression of previously silenced genes offers significant promise toward new avenues in treatment options and thus guides clinical decision-making. In these cases, epidrugs might find uses as stand-alone therapies or may be used in conjunction with more conventional therapeutic options [3].

Central Neurocytomas

Introduction

Central neurocytoma (CN) is a rare neuronal tumor of the CNS, which was recognized in the early 1980s. These tumors, though mostly benign (WHO grade II), are more often likely to recur after surgery than previously thought.

In 1982 Hassoun and co-workers described two cases of primary intraventricular tumor with features of neuronal differentiation and a benign clinical behavior [39]. In 1985, Wilson et al. also reported a rare case of lateral ventricular tumor that resembled oligodendroglioma on a light microscope [40]. However, it was Hassoun who first used the term "central neurocytoma" [39]. With its indolent course and nonaggressive behavior, the tumor has often been called "benign central neurocytoma." It is believe to arise in young adults from the neuronal cells of the septum pellucidum and the subependymal cells of the lateral ventricles. However, as more information emerged, it has been recognized that these tumors are neither always benign nor are they necessarily centrally located [35]. More recent data suggests that their location, biological potential, and clinical behavior are more variable than previously thought. In addition, cases of extraventricular and parenchymal neurocytomas as well as tumor cell dissemination through cerebrospinal fluid (CSF) have been reported [77]. Recent studies indicating their atypical location, aggressive biological behavior, and frequent recurrences after subtotal/total surgical resection have generated significant interest in various adjunctive treatment modalities and also in their nomenclature, lineage potential, and molecular regulation [35].

Clinical Features of Central Neurocytoma

Central neurocytomas represent approximately 0.1–0.5 % of all primary brain tumors, and more than 500 cases have been reported since Hassoun's original report. These tumors are more common among Asians and Japanese as compared to Western population. The majority of central neurocytomas are located in the lateral ventricle, most in the anterior half, with a preference for the left. Some may extend into the third ventricle. In a classic case of central neurocytoma, the patient presents with an insidious onset of symptoms related to increased intracranial pressure, due to the obstructive hydrocephalus caused by blocking the CSF flow to the foramen of Monroe. The patient may have headaches, seizures, nausea and vomiting, visual impairment, and gait, bladder, and memory disturbances. Lateralizing signs were reported in cases of parenchymal lesions. Rarely, acute presentation with intraventricular hemorrhage has been reported [35].

Pathology of Central Neurocytoma

Pathological Diagnosis of Central Neurocytoma

Although rare, central neurocytomas usually do not pose too much of diagnostic challenge in practice. The unique location and morphology are helpful for making a correct diagnosis. Some points that need to be mentioned here are major differential diagnosis and atypical central neurocytoma.

Differential Diagnosis of Central Neurocytoma

Due to its unique low-grade nuclear morphology and commonly calcified background, major differential diagnosis may include low-grade oligodendroglioma and clear cell ependymoma.

Oligodendroglioma, especially those low-grade ones, carries low-grade nuclei, most often with perinuclear halos, and occasionally happens in an intraventricular location. It also usually has focally calcified areas. Differential diagnosis between those two tumors is important since they have different clinical outcomes and different treatment options. Perry et al. found no 1p/19q deletion in a series of 22 central neurocytomas [52].

Currently, chromosome 1p/19q co-deletion becomes a key marker for the diagnosis of oligodendroglioma, either by FISH (fluorescence in situ hybridization) or by LOH (loss of heterozygosity). In addition, positive for multiple neuronal markers will be helpful for central neurocytoma diagnosis.

In addition, a recent study indicates that central neurocytomas are not reactive to IDH-1 (isocitrate dehydrogenase enzyme isoform 1) and p53 [37], two markers that are usually positive in most oligodendrogliomas and low-grade astrocytomas by immunohistochemical stain.

Clear cell ependymomas are even rarer, and it is primarily a pediatric tumor. Intraventricular ones are usually without calcified background but with perivascular pseudorosettes, which can be identified by careful histological evaluation. The immunohistochemical stainings will be helpful for making a correct diagnosis.

As usual, no markers are perfect, and as such a careful histological evaluation and review of those neuroimaging studies and clinical information are still the key points for making an accurate diagnosis in our daily practice.

Additionally, almost all isolated central neurocytomas of the 4th ventricle were actually cerebellar liponeurocytomas, and those of the posterior part of the 3rd ventricle were low-grade pineal parenchymal tumors; thus, the diagnostic of central neurocytomas should be robustly argued in these two locations based on radiological images [35].

Atypical Central Neurocytomas (WHO Grade II)

The majority of central neurocytomas has low-grade histological features and has been designated as WHO grade II. A smaller subset is occasionally encountered that either has histopathological features suggestive of aggressive behavior or demonstrate an unusually elevated MIB-1 (Ki-67) proliferation index, warranting the diagnosis of "atypical central neurocytoma." However, this diagnostic variant has not been assigned a higher WHO grade yet. Microvascular proliferation, focal necrosis, and elevated mitotic activity (more than just occasional mitosis) are the histological features of atypical central neurocytomas and for atypical neurocytomas that occur in an extraventricular location. In a study of 36 central neurocytomas, the proliferative potential and histological criteria of anaplasia were inversely correlated with patients' survival. Since an MIB-1 index of greater than 2 % was associated with vascular proliferation and shorter recurrence-free interval, this threshold of proliferation was proposed for the designation of "atypical central neurocytomas." The same criteria are also used for atypical extraventricular neurocytomas [53]. Approximately 15 cases of central neurocytomas have been reported as disseminated through cerebrospinal fluid (CSF), and almost all those tumors were recurrent and labeled with higher proliferation index of MIB-1 by immunohistochemically staining (>2 %) and should be designated as atypical central neurocytomas [77].

Histogenesis

There has been a long time debate over whether central neurocytoma arises from cells committed to neuronal phenotype or from bipotential cells in the periventricular matrix [36]. The precise origin, phenotypic potential, and molecular regulation of central neurocytoma have remained largely unanswered. It is well established that the ventricular wall of human forebrain harbors a persistent pool of neural stem cells that remains mitotically active throughout life and retains the capacity to produce both neurons and glia [35].

Neural Cell of Origin

Central neurocytoma, in its purest form, was initially considered a tumor of neural origin, as the morphological pathology demonstrated the tumor with an expression pattern consistent with neurons. As by immunohistochemical studies, the tumor is consistently positive for those neural markers of synaptophysin, neuron-specific enolase (NSE), neuronal specific nuclear protein (NeuN), neuron-specific class III beta tubulin (Tuj-1) and neurofilament (NF), and negative for the glial marker of IDH-1 as well as p53 [37], although immunohistochemical markers for cell types are not specific enough to draw conclusions. In addition, ultrastructural studies demonstrated thin cell processes, parallel microtubules, and dense core vesicles [42]. Additional research found that tumor cells with sodium and calcium channels produced similar neuron-like electrophysiology [44].

Multipotential Central Neurocytoma Cells

Additional studies showed that the central neurocytoma cells can be labeled by both neural and glial markers of GFAP (glial fibrillary acidic protein) [45].

Neural Stem Cells

Neural stem cells have been shown to exist in the adult mammalian brain in the subventricular zone (SVZ) or subependymal zone [41]. Due to the frequent intraventricular location of central neurocytomas, several lines of evidence support that central neurocytomas might arise from neural stem cells. The tumor specimens can demonstrate a variety of cell types, similar to subependymal plate cells, and contain high levels of choline, cholinergic receptors, and gamma-aminobutyric acid, while containing normal or low levels of glutamate and catecholamines [49, 50]. In culture, the growth of tumor cells can be stimulated by stem cell trophic factors such as basic fibroblast growth factor [43] and epidermal growth factor [46]. Various studies have reported the presence of musashi-1, a neural stem cell marker, on central neurocytoma cells as well as expression of the neuroepithelial enhancer gene nestin, also seen in neural stem cells [43, 47, 48, 50]. Kim et al. exposed CN cells to forskolin and observed a synchronous decrease in nestin expression with adoption of a glial phenotype and an increase in GFAP staining, indicating an important correlation between genetic expression and cellular differentiation [43].

Those lines of evidence support that CN may be derived from stem cells preferentially committed toward the neuronal phenotype. It is important to note that there must be a tumor stem cell present to make the final tumor formation, which should be different from those of neural stem cells, since the tumor stem cells would give the uncontrolled proliferation ability to the tumor. It is possible that one or several neural stem cells, under some unknown factors, mutated to tumor stem cells, which finally drive the formation of a central neurocytoma.

Chromosomal Abnormalities

1p/19q

Central neurocytoma often presents a diagnostic dilemma both radiographically and histopathologically, due to its similarity to oligodendrogliomas. A current approach is to perform a chromosomal analysis to identify chromosome 1p/19q co-deletion (by FISH or LOH) as a marker for diagnosis of oligodendrogliomas. Most pathologists have advocated this technique to help finalize the diagnosis of oligodendrogliomas in difficult cases.

However, some researchers have found that some central neurocytomas, especially extraventricular ones, have the similar chromosome 1p/19q deletion [52, 55]. In addition, these studies demonstrated that those central neurocytomas with 1p/19q co-deletion were with more atypia and mitosis on histology and that all of these patients developed tumor recurrence following surgical resection. This suggests that while 1p/19q deletion in oligodendrogliomas is a good prognostic indicator for treatment response, it may be either inconsequential or possibly a predictor of poor outcome in neurocytomas [55].

Other Chromosomal Abnormalities

There are several reports of chromosomal abnormalities in central neurocytomas, including gains in 2p, 10q, and 18q. There is no functional molecular correlation identified so far. In addition, gains of chromosome 7 were identified [58]. Polysomy 7 has been implicated in the development of various tumors; for example, polysomy 7 is found in glioblastoma multiforme (GBM) and has correlated with overexpression of ErbB and MET oncogenes [59]. Trisomy 7q is also found in hereditary papillary renal cell carcinoma due to the overexpression of the MET oncogene [60].

Genetic and Oncogenesis Pathways

Genetic expression and proteomics are at the center of understanding the specific molecular genesis of tumors, and the demonstration of abnormal expression patterns in tumors creates potential for targeted and novel therapeutics [36, 38].

N-MYC and BIN-1

N-MYC is an oncogene implicated in the development of several cancers, as it is overexpressed in approximately 22 % of neuroblastomas and predicts worse outcomes [51, 61]. In a study of 55 central neurocytomas, 27 (49 %) were found to harbor N-MYC amplification [62]. In addition, BIN-1, a tumor suppressor, was found to have reduced expression in 12/20 (60 %) central neurocytomas, and the level of BIN-1 was inversely related to the level of N-MYC, suggesting that most central neurocytomas possess mutations at some point in this pathway [57]. N-MYC is required for neural proliferation and inhibits its complete neural differentiation [63]. Thus, overexpression of this oncogene could help explain both the tumorigenic characteristics of central neurocytoma and their preferential neuronal phenotype. This pathway could be an important area for the therapeutic innovation to inhibit or suppress the activity of the N-MYC gene and its product [64].

PTEN

PTEN, a tumor suppressor located in chromosome 10, was shown to be overexpressed in 12/20 (60 %) of central neurocytomas [57]. The overexpression of PTEN, a tumor suppressor gene, would appear to be protective against oncogenesis. However, PTEN overexpression has been shown to inhibit neural differentiation in pheochromocytoma via the PI3K and Map-K pathways [65]. It may help to explain the lack of full neural differentiation commonly found in these tumors.

Insulin-Like Growth Factor 2

Sim et al. compared the gene expression levels of insulin-like growth factor 2 (IGF2) in subventricular zone cells to central neurocytoma and found a 50-fold increase in central neurocytoma cells [50]. Further study demonstrated overexpression of IGF2 downstream mediators, including insulin receptors substrate 2 and PI3KR3. IGF2 has been implicated in the pathogenesis of other tumors, including other CNS neoplasms. More specifically, IGF has been shown to be involved in medulloblastoma and glioblastoma pathogenesis [66, 67]. Inhibition of the IGF2 receptor overexpression in central neurocytomas provides another potential method to prevent tumor growth and has been demonstrated in other tumor models [68, 69].

Platelet-Derived Growth Factor (PDGF) and Neuregulin (NRG)

PDGF-D and NRG-2 are two growth factor ligands that are overexpressed approximately five- and tenfold, respectively, in central neurocytoma cells as compared to controls [50]. These ligands are both particularly interesting as they have been demonstrated to contribute to cancer formation. PDGF-D acts through the PDGF receptor, and it regulates mitogenic and survival pathways in glioblastomas via the AKT/

MAP-K pathway. Its blockade significantly reduces tumor genesis in vivo [70]. Overexpression of PDGF-D has been demonstrated to play a role in the development and maintenance of a variety of other tumors as well [71]. PDGF receptor inhibitors already exist in the form of small molecules CT52923 [70] and sunitinib [72], as well as the antibody imatinib, and have been used as antineoplastic agents in other tumor types.

NRG-2 is an erbB-3/erbB-4 agonist [73]. ErbB molecules are members of the epidermal growth factor receptor family. NRG-2 acts through erbB-4 to promote proliferation of neuroblasts and GFAP-positive stem cells in the SVZ [74] and represents another target for therapeutic inhibition. Other NRGs have also been shown to promote neural stem cell growth [75]. Study on breast carcinoma suggests that high expression of NRG-2 is related to the aggressiveness of breast cancer [76]. Thus, PDGF-D and NRG-2 growth factors could explain induction of tumorigenesis in neural progenitor cells.

Others

Several genes and proteins commonly altered in brain neoplasms have been examined in central neurocytoma and found to be normal, including EGFR, BCL-2, and p53 [51, 54, 56].

Summary

Central neurocytomas are uncommon but challenging tumors of neuronal origin usually seen in young adults. Though mostly benign with indolent course, aggressive clinical behavior and recurrences after surgery are well known. So far, the exact etiological origin and behavior of these tumors are difficult to predict. Gross total surgical resection (GTR) is still the treatment of choice, with radiotherapy as a useful adjuvant in progressive residual and recurrent cases. As new molecular evidence unfolds, stereotactic radiosurgery and chemotherapy are likely to play important roles in the management of these patients in future. Recent advances in molecular regulation of these tumors indicate a future possibility of target gene therapy for these tumors [35].

Pineal Region Tumors

Introduction

The pineal gland is a unique organ with midline location, posterior to the third ventricle, and is surrounded by the splenium of the corpus callosum, thalami, corpora quadrigemina, and vermis, which defines the pineal region [78]. The human pineal gland parenchyma consists mainly of pineocytes, admixed with a few supportive astrocytes and forming a lobular pattern. The pineal gland can undergo cystic change with hemorrhagic foci, sometimes forming the pineal cyst. The cyst wall displays three-layered structure: inner gliosis layer usually with Rosenthal fiber formation, hemosiderin deposition, and macrophages, pineal parenchymal layer, and outer sclerotic leptomeningeal layer [79].

The pineal region tumors represent less than 1 % of all intracranial neoplasms of the central nervous system [80, 81]. However, it shows broad spectrum of neoplasms within this small region, e.g., gliomas (pilocytic astrocytoma, ependymoma, papilloma of choroid plexus), meningiomas, germ cell tumors (germinoma, yolk sac tumor, embryonal carcinoma, teratoma, mixed germ cell tumor), and pineal parenchymal tumors (PPT) [81, 82]. Pineal parenchymal tumors account for approximately 14–27 % of tumors originated from the pineal region [83, 84]. According to the WHO classification of CNS tumors (2007), pineal region tumors mainly can be further categorized into the following subgroups: pineocytoma, pineal parenchymal tumor of intermediate differentiation (PPTID), pineoblastoma, and papillary tumor of the pineal region (PTPR) [8]. PTPR occurs in pineal region exclusively, currently assumed originating from specialized ependymocytes of the subcommissural organ with close anatomical relation to the pineal gland [85–87]. The first three subgroups of tumors have been demonstrated bearing a strong relationship with pineocytes in the view of histogenesis. Pineocytes, a type of neuroendocrine cells, which can produce and secrete serotonin and various neurotransmitters or hormones, as well as melatonin, involved in the regulation of sleep patterns [88]. However, the papillary tumor of the pineal region has a different histogenic origin, possibly deriving from residues of the specialized ependymal cells of the subcommissural organ [87].

The incidence of the first three subgroups varies with age based on the current epidemiological investigations. In adults, pineocytoma is the most frequent parenchymal tumor with a mean age of 38 years old, whereas pineoblastoma mostly occurs in the first two decades of life with a mean age of 18.5 years old. PPTID can appear in all age groups ranging from 1 to 69, with a peak onset in early adults (38 years) [84, 88–93]. However, the papillary tumor of the pineal region was found in both adults and children, mostly affecting young adults of the third decade of life [94, 95]. But the epidemiological evidences are not very convincing due to the rareness of the PTPR. Until now, there are less than 100 cases reported in English literatures [87, 93–97].

Clinical Features of Pineal Region Tumors

Similar to other lesions in the pineal region, all pineal parenchymal tumors share the common clinical symptoms. Since the tumors are adjacent to the structures of cerebral aqueduct, they can obstruct the pathway of cerebrospinal fluid (CSF) circulation, forming hydrocephalus and elevating the intracranial pressure. Neuro-ophthalmological dysfunction, characterized as Parinaud's syndrome, includes paralysis of upward gaze and convergence, due to the compression/invasion of midbrain tectum by the tumors. In addition, hypothalamic-based endocrine abnormalities (e.g., precocious puberty) can also appear in some cases due to the secretion of hormones (melatonin) or other neurotransmitters of the neoplastic cells [80, 98, 99].

Neuroimaging Study of Pineal Region Tumors

The neuroimaging of CT scanning of pineal tumors shows different neuroimaging features: the pineocytoma presents with a globular, well-demarcated, homogeneous mass, whereas the pineoblastoma usually presents with a large, lobulated, or poorly demarcated, heterogeneous mass and with enhancement in imaging [100]. Calcification and cystic change in tumors can appear in pineocytoma occasionally [101]. Hydrocephalus is a common sign of imaging finding in both pineocytoma and pineoblastoma [100–102].

On magnetic resonance imaging (MRI), both pineocytoma and pineoblastoma may appear hypointense or isointense on T1-weighted images and hyperintense on T2-weighted images. But after contrast enhancement pineocytoma will present as an homogeneous mass, whereas pineoblastoma will exhibit an heterogeneous pattern of signal [103] (Fig. 1).

Furthermore, the imaging findings of PTPR on CT and MRI scanning are similar to that seen in pineocytoma. There is no specific neuroimaging characteristic which is helpful in distinguishing PPTID from other pineal parenchymal tumors [86].

Pathology of Pineal Region Tumors

The pineal parenchymal tumor grading parameters include tumor architecture, cell size, nuclear atypia, and counting on mitotic figures in tumor tissue [81, 82, 104]. Based on the histomorphology and its biological behavior, the pineal tumors can be graded into the following categories: pineocytoma (WHO grade I), PPTID (WHO grades II/III), and pineoblastoma (WHO grade IV), respectively. Since the rare incidence and seldom reported cases of the PTPRs, it is undetermined whether it corresponds to WHO grade II or grade III. The malignant biological behavior of this tumor was suggested in WHO Classification (2007), although more experiences and/or accumulating case series on this tumor are still needed [85].

Grossly, pineocytoma is in gray-tan color and homogeneous mass with a distinct boundary from the peripheral tissues. Cystic degeneration and hemorrhagic foci can occur [93]. But necrosis is unusually seen. In contrast, pineoblastoma, a soft, friable, and poorly demarcated tissue, usually invades the adjacent tissue with hemorrhagic and/or necrotic foci. Leptomeningeal diffusion and craniospinal dissemination via the CSF pathway occur frequently. The gross pathology of PPTIDs and PTPRs

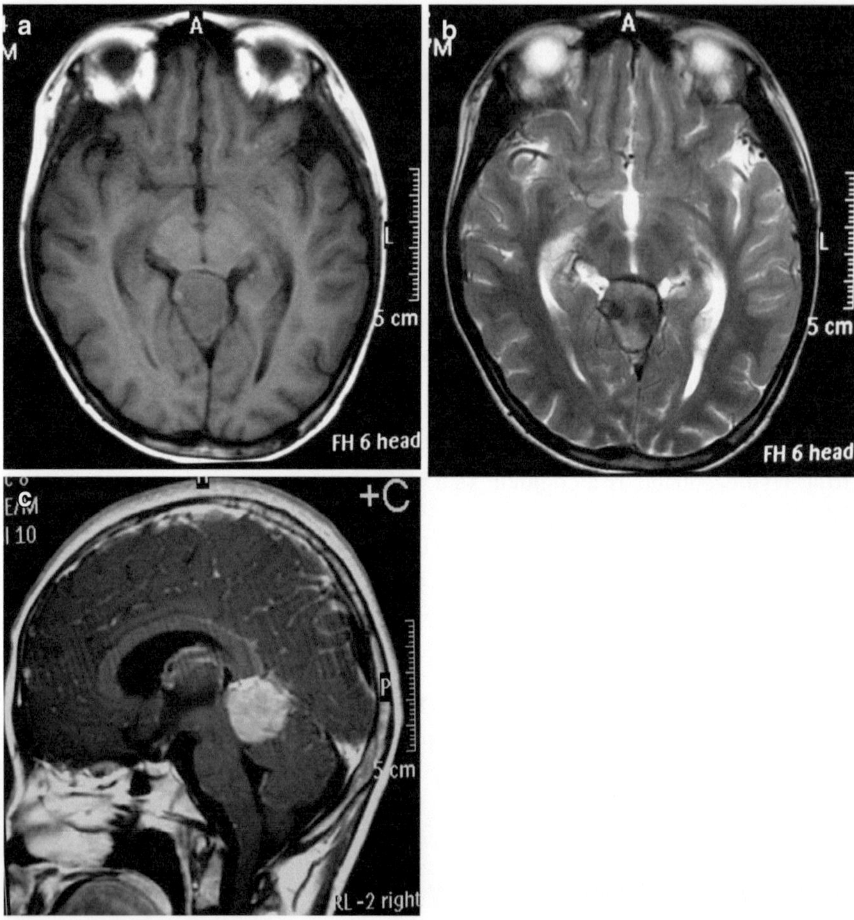

Fig. 1 The MRI characteristics of pineoblastoma. (**a**) T1-weighted image (T1WI) of pineoblastoma showed the pineal region location of the tumor, with heterogeneous signal of the tumor. (**b**) T2-weighted image (T2WI) displayed unevenly edematous pattern of the tumor. (**c**) Diffuse enhancement signal of the tumor was observed

is mostly similar to pineocytoma, with well-circumscribed masses from the surrounding structures [92, 93, 105].

On microscopic examination, pineocytoma is a well-differentiated tumor consisting mainly of small, uniform, and mature tumor cells resembling the pineocytes. The neoplastic cells are arranged in sheets or ill-defined lobules with a medium cellular density. The nuclei are round, oval, or indented, with thin or "salt-and-pepper" chromatin. The characteristic structure is known as the pineocytomatous rosettes, formed by the club-shaped cytoplasmic processes of tumor cells, oriented toward the center, which is more prominently seen with silver staining or neurofilament protein immunostaining. Mitotic figures are rarely seen, and necrosis is absent in pineocytoma.

Pineoblastoma, on the other hand, like other primitive neuroectodermal tumors (PNET) of the CNS, consists of highly cellular, small, disarranged, and poorly differentiated tumor cells with scant cytoplasm. Instead of the presence of pineocytomatous rosettes, Homer-Wright and Flexner-Wintersteiner rosettes may be appreciated occasionally in this tumor. And the appearance of Flexner-Wintersteiner rosettes usually suggests the possible differentiation towards retinoblasts. The tumor cells are small and round with high nuclear-to-cytoplasmic ratio (N/C ratio) and nuclear molding. Necrosis is commonly seen, and mitotic activity is usually high, demonstrated by Ki-67-labeling index ranging from 16.9 to 40.2 % (average 27.2 %) [104] (Fig. 2).

The histopathological features of PPTID are somewhere between the pineocytoma and the pineoblastoma, with mixed diffuse and pseudo-lobular patterns. The interstitial vessels are hyalinized. Neoplastic cells are with moderate to high cellularities, having less cytoplasm than in PCs. The round and uniform nuclei and "salt-and-pepper" chromatin are also appreciated. The mitotic figure counting are variable, usually low to moderate mitotic activity, demonstrated by Ki-67-labeling index ranging from 3 to 10 % [98, 106]. Furthermore, the grading of PPTID is based on mitotic activity and immunoreactivity of neurofilament protein even though the definite criteria have not yet been well established. In general, when PPTID shows strong neurofilament protein expression and fewer than 6 mitoses/10 HPFs, it tends to be a low-grade tumor, usually WHO grade II; otherwise if the tumor shows limited neurofilament immunohistochemical expression and increased mitoses (≥6 mitoses /10 HPF), this strongly suggests a high-grade biological behavior and should be classified as WHO grade III [90] (Fig. 3).

Unlike the above three tumors, PTPR has been recognized as a distinct tumor entity with papillary architecture, the neoplastic cells showing ependymal-like differentiation frequently, with columnar cells, covering the microvessels and forming the papillary architecture, are large in size with pale to eosinophilic cytoplasm. In the non-papillary areas, cellularity is increased, and the cytoplasm sometimes is a sort of clear or vacuolated. Variable perivascular pseudorosettes and true rosettes can be seen in the solid areas of the tumor parenchyma. Moreover, necrotic foci usually appear in this tumor. Immunostaining detects the expression of pan-cytokeratin and CK18 in tumor cells. Focal expression of synaptophysin and chromogranin A is also seen in this tumor [85, 86].

Immunohistochemistry of Pineal Tumors

The expression of synaptophysin, NSE, and NFP is strongly positive in most pineocytomas. Other neuronal markers like class III ß-tubulin, tau protein, PGP 9.5, chromogranin, and the neuropeptide serotonin were also reported in some of the cases [107, 108]. For the photosensory differentiation potential of the tumor cells, retinal S-antigen and rhodopsin staining may appear in the tumor tissue [104, 109]. Similar to pineocytoma, pineoblastoma cells also show immunoreactivity to neuronal, glial, and photoreceptor markers mentioned above. But the average Ki-67 proliferation indices are much higher than that of pineocytoma [110]. PPTID expresses synaptophysin and NSE as well, but the expression of NFP, chromogranin A, retinal

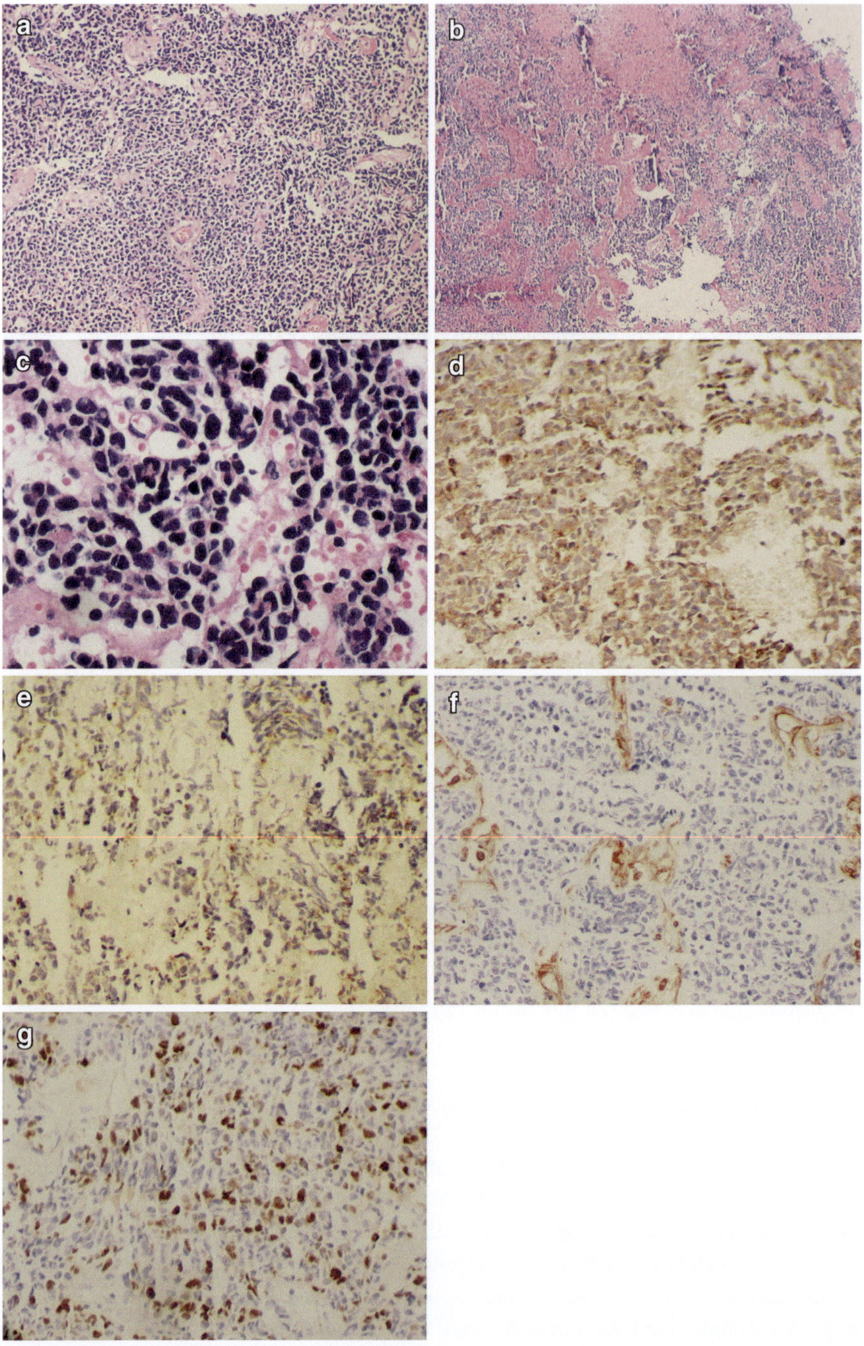

Fig. 2 Histopathological features of pineoblastoma. (**a**) Highly cellular, densely packed small cells with patternless sheets. (**b**) Necrosis is commonly seen. (**c**) Small tumor cells with round to somewhat irregular nuclei and scant cytoplasm. (**d**) Diffuse and strong expression of Syn. (**e**) The positive immunostaining of CgA is commonly seen. (**f**) Negative expression of GFAP. (**g**) The Ki-67 labeling index of pineoblastoma is usually high

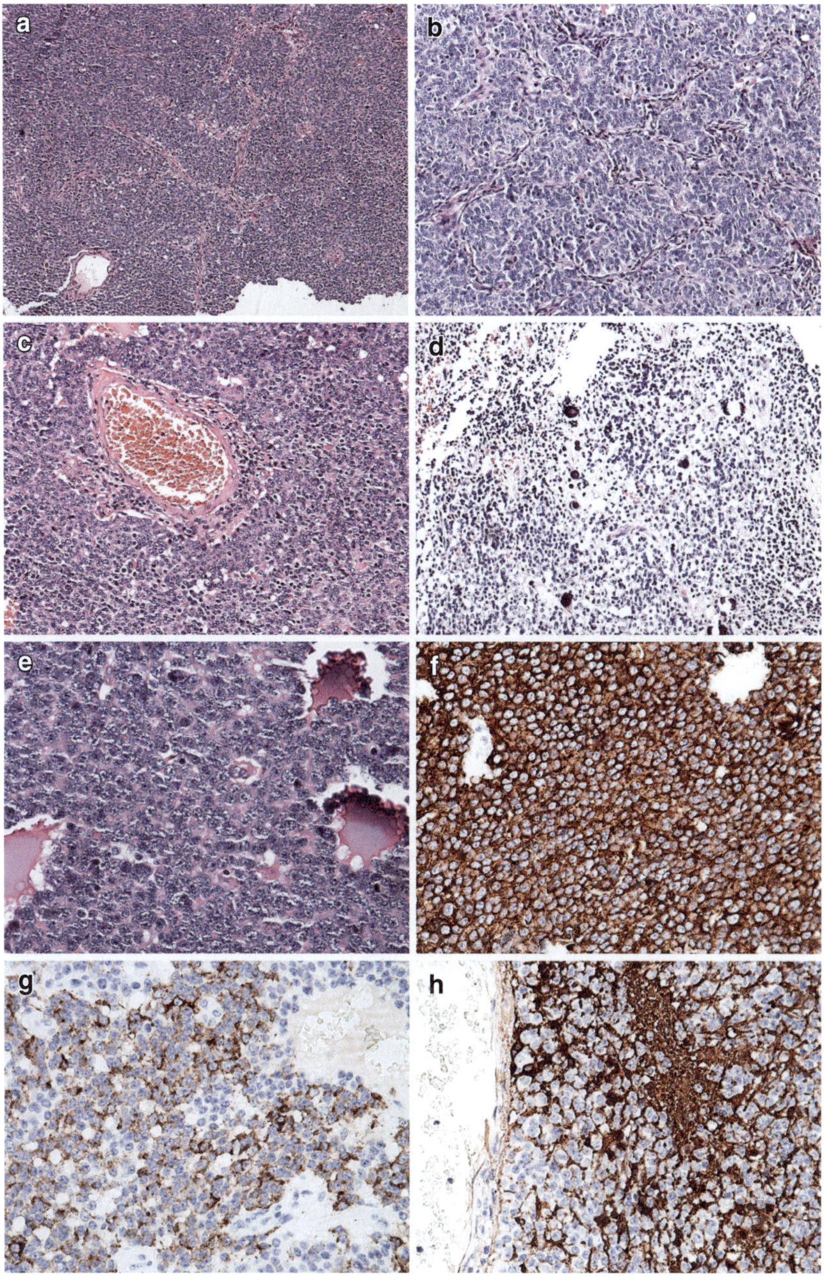

Fig. 3 Histopathological features of PPTID. (**a**) Moderate to high cellularity diffusely solid pattern. (**b**) Cells in a pseudo-lobular pattern are also seen in this tumor. (**c**) The interstitial vessel wall is hyalinized. (**d**) Microcalcifications are occasionally seen. (**e**) The round and uniform nuclei with "salt-and-pepper" chromatin are also appreciated. (**f**) Diffuse and strong expression of synaptophysin. (**g**) Focal/partial expression of chromogranin A. (**h**) A few tumor cells express GFAP, suggesting the existence of glial differentiation. (**i**) Negative expression of CK8/18. (**j**) The Ki-67 labeling index of PPTID in this case is approximately 5 %

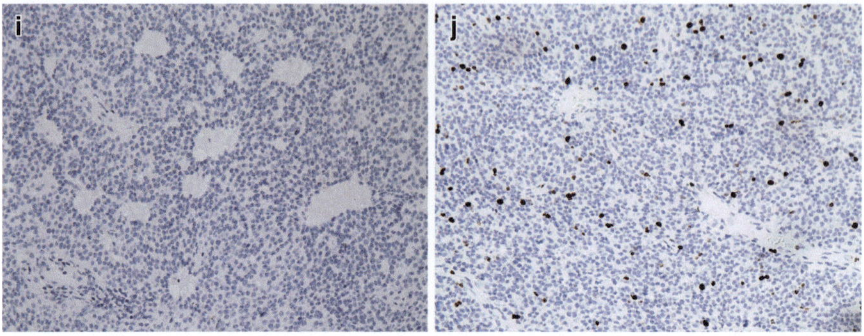

Fig. 3 (continued)

S-antigen, and S-100 is variable [111, 112]. In contrast to the three tumors above, PTPR almost never shows NFP immunohistochemical staining, only weak expression of synaptophysin, chromogranin A, and pan-cytokeratin and strong expression of cytokeratin 18 [113], suggesting the epithelioid nature of this tumor.

Electron Microscopic Study

Ultrastructural examination not only can help to identify the pineal parenchymal lineage of these neoplastic cells but also reflect the degree of tumor differentiation. The well-differentiated pineocytoma cells comprise moderate-sized and round to oval nuclei, containing moderate amounts of heterochromatin, without prominent nucleoli. They also contain abundant cytoplasm and well-developed organelles, including smooth and rough endoplasmic reticulum, Golgi complex, mitochondria, multivesicular bodies, and lysosomes. In addition, numerous processes can be present in the cytoplasm, occasionally terminating in perivascular bulbous ends. Their ultrastructural appearances in part overlap with that of normal pineocytes, suggesting the neurosensory/photoreceptor differentiation of the tumor cells, such as synaptic ribbons, paired twisted filaments, and fibrous bodies. Both dense core vesicles and clear vesicles can be seen in pineocytoma cells, the former manifesting neuroendocrine differentiation and latter showing occasional synapse-like junction [91, 99, 114]. However, as a poorly differentiated tumor, the ultrastructures of pineoblastoma cells are similar to that of other primitive neuroectodermal tumors (PNET), bearing scant cytoplasm and poorly formed or absent processes, junctions, and organelles [91]. PPTID shows intermediate ultrastructural characteristics, including short processes and rare bulbous endings.

Genetics of Pineal Tumors

Genetic studies on tumors of the pineal parenchyma present both numerical and structural abnormalities, but the results of all studies are not highly congruent and no characteristic aberrations are found in all categories of PPTs due to the rarity of the cases. Thus, genetic analyses on PPTs are not sufficient to be routine diagnostic approaches in current practice. As far as we know, the association between the genetic abnormalities and prognosis is not discovered yet. In order to better understanding the essence of these tumors on molecular biological level, studies on larger cohorts are still needed.

Cytogenetic analyses of pineocytomas have displayed numerical alterations of chromosomes 8, 11, X, 10, 18, 21, and Y as well as structural changes of 1, 3, 2, 6, and 11 [115, 116]. In addition, an ultrastructural and cytogenetic research of a pineocytoma has also reported abnormalities including losses of chromosomes 4, 5, 14, 13, and 5 and gains in chromosome 19 [117]. Conventional cytogenetic studies of pineocytoma have revealed aberrations involving monosomy or losses of chromosome 22, deletions in the distal 12q region, as well as partial deletion or losses of chromosome 11, which were demonstrated to relate to tumor progression [115, 116]. However, in a comparative genomic hybridization (CGH) study of PPT, neither gains nor losses were discovered in pineocytomas, and in contrast, gains of 12q were found in higher-grade PPTs [118]. Pineoblastomas, on the other hand, were reported to have aberrations of der (10) t(10;17) and der(16)t(1;16) [119], deletion of 11q, and an isochromosome 17q [120, 121]. In a conventional cytogenetic study of 4 pineoblastomas, the tumors showed that karyotypes vary from hypodiploid to hypertetraploid, and three of four cases showed structural rearrangements in chromosome 1 and two cases presented unbalanced gains of chromosome 17q [122]. The CGH study has shown an average 5.6 chromosomal changes per pineoblastoma (2.3 gains vs. 3.3 losses) [118]. In the cytogenetic analyses of PPTIDs, gains in chromosomes 4q and 12q and losses of chromosome 22 were found to be the most common chromosomal imbalances. And CGH study has identified 3.3 gains and 2.0 losses with average of 5.3 chromosomal changes per PPTID [118]. In PTPRs, one CGH study performed on 5 cases has mainly presented the alterations including losses of chromosome 10 and 22q and gains affecting chromosome 4, 8, 9, and 12 [123]. Another CGH analysis conducted on PTPRs revealed that both primary and recurrent tumors shared the common chromosome imbalance with gain at 9p, and additionally, the primary and recurrent neoplasms in the same case presented clonal chromosomal relation with gains in chromosomes 4, 8, 9p, and 12p12q21 and losses in chromosome 10 [96].

In view of the photosensory differentiation potential of the PPTs, the retinoblastoma gene Rb was also investigated in a series of studies. However, no specific mutations of Rb gene were found in genetic studies on pineocytomas. But in a retrospective analysis on pineoblastomas, mutated Rb gene occurred which suggests that the inheritance of this gene not only is causal in the generation of familial retinoblastoma developed pineoblastomas but also renders highly worse prognosis compared with sporadic cases [124]. In a microarray analysis of PPTs, the genes coding for enzymes contributing to melatonin synthesis (TPH1, a subtype of tryptophan hydroxylase, and HIOMT, hydroxyindole O-methyltransferase) as well as genes related to phototransduction in the retina (OPN4, melanopsin; RGS16, regulator of G-protein signaling 16; and CRB3, crumbs family member 3) were demonstrated to express in a high level in pineocytomas with potential bi-differentiation of neurosecretory and photosensory, whereas ubiquitin-conjugating enzyme E2 C (UBEC2), SRY (sex determining region Y)-box 4 (SOX4), telomerase reverse transcriptase (TERT), telomerase protein component 1 (TEP1), preferentially expressed antigen in melanoma (PRAME), CD24, POU class 4 homeobox 2(POU4F2), and homeobox D13 (HOXD13) were identified highly expressing in pineoblastomas [125]. Another study using Atlas plastic human 8 K microarray analysis displayed that puromycin-sensitive aminopeptidase and teratocarcinoma-derived growth factor 3 were upregulated in PPT and in medulloblastomas and adenomatous polyposis coli-like was downregulated only in PPT [126]. Genome-wide molecular study has reported alterations of gene copy number with gains of protocadherin gamma-A3 (PCDHGA3) (5q31.3) and family with sequence similarity 129, member A (FAM129A) (1q25) [127]. The features of gene mutations of PPTIDs are similar to that of pineoblastomas with distinctly high-level expression of PRAME, CD24, POU4F2, and HOXD13 [125]. One study of gene expression of PTPR has found that one case had a homozygous PTEN deletion, and 2-point mutations in exon 7 of PTEN (G251D and Q261stop), implicating the PTEN mutations and PI3K/Akt/mTOR signaling pathway activation may play a role in the development of PTPR. PI3K/Akt/mTOR inhibitors may be considered as a possible treatment option for such tumors [128].

Prognosis

The prognosis of PPTs is affected by numerous factors, including the histopathological category and grading of the tumors, clinicopathologic staging at diagnosis, and the individual reactions to initial treatments. As a low-grade subtype of PPTs, the pineocytoma is characterized by a longer clinical course and a better prognosis. Recurrence and metastasis are rarely seen after gross total resection of the tumor. The 5-year survival rate of patients suffering from pineocytomas is the highest in all PPTs with a range of 86–100 % [92, 129]. Additionally, the divergent differentiations of this tumor with retinoblastic, neuronal, or glial differentiation scarcely influence the outcome of the patients [93]. The PPTID has a worse outcome than pineocytoma with a lower 5-year survival rate ranging from 39 to 74 % [92]. Although the genetic aberrations of PPTIDs are similar to that of pineoblastomas, the prognosis of PPTIDs more parallels with pineocytomas, with recurrence and metastasis occurring occasionally. For pineoblastoma, the outcome of patient is actually dismal with a 5-year survival rate of only 10 %, especially in patients of very young ages [92, 130]. Compared with other PNET of CNS, the prognosis of pineoblastoma is worse than that of medulloblastoma [131]. The main cause of death in pineoblastoma patients is intracranial and spinal metastasis. The outcome of PTPR varies, and no consensus on the treatment and prognosis of this tumor has been estimated to date. PTPRs with both higher mitotic activity (5 or more mitoses per 10 HPF) and incomplete resection may suggest a decreased survival rate [94].

Conclusion

Pineal region tumors are real challenge to both neurosurgeons and pathologists due to its specific anatomic location, bleeding potential, rareness of the disease, as well as limited tissue specimen. As more cases are reported and more and more knowledge about its pathogenesis accumulated, the diagnosis of this type of neoplasms should be becoming less stressful. When molecular information about this tumor becomes available, target treatment may provide our patients with more therapeutic options and better prognosis.

Abbreviations

ACTH	Adrenocorticotropic hormone
CD24	Cluster of differentiation 24 or heat-stable antigen CD24 (HSA)
CGH	Comparative genomic hybridization
CN	Central neurocytoma
CRB3	Crumbs family member 3
CSF	Cerebrospinal fluid
CT	Computerized tomography
EVN	Extraventricular neurocytoma
FAM129A	Family with sequence similarity 129, member A
FISH	Florescent in situ hybridization
FSH	Follicle-stimulating hormone
GH	Growth hormone
HIOMT	Hydroxyindole O-methyltransferase
HOXD13	Homeobox D13
IDH	Isocitrate dehydrogenase
IGF2	Insulin-like growth factor 2
LH	Luteinizing hormone
LOH	Loss of heterozygosity
MEN1	Multiple endocrine neoplasm type 1
miRNA	microRNA
MRI	Magnetic resonance image
NFP	Neurofilament protein
NRG	Neuregulin
NSE	Neuron-specific enolase
OPN4	Melanopsin
PCDHGA3	Protocadherin gamma-A3
PDGF	Platelet-derived growth factor
PNET	Primitive neuroectodermal tumor

POU4F2	POU class 4 homeobox 2
PPT	Pineal parenchymal tumor
PPTID	Pineal parenchymal tumor of intermediate differentiation
PRAME	Preferentially expressed antigen in melanoma
PTEN	Phosphatase and tensin homolog
PTPR	Papillary tumor of pineal region
PTTG	Pituitary tumor transforming gene
Rb	Retinoblastoma susceptibility gene
RGS16	Regulator of G-protein signaling 16
SOX4	SRY (sex determining region Y)-box 4
TEP1	Telomerase protein component 1
TERT	Telomerase reverse transcriptase
TPH1	A subtype of tryptophan hydroxylase
TSG	Tumor suppressor gene
UBE2C	Ubiquitin-conjugating enzyme E2 C
WHO	World Health Organization

References

1. Farrell WE, Clayton RN. Molecular pathogenesis of pituitary tumors. Front Neuroendocrinol. 2000;21:174–98.
2. Lloyd RV. Molecular pathology of pituitary adenomas. J Neurooncol. 2001;54:111–9.
3. Farrell WE. Epigenetics of pituitary tumors: an update. Curr Opin Endocrinol Diabetes Obes. 2014;21(4):299–305.
4. Simpson DJ, Magnay J, Bicknell JE, Barkan AL, McNicol AM, Clayton RN, Farrell WE. Chromosome 13q deletion mapping in pituitary tumors: infrequent loss of the retinoblastoma susceptibility gene (RB1) despite loss of RB1 protein product in somatotropinomas. Cancer Res. 1999;59:1562–6.
5. Zamore PD, Haley B. Rebo-genome: the big world of small RNAs. Science. 2005;309:1519–24.
6. Huntzinger E, Izaurralde E. Gene silencing by microRNAs: contributions of translational repression and mRNA decay. Nat Rev Genet. 2011;12:99–110.
7. Bates AS, Farrell WE, Bicknell EJ, Talbot AJ, Broome JC, Perrett CW, Thakker RV, Clayton RN. Allelic deletion in pituitary adenomas reflects aggressive biological activity and has potential value as a prognostic marker. J Clin Endocrinol Metab. 1997;82:818–24.
8. Duong CV, Emes RD, Wessely F, et al. Quantitative, genome-wide analysis of the DNA methylome in sporadic pituitary adenomas. Endocr Relate Cancer. 2012;19:805–16.
9. Pei L, Melmed S. Isolation and characterization of a pituitary tumor-transforming gene (PTTG). Mol Endocrinol. 1997;11:433–41.
10. Zhang X, Horwitz GA, Heaney AP, Nakashima M, Bronotein M, Melmed S. Pituitary tumor-transforming gene expression in human pituitary adenomas. J Clin Endocrinol Metab. 1999;84:761–7.
11. Spade A, Vallar L, Faglia G. G protein oncogenes in pituitary tumors. Trans Endocrnol Metab. 1992;3:355–60.
12. Herman V, Fagin J, Gonsky R, Kovacs K, Melmed S. Clonal origin of pituitary adenomas. J Clin Endocrinol Metab. 1990;71:1427–33.
13. Alexander JM, Biller BMK, Bakkal H, Zervas NT, Arnold A, Klibanski A. Clinically non-functioning pituitary tumors are monoclonal in origin. J Clin Invest. 1990;86:336–40.

14. Levy A, Hall S, Yendall WA, Lightman SL. p53 gene mutations in pituitary adenoma: rare events. Clin Endocrinol. 1994;41:809–14.
15. Lloyd RV, Jin L, Kulig E. Aberrant p27/kip1 expression in endocrine and other tumors. Am J Pathol. 1997;150(2):401–7.
16. Thapar K, Scheithauer BW, Kovacs K, Pernicome PJ, Laws ER. P53 expression in pituitary adenomas and carcinoma. Correlation with invasiveness and tumor growth fractions. Neurosurgery. 1996;38:765–71.
17. Lyons J, Landis CA, Harsh G, Vallar L, Grunewald K, Feichtinger H, Duh OY, Clark OH, Kawasaki E, Brourne HR, McCormick F. Two G protein oncogenes in human endocrine tumors. Science. 1990;249:655–9.
18. Takino H, Herman V, Weiss M, Melmed S. Purine binding factor (nm23) gene expression in pituitary tumors: markers of adenoma invasiveness. J Clin Endocrinol Metab. 1995;80:1733–8.
19. Hunter T, Pines J. Cyclins and cancer II C cyclin D and CDK inhibitors come of age. Cell. 1994;79:573–82.
20. Yang I, Park S, Ryu M, Woo J, Kim S, Kim Y, Choi Y. Characteristics of gsp-positive growth hormone-secreting pituitary tumors in Korean acromegalic patients. Eur J Endocrinol. 1996;134:720–6.
21. Karger HJ, Alexander JM, Hedley-Whte ET, Klibansky A, Jameson LJ. Ras mutations in human pituitary tumors. J Clin Endocrinol Metab. 1992;74:914–9 (Add'l 07/28/14).
22. Jordan S, Lidher K, Korbonits M, Lowe DG, Grossman AB. Cyclin D and cyclin E expression in normal and adenomatous pituitary. Eur J Endocrinol. 2000;143:R1–6.
23. Qian X, Kulig E, Jin L, Lloyd RV. Expression of D-type cyclins in normal and neoplastic rat pituitary. Endocrinology. 1998;139:2058–67.
24. Pei L, Melmed S, Scheithauer B, Kovacs K, Benedict WE, Prager D. Frequent loss of heterozygosity at the retinoblastoma susceptibility gene (RB) locus in aggressive pituitary tumors. Evidence for a chromosomal 13 tumor suppressor gene other than RB. Cancer Res. 1995;55:644–6.
25. Woloschak M, Yu A, Xiao J, Post KD. Frequent loss of the p16/INK4a gene product in human pituitary tumors. Cancer Res. 1996;56:2493–6.
26. Woloschak M, Yu A, Post KD. Frequent inactivation of the p16 gene in human pituitary tumors by gene methylation. Mol Carcinogen. 1997;19:221–4.
27. Simpson DJ, Bicknell JE, McNicol AM, Clayton RN, Farrell WE. Hypermethylation of the p16/CDKN2A/MTSI gene and loss of protein expression is associated with nonfunctional pituitary adenomas but not somatotrophinomas. Genes Chrom Cancer. 1999; 24:328–36.
28. Qian X, Jin L, Kulig E, Lloyd RV. DNA methylation regulates p27kip1 expression in rodent pituitary cell lines. Am J Pathol. 1998;153(5):1475–82.
29. Franklin DS, Godfrey VL, Lee H, Kovales GL, Schoonhoven R, Chen-Kiang S, Su I, Xiong Y. CD inhibitors p18INK4C and p27kip1 mediate two separate pathways to collaboratively suppress pituitary tumorigenesis. Gene Dev. 1998;12:2899–911.
30. Farrell WE, Simpson D, Bates AS, Talbot JA, Bicknell J, Clayton RN. Chromosome 9p deletions in invasive and noninvasive nonfunctional pituitary adenomas. The deleted region involves markers outside the MTS1 and MTS2 gene. Cancer Res. 1999;57: 2703–9.
31. Metzger AK, Mohapatra G, Minn YA, Bollen AW, Lamborn K, Waldman F, Wilson CB, Feuerstein BG. Multiple genetic aberrations including evidence of chromosome 11q13 rearrangement detected in pituitary adenomas by comparative genomic hybridization. J Neurosurg. 1999;90:306–14.
32. Franklin D, Godfrey VL, O'Brien DP, Deng C, Xiang Y. Functional collaboration between different cyclin-dependent kinase inhibitors suppress tumor growth with distinct tissue specificity. Mol Cell Biol. 2000;20:6147–58.
33. Zamore PD, Haley B. Ribo-gnome: the big world of small RNAs. Sciences. 2005;309:1519–24.

34. Hibberts NA, Simpson DJ, Bicknell JE, Broome JC, Hoban PR, Clayton RN, Farrell WE. Analysis of cyclin D1 (CCND1) allelic imbalance and overexpression in sporadic pituitary adenomas. Clin Cancer Res. 1995;5:2133–9.
35. Choudhari KA, Kaliaperumal C, Jain A, Sarkar C, Soo MYS, Rades D, Singh J. Central neurocytoma: a multi-disciplinary review. Br J Neurosurg. 2009;23(6):585–95 (RR).
36. Kane AJ, Surhrue ME, Rutkowski MJ, Parsa AT. The molecular pathology of central neurocytomas. J Clin Neurosci. 2011;18:1–6 (M).
37. Myung JK, Cho HJ, Park CK, Chung CK, Choi SH, Kim SK, Park SH. Clinicopathological and genetic characteristics of extraventricular neurocytoma. Neuropathology. 2013;33:111–21.
38. Vasiljevic A, Champier J, Figarella-Branger D, Wierinckx A, Jouvet A, Fevre-Montange F. Molecular characterization of central neurocytomas: potential markers for tumor typing and progression. Neuropathology. 2013;33:149–61.
39. Hassoun J, Gambarelli D, Grisoli F, Pellet W, Salamon G, Pellissier JF, Toga M. Central neurocytoma. An electron-microscopic study of two cases. Acta Neuropathol. 1982;56:151–6.
40. Wilson AJ, Leaffer DH, Kohout ND. Differentiated cerebral neuroblastoma: a tumor in need of discovery. Human Pathol. 1985;16:647–9.
41. Sanai N, Tramotin AD, Quinones-Hinojosa A, Barbaro NM, Gupta N, Kunwar S, Lawton MT, McDermott MW, Parsa AT, Manuel-García Verdugo J, Berger MS, Alvarez-Buylla A. Unique astrocyte ribbon in adult human brain contains neural stem cells but lacks chain migration. Nature. 2004;427:740–4.
42. Patt S, Schmidt H, Labrakakis C, Weydt P, Fritsch M, Cervós-Navarro J, Kettenmann H. Human central neurocytoma cells show neuronal physiological properties in vitro. Acta Neuropathol. 1996;91:209–14.
43. Kim BJ, Kim SS, Kim JI, et al. Forskolin promotes astroglial differentiation of human central neurocytoma cells. Exp Mol Med. 2004;36:52–6.
44. Ishiuchi S, Nakazato Y, Lino M, et al. In vitro neuronal and glial production and differentiation of human central neurocytoma cells. J Neurosci Res. 1998;51:526–35.
45. von Deimling A, Kleihues P, Saremaslani P, Yasargil MG, Spoerri O, Südhof TC, Wiestler OD. Histogenesis and differentiation potential of central neurocytomas. Lab Invest. 1991;64:585–91.
46. Westphal M, Stavrou D, Nausch H, Valdueza JM, Herrmann HD. Human neurocytoma cells in culture show characteristics of astroglial differentiation. J Neurosci Res. 1994;38:698–704.
47. Yano H, Ohe N, Shinoda J, et al. Immunohistochemical study concerning the origin of neurocytoma – a case report. Pathol Oncol Res. 2009;15:301–5.
48. You H, Kim YI, Im SY, Yoshimura S, Iwama T. Immunohistochemical study of central neurocytoma, subependymoma, and subependymal giant cell astrocytoma. J Neurooncol. 2005;74:1–8.
49. Sugita Y, Yamada S, Sugita S, Sakata K, Morimatsu M, Shigemori M. The biochemical analysis of neurotransmitters in central neurocytomas. Int J Mol Med. 2001;7:521–5.
50. Sim FJ, Keyoung HM, Goldman JE, Kim DK, Jung HW, Roy NS, Goldman SA. Neurocytoma is a tumor of adult neuronal progenitor cells. J Neurosci. 2006;26:12544–55.
51. Fujisawa H, Marukawa K, Hasegawa M, Tohma Y, Hayashi Y, Uchiyama N, Tachibana O, Yamashita J. Genetic differences between neurocytoma and dysembryoplastic neuroepithelial tumor and oligodendroglial tumors. J Neurosurg. 2002;97:1350–5.
52. Perry A, Fuller CE, Banerjee R, Brat DJ, Scheithauer BW. Ancillary FISH analysis for 1p and 19q status: preliminary observations in 287 gliomas and oligodendrogliomas mimics. Front Biosci. 2003;8:a1–9.
53. Brat DJ. Neuronal and glioneuronal neoplasms. In: Perry A, Brat DJ, editors. Practical surgical neuropathology, a diagnostic approach. 1st ed. Philadelphia: Churchill Livingston Elsevier; 2010. p. 125–63.

54. Tong CY, Ng HK, Pang JC, Hu J, Hui AB, Poon WS. Central neurocytomas are genetically distinct from oligodendrogliomas and neuroblastomas. Histopathology. 2000;37:160–5.
55. Rodriguez FJ, Mota RA, Scheithauer BW, Giannini C, Blair H, New KC, Wu KJ, Dickson DW, Jenkins RB. Interphase cytogenetics for 1p19q and t(1:19)(q10;p10) may distinguish prognostically relevant subgroups in extraventricular neurocytoma. Brain Pathol. 2009;19:623–9.
56. Yin XL, Pang JC, Hui AB, et al. Detection of chromosomal imbalances in central neurocytomas by using comparative genomic hybridization. J Neurosurg. 2007;113:303–12.
57. Korshunov A, Sycheva R, Golanov A. Recurrent cytogenetic aberrations in central neurocytomas and their biological relevance. Acta Neuropathol. 2007;113:303–12.
58. Taruscio D, Danesi R, Montaldi A, Cerasoli S, Cenacchi G, Giangaspero F. Nonrandom gain of chromosome 7 in central neurocytoma: a chromosomal analysis and fluorescence in situ hybridization study. Virchows Arch. 1997;430:47–51.
59. Wullich B, Sattler HP, Fischer U, Meese E. Two independent amplification events on chromosome 7 in glioma: amplification of the epidermal growth factor receptor gene and amplification of the oncogene MET. Anticancer Res. 1994;14:577–9.
60. Zhuang Z, Park WS, Pack S, Schmidt L, Vortmeyer AO, Pak E, Pham T, Weil RJ, Candidus S, Lubensky IA, Linehan WM, Zbar B, Weirich G. Trisomy 7 harboring non-random duplication of the mutant MET allele in hereditary papillary renal cell carcinomas. Nat Genet. 1998;20:66–9.
61. Brodeur GM. Neuroblastoma: biological insights into a clinical enigma. Nat Rev Cancer. 2003;3:203–16.
62. Malakho SG, Korshunov A, Stroganova AM, Poltaraus AB. Fast detection of MYCN copy number alterations in brain neuronal tumors by real-time PCR. J Clin Lab Anal. 2008;22:123–30.
63. Knoepfler PS, Cheng PF, Eisenman RN. N-myc is essential during neurogenesis for the rapid expansion of progenitor cell populations and inhibition of neuronal differentiation. Genes Dev. 2002;16:2699–712.
64. Pession A, Tonelli R. The MYCN oncogene as a specific and selective drug target for peripheral and central nervous system tumors. Curr Cancer Drug Targets. 2005;5:273–83.
65. Musatov S, Robers J, Brook AI, Pena J, Betchen S, Pfaff DW, Kaplitt MG. Inhibition of neuronal phenotype by PTEN in PC12 cells. Proc Natl Acad Sci U S A. 2004;101:3627–31.
66. Rao G, Pedone CA, Del Valle L, Reiss K, Holland EC, Fults DW. Sonic hedgehog and insulin-like growth factor signaling synergize to induce medulloblastoma formation from nestin expressing neural progenitors in mice. Oncogene. 2004;23:6156–62.
67. Soroseanu L, Kharbanda S, Chen R, Soriano RH, Aldape K, Misra A, Zha J, Forrest WF, Nigro JM, Modrusan Z, Feuerstein BG, Phillips HS. Identification of IGF2 signaling through phosphoinositide-3-kinase regulatory subunit 3 as a growth-promoting axis in glioblastoma. Proc Natl Acad Sci U S A. 2007;104:3466–71.
68. Cororan RB, Bachar Raven T, Barakat MT, Lee EY, Scott MP. Insulin-like growth factor 2 is required for progression to advanced medulloblastoma in patched 1 heterozygous mice. Cancer Res. 2008;68:8788–95.
69. Yao X, Hu JF, Daniels M, Shiran H, Zhou X, Yan H, Lu H, Zeng Z, Wang Q, Li T, Hoffman AR. A methylated oligonucleotide inhibits IGF2 expression and enhances survival in a model of hepatocellular carcinoma. J Clin Invest. 2003;111:265–73.
70. Lokker NA, Sullivan CM, Hollenback SJ, Israel MA, Giese NA. Platelet-derived growth factor)(PDGF) autocrine signaling regulates survival and mitogenic pathways in glioblastoma cells: evidence that the novel PDGF-C and PDGF-D ligands may play a role in the development of brain tumors. Cancer Res. 2002;62:3729–35.
71. LaRochelle WJ, Jeffers M, Corvalan JR, Jia XC, Feng X, Vanegas S, Vickroy JD, Yang XD, Chen F, Gazit G, Mayotte J, Macaluso J, Rittman B, Wu F, Dhanabal M, Herrmann J, Lichenstein HS. Platelet-derived growth factor D: tumorigenicity in mice and dysregulated expression in human cancer. Cancer Res. 2002;62:2468–73.

72. Mendel DB, Laird AD, Xin X, Louie SG, Christensen JG, Li G, Schreck RE, Abrams TJ, Ngai TJ, Lee LB, Murray LJ, Carver J, Chan E, Moss KG, Haznedar JO, Sukbuntherng J, Blake RA, Sun L, Tang C, Miller T, Shirazian S, McMahon G, Cherrington JM. Antitumor activity of SU11248, a novel tyrosine kinase inhibitor targeting vascular endothelial growth factor and platelet-derived growth factor receptors: determination of a pharmacokinetic/pharmacodynamics relationship. Clin Cancer Res. 2003;9:327–37.
73. Carraway 3rd KL, Weber JL, Unger MJ, Ledesma J, Yu N, Gassmann M, Lai C. Neuregulin-2, a new ligand of ErbB3/ErbB4-receptor tyrosine kinases. Nature. 1997;387:512–6.
74. Ghashghaei HT, Weber J, Pevny L, Schmid R, Schwab MH, Lloyd KC, Eisenstat DD, Lai C, Anton ES. The role of neuregulin-ErbB4 interaction on the proliferation and organization of cells in the subventricular zone. Proc Natl Acad Sci U S A. 2006;103:1930–5.
75. Edwards JM, Bottenstein JE. Neuregulin 1 growth factor regulate proliferation but no apoptosis of a CNS neuronal progenitor cell line. Brain Res. 2006;1108:63–75.
76. Revillion F, Lhotellier V, Hornez L, Bonneterre J, Peyrat JP. ErbB/HER ligands in human breast cancer, and relationships with their receptors, the bio-pathological features and prognosis. Ann Oncol. 2008;19:73–80.
77. Tran H, Medina-Flores R, Cerilli LA, Phelps J, Lee FC, Wong G, Turner P. Primary disseminated central neurocytoma: cytology and MRI evidence of tumor spread prior to surgery. J Neurooncol. 2010;100:291–8.
78. Yamamoto I. Pineal region tumor: surgical anatomy and approach. J Neurooncol. 2001;54(3):263–75.
79. Jouvet A, Vasiljevic A, Champier J, Fevre Montange M. Pineal parenchymal tumours and pineal cysts. Neurochirugie. 2015;61(2–3):123–9. doi: 10.1016/j.neuchi.2013.04.003. Epub 2014 Jun 27.
80. Schild SE, Scheithauer BW, Schomberg PJ, Hook CC, Kelly PJ, Frick L, Robinow JS, Buskirk SJ. Pineal parenchymal tumors. Clinical, pathologic, and therapeutic aspects. Cancer. 1993;72:870–80.
81. Han SJ, Clark AJ, Ivan ME, Parsa AT, Perry A. Pathology of pineal parenchymal tumors. Neurosurg Clin N Am. 2011;22(3):335–40.
82. Hirato J, Nakazato Y. Pathology of pineal region tumors. J Neurooncol. 2001;54(3): 239–49.
83. Konovalov AN, Pitskhelauri DI. Principles of treatment of the pineal region tumors. Surg Neurol. 2003;59(4):250–68.
84. Whittle IR, Signorini DF. Pineal region tumors and the role of stereotactic biopsy: review of the mortality, morbidity, and diagnostic rates in 370 cases. Neurosurgery. 1998;42(3):676–7.
85. Nakazato Y, Jouvet A, Scheithauer BW. Tumours of the pineal region. In: Louis DN, Ohgaki H, Wiestler OD, Cavenee WK, editors. WHO classification of tumours of the central nervous system. 4th ed. Lyon: IARC, WHO Press; 2007. p. 123–7.
86. Vandergriff C, Opatowsky M, O'Rourke B, Layton K. Papillary tumor of the pineal region. Proc (Bayl Univ Med Cent). 2012;25(1):78–9.
87. Rickard KA, Parker JR, Vitaz TW, Plaga AR, Wagner S, Parker Jr JC. Papillary tumor of the pineal region: two case studies and a review of the literature. Ann Clin Lab Sci. 2011;41(2):174–81.
88. Macchi MM, Bruce JN. Human pineal physiology and functional significance of melatonin. Front Neuroendocrinol. 2004;25(3–4):177–95.
89. Cho BK, Wang KC, Nam DH, Kim DG, Jung HW, Kim HJ, Han DH, Choi KS. Pineal tumors: experience with 48 cases over 10 years. Childs Nerv Syst. 1998; 14(1–2):53–8.
90. Jouvet A, Saint-Pierre G, Fauchon F, Privat K, Bouffet E, Ruchoux MM, Chauveinc L, Fèvre-Montange M. Pineal parenchymal tumors: a correlation of histological features with prognosis in 66 cases. Brain Pathol. 2000;10(1):49–60.
91. Min KW, Scheithauer BW, Bauserman SC. Pineal parenchymal tumors: an ultrastructural study with prognostic implications. Ultrastruct Pathol. 1994;18(1–2):69–85.

92. Fauchon F, Jouvet A, Paquis P, Saint-Pierre G, Mottolese C, Ben Hassel M, Chauveinc L, Sichez JP, Philippon J, Schlienger M, Bouffet E. Parenchymal pineal tumors: a clinicopathological study of 76 cases. Int J Radiat Oncol Biol Phys. 2000;46(4):959–68.
93. Mena H, Rushing EJ, Ribas JL, Delahunt B, McCarthy WF. Tumors of pineal parenchymal cells: a correlation of histological features, including nucleolar organizer regions, with survival in 35 cases. Hum Pathol. 1995;26(1):20–30.
94. Fèvre-Montange M, Hasselblatt M, Figarella-Branger D, Chauveinc L, Champier J, Saint-Pierre G, Taillandier L, Coulon A, Paulus W, Fauchon F, Jouvet A. Prognosis and histopathologic features in papillary tumors of the pineal region: a retrospective multicenter study of 31 cases. J Neuropathol Exp Neurol. 2006;65(10):1004–11.
95. Fevre Montange M, Vasiljevic A, Champier J, Jouvet A. Papillary tumor of the pineal region: Histopathological characterization and review of the literature. Neurochirurgie. 2015;61(2–3):138–42. doi: 10.1016/j.neuchi.2013.04.011. Epub 2014 Feb 18.
96. Gutenberg A, Brandis A, Hong B, Gunawan B, Enders C, Schaefer IM, Burger R, Ostertag H, Gaab M, Krauss JK, Füzesi L. Common molecular cytogenetic pathway in papillary tumors of the pineal region (PTPR). Brain Pathol. 2011;21(6):672–7.
97. Sharma MC, Jain D, Sarkar C, Suri V, Garg A, Sharma BS, Mehta VS. Papillary tumor of the pineal region–a recently described entity: a report of three cases and review of the literature. Clin Neuropathol. 2009;28(4):295–302.
98. Tsumanuma I, Tanaka R, Washiyama K. Clinicopathological study of pineal parenchymal tumors: correlation between histopathological features, proliferative potential, and prognosis. Brain Tumor Pathol. 1999;16(2):61–8.
99. Herrick MK, Rubinstein LJ. The cytological differentiating potential of pineal parenchymal neoplasms (true pinealomas). A clinicopathological study of 28 tumours. Brain. 1979;102(2):289–320.
100. Chiechi MV, Smirniotopoulos JG, Mena H. Pineal parenchymal tumors: CT and MR features. J Comput Assist Tomogr. 1995;19(4):509–17.
101. Fakhran S, Escott EJ. Pineocytoma mimicking a pineal cyst on imaging: true diagnostic dilemma or a case of incomplete imaging? AJNR Am J Neuroradiol. 2008;29(1):159–63.
102. Reis F, Faria AV, Zanardi VA, Menezes JR, Cendes F, Queiroz LS. Neuroimaging in pineal tumors. J Neuroimaging. 2006;16(1):52–8.
103. Satoh H, Uozumi T, Kiya K, Kurisu K, Arita K, Sumida M, Ikawa F. MRI of pineal region tumours: relationship between tumours and adjacent structures. Neuroradiology. 1995;37(8):624–30.
104. Sato K, Kubota T. Pathology of pineal parenchymal tumors. Prog Neurol Surg. 2009;23:12–25.
105. Lee JY, Wakabayashi T, Yoshida J. Management and survival of pineoblastoma: an analysis of 34 adults from the brain tumor registry of Japan. Neurol Med Chir (Tokyo). 2005;45(3):132–41.
106. Numoto RT. Pineal parenchymal tumors: cell differentiation and prognosis. J Cancer Res Clin Oncol. 1994;120(11):683–90.
107. Coca S, Vaquero J, Escandon J, Moreno M, Peralba J, Rodriguez J. Immunohistochemical characterization of pineocytomas. Clin Neuropathol. 1992;11(6):298–303.
108. Yamane Y, Mena H, Nakazato Y. Immunohistochemical characterization of pineal parenchymal tumors using novel monoclonal antibodies to the pineal body. Neuropathology. 2002;22(2):66–76.
109. Perentes E, Rubinstein LJ, Herman MM, Donoso LA. S-antigen immunoreactivity in human pineal glands and pineal parenchymal tumors. A monoclonal antibody study. Acta Neuropathol. 1986;71(3–4):224–7.
110. Fèvre-Montange M, Vasiljevic A, Frappaz D, Champier J, Szathmari A, Aubriot Lorton MH, Chapon F, Coulon A, Quintin Roué I, Delisle MB, Figarella-Branger D, Laquerrière A, Miquel C, Michiels JF, Péoch M, Polivka M, Fauchon F, Jouvet A. Utility of Ki67 immunostaining in the grading of pineal parenchymal tumours: a multicentre study. Neuropathol Appl Neurobiol. 2012;38(1):87–94.

111. Fang J, Luo L, Li J, Sun S, Yuan Y. Pathological and immunohistochemical study of pineal parenchymal tumors. Zhonghua Bing Li Xue Za Zhi. 2002;31(1):8–11.
112. Ito T, Kanno H, Sato K, Oikawa M, Ozaki Y, Nakamura H, Terasaka S, Kobayashi H, Houkin K, Hatanaka K, Murata J, Tanaka S. Clinicopathologic study of pineal parenchymal tumors of intermediate differentiation. World Neurosurg. 2014;81(5–6):783–9.
113. Jouvet A, Fauchon F, Liberski P, Saint-Pierre G, Didier-Bazes M, Heitzmann A, Delisle MB, Biassette HA, Vincent S, Mikol J, Streichenberger N, Ahboucha S, Brisson C, Belin MF, Fèvre-Montange M. Papillary tumor of the pineal region. Am J Surg Pathol. 2003;27(4):505–12.
114. Jouvet A, Fèvre-Montange M, Besançon R, Derrington E, Saint-Pierre G, Belin MF, Pialat J, Lapras C. Structural and ultrastructural characteristics of human pineal gland, and pineal parenchymal tumors. Acta Neuropathol. 1994;88(4):334–48.
115. Rainho CA, Rogatto SR, de Moraes LC, Barbieri-Neto J. Cytogenetic study of a pineocytoma. Cancer Genet Cytogenet. 1992;64(2):127–32.
116. Bello MJ, Rey JA, de Campos JM, Kusak ME. Chromosomal abnormalities in a pineocytoma. Cancer Genet Cytogenet. 1993;71(2):185–6.
117. Dario A, Cerati M, Taborelli M, Finzi G, Pozzi M, Dorizzi A. Cytogenetic and ultrastructural study of a pineocytoma case report. J Neurooncol. 2000;48(2):131–4.
118. Rickert CH, Simon R, Bergmann M, Dockhorn-Dworniczak B, Paulus W. Comparative genomic hybridization in pineal parenchymal tumors. Genes Chromosomes Cancer. 2001;30(1):99–104.
119. Kees UR, Spagnolo D, Hallam LA, Ford J, Ranford PR, Baker DL, Callen DF, Biegel JA. A new pineoblastoma cell line, PER-480, with der(10)t(10;17), der(16)t(1;16), and enhanced MYC expression in the absence of gene amplification. Cancer Genet Cytogenet. 1998;100(2):159–64.
120. Kees UR, Biegel JA, Ford J, Ranford PR, Peroni SE, Hallam LA, Parmiter AH, Willoughby ML, Spagnolo D. Enhanced MYCN expression and isochromosome 17q in pineoblastoma cell lines. Genes Chromosomes Cancer. 1994;9(2):129–35.
121. Sreekantaiah C, Jockin H, Brecher ML, Sandberg AA. Interstitial deletion of chromosome 11q in a pineoblastoma. Cancer Genet Cytogenet. 1989;39(1):125–31.
122. Brown AE, Leibundgut K, Niggli FK, Betts DR. Cytogenetics of pineoblastoma: four new cases and a literature review. Cancer Genet Cytogenet. 2006;170(2):175–9.
123. Hasselblatt M, Blümcke I, Jeibmann A, Rickert CH, Jouvet A, van de Nes JA, Kuchelmeister K, Brunn A, Fevre-Montange M, Paulus W. Immunohistochemical profile and chromosomal imbalances in papillary tumours of the pineal region. Neuropathol Appl Neurobiol. 2006;32(3):278–83.
124. Plowman PN, Pizer B, Kingston JE. Pineal parenchymal tumours: II. On the aggressive behaviour of pineoblastoma in patients with an inherited mutation of the RB1 gene. Clin Oncol (R Coll Radiol). 2004;16(4):244–7.
125. Fèvre-Montange M, Champier J, Szathmari A, Wierinckx A, Mottolese C, Guyotat J, Figarella-Branger D, Jouvet A, Lachuer J. Microarray analysis reveals differential gene expression patterns in tumors of the pineal region. J Neuropathol Exp Neurol. 2006;65(7):675–84.
126. Champier J, Jouvet A, Rey C, Brun V, Bernard A, Fèvre-Montange M. Identification of differentially expressed genes in human pineal parenchymal tumors by microarray analysis. Acta Neuropathol. 2005;109(3):306–13.
127. Miller S, Rogers HA, Lyon P, Rand V, Adamowicz-Brice M, Clifford SC, Hayden JT, Dyer S, Pfister S, Korshunov A, Brundler MA, Lowe J, Coyle B, Grundy RG. Genome-wide molecular characterization of central nervous system primitive neuroectodermal tumor and pineoblastoma. Neuro Oncol. 2011;13(8):866–79.
128. Goschzik T, Gessi M, Denkhaus D, Pietsch T. PTEN mutations and activation of the PI3K/Akt/mTOR signaling pathway in papillary tumors of the pineal region. J Neuropathol Exp Neurol. 2014;73(8):747–51.

129. Schild SE, Scheithauer BW, Haddock MG, Wong WW, Lyons MK, Marks LB, Norman MG, Burger PC. Histologically confirmed pineal tumors and other germ cell tumors of the brain. Cancer. 1996;78(12):2564–71. The long-term postsurgical prognosis of patients with pineoblastoma. Cancer. 2012;118(1):173–9.
130. Tate M, Sughrue ME, Rutkowski MJ, Kane AJ, Aranda D, McClinton L, Barani IJ, Parsa AT. The long-term postsurgical prognosis of patients with pineoblastoma. Cancer, 2012; 118(1):173–9. doi: 10.1002/cncr.2630. Epub 2011 Jun 29.
131. Duffner PK, Horowitz ME, Krischer JP, Burger PC, Cohen ME, Sanford RA, Friedman HS, Kun LE. The treatment of malignant brain tumors in infants and very young children: an update of the Pediatric Oncology Group experience. Neuro Oncol. 1999;1(2):152–61.
132. Kleinschmidt-DeMasters BK, Lopes MBS, Prayson RA. An algorithmic approach to sellar region masses. Arch Patho Lab Med. 2015;139:356–72.

Medullary Thyroid Carcinoma

Pablo Valderrabano, Stacey Simons, Jaime Montilla-Soler, Tuya Pal, Victor Zota, Kristen Otto, Bryan McIver, Domenico Coppola, and Marino E. Leon

Introduction

Medullary thyroid carcinoma (MTC) represents 4–10 % of all thyroid carcinomas [1–3] and originate from parafollicular cells (C cells) [4]. Around 20–25 % of MTCs are part of inherited multiple endocrine neoplasia type 2 (MEN2) syndromes [3, 5], while the rest are sporadic.

Inherited Forms of MTC

These syndromes are due to germline point mutations in the *RET* (Rearranged during transfection) proto-oncogene that are transmitted in an autosomal dominant fashion. *RET* is a cell membrane receptor with tyrosine kinase function involved in growth

P. Valderrabano, MD • K. Otto, MD • B. McIver, MD
Head and Neck, and Endocrine Oncology Oncology Program, H. Lee Moffitt Cancer Center and Research Institute, Tampa, FL, USA

S. Simons, MD • V. Zota, MD • D. Coppola, MD • M.E. Leon, MD (✉)
Department of Anatomic Pathology, H. Lee Moffitt Cancer Center and Research Institute, Tampa, FL, USA
e-mail: Marino.Leon@Moffitt.org

J. Montilla-Soler, MD
Department of Diagnostic Imaging, H. Lee Moffitt Cancer Center and Research Institute, Tampa, FL, USA

T. Pal, MD
Department of Infectious Disease and Genetics, H. Lee Moffitt Cancer Center and Research Institute, Tampa, FL, USA

A. Nasir, D. Coppola (eds.), *Neuroendocrine Tumors: Review of Pathology, Molecular and Therapeutic Advances*, DOI 10.1007/978-1-4939-3426-3_7

and differentiation signals in several developing tissues, including those derived from the neural crest. Mutations associated with MEN2 result in a gain of function and lead to multicentric tumor formation in all organs where *RET* proto-oncogene is expressed. In MEN2, MTCs develop from primary C-cell hyperplasia (CCH) and are frequently multifocal and bilateral [6]. Characteristically, the phenotype is strongly associated with genotype in all MEN2 syndromes [7]. MEN2 syndromes are clinically divided in MEN2A and MEN2B [7].

MEN2A represents 95 % of all MEN2 cases and is subdivided in 4 variants according to the clinical picture [7]: classical MEN2A, MEN2A with cutaneous lichen amyloidosis (CLA), MEN2A with Hirschsprung's disease (HD), and familial MTC [7]. Classical MEN2A syndrome is characterized by the development of MTC during the adolescence or early adulthood; MTC is associated with pheochromocytoma or primary hyperparathyroidism or both in a proportion of cases. The penetrance of each of these conditions is 90–100 %, 40–50 %, and 10–20 %, respectively [5], although it is influenced by the specific mutation acquired (see Table 2) [7]. In the 2015 American Thyroid Association guidelines, familial MTC is characterized by the presence of an *RET* germline mutation in families with MTC with 0 % penetrance for pheochromocytoma and hyperparathyroidism [7].

Most mutations in MEN2A involve the cysteine residues in the RET protein's extracellular domain encoded in exons 10 and 11. Codon 634 in exon 11 is mutated in 80–93 % of MEN2A patients [8–11]. Mutations in this codon are associated with more aggressive and earlier development of MTC (40 % present by age 20), higher penetrance of pheochromocytoma, and primary hyperparathyroidism [7] and are associated with cutaneous lichen amyloidosis in one third of the patients [12]. On this codon, the most common mutations are C634R (52.1 %), C634Y (26.0 %), and C634G (9.5 %) [11].

Other less common and less aggressive *RET* mutations occur in codons 609, 611, 618, 620, 630, 790, and 791 [10]. *RET m*utations in exon 10 (codons 609, 611, 618, and 620) may also be associated with Hirschsprung's disease (see Table 2) [7, 13].

MEN2B represents 5 % of all patients with MEN2 syndrome, and it is due to a *de novo* mutation in 75 % of the cases [11]. It is characterized by the presence of MTC, pheochromocytoma, ganglioneuromatosis of the intestine and oral mucosa, neuromas of the tongue, marfanoid habitus, and medullated corneal nerve fibers [5]. MTC has a 100 % penetrance; presents earlier in age, often during infancy or early childhood; and is highly aggressive developing early regional and distant metastases. Pheochromocytoma presents in 50 % of these patients [7]. The single point mutation Met to Thr in codon 918 (M918T) in exon 16 is seen in 95–100 % of MEN2B cases [9–11].

Sporadic MTC

Sporadic MTC typically presents as a solitary thyroid nodule, preferentially located in the upper poles of the thyroid gland, where C cells are more abundant. Sporadic MTCs usually present during the 4th and 6th decade of life and have a slight female predominance [2]. Two thirds of sporadic MTCs have somatic mutations in *RET*, being M918T in exon 16 the most common one [14]; 8–68 % of the *RET* mutation-negative cases have somatic mutations in *HRAS and KRAS* [15, 16].

Clinical Presentation

Sporadic MTC and index cases of hereditary syndromes are diagnosed as an incidental finding during radiologic evaluation for other reasons or on physical exam when it becomes palpable. Thyroid function tests are normal; and MTCs are seen as cold nodules in the scintigraphy as C cells do not uptake iodine. With ultrasound, MTC usually appear as a solid nodule, frequently hypoechoic, and often with micro- and/or macrocalcifications [17]. However, these features associated with thyroid malignancies are not always present, and none of them are pathognomonic (see Figs. 1a–c) [18, 19].

At diagnosis, over 50 % of MTCs have local or distant metastases; and 15 % have local symptoms of compression or invasion of the aerodigestive tract such as hoarseness or dysphagia [3]. Distant metastases occur preferentially to the

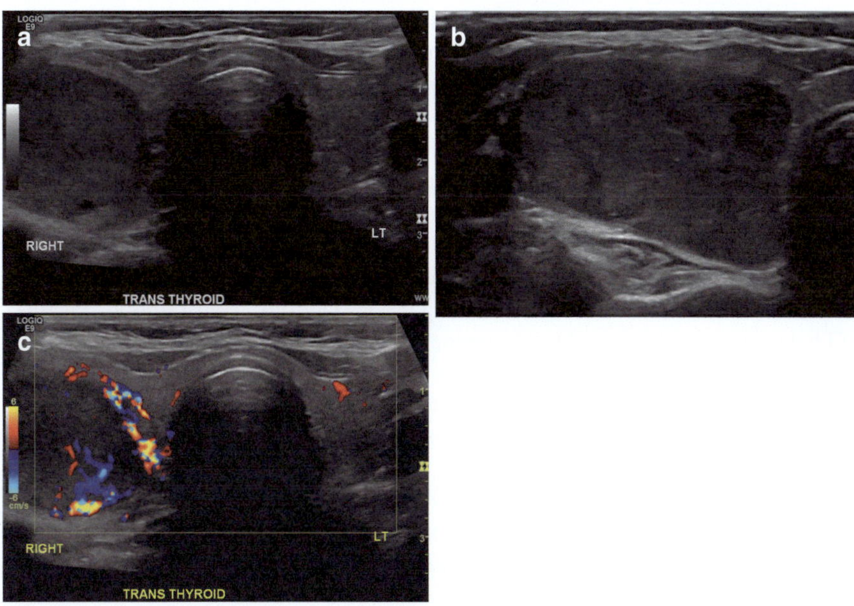

Fig. 1 (**a**, **b**) A 70-year-old woman with a palpable right thyroid nodule on physical exam who underwent an ultrasound-guided FNA, consistent with MTC. Grayscale images of the thyroid gland show a heterogeneous large thyroid nodule. (**c**) Color Doppler sonographic interrogation shows increased peripheral and central nodule vascularity

lungs, liver, and bones but can sometimes metastasize to the brain and other soft tissues. Systemic symptoms such as diarrhea and flushing may occur as a consequence of hormone secretion – calcitonin and other peptides like serotonin – and typically present when there is a high burden of disease. Paraneoplastic ACTH secretion has been documented in MTC resulting in Cushing's syndrome [20]. The clinical course is usually progressive and the 10-year overall survival rate is around 75 % [1].

Presurgical Diagnosis and Initial Evaluation

Fine-Needle Aspiration (FNA) Cytology

MTC may be diagnosed by FNA. The sensitivity of FNA cytology for the diagnosis of MTC is generally low, around 60 %, although it can be higher, close to 90 %, in experienced centers [21–23]. Additionally, FNA cytology may be used in the diagnosis of recurrence in the thyroid bed [24].

FNA yields a cellular specimen composed of numerous noncohesive cells and loose clusters. The cells show eccentrically located nucleus giving them a plasmacytoid appearance (see Fig. 2a and 2b). Epithelioid and spindle cell morphologies may be observed as well (see Fig. 2c). The nuclei are round to oval with finely stippled chromatin and inconspicuous nucleoli. Multinucleation is common (see Fig. 2b). Occasionally, intranuclear pseudoinclusions may be present (see Fig. 2c). Tridimensional clusters and rarely papillary formations are sometimes encountered; and rosette-like formation may be seen. Oncocytic features are rarely present (see Fig. 2d) [25]. The tumor cells cytoplasm is moderate and faintly granular but may show conspicuous red granules in air-dried Giemsa stained smears. Small clumps of amorphous, glassy, eosinophilic material may be seen in the background, representing amyloid (see Table 1).

Cell block preparations are helpful and facilitate the use of routine IHC stains (see Fig. 2e). IHC studies increase the sensitivity of the cytology. MTC cells are immunoreactive for calcitonin (see Fig. 2f), Thyroid Transcription Factor-1 (TTF-1), synaptophysin, chromogranin, and Carcinoembryonic antigen (CEA) stains and therefore can be used to confirm diagnosis in challenging cases. Measuring calcitonin in the washout of the nodule aspirate also increases the sensitivity and specificity of the cytology and may be especially useful when immunostaining is not feasible or inconclusive [26–29].

The differential diagnosis in FNA cytology includes the following discussed lesions. Occasionally, the FNA material may be interpreted as follicular neoplasm [30]. The cytologic features may help to distinguish these lesions. MTC shows plasmacytoid cells with an eccentric round to oval nuclei with a finely stippled chromatin. Rarely, a predominantly small cell pattern in MTC with nuclear molding raises the differential diagnosis of malignant lymphoma, poorly differentiated thyroid carcinoma (insular carcinoma), or metastatic small cell carcinoma. Absence of lym-

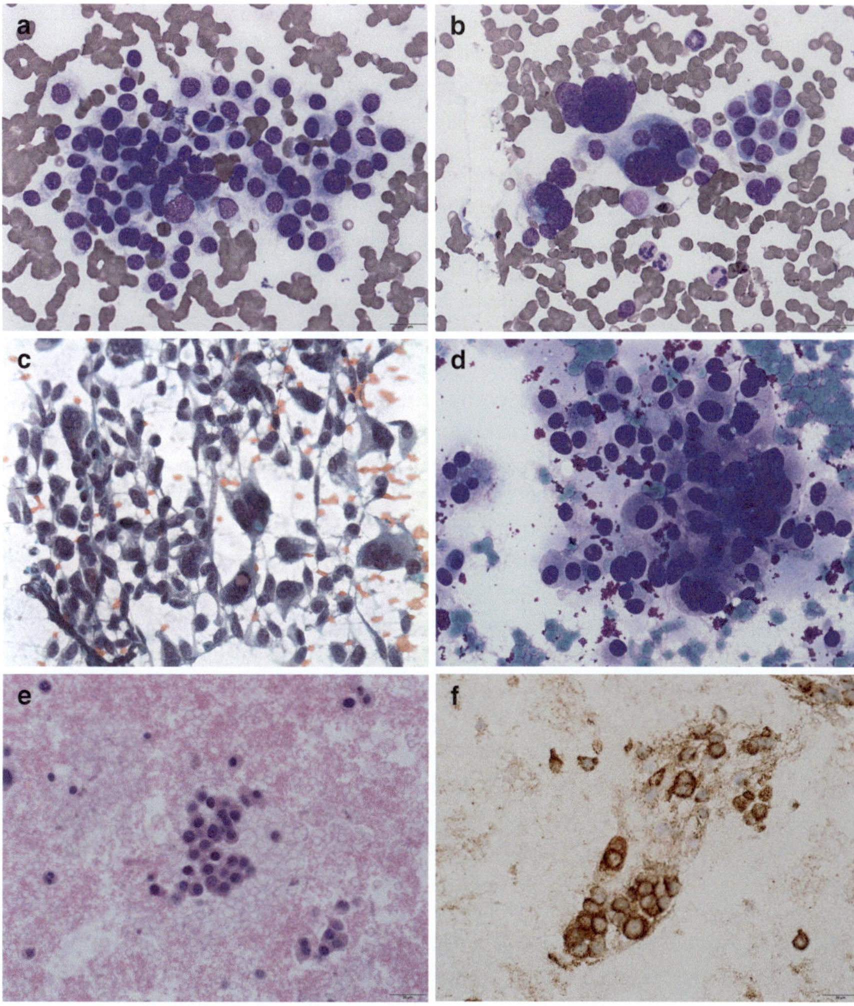

Fig. 2 (**a**) Material from a fine-needle aspiration of a thyroid mass showing MTC cells with the classic plasmacytoid morphology and round to oval nuclei (Diff-Quik stain, original magnification 400×). (**b**) MTC FNA cytology material showing multinucleated cells (Diff-Quik stain, original magnification 400×). (**c**) MTC cell showing spindle cell and epithelioid morphology with rare cells with intranuclear pseudoinclusions (Papanicolaou stain, original magnification 400×). (**d**) FNA material showing MTC cells with oncocytic appearance; this finding may be a pitfall in FNA cytology interpretation (Diff-Quik stain, original magnification 400×). (**e**) Cell block section showing clusters of MTC cells (H&E, original magnification 200×). (**f**) Cell block cells stained with calcitonin confirming the diagnosis of MTC (original magnification 400×)

phoglandular bodies argues against a lymphoproliferative disorder, whereas detection of amyloid and elevated serum calcitonin level will aid in the diagnosis of MTC. Poorly differentiated thyroid carcinomas show high cellularity with small to intermediate cells with occasionally microfollicular architecture and scant colloid.

Table 1 Cytologic features of medullary thyroid carcinoma

Numerous noncohesive cells
Loose clusters
Epithelioid, plasmacytoid, and/or spindle-shaped cells
Dense cytoplasm with metachromatic granules (seen in 70 % of cases)
Nuclei round or elongated with granular chromatin
Inconspicuous nucleoli
Intranuclear pseudoinclusions (seen in 50 % of cases)
Amyloid in the background
Oncocytic features, rarely

The nuclei may be bland with fine chromatin and small nucleoli; mitotic figures and necrosis may be seen. Small cell carcinoma shows nuclear molding, nuclear crushing, nuclear material stranding, focal necrosis, and numerous mitotic figures. Usually, small cell carcinoma has a high proliferation index on a Ki67 immunostain, and MTC has a low proliferative rate [31].

Papillary thyroid carcinoma, undifferentiated thyroid carcinoma (anaplastic thyroid carcinoma), and metastatic tumors, such as malignant melanoma, are also in the differential diagnosis [32]. Papillary thyroid carcinomas show papillary architecture and the usual nuclear features with nuclear grooves, nuclear clearing, single small nucleoli, nuclear irregular outlines, and nuclear pseudoinclusions. Undifferentiated thyroid carcinoma (anaplastic thyroid carcinoma) may show spindle cells or may display epithelioid cells with large pleomorphic nuclei. IHC stains, such as calcitonin and thyroglobulin, are helpful in the characterization of these tumors.

Paragangliomas are rare but may be a pitfall in FNA cytology and intraoperative cytology [33], as they show features suggestive of a neuroendocrine neoplasm [34]. Paragangliomas also express neuroendocrine markers, such chromogranin and synaptophysin, and are negative for cytokeratin AE1/AE3, calcitonin, and thyroglobulin [33]. FNA aspiration of suspected paragangliomas must be performed in an area equipped with the therapeutic tools to handle a possible hypertensive crisis [35].

A plasmacytoma involving the thyroid may have plasmacytoid noncohesive cells and amyloid; and they should be considered and excluded with the use of IHC stains [36]; plasmacytoma cells are positive for CD138 and show a monoclonal expression of either kappa or lambda light chains [37].

Mucosa-associated lymphoid tissue (MALT) lymphoma with prominent plasma cells and associated amyloid protein deposition may pose another possible pitfall [38]. Awareness of these pitfalls should help in the recognition of these lesions.

Serum Calcitonin and CEA

Routine measurement of serum calcitonin levels, for the evaluation of thyroid nodules to complement FNA, has some proven utility; however, it remains controversial [7, 21, 32, 39, 40]. Although elevated levels of serum or stimulated calcitonin may help identify patients with MTC, cutoff levels and cost-effectiveness are unclear [41]. Falsely elevated calcitonin can be observed in numerous situations, including hypercalcemia, hypergastrinemia, renal insufficiency, goiter, chronic lymphocytic thyroiditis, papillary and follicular thyroid carcinomas, and other neuroendocrine tumors. However, a non-stimulated serum calcitonin >100 pg/ml is likely associated to MTC [42]. Serum calcitonin should be measured in cases in which MTC is suspected during cytology evaluation and in nodules with indeterminate cytology, where finding an elevated calcitonin would modify management. Besides aiding in the diagnosis of MTC when the cytology results are inconclusive; serum calcitonin and CEA levels are useful to identify patients that need evaluation for distant metastases, to guide the extent of initial surgery in the neck, and to establish the capacity of the tumor to secrete these hormones, setting a baseline to assess the response to the initial surgery [43]. Additionally, serum calcitonin and serum CEA have a direct correlation with the tumor size [44]. For all these reasons, serum calcitonin and CEA levels should be measured in every patient with a diagnosis of MTC during the preoperative evaluation [7].

RET *Germline Mutation*

RET germline mutations should be offered to all patients with CCH, familial MTC, and apparently sporadic MTC, since germline mutations are also detected in around 7 % of these patients [45]. In MEN2A patients, exons 8, 10, 11, 13, 14, 15, and 16 of the *RET* gene are initially tested. Patients with MEN2B phenotype are tested initially for the mutation M918T in exon 16 and, if negative, for the mutation A883F in exon 15. In cases that are clinically hereditary with negative results in the prior analysis, or when there is discrepancy between the MEN2 phenotype and the expected genotype, the entire *RET* coding region should be sequenced [7]. *RET* germline mutation should also be offered to every family member at risk and patients with Hirschsprung's disease or cutaneous lichen amyloidosis [7]. Currently, the routine evaluation for somatic mutation in sporadic MTC is not recommended [7].

If an *RET* germline mutation is identified or suspected or results are unavailable, the patient should be preoperatively screened for pheochromocytoma and primary hyperparathyroidism [7]. MTC should not be resected until pheochromocytoma has been appropriately ruled out; and if present, the pheochromocytoma should be resected before the MTC to avoid hypertensive crisis during surgery [7] (Table 2).

Preoperative Imaging Studies

Cervical lymph node metastases are present in half of the patients with MTC at the time of presentation and in 70 % if the tumor is already palpable [46–48]. For this reason, the American Thyroid Association recommends screening with a

Table 2 Relationship of common *RET* mutations to risk of aggressive MTC in MEN2A and MEN2B and to the incidence of PHEO, HPTH, CLA, and HD in MEN2A

RET mutation	Exon	MTC risk level[a]	PHEO[b]	HPTH[b]	CLA[c]	HD[c]
G533C	8	MOD	+	–	N	N
C609F/G/R/S/Y	10	MOD	+/++	+	N	Y
C611F/G/S/Y/W	10	MOD	+/++	+	N	Y
C618F/R/S	10	MOD	+/++	+	N	Y
C620F/R/S	10	MOD	+/++	+	N	Y
C630R/Y	11	MOD	+/++	+	N	N
D631Y	11	MOD	+++	–	N	N
C634F/G/R/S/W/Y	11	H	+++	++	Y	N
K666E	11	MOD	+	–	N	N
E768D	13	MOD	–	–	N	N
L790F	13	MOD	+	–	N	N
V804L	14	MOD	+	+	N	N
V804M	14	MOD	+	+	Y	N
A883F	15	H	+++	–	N	N
S891A	15	MOD	+	+	N	N
R912P	16	MOD	–	–	N	N
M918T	16	HST	+++	–	N	N

With permission from Wells et al. [7]
[a]Risk of aggressive MTC: *MOD* moderate; *H* high, *HST* highest
[b]Incidence of PHEO and HPTH: + = *10 %; ++ = *20 %–30 %; +++ = *50 %
[c]*Y* positive occurrence, *N* negative occurrence

neck ultrasound every patient diagnosed with MTC before surgery [7]. This evaluation should include the superior mediastinum, central and bilateral neck compartments. Neck Computerized tomography (CT) may be useful if the tumor is large and there are symptoms suggestive of local invasion or bulky lymphadenopathy on ultrasound. In the presence of clinically evident lateral lymph node metastasis or serum calcitonin >500 pg/ml, further imaging is required to assess for distant metastases, including contrast-enhanced (CE) neck and chest CT, three-phase Contrast-enhanced computed tomography (CECT) or Contrast-enhanced magnetic resonance imaging (CEMRI) of the liver, and axial MRI and bone scintigraphy (see Fig. 3a-3d and 4a–d) [7, 49]. Neither 2-[Fluorine-18]fluoro-2-deoxy-D-glucose positron emission tomography (FDG-PET) scan nor 18F-dihydroxyphenylalanine-Positron Emission Tomography – Computed Tomography (PET/CT) is recommended to screen for distant metastases due to low sensitivity of these techniques for MTC during initial evaluation [7, 49]. However, functional studies may play a role in specific clinical scenarios, especially when a recurrence is suspected and no lesion can be found with the standard techniques (see Figs. 5a–c and 6a–d) [19, 50–52].

Histopathology Findings

On examination, the excised tumors are well circumscribed, with white-gray to tan surfaces and gritty consistency [53]. The tumors vary in size from less than 1 cm to several centimeters [54]. Sporadic tumors are unilateral, and familial tumors are multiple and bilateral. Histologically, the MTC tumors show a variable appearance. The tumor cells infiltrate the thyroid gland and may show sheets, nests, and trabeculae of polygonal, round, or spindle cells [53]. The cells are embedded in varying amounts of fibrovascular stroma, creating the organoid or trabecular architecture (see Fig. 7a, b). The stroma may be very vascular or hyalinized. Some tumors resemble carcinoid tumors, and the cell nests vary in size and configuration. Noncohesive morphologic features are frequent; the MTC tumor cells show round to oval nuclei with homogeneous delicate and finely stippled to coarse chromatin

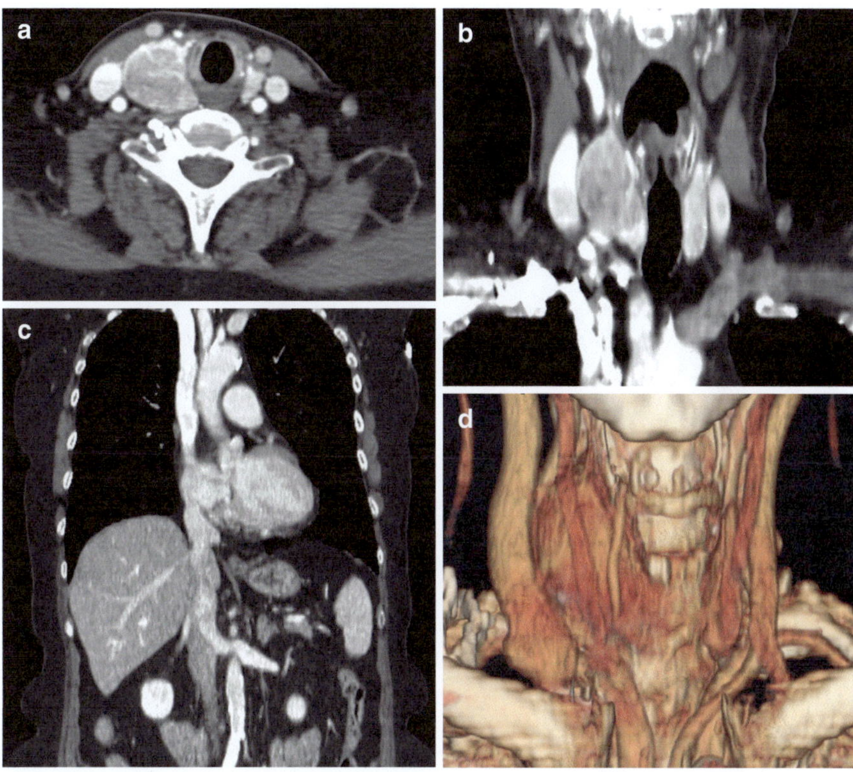

Fig. 3 (**a–c**) Axial (**a**) and coronal (**b**) CECT of the neck shows a heterogeneous enhancement of a complex right thyroid nodule. (**c**) CECT is used for systemic staging with multiphasic, multiplanar body imaging capabilities. (**d**) Tridimensional (3D) CECT reconstruction of the neck with interest over the right thyroid nodule

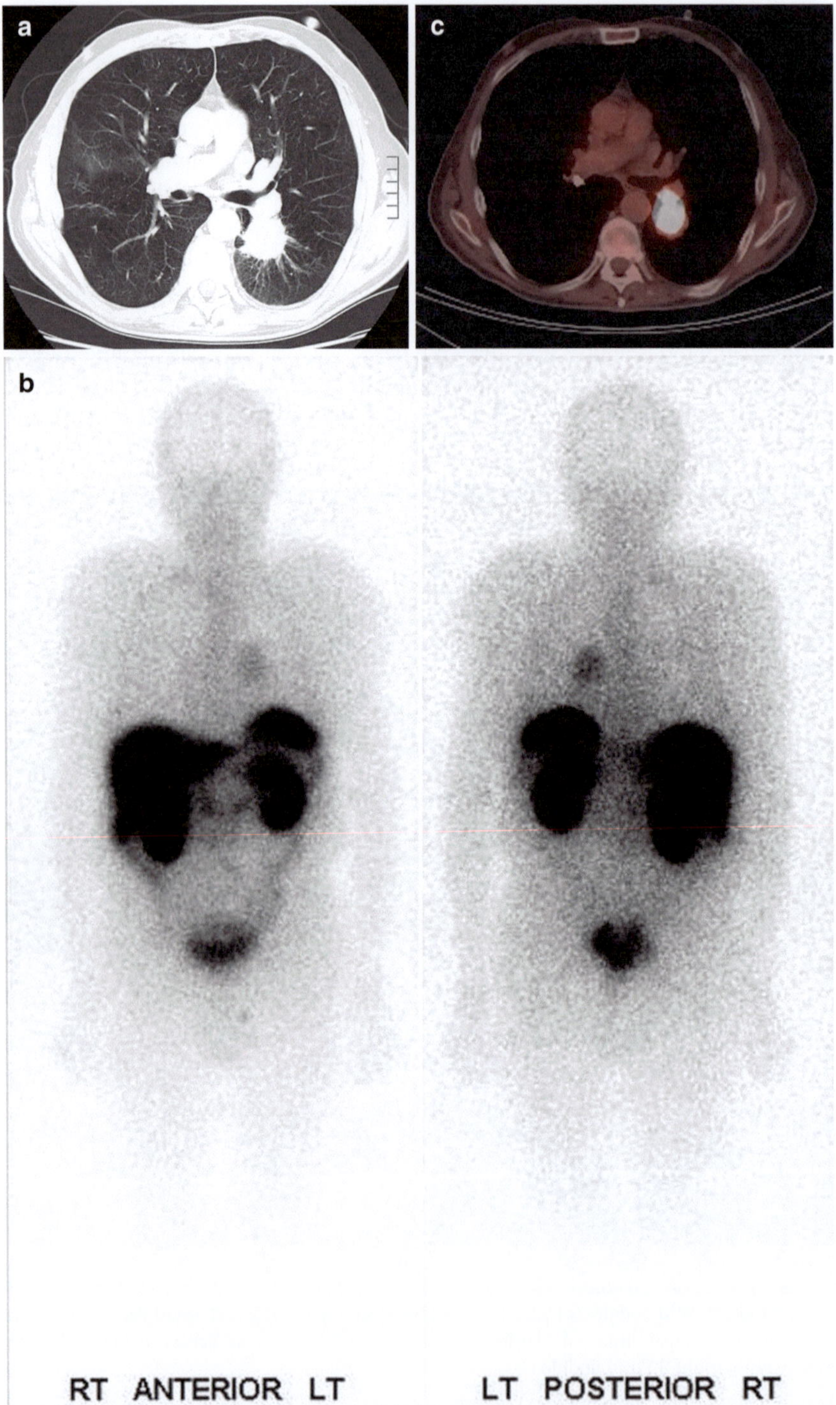
a
c
b
RT ANTERIOR LT
LT POSTERIOR RT

Fig. 4 continued

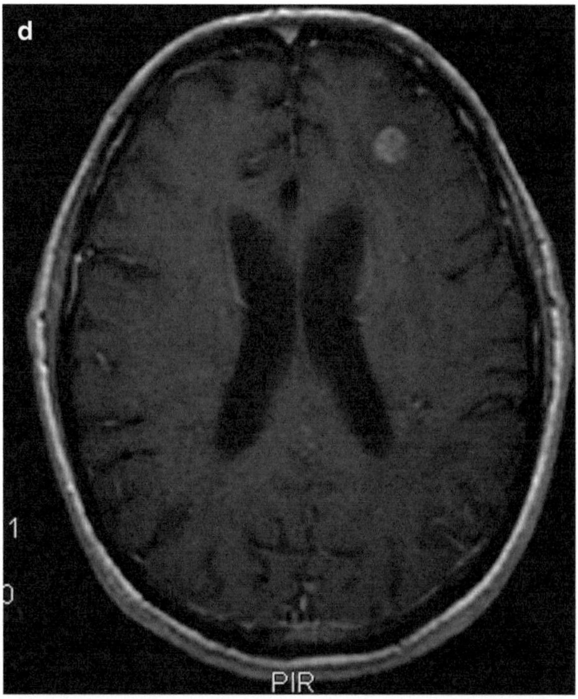

Fig. 4 (**a**) CECT of the chest shows a left lung perihilar mass on a patient with diagnosed MTC. Histologic evaluation was consistent with MTC pulmonary metastasis. (**b**) Somatostatin receptor imaging with 111-In-octreotide single-photon emission computerized tomography (SPECT)/CT shows mild increased somatostatin receptor within this mass. (**c**) 18-F-FDG-PET/CT exam shows marked increased metabolic activity within the pulmonary metastasis. (**d**) CE brain MRI shows a left frontal lobe-enhancing brain metastasis on this patient. As discussed, these patients often require a comprehensive, multimodality radiologic workup

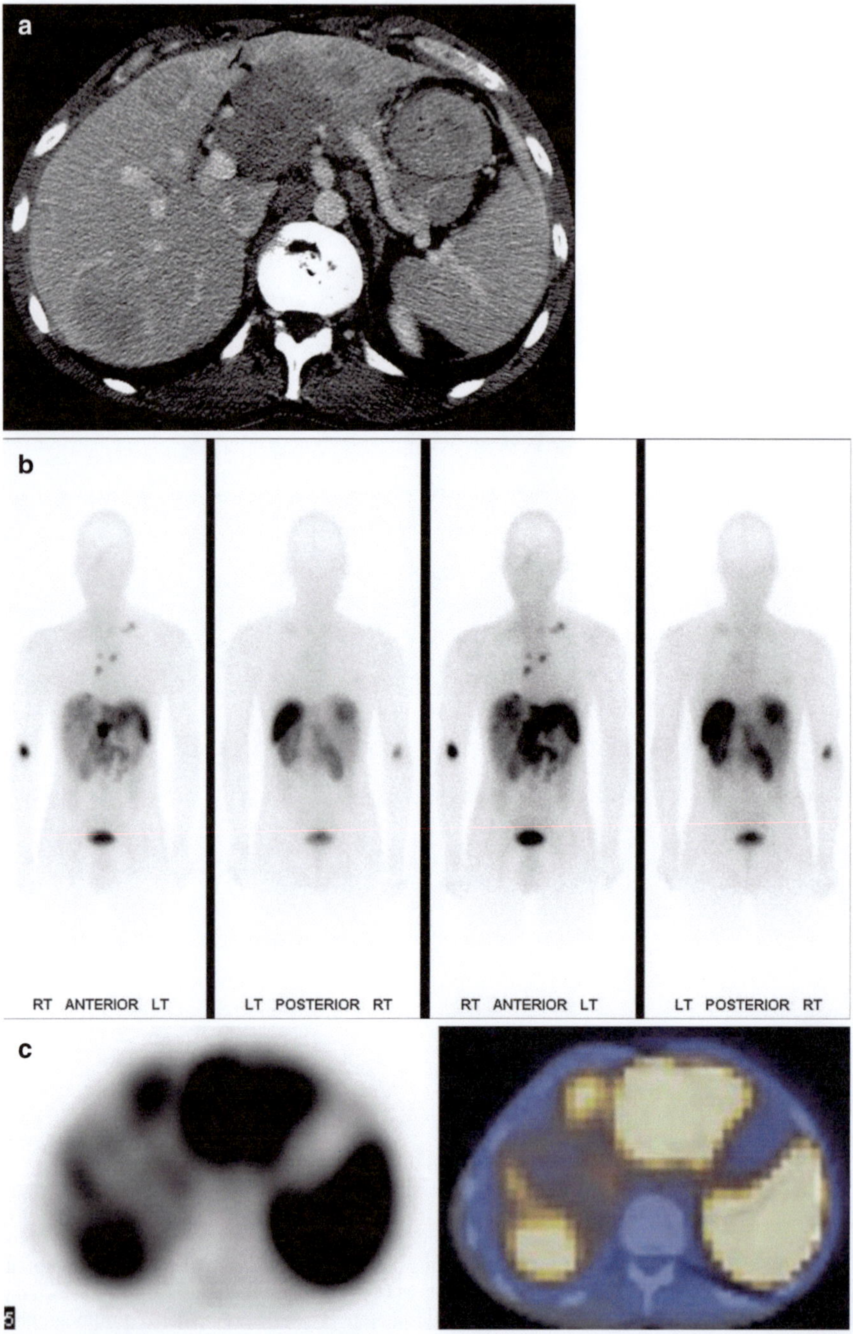

Fig. 5 (**a**) Multiphasic CECT of the liver showed multiple liver masses with variable enhancement characteristics on a patient with a history of MTC and rising calcitonin. (**b**, **c**) Planar (4B) and tomographic (4C) SPECT/CT images 24 h after 111-In-octreotide administration show markedly increased somatostatin receptor expression within numerous MTC hepatic metastases

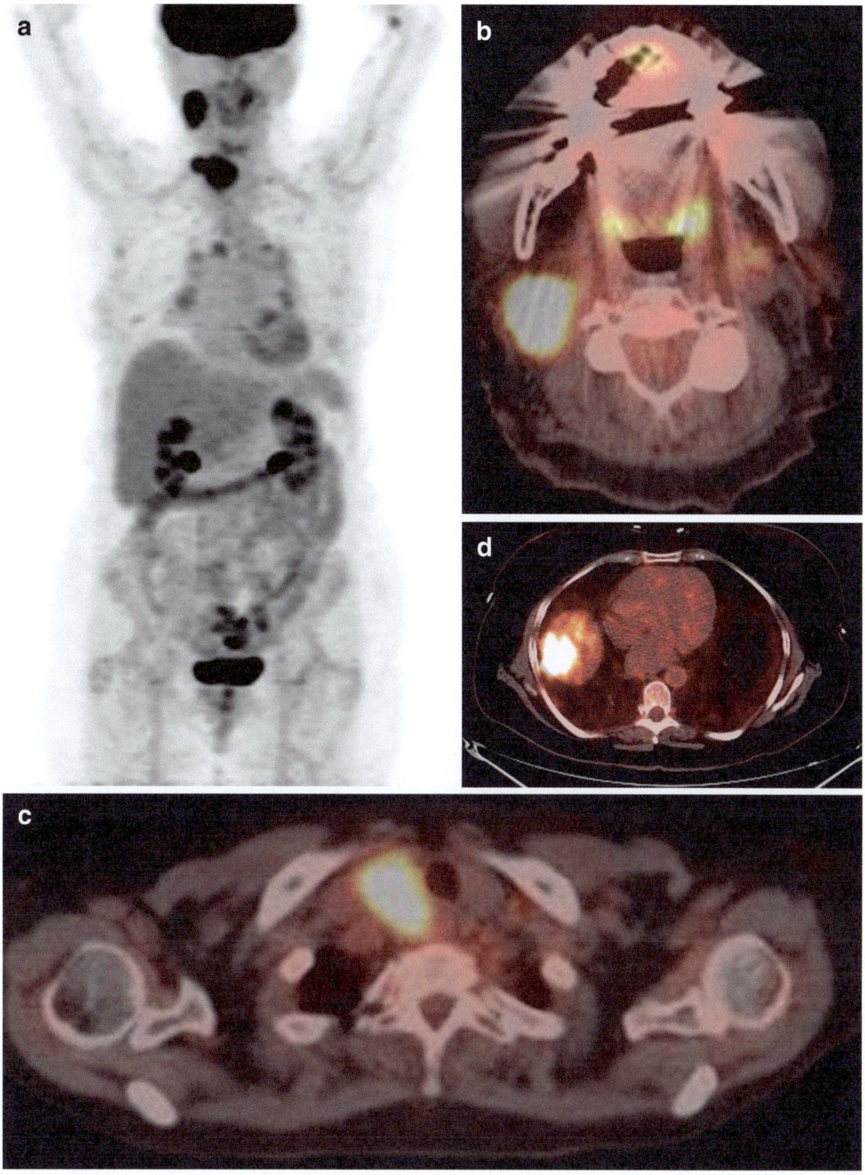

Fig. 6 (**a**) 18-F-FDG-PET/CT images on a patient with the diagnosis of MTC and rising calcitonin show hypermetabolic masses in the neck and chest. (**b**, **c**) Axial images through the neck (5B) and chest (5C) demonstrate the hypermetabolic MTC metastases. (**d**) Axial images through the liver on a different patient show hypermetabolic MTC liver metastases

with a "salt and pepper" appearance. Nucleoli are inconspicuous, except in the oncocytic variant. Intranuclear pseudoinclusions may be seen; and the nuclei may be enlarged and pleomorphic. The cytoplasm is amphophilic to granular eosinophilic; plasmacytoid morphologic features are sometimes seen. Necrosis and hemorrhage are rare. Lymphatic invasion is frequent. Focal pseudopapillary pattern may be seen. Occasionally, a tumor that measures less than 1 cm is found; these lesions are so denominated "micro-MTC" [54].

Amorphous acellular materials positive for Congo red consistent with amyloid deposits are noted in 80 % of MTC cases (see Fig. 7c) [4]. MTC tumor cells are positive for calcitonin; CEA; neuroendocrine markers, such as chromogranin and synaptophysin; TTF-1; and keratins (see Fig. 7d–g). S100 protein-positive sustentacular cells may be seen surrounding tumor cell nests. The tumor cells are negative for thyroglobulin and PAX-8 [55]. The proliferation index of these cells on a Ki67 immunostain is usually low [31].

MTC may present with different histologic patterns or variants including follicular, papillary, and pseudopapillary, small cell variant, giant cell, clear cell oncocytic, mixed or composite mucin producing, and paraganglioma like [25, 56]. Rarely, a melanotic variant is encountered [57].

C-Cells

C cells have been traditionally thought to derive from the neural crest and to migrate to the ultimobranchial bodies before the incorporation of the latter in the thyroid. However, recent research points into a possible endodermal origin in the ultimobranchial bodies for the C-cells [58–60]. In humans, the incorporation from the ultimobranchial bodies into thyroid distributes the cells to the middle and upper thirds of the outer lobes [61–63]. Ultrastructurally, the C-cells are characterized by the presence of dense core neurosecretory granules. C-cells secrete several hormones, biogenic amines, and proteins such as calcitonin, chromogranin, neurotensin, histamine, synaptophysin, and CEA. Of these secretory products, calcitonin and CEA are the most useful markers in patients with MTC; their serum levels are related with tumor burden and may be identified by IHC stains [70].

Fig. 7 (**a**, **b**) MTC tumor section showing trabecular pattern (H&E, original magnifications 100× and 400×, respectively). (**c**) MTC stained with Congo red and photographed using polarized light. The amyloid deposits show the characteristic green birefringence (Congo red stain, original magnification 200×). (**d**) MTC tumor cells positive for calcitonin (calcitonin IHC stain, original magnification 400×). (**e**) Tumor cells expressing chromogranin consistent with the neuroendocrine differentiation (chromogranin IHC stain, original magnification 400×). (**f**) MTC tumor cells expressing CEA. This is a characteristic finding in MTC cells (CEA IHC stain, original magnification 400×). (**g**) MTC tumor cells express AE1/AE3; this finding may be helpful in the differential diagnosis with paraganglioma as these tumors are negative for cytokeratins (AE1/AE3 IHC stain, original magnification 400×)

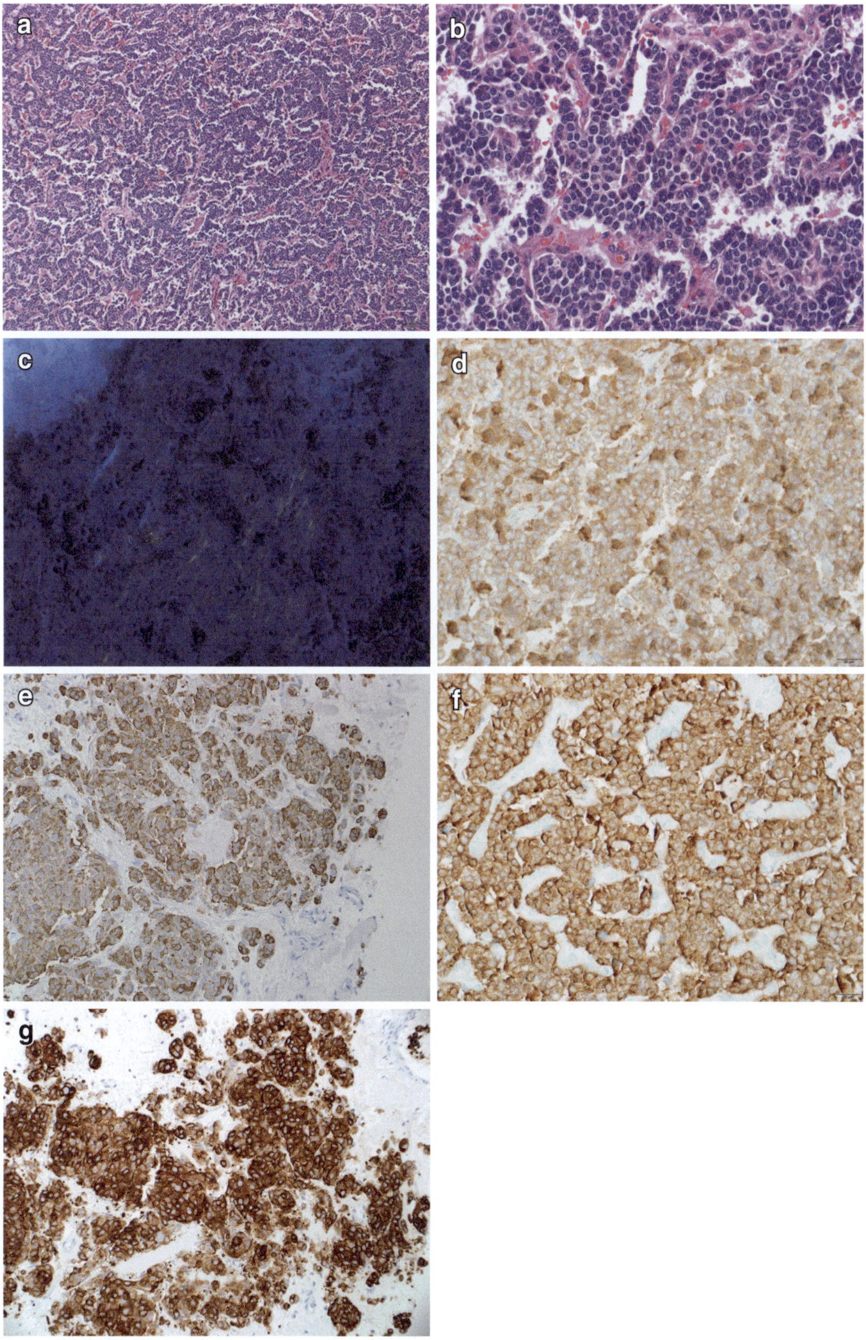
a
b
c
d
e
f
g

C-Cell Proliferations

C-cell proliferations may be reactive, "truly hyperplastic," or neoplastic [7, 64]. Reactive CCH may be associated with chronic lymphocytic thyroiditis [65] and in the nonneoplastic thyroid tissue associated with other thyroid tumors such as papillary thyroid carcinomas, follicular adenomas, and follicular carcinomas [64]; and it is not easily identified on routine stains. IHC stains for calcitonin show an increased number of normal appearing with a diffuse distribution [66].

The criteria for CCH are controversial [7]. Some authors propose that neoplastic CCH is defined as aggregates of more than 50 cells per one low high-power field and if the tumor cells are found in nodules, bilaterally, and diffusely and easily identified on Hematoxylin and Eosin (H&E) stains [64, 66, 67]. Other authors propose that a diagnosis may be warranted if there are more than seven C-cells per cluster, if they completely surround a thyroid follicle and the distribution of C-cells is beyond the normal anatomical location [68]. Usually, these clusters of C-cells are confined within the follicle [66, 69]; and cells show mild to moderate atypia with nuclear pleomorphism resembling those of MTC [66]. "C-cell hyperplasia" is a misnomer because, on molecular studies, these cells are monoclonal; and therefore, they should be considered a preneoplastic condition, similar to intraepithelial lesions elsewhere in the body [65]. For this reason, it may be more appropriate, as some authors support, to use the denomination of "C-cell carcinoma in situ" or "C-cell neoplasia" [7, 66, 70]. Invasion through the basement membrane is consistent with a MTC [69, 71, 72].

Differential Diagnosis

The differential diagnosis includes CCH; hyalinizing trabecular tumor; follicular neoplasms with trabecular growth patterns; poorly differentiated carcinomas with solid, trabecular, or insular patterns; undifferentiated thyroid carcinoma (anaplastic thyroid carcinoma); papillary thyroid carcinoma, solid variant; intrathyroidal parathyroid tumors; paraganglioma; metastatic neuroendocrine tumor from other sites; other metastatic malignancies, including metastatic malignant melanoma; and tumors with spindle cell and plasmacytoid morphology.

In CCH, the proliferating cells are confined within the follicle basement membrane. Invasion through the follicular basement membrane and beyond demonstrates a micro-MTC; however, this examination may be challenging to identify on a routine H&E stain (see Fig. 8a, b) [69, 71, 72]. A collagen IV IHC stain may be useful to reveal the microinvasion [71]. Tumor-induced reduplication of the basement membrane may also be seen [71].

Hyalinizing trabecular tumors show cells with trabecular arrangements an epithelial cell appearance, with palisading cells embedded in a dense hyalinized stroma. The cells may show nuclear grooves and intranuclear pseudoinclusions and express

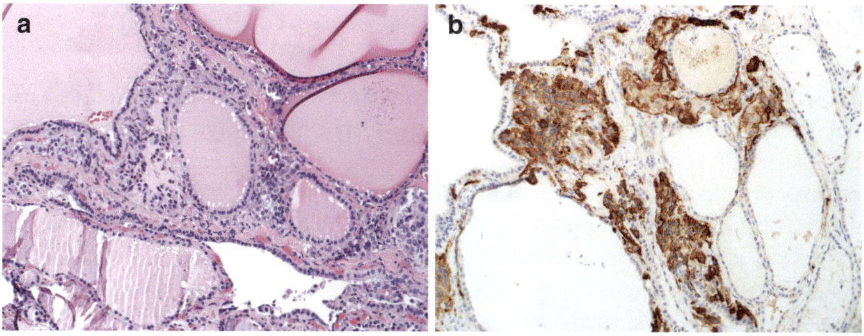

Fig. 8 (**a**, **b**) C-cell proliferation most consistent with MTC microcarcinoma. These lesion cells are better visualized in the calcitonin IHC; this stain shows tumor cells in the thyroid stroma beyond the thyroid follicle basement membrane (**a,** H&E stain, original magnification 200×; **b**, calcitonin IHC stain, original magnification 200×)

cytokeratin, thyroglobulin, and TTF-1; they may show membranous expression of MIB-1 and are negative for calcitonin, polyclonal CEA, and neuroendocrine markers such as chromogranin and synaptophysin.

Follicular adenomas are encapsulated, noninvasive follicle-derived neoplasms, while follicular carcinomas are encapsulated, follicle-derived neoplasms with capsular and/or vascular invasion within or beyond the capsule. Both of these latter follicle-derived neoplasms may show a focal trabecular pattern, with conspicuous follicular thyroid histologic features with follicular cells and colloid. These tumor cells usually lack intranuclear pseudoinclusions and the finely stippled chromatin seen in MTC. Occasionally, they may show oncocytic features (Hürthle cell tumors).

The solid variant of papillary thyroid carcinoma should also be considered in the differential diagnosis. All tumor cells of follicle-derived neoplasms, including papillary thyroid carcinomas (PTC), express cytokeratin, thyroglobulin, TTF-1, and PAX-8 and are negative for calcitonin, CEA, and neuroendocrine markers such as chromogranin and synaptophysin.

Paraganglioma rarely involves the thyroid [34]. Paraganglioma tumors show an organoid (nesting) pattern with delicate stroma [34]; the cells are epithelioid with bland to atypical morphologic features [34]. They may appear oncocytic [33, 73]. Paraganglioma shows neuroendocrine differentiation, with expression of chromogranin, synaptophysin, and CD56. These cells in the organoid nests are surrounded by S100 protein-positive sustentacular cells and are negative for cytokeratin, thyroglobulin, TTF-1, and calcitonin [33, 34].

Spindle cell tumors, such as leiomyosarcoma, rarely present in the thyroid but may be included in differential diagnosis [74]; these tumors express actin and are usually negative for cytokeratins. Plasmacytomas are rarely encountered and easily identified with IHC stains [37].

An appropriate panel of IHC stains, including but not limited to cytokeratins, calcitonin, thyroglobulin, and PAX-8, would be helpful in excluding all the other histologic mimickers.

Treatment

Total thyroidectomy with bilateral central lymph node dissection is the preferred initial treatment for patients with MTC and no evidence of neck lymph node or distant metastases [7]. If the tumor is confined to the neck, any other cervical compartments involved should also be resected at the initial surgery [7]. Prophylactic lateral lymph node dissection may be considered if extensive lymph node metastases are present in the central compartment or based on serum calcitonin levels [7, 43]. Postoperative levothyroxine is indicated to maintain TSH Thyroid-stimulating hormone within the normal range, but TSH suppression is inappropriate. Radioactive iodine is not effective and conventional chemotherapy is generally not effective. Postoperative adjuvant external beam radiotherapy can be used in patients with extensive extrathyroidal extension and macroscopic positive margins after resection. Palliative radiation therapy can be used for unresectable cases to control disease in the neck and also for bone metastases to palliate pain, control growth, and prevent fractures [7].

Patients with progressive or symptomatic unresectable locally advanced or metastatic disease can be considered for treatment with tyrosine kinase inhibitors [7]. Currently, vandetanib and cabozantinib are approved for treatment of MTC. Although these drugs have demonstrated prolongation of progression-free survival, their effect of overall survival is unknown. Complete responses are rare and partial responses are achieved in 20–50 % of the patients. Side effects are common and occur in >20 % of the patients and are severe in >5 % [75, 76]. There might be a role in the future for radiopharmaceuticals like somatostatin receptor analogs combined with beta radiation emitter agents like 131-Iodine, 90-Ytrium, or 177-Lutetium, but their use is still experimental [77].

For MEN2 patients, prophylactic total thyroidectomy should be considered at different times depending on the specific mutation inherited [7]. All children should be operated on by an experienced pediatric/endocrine surgeon. For infants with M918T mutation, total thyroidectomy should be performed during the first year of life; and bilateral central lymph node dissection considered even in the absence of suspicious lymph nodes [7]. Patients with mutations in codon 634 or mutation A883F should have a total thyroidectomy at age 5 years or before based on serum calcitonin levels and a bilateral central lymph node dissection if there are suspicious lymph nodes or serum calcitonin levels are >40 pg/ml [7]. In patients with other mutations, screening should start around 5 years of age and the timing for total thyroidectomy guided by the detection of elevated serum calcitonin levels; or if preferred, prophylactic thyroidectomy may be done around 5 years of age [7].

Prognostic Factors

Several factors have been found to determine the prognosis of the disease. Specific mutations are associated with rapid progression and spread such as M918T, A883F, and mutations in codon 634 [78]. Age at diagnosis may have an impact on mortality rates. In one study, the disease-specific survival at 10 years was 75 % for patients younger than 40 years compared to 50 % in those older than 40 years [79]. However, this has not been found in all studies [80]. An incomplete biochemical response – persistence of elevated calcitonin – after initial surgery is also associated with higher risk for recurrence and mortality [81]. However, postoperative serum calcitonin and CEA doubling times provide more relevant prognostic information being the worse prognosis associated with shorter doubling time periods [82–85]. Doubling times under 6 months, between 6 months, and 2 years or >2 years are associated with 10-year survival rates of 8 %, 37 %, and 100 %, respectively [82]. Rapidly increasing CEA level, particularly in the setting of a stable calcitonin level, and paucity of calcitonin IHC staining of the tumor might be seen in poorly differentiated tumors with worse prognosis [86, 87]. AJCC staging system has also proved to stratify patients according to cause-specific mortality rates. In one study with 4 years of median follow-up time, the cause-specific mortality was 0 %, 13 %, 56 %, and 100 % for stage I, II, III, and IV, respectively [81].

Abbreviations

ACTH	Adrenocorticotropic hormone
AJCC	American Joint Committee on Cancer
CCH	C-cell hyperplasia
CE	Contrast enhanced
CEA	Carcinoembryonic antigen
CECT	Contrast-enhanced computed tomography
CEMRI	Contrast-enhanced magnetic resonance imaging
CLA	Cutaneous lichen amyloidosis
CT	Computerized tomography
FDG-PET	2-[Fluorine-18]fluoro-2-deoxy-D-glucose positron emission tomography
F-DOPA	18F-dihydroxyphenylalanine
FNA	Fine-needle aspiration
H&E	Hematoxylin and eosin
HD	Hirschsprung's disease
HPTH	Hyperparathyroidism
IHC	Immunohistochemical stain
MEN	Multiple endocrine neoplasia
MRI	Magnetic resonance imaging
MTC	Medullary thyroid carcinoma
PET	Positron emission tomography
PHEO	Pheochromocytoma
RET	Rearranged during transfection proto-oncogene
TSH	Thyroid-stimulating hormone or thyrotropin
TTF-1	Thyroid Transcription Factor-1

References

1. Hundahl SA, Fleming ID, Fremgen AM, Menck HR. A National Cancer Data Base report on 53,856 cases of thyroid carcinoma treated in the U.S., 1985–1995 [see comments]. Cancer. 1998;83(12):2638–48.
2. Matias-Guiu X, DeLellis RA, Moley JF, et al. Medullary thyroid carcinoma. In: DeLellis RA, Lloyd RV, Heitz PU, Eng C, editors. Pathology and genetics of tumours of endocrine organs. Lyon: IARC Press; 2004. p. 86–91.
3. Saad MF, Ordonez NG, Rashid RK, et al. Medullary carcinoma of the thyroid. A study of the clinical features and prognostic factors in 161 patients. Medicine (Baltimore). 1984;63(6):319–42.
4. Williams ED. Histogenesis of medullary carcinoma of the thyroid. J Clin Pathol. 1966;19(2):114–8.
5. Gimm O, Morrison CD, Suster S, Komminoh P, Mulligan L, Sweet KM. Multiple endocrine neoplasia type 2. In: DeLellis RA, Lloyd RV, Heitz PU, Eng C, editors. Pathology and genetics of tumours of endocrine organs. Lyon: IARC Press; 2004. p. 211–7.
6. Machens A, Dralle H. Genotype-phenotype based surgical concept of hereditary medullary thyroid carcinoma. World J Surg. 2007;31(5):957–68.
7. Wells Jr SA, Asa SL, Dralle H, et al. Revised american thyroid association guidelines for the management of medullary thyroid carcinoma. Thyroid (Official Journal of the American Thyroid Association). 2015;25(6):567–610.
8. Mulligan LM, Eng C, Healey CS, et al. Specific mutations of the RET proto-oncogene are related to disease phenotype in MEN 2A and FMTC. Nat Genet. 1994;6(1):70–4.
9. Mulligan LM, Marsh DJ, Robinson BG, et al. Genotype-phenotype correlation in multiple endocrine neoplasia type 2: report of the International RET Mutation Consortium. J Intern Med. 1995;238(4):343–6.
10. Eng C, Clayton D, Schuffenecker I, et al. The relationship between specific RET proto-oncogene mutations and disease phenotype in multiple endocrine neoplasia type 2. International RET mutation consortium analysis. JAMA. 1996;276(19):1575–9.
11. Romei C, Tacito A, Molinaro E, et al. Twenty years of lesson learning: how does the RET genetic screening test impact the clinical management of medullary thyroid cancer? Clin Endocrinol (Oxf). 2015;82(6):892–9.
12. Verga U, Fugazzola L, Cambiaghi S, et al. Frequent association between MEN 2A and cutaneous lichen amyloidosis. Clin Endocrinol (Oxf). 2003;59(2):156–61.
13. Mulligan LM, Eng C, Attie T, et al. Diverse phenotypes associated with exon 10 mutations of the RET proto-oncogene. Hum Mol Genet. 1994;3(12):2163–7.
14. Dvorakova S, Vaclavikova E, Sykorova V, et al. Somatic mutations in the RET proto-oncogene in sporadic medullary thyroid carcinomas. Mol Cell Endocrinol. 2008;284(1–2):21–7.
15. Ciampi R, Mian C, Fugazzola L, et al. Evidence of a low prevalence of RAS mutations in a large medullary thyroid cancer series. Thyroid (Official Journal of the American Thyroid Association). 2013;23(1):50–7.
16. Boichard A, Croux L, Al Ghuzlan A, et al. Somatic RAS mutations occur in a large proportion of sporadic RET-negative medullary thyroid carcinomas and extend to a previously unidentified exon. J Clin Endocrinol Metab. 2012;97(10):E2031–5.
17. Trimboli P, Nasrollah N, Amendola S, et al. Should we use ultrasound features associated with papillary thyroid cancer in diagnosing medullary thyroid cancer? Endocr J. 2012;59(6):503–8.
18. Moon WJ, Jung SL, Lee JH, et al. Benign and malignant thyroid nodules: US differentiation–multicenter retrospective study. Radiology. 2008;247(3):762–70.
19. Lee S, Shin JH, Han BK, Ko EY. Medullary thyroid carcinoma: comparison with papillary thyroid carcinoma and application of current sonographic criteria. AJR Am J Roentgenol. 2010;194(4):1090–4.

20. Ilias I, Torpy DJ, Pacak K, Mullen N, Wesley RA, Nieman LK. Cushing's syndrome due to ectopic corticotropin secretion: twenty years' experience at the National Institutes of Health. J Clin Endocrinol Metab. 2005;90(8):4955–62.
21. Bugalho MJ, Santos JR, Sobrinho L. Preoperative diagnosis of medullary thyroid carcinoma: fine needle aspiration cytology as compared with serum calcitonin measurement. J Surg Oncol. 2005;91(1):56–60.
22. Trimboli P, Treglia G, Guidobaldi L, et al. Detection rate of FNA cytology in medullary thyroid carcinoma: a meta-analysis. Clin Endocrinol (Oxf). 2015;82(2):280–5.
23. Papaparaskeva K, Nagel H, Droese M. Cytologic diagnosis of medullary carcinoma of the thyroid gland. Diagn Cytopathol. 2000;22(6):351–8.
24. Webster N, Fox C, Fan F. Thyroid bed fine needle aspiration in patients after thyroidectomy–a useful follow-up tool with proposed diagnostic categories. Ann Diagn Pathol. 2014;18(3):177–80.
25. Tranchida P, Estigarribia J, Sethi S, Giorgadze T. Cytologic diagnosis of recurrent medullary thyroid carcinoma with oncocytic change twenty-one years post-thyroidectomy: case report and review of the literature. Diagn Cytopathol. 2011;39(9):641–6.
26. Giovanella L, Ceriani L, Bongiovanni M. Calcitonin measurement on fine needle washouts: preanalytical issues and normal reference values. Diagn Cytopathol. 2013;41(3):226–9.
27. Mousa U, Gursoy A, Ozdemir H, Moray G. Medullary thyroid carcinoma in a patient with Hashimoto's thyroiditis diagnosed by calcitonin washout from a thyroid nodule. Diagn Cytopathol. 2013;41(7):644–6.
28. Trimboli P, Nigri G, Romanelli F, et al. Medullary thyroid nodules by measurement of calcitonin (Ct) in aspiration needle washout in patients with multinodular goiter and moderately elevated serum Ct. Exp Clin Endocrinol Diabetes (Official Journal, German Society of Endocrinology [and] German Diabetes Association). 2012;120(4):234–7.
29. Trimboli P, Rossi F, Baldelli R, et al. Measuring calcitonin in washout of the needle in patients undergoing fine needle aspiration with suspicious medullary thyroid cancer. Diagn Cytopathol. 2012;40(5):394–8.
30. Baloch ZW, Fleisher S, LiVolsi VA, Gupta PK. Diagnosis of "follicular neoplasm": a gray zone in thyroid fine-needle aspiration cytology. Diagn Cytopathol. 2002;26(1):41–4.
31. Tisell LE, Oden A, Muth A, et al. The Ki67 index a prognostic marker in medullary thyroid carcinoma. Br J Cancer. 2003;89(11):2093–7.
32. Ozgen AG, Hamulu F, Bayraktar F, et al. Evaluation of routine basal serum calcitonin measurement for early diagnosis of medullary thyroid carcinoma in seven hundred seventy-three patients with nodular goiter. Thyroid (Official Journal of the American Thyroid Association). 1999;9(6):579–82.
33. Armstrong MJ, Chiosea SI, Carty SE, Hodak SP, Yip L. Thyroid paragangliomas are locally aggressive. Thyroid (Official Journal of the American Thyroid Association). 2012;22(1):88–93.
34. Kronz JD, Argani P, Udelsman R, Silverberg L, Westra WH. Paraganglioma of the thyroid: two cases that clarify and expand the clinical spectrum. Head Neck. 2000;22(6):621–5.
35. Jimenez-Heffernan JA, Vicandi B, Lopez-Ferrer P, Gonzalez-Peramato P, Perez-Campos A, Viguer JM. Cytologic features of pheochromocytoma and retroperitoneal paraganglioma: a morphologic and immunohistochemical study of 13 cases. Acta Cytol. 2006;50(4):372–8.
36. Bourtsos EP, Bedrossian CW, De Frias DV, Nayar R. Thyroid plasmacytoma mimicking medullary carcinoma: a potential pitfall in aspiration cytology. Diagn Cytopathol. 2000;23(5):354–8.
37. Avila A, Villalpando A, Montoya G, Luna MA. Clinical features and differential diagnoses of solitary extramedullary plasmacytoma of the thyroid: a case report. Ann Diagn Pathol. 2009;13(2):119–23.
38. Nobuoka Y, Hirokawa M, Kuma S, et al. Cytologic findings and differential diagnoses of primary thyroid MALT lymphoma with striking plasma cell differentiation and amyloid deposition. Diagn Cytopathol. 2014;42(1):73–7.

39. Pacini F, Fontanelli M, Fugazzola L, et al. Routine measurement of serum calcitonin in nodular thyroid diseases allows the preoperative diagnosis of unsuspected sporadic medullary thyroid carcinoma. J Clin Endocrinol Metab. 1994;78(4):826–9.
40. Gharib H, Papini E, Paschke R, et al. American Association of Clinical Endocrinologists, Associazione Medici Endocrinologi, and European Thyroid Association Medical Guidelines for clinical practice for the diagnosis and management of thyroid nodules. Endocr Pract. 2010;16 Suppl 1:1–43.
41. Cheung K, Roman SA, Wang TS, Walker HD, Sosa JA. Calcitonin measurement in the evaluation of thyroid nodules in the United States: a cost-effectiveness and decision analysis. J Clin Endocrinol Metab. 2008;93(6):2173–80.
42. Costante G, Meringolo D, Durante C, et al. Predictive value of serum calcitonin levels for preoperative diagnosis of medullary thyroid carcinoma in a cohort of 5817 consecutive patients with thyroid nodules. J Clin Endocrinol Metab. 2007;92(2):450–5.
43. Machens A, Dralle H. Biomarker-based risk stratification for previously untreated medullary thyroid cancer. J Clin Endocrinol Metab. 2010;95(6):2655–63.
44. Yip DT, Hassan M, Pazaitou-Panayiotou K, et al. Preoperative basal calcitonin and tumor stage correlate with postoperative calcitonin normalization in patients undergoing initial surgical management of medullary thyroid carcinoma. Surgery. 2011;150(6):1168–77.
45. Elisei R, Romei C, Cosci B, et al. RET genetic screening in patients with medullary thyroid cancer and their relatives: experience with 807 individuals at one center. J Clin Endocrinol Metab. 2007;92(12):4725–9.
46. Moley JF, DeBenedetti MK. Patterns of nodal metastases in palpable medullary thyroid carcinoma: recommendations for extent of node dissection. Ann Surg. 1999;229(6):880–7; discussion 887–88.
47. Moley JF. Medullary thyroid carcinoma: management of lymph node metastases. J Natl Compr Canc Netw. 2010;8(5):549–56.
48. Weber T, Schilling T, Frank-Raue K, et al. Impact of modified radical neck dissection on biochemical cure in medullary thyroid carcinomas. Surgery. 2001;130(6):1044–9.
49. Giraudet AL, Vanel D, Leboulleux S, et al. Imaging medullary thyroid carcinoma with persistent elevated calcitonin levels. J Clin Endocrinol Metab. 2007;92(11):4185–90.
50. Pestourie C, Theze B, Kuhnast B, et al. PET imaging of medullary thyroid carcinoma in MEN2A transgenic mice using 6-[(18)F]F-L-DOPA. Eur J Nucl Med Mol Imaging. 2010;37(1):58–66.
51. Conry BG, Papathanasiou ND, Prakash V, et al. Comparison of (68)Ga-DOTATATE and (18) F-fluorodeoxyglucose PET/CT in the detection of recurrent medullary thyroid carcinoma. Eur J Nucl Med Mol Imaging. 2010;37(1):49–57.
52. Ambrosini V, Marzola MC, Rubello D, Fanti S. (68)Ga-somatostatin analogues PET and (18) F-DOPA PET in medullary thyroid carcinoma. Eur J Nucl Med Mol Imaging. 2010;37(1):46–8.
53. Williams ED, Brown CL, Doniach I. Pathological and clinical findings in a series of 67 cases of medullary carcinoma of the thyroid. J Clin Pathol. 1966;19(2):103–13.
54. Samulski TD, Livolsi VA, Montone K, Baloch Z. The variable pathologic presentations of medullary and micro-medullary thyroid carcinoma: an institutional experience. Pathol Res Pract. 2014;210(3):182–5.
55. Puglisi F, Cesselli D, Damante G, Pellizzari L, Beltrami CA, Di Loreto C. Expression of Pax-8, p53 and bcl-2 in human benign and malignant thyroid diseases. Anticancer Res. 2000;20(1A):311–6.
56. Bockhorn M, Sheu SY, Frilling A, Molmenti E, Schmid KW, Broelsch CE. Paraganglioma-like medullary thyroid carcinoma: a rare entity. Thyroid (Official Journal of the American Thyroid Association). 2005;15(12):1363–7.
57. Ikeda T, Satoh M, Azuma K, Sawada N, Mori M. Medullary thyroid carcinoma with a paraganglioma-like pattern and melanin production: a case report with ultrastructural and immunohistochemical studies. Arch Pathol Lab Med. 1998;122(6):555–8.

58. Fagman H, Nilsson M. Morphogenesis of the thyroid gland. Mol Cell Endocrinol. 2010;323(1):35–54.
59. Westerlund J, Andersson L, Carlsson T, Zoppoli P, Fagman H, Nilsson M. Expression of Islet1 in thyroid development related to budding, migration, and fusion of primordia. Dev Dyn. 2008;237(12):3820–9.
60. Kameda Y, Nishimaki T, Miura M, Jiang SX, Guillemot F. Mash1 regulates the development of C cells in mouse thyroid glands. Dev Dyn. 2007;236(1):262–70.
61. McMillan PJ, Hooker WM, Deptos LJ. Distribution of calcitonin-containing cells in the human thyroid. Am J Anat. 1974;140(1):73–9.
62. Wolfe HJ, DeLellis RA, Voelkel EF, Tashjian Jr AH. Distribution of calcitonin-containing cells in the normal neonatal human thyroid gland: a correlation of morphology with peptide content. J Clin Endocrinol Metab. 1975;41(06):1076–81.
63. Wolfe HJ, Melvin KE, Cervi-Skinner SJ, et al. C-cell hyperplasia preceding medullary thyroid carcinoma. N Engl J Med. 1973;289(9):437–41.
64. Albores-Saavedra J, Monforte H, Nadji M, Morales AR. C-cell hyperplasia in thyroid tissue adjacent to follicular cell tumors. Hum Pathol. 1988;19(7):795–9.
65. Diaz-Cano SJ, de Miguel M, Blanes A, Tashjian R, Wolfe HJ. Germline RET 634 mutation positive MEN 2A-related C-cell hyperplasias have genetic features consistent with intraepithelial neoplasia. J Clin Endocrinol Metab. 2001;86(8):3948–57.
66. Perry A, Molberg K, Albores-Saavedra J. Physiologic versus neoplastic C-cell hyperplasia of the thyroid: separation of distinct histologic and biologic entities. Cancer. 1996;77(4):750–6.
67. Thompson LDR. Malignant neoplasms of the thyroid gland. In: Thompson LDR, editor. Head and neck pathology. 2nd ed. Philadelphia: Elsevier Saunders; 2012. p. 598–608.
68. Mete O, Asa SL. Precursor lesions of endocrine system neoplasms. Pathology. 2013;45(3):316–30.
69. Hinze R, Holzhausen HJ, Gimm O, Dralle H, Rath FW. Primary hereditary medullary thyroid carcinoma–C-cell morphology and correlation with preoperative calcitonin levels. Virchows Arch. 1998;433(3):203–8.
70. Guyetant S, Josselin N, Savagner F, Rohmer V, Michalak S, Saint-Andre JP. C-cell hyperplasia and medullary thyroid carcinoma: clinicopathological and genetic correlations in 66 consecutive patients. Mod Pathol. 2003;16(8):756–63.
71. McDermott MB, Swanson PE, Wick MR. Immunostains for collagen type IV discriminate between C-cell hyperplasia and microscopic medullary carcinoma in multiple endocrine neoplasia, type 2a. Hum Pathol. 1995;26(12):1308–12.
72. Etit D, Faquin WC, Gaz R, Randolph G, DeLellis RA, Pilch BZ. Histopathologic and clinical features of medullary microcarcinoma and C-cell hyperplasia in prophylactic thyroidectomies for medullary carcinoma: a study of 42 cases. Arch Pathol Lab Med. 2008;132(11):1767–73.
73. Baloch ZW, LiVolsi VA. Oncocytic lesions of the neuroendocrine system. Semin Diagn Pathol. 1999;16(2):190–9.
74. Tanboon J, Keskool P. Leiomyosarcoma: a rare tumor of the thyroid. Endocr Pathol. 2013;24(3):136–43.
75. Elisei R, Schlumberger MJ, Muller SP, et al. Cabozantinib in progressive medullary thyroid cancer. J Clin Oncol. 2013;31(29):3639–46.
76. Wells Jr SA, Robinson BG, Gagel RF, et al. Vandetanib in patients with locally advanced or metastatic medullary thyroid cancer: a randomized, double-blind phase III trial. J Clin Oncol. 2012;30(2):134–41.
77. Sharkey RM, Hajjar G, Yeldell D, et al. A phase I trial combining high-dose 90Y-labeled humanized anti-CEA monoclonal antibody with doxorubicin and peripheral blood stem cell rescue in advanced medullary thyroid cancer. J Nucl Med (Official Publication, Society of Nuclear Medicine). 2005;46(4):620–33.
78. Romei C, Elisei R, Pinchera A, et al. Somatic mutations of the ret protooncogene in sporadic medullary thyroid carcinoma are not restricted to exon 16 and are associated with tumor recurrence. J Clin Endocrinol Metab. 1996;81(4):1619–22.

79. Kebebew E, Ituarte PH, Siperstein AE, Duh QY, Clark OH. Medullary thyroid carcinoma: clinical characteristics, treatment, prognostic factors, and a comparison of staging systems. Cancer. 2000;88(5):1139–48.
80. de Groot JW, Plukker JT, Wolffenbuttel BH, Wiggers T, Sluiter WJ, Links TP. Determinants of life expectancy in medullary thyroid cancer: age does not matter. Clin Endocrinol (Oxf). 2006;65(6):729–36.
81. Dottorini ME, Assi A, Sironi M, Sangalli G, Spreafico G, Colombo L. Multivariate analysis of patients with medullary thyroid carcinoma. Prognostic significance and impact on treatment of clinical and pathologic variables. Cancer. 1996;77(8):1556–65.
82. Barbet J, Campion L, Kraeber-Bodere F, Chatal JF, Group GTES. Prognostic impact of serum calcitonin and carcinoembryonic antigen doubling-times in patients with medullary thyroid carcinoma. J Clin Endocrinol Metab. 2005;90(11):6077–84.
83. Gawlik T, d'Amico A, Szpak-Ulczok S, et al. The prognostic value of tumor markers doubling times in medullary thyroid carcinoma – preliminary report. Thyroid Res. 2010;3(1):10.
84. Miyauchi A, Onishi T, Morimoto S, et al. Relation of doubling time of plasma calcitonin levels to prognosis and recurrence of medullary thyroid carcinoma. Ann Surg. 1984;199(4):461–6.
85. Laure Giraudet A, Al Ghulzan A, Auperin A, et al. Progression of medullary thyroid carcinoma: assessment with calcitonin and carcinoembryonic antigen doubling times. Eur J Endocrinol. 2008;158(2):239–46.
86. Mendelsohn G, Wells Jr SA, Baylin SB. Relationship of tissue carcinoembryonic antigen and calcitonin to tumor virulence in medullary thyroid carcinoma. An immunohistochemical study in early, localized, and virulent disseminated stages of disease. Cancer. 1984;54(4):657–62.
87. Lippman SM, Mendelsohn G, Trump DL, Wells Jr SA, Baylin SB. The prognostic and biological significance of cellular heterogeneity in medullary thyroid carcinoma: a study of calcitonin, L-dopa decarboxylase, and histaminase. J Clin Endocrinol Metab. 1982;54(2):233–40.

Neuroendocrine Tumors (NETs) of the Mediastinum and Thymus

Sameer Al Diffalha and Farah Khalil

Introduction

Neuroendocrine tumors (NETs) of the mediastinum and thymus are rare, and as such they have received far less attention from investigators, compared to their gastrointestinal (GI) and lung counterparts. Where research over the last several years has proven reproducible molecular alterations in GI and lung cancers, there have only been a handful of studies investigating the findings in mediastinal and thymic NETs. Diagnosis of mediastinal and thymic NETs, description of the predictive molecular markers in NET tumors with background on the role in tumorigenesis, and evidence for their value as productive markers will be discussed in this chapter.

Terminology

The term carcinoid was first presented in 1907 by Oberndorfer [1]. Later, Gosset and Masson established the existence of argentaffin granules in the tumor cells. In due time, the occurrence of these tumors in other anatomic areas was recognized [2]. Rosai and Higa were the first to acknowledge the existence of carcinoid tumors in the thymus and to separate them from more common tumors arising in this

S. Al Diffalha, MD (✉)
Department of Pathology, H. Lee Moffitt Cancer Center and Research Institute, University of South Florida, Tampa, FL, USA
e-mail: sameer.aldiffalha@moffitt.org

F. Khalil, MD
H. Lee Moffitt Cancer Center and Research Institute, University of South Florida, Tampa, FL, USA

Department of Pathology and Cell Biology, University of South Florida, Tampa, FL, USA

A. Nasir, D. Coppola (eds.), *Neuroendocrine Tumors: Review of Pathology, Molecular and Therapeutic Advances*, DOI 10.1007/978-1-4939-3426-3_8

location, such as thymoma [3]. Since there is obvious variability in the histologic and biologic range of these lesions, Rosai et al. proposed a nomenclature [4] in 1976 for mediastinal NETs that included carcinoid grade I, for the well-differentiated tumors (conventional carcinoids); carcinoid grade II, for the moderately differentiated lesions (atypical carcinoid); and carcinoid grade III, for poorly differentiated lesions (small cell carcinoma/oat cell carcinoma). Thymic neuroendocrine tumors (neuroendocrine carcinoma) can be separated adequately based on their histopathologic features into well-differentiated, moderately differentiated, and poorly differentiated neoplasms.

According to the World Health Organization (WHO), they are classified into four histological types: typical carcinoid (TC), atypical carcinoid (AC), small cell neuroendocrine cell carcinoma (SCNEC), and large cell neuroendocrine cell carcinoma (LCNEC) [5].

Epidemiology

Primary neuroendocrine tumors of the mediastinum and thymus are uncommon neoplasms [6] with an annual incidence of 0.01/100,000 in the USA [7] with ~400 cases reported in the literature to date [8]. The prevalence of thymic NET is ~3 % of the total number of NETs at all sites [9] and estimated to account for approximately 2–4 % of all anterior mediastinal neoplasms [6, 10]. Both bronchial and thymic NETs may be part of the multiple endocrine neoplasia type 1 syndrome (MEN-1, 5–15 %) [6, 7, 9, 11, 12]. The median age at diagnosis for bronchial NETs is 64 years and for thymic NETs 59 years [9]. They are more common in males (M:F ratio, 3:1) [6, 9].

Location

The neuroendocrine tumors are generally located in parenchymal organs [13, 14] and are the most frequently reported tumors which include neuroendocrine tumors of the lung, thymus, and parathyroid [3, 9]. Rare cases of neuroendocrine tumors located in the mesentery, retroperitoneum, inferior vena cava, presacral region, and posterior mediastinum have been reported [3, 15–18]. One NET case has been described arising from a foregut cyst [19].

Diagnostic Radiology

Chest X-ray may suggest a diagnosis of both bronchial and thymic NETs, but CT scan is the recommended investigation, and magnetic resonance imaging (MRI) is recommended to detect tumor metastases. ^{18}F-FDG PET generally demonstrates significantly increased glucose metabolism in the poorly differentiated tumors, but it is limited in NETs [20]. However, 68Ga-DOTATOC is a somatostatin analog for highly sensitive and specific PET imaging of NETs, with a high affinity for the human SSTR2 (somatostatin receptor subtype-2) [21].

Symptoms

Most NETs of the mediastinum and the thymus are asymptomatic and are usually discovered incidentally. Clinical symptoms generally occur at an advanced stage. The patient may complain of chest discomfort, dyspnea, and cough or may present with superior vena cava syndrome. NETs may be accompanied by hormonal hypersecretion, and the patient may present with Cushing's syndrome due to ACTH secretion or may have acromegaly due to growth hormone-releasing hormone (GHRH) hypersecretion [6, 22–25]. Not infrequently, distant metastases are present at the time of diagnosis.

Tumorigenesis

The source of the primary NETs of the mediastinum is not clear; however, there are two main hypotheses. The first hypothesis proposes that the NET tumor cells arise from ectopic tissues (migratory abnormalities), and the other hypothesis suggests that they form teratomatous components [15, 16]. The source of the primary NETs of the thymus has been proposed that they are derived from Kulchitsky cells. It has been mentioned in old reports that in the high-grade NETs, you might see areas showing well-differentiated neuroendocrine tumor of the thymus in direct transition with areas of poorly differentiated neuroendocrine carcinoma indistinguishable from those of small cell carcinoma of the lung [26] which has been used to support that these tumors represent part of a continuous spectrum of differentiation that ranges from well-differentiated through poorly differentiated neuroendocrine neoplasms.

Morphology

Gross Features

Usually the neuroendocrine tumors (NETs) of the mediastinum and the thymus are well circumscribed, large (ranging from 2 to 20 cm), soft, tan brown, and with a lobulated homogeneous rubbery cut surface. Focal areas of hemorrhage, necrosis, or both might be seen.

Microscopic Features

The NETs are composed of small to medium-sized cells that are usually arranged in solid and trabecular pattern with scant cytoplasm, granular nuclear chromatin, and indistinct nucleoli (Fig. 1). You may observe pseudo-rosette formation as well. The tumors may or may not have tumor necrosis, and the mitotic rate may be less than 2, 2–10 or more than 10/10 HPF). Small cell carcinoma shows small round blue cells, with scant cytoplasm, high N:C ratio, apoptosis, necrosis, and brisk mitosis. By electron microscopy, the tumor cells demonstrate numerous desmosomes and neurosecretory granules [15].

Immunohistochemical Stains

The tumor cells express both epithelial and neuroendocrine markers. Most NETs are positive for CAM 5.2 low-molecular-weight cytokeratins (100 %), broad-spectrum keratin (AE1/3) (88 %), chromogranin (75 %), synaptophysin

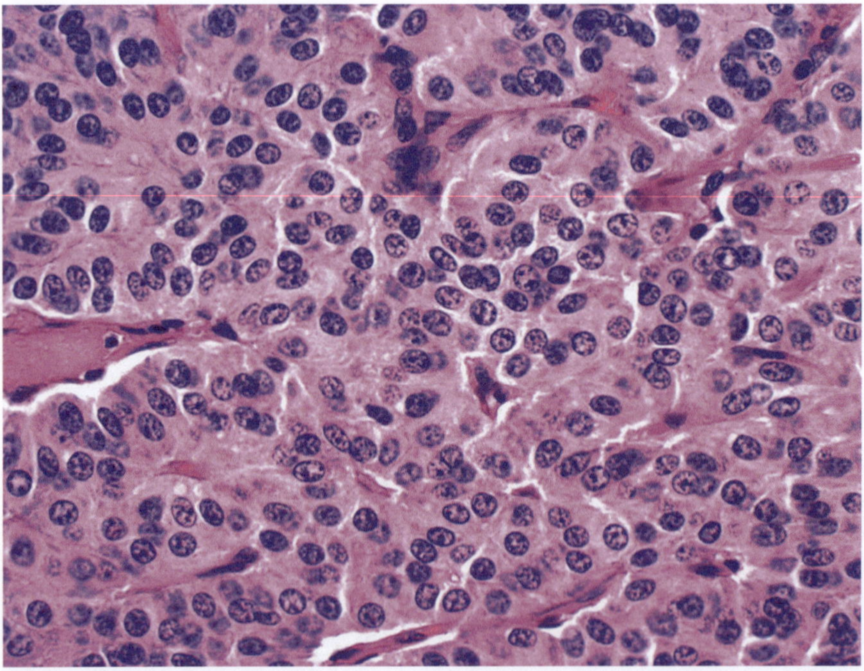

Fig. 1 Typical carcinoid (well-differentiated neuroendocrine tumor) shows nesting pattern. The nests are composed of medium-sized cells with eosinophilic cytoplasm, round to oval nuclei with granular chromatin, and no minimal mitotic activity (<2/10 HPF). There is no necrosis present in the additional section.

(72 %), and Leu-7 (68 %) [27] but negative for thyroid transcription factor-1 (TTF-1) [28].

Classification

The tumors were classified into four types: typical carcinoid (TC), atypical carcinoid (AC), large cell neuroendocrine carcinoma (LCNEC), and small cell neuroendocrine carcinoma (SCNEC). The WHO criteria based on the histopathologic differentiation are shown below:

1. TC: A well-differentiated tumor with mitotic figures, fewer than 2 mitoses per 10 high-power fields (HPFs) and no necrosis (Fig. 1)
2. AC: A well-differentiated tumor with mitotic figures, 2–10 mitoses per 10 HPFs and/or presence of necrosis
3. SCNEC: A poorly differentiated tumor with small cell cytology, mitotic figures with more than 10 mitoses per 10 HPFs and extensive areas of necrosis
4. LCNEC: A poorly differentiated tumor with non-small cell NEC, mitotic figures with more than 10 mitoses per 10 HPFs and extensive areas of necrosis [5]

LCNEC is extremely rare, with only few cases that have been reported so far [28, 29]. It is a relatively new category of NECs that was first described by Travis et al. [29, 30]. The majority of the reported causes of mediastinal LCNEC originated from the thymus [29, 31–33]. However, there is a case report of mediastinal LCNEC in a young patient with increase in the serum AFP which includes embryonal carcinoma in the differential diagnosis. LCNEC is strongly positive for CK7 and neuroendocrine markers (CD56, synaptophysin, and chromogranin) and negative for CD5, CD30, HCG, and PLAP, also for hepatocyte antigen [29].

Differential Diagnosis

The differential diagnosis for NECs includes other primary mediastinal tumors, which include thymoma particularly the spindle type, paraganglioma, lymphoma, parathyroid adenoma or parathyroid carcinoma, and medullary carcinoma of the thyroid arising in the mediastinum. The differential diagnosis also includes a group of small round cell tumors as PNET/Ewing sarcoma, neuroblastoma, lymphoma, and rhabdomyosarcoma [3, 15]. Spindle cell thymomas may display zones with neuroendocrine appearance and epithelial pseudo-rosettes [34, 35], like NETs, and both lesions share strong CAM 5.2 reactivity, but thymomas are negative for the neuroendocrine markers. Mediastinal paraganglioma is a real pitfall when mediastinal biopsy is performed for NETs, because they often have large hyperchromatic atypical nuclei and demonstrate prominent organoid or neuroendocrine growth pattern. They are reactive for neuroendocrine markers, but they usually are not mitotically active and most often do not have necrosis or vascular invasion [36]. Ectopic mediastinal parathyroid tumors (adenomas and carcinomas) have intracellular glycogen that is positive with periodic acid–Schiff [37]. Immunohistochemical stains for parathyroid hormones also may be useful. Medullary thyroid carcinoma arising in ectopic mediastinal location is positive for calcitonin and carcinoembryonic antigen (CEA).

Molecular Pathology

The genetic abnormalities in thymic NETs have not been as well characterized as the other foregut NETs, but carcinoids have a distinct gene expression pattern from the normal thymus, and they are characterized by deregulations of a series of bio-functions, which may be involved in the development of NETs. Literature shows that the development of NETs may involve different genes, each of which may be associated with several different abnormalities that include point mutations, gene deletions, DNA methylation, chromosomal losses, and chromosomal gains. The foregut, midgut, and hindgut NETs have different molecular pathways. Foregut NETs have frequent deletions and mutations of the MEN-1 gene, midgut NETs have losses of chromosome 18, 11q, and 16q, and hindgut NETs express transforming growth factor alpha and the epidermal growth factor receptor. On the other hand, the most common abnormality in lung NETs is loss of chromosome 3p. Moreover, p53 mutations and 5q21 loss have more aggressive behavior and are associated with poor survival [38].

There are chromosomal imbalances that have been found by some investigators in thymic tumors, which include gains of chromosome Xp, 7p, 7q, 11q, 12q, and 20q and losses at 6q, 6p, 4q, 3p, 10q, 11q, and 13q [39, 40]. Loss of heterozygosity (LOH) at chromosome 1p has been reported in two thymic neuroendocrine tumors [39, 41]. Loss of chromosomes 3, 9p21, and Y and gain of chromosome 19p were discovered in one case [38, 39]. Although 25 % of the reported thymic NETs are from MEN-1 patients [39, 41], LOH of the MEN-1 locus on chromosome 11q13 has not been reported in thymic NETs, except in one patient [39].

Of the abnormal expression of genes that involve in cell differentiation, Wnt-signaling pathway was shown as being tightly associated with thymic carcinoids. Bi Y.F. et al. examined the b-catenin target genes MYC (c-Myc) and CCND1 (cyclin D1) expression in AC tissues to search for more evidence of Wnt pathway activation and found consistently elevated level of cyclin D1 in AC tumors, but c-Myc expression changed only moderately.

Management, Response Evaluation, and Follow-Up

The NETs of the mediastinum and thymus are characterized by more atypical histologic features and more aggressive behavior than conventional carcinoid tumor of the lung [42, 43]. It is not uncommon to find lymph node metastases even with the low-grade NETs. A standard therapeutic approach for mediastinal NETs has not yet been defined. However, surgery remains the typical way for the management for thymic tumors [7, 8]. Localized NETs should, whenever possible, be subjected to radical surgical resection. Unfortunately, the percentage of recurrence remains remarkably elevated, higher than in bronchial NETs counterparts [44]. Surgical resection followed by cytotoxic drug therapy has become standard for metastatic bronchial and thymic NETs. Somatostatin analogs may be an option for low-grade NETs, and alpha interferon might be an option for functional tumors. Tyrosine kinase inhibitors (e.g., sunitinib) and TOR inhibitor everolimus have been stated to show better prognosis in a small series, and cisplatin-based regimens have also been of value in thymic NETs [44]. Also temozolomide-based treatment is reported to provide some advantage [45, 46]. The role of neoadjuvant/adjuvant treatment for mediastinal LCNEC has not been sufficiently evaluated because of the limited number of reported cases. SCLC is sensitive to chemotherapy, and since the biological characteristics of LCNEC are similar to those of SCLC [3], both are treated with chemotherapy regimens.

After primary surgery, patients with NETs should be followed at least yearly, up to 15 years, to detect surgically manageable recurrences. CT scan should typically be performed once a year in AC and every 2 or 3 years in TC. Patients with metastatic or recurrent disease should be followed during treatment with cytotoxic or biological agents more often, at 3–6-month intervals with imaging, preferably by CT and biological markers to assess possible benefits of the treatment administered [44, 47].

Prognosis

NETs arising in the thymus may show a more aggressive behavior than their pulmonary equivalents [5]. The most important prognostic factors with validated significance are tumor size, histological grade, paraneoplastic symptoms, thymic Masaoka staging, and surgical resection [7, 8, 48, 49]. Ki67 proliferation index is the key player in the stratification of patients with good and bad prognosis in other neuroendocrine tumors [50], but it has yet to be validated for use in thymic carcinoids [42]. Regional lymph nodes are often affected and distant metastases are common [11].

Thymic neuroendocrine tumors must be regarded as malignant neoplasms that are prone to metastasize to mediastinal lymph nodes and to distant sites, even after total excision [3, 6, 51–54], and follow-up is therefore recommended. LCNEC is associated with a 5-year survival rate of 15–57 % and the 5-year survival rate for SCLC is ~5 % [22, 44, 55–57]. Very poor prognosis is due to high propensity for early distant hematogenous metastases [58].

Abbreviations

AC	Atypical carcinoid
LCNEC	Large cell neuroendocrine cell carcinoma
NET	Neuroendocrine tumor
SCNEC	Small cell neuroendocrine cell carcinoma
TC	Typical carcinoid

References

1. Oberndorfer S, Oberndorfer S. Karzinoide Tumoren des Duenndarns. Frankfurt Z Pathol. 1907;1:426–30.
2. Gosset A, Masson P. Tumeurs endocrines de l'appendice. Presse Med. 1914;22:37–40.
3. Rosai J, Higa E. Mediastinal endocrine neoplasm, of probable thymic origin, related to carcinoid tumor. Clinicopathologic study of 8 cases. Cancer. 1972;29(4):1061–74. PubMed PMID: 4111691.
4. Rosai J, Levine G, Weber WR, Higa E. Carcinoid tumors and oat cell carcinomas of the thymus. Pathol Annu. 1976;11:201–26. PubMed PMID: 188002, Review.
5. Travis WD, Brambilla E, Müller-Hermelink HK, Harris CC. World Health Organization classification of tumours: pathology and genetics of tumours of the lung, pleura, thymus and heart. Lyon: IARC Press; 2004.
6. Ahn S, Lee JJ, Ha SY, Sung CO, Kim J, Han J. Clinicopathological analysis of 21 thymic neuroendocrine tumors. Korean J Pathol. 2012;46(3):221–5. doi:10.4132/KoreanJPathol.2012.46.3.221. PubMed PMID: 23110006, PubMed Central PMCID: PMC3479770, Epub 2012 Jun 22.
7. Gaur P, Leary C, Yao JC. Thymic neuroendocrine tumors: a SEER database analysis of 160 patients. Ann Surg. 2010;251(6):1117–21. doi:10.1097/SLA.0b013e3181dd4ec4. PubMed PMID: 20485130.
8. Song Z, Zhang Y. Primary neuroendocrine tumors of the thymus: clinical review of 22 cases. Oncol Lett. 2014;8(5):2125–9. PubMed PMID: 25295099, PubMed Central PMCID: PMC4186590, Epub 2014 Sep 1.
9. Öberg K, Hellman P, Ferolla P, Papotti M, ESMO Guidelines Working Group. Neuroendocrine bronchial and thymic tumors: ESMO Clinical Practice Guidelines for diagnosis, treatment and follow-up. Ann Oncol. 2012;23(Suppl 7):vii120–3. PubMed
10. Viebahn R, Hiddemann W, Klinke F, von Bassewitz DB. Thymus carcinoid. Pathol Res Pract. 1985;180(4):445–51. PubMed.
11. Crona J, Björklund P, Welin S, Kozlovacki G, Oberg K, Granberg D. Treatment, prognostic markers and survival in thymic neuroendocrine tumours. A study from a single tertiary referral centre. Lung Cancer. 2013;79(3):289–93. doi:10.1016/j.lungcan.2012.12.001. PubMed PMID: 23286964, Epub 2013 Jan 1.
12. Falchetti A, Marini F, Brandi ML. Multiple endocrine neoplasia Type 1; 1993.
13. Modlin IM, Sandor A. An analysis of 8305 cases of carcinoid tumors. Cancer. 1997;79(4):813–29. PubMed PMID: 9024720.
14. Wick MR, Scheithauer BW. Thymic carcinoid. A histologic, immunohistochemical, and ultrastructural study of 12 cases. Cancer. 1984;53(3):475–84. PubMed PMID: 6141000.
15. Horie Y, Kato M. Neuroendocrine carcinoma of the posterior mediastinum: a possible primary lesion. Arch Pathol Lab Med. 1999;123(10):933–6. PubMed PMID: 10506448.
16. Yajima A, Toki T, Morinaga S, Sasano H, Sasano N. A retroperitoneal endocrine carcinoma. Cancer. 1984;54(9):2040–2. PubMed PMID: 6478437.

17. Horenstein MG, Erlandson RA, Gonzalez-Cueto DM, Rosai J. Presacral carcinoid tumors: report of three cases and review of the literature. Am J Surg Pathol. 1998;22(2):251–5. PubMed PMID: 9500228.
18. Enzinger FM, Weiss SW. Peripheral neuroepithelioma. In: Soft tissue tumors. 3rd ed. New York: Mosby; 1995. p. 945–51.
19. Yamashita A, Marutsuka K, Moriguchi S, Shimizu T, Matsuzaki Y, Onitsuka T, Asada Y. Neuroendocrine carcinoma of the posterior mediastinum arising from a foregut cyst. Pathol Int. 2005;55(5):285–9. PubMed.
20. Adams S, Baum R, Rink T, Schumm-Dräger PM, Usadel KH, Hör G. Limited value of fluorine-18 fluorodeoxyglucose positron emission tomography for the imaging of neuroendocrine tumours. Eur J Nucl Med. 1998;25(1):79–83. PubMed PMID:9396878.
21. Maecke HR, Hofmann M, Haberkorn U. (68)Ga-labeled peptides in tumor imaging. J Nucl Med. 2005;46 Suppl 1:172S–8. Review. PubMed PMID: 15653666.
22. Phan AT, Oberg K, Choi J, Harrison Jr LH, Hassan MM, Strosberg JR, Krenning EP, Kocha W, Woltering EA, Maples WJ, North American Neuroendocrine Tumor Society (NANETS). NANETS consensus guideline for the diagnosis and management of neuroendocrine tumors: well-differentiated neuroendocrine tumors of the thorax(includes lung and thymus). Pancreas. 2010;39(6):784–98. doi:10.1097/MPA.0b013e3181ec1380. PubMed PMID: 20664476.
23. Van Brandt V, Heyman S, Van Marck E, Hendriks J, Van Schil P. Atypical presentation of an atypical carcinoid. Ann Thorac Surg. 2009;88(6):2004–6. doi:10.1016/j.athoracsur.2009.04.124. PubMed PMID: 19932277.
24. Wang WQ, Ye L, Bi YF, Zhao HY, Sun SY, Tang ZY, Zhao YJ, Fang WQ, Chen ZY, Chen KM, Jin XL, Ning G. Six cases of ectopic ACTH syndrome caused by thymic carcinoid. J Endocrinol Invest. 2006;29(4):293–7. PubMed PMID: 16699293, Review.
25. Simsek I, Pay S, Dinc A, Erdem H, Kurt B. Atypical carcinoid tumor of the thymus with ectopic ACTH production developed during the course of etanercept treatment–case report. Clin Rheumatol. 2007;26(9):1561–2. PubMed PMID: 17061154, Epub 2006 Oct 24.
26. Wick MR, Scheithauer BW. Oat-cell carcinoma of the thymus. Cancer. 1982;49(8):1652–7. PubMed PMID: 6279270.
27. Kacar F, Meteoglu I, Sen S, Levi E. Primary neuroendocrine carcinoma of the mediastinum. Pathol Oncol Res. 2002;8(3):200–1. PubMed PMID: 12516001, Epub 2003 Jan 6.
28. Maeda A, Nakata M, Yasuda K, Yukawa T, Saisho S, Okita R, Hirami Y, Shimizu K. Unknown primary large cell neuroendocrine carcinoma (LCNEC) in the mediastinum. Gen Thorac Cardiovasc Surg. 2013;61(9):542–5. doi:10.1007/s11748-012-0157-5. PubMed PMID: 23011520, Epub 2012 Sep 26.
29. Takezawa K, Okamoto I, Fukuoka J, Tanaka K, Kaneda H, Uejima H, Yoon HE, Imakita M, Fukuoka M, Nakagawa K. Large cell neuroendocrine carcinoma of the mediastinum with alpha-fetoprotein production. J Thorac Oncol. 2008;3(2):187–9. doi:10.1097/JTO.0b013e3181623359. PubMed PMID: 18303442.
30. Travis WD, Linnoila RI, Tsokos MG, Hitchcock CL, Cutler Jr GB, Nieman L, Chrousos G, Pass H, Doppman J. Neuroendocrine tumors of the lung with proposed criteria for large-cell neuroendocrine carcinoma. An ultrastructural, immunohistochemical, and flow cytometric study of 35 cases. Am J Surg Pathol. 1991;15(6):529–53. PubMed PMID: 1709558.
31. Natsuhara A, Iwasaki Y, Minagawa T, Takemura Y, Nakanisi M, Nagata K, Harada H, Kubota Y, Yokomura I, Nakagawa M. Aggressively metastatic neuroendocrine carcinoma in the middle mediastinum. Nihon Kokyuki Gakkai Zasshi. 2001;39(9):705–9. Japanese. PubMed PMID: 11729693.
32. Nojima D, Kiura K, Hotta K, Takigawa N, Tabata M, Tanimoto M. Large cell neuroendocrine carcinoma of the mediastinum. Nihon Kokyuki Gakkai Zasshi. 2010;48(7):506–10. Japanese. PubMed PMID: 20684214.
33. Lukina O, Gorbunkov S, Dvorakovskaja I, Varlamov V, Akopov A. Fast-growing large cell neuroendocrine carcinoma of mediastinum. Ann Thorac Surg. 2011;91(5):1618–20. doi:10.1016/j.athoracsur.2010.09.065. PubMed PMID: 21524479.

34. Rosai J, Levine GD. Tumors of the thymus. In: Atlas of tumor pathology. Second series, Fascicle 13. Washington, DC: Armed Forces Institute of Pathology; 1976. p. 34–161.
35. Suster S. Mediastinal pathology. In: Weidner N, editor. The difficult diagnosis in surgical pathology. Philadelphia: Saunders; 1995. p. 143–76.
36. Moran CA, Suster S, Fishback N, Koss MN. Mediastinal paragangliomas. A clinicopathologic and immunohistochemical study of 16 cases. Cancer. 1993;72(8):2358–64. PubMed PMID: 8402449.
37. Wick MR, Rosai J. Neuroendocrine neoplasms of the mediastinum. Semin Diagn Pathol. 1991;8(1):35–51. PubMed PMID: 1646476, Review.
38. Leotlela PD, Jauch A, Holtgreve-Grez H, Thakker RV. Genetics of neuroendocrine and carcinoid tumours. Endocr Relat Cancer. 2003;10(4):437–50. Review. PubMedPMID: 14713256.
39. Bi YF, Liu RX, Ye L, Fang H, Li XY, Wang WQ, Zhang J, Wang KK, Jiang L, Su TW, Chen ZY, Ning G. Gene expression profiles of thymic neuroendocrine tumors(carcinoids) with ectopic ACTH syndrome reveal novel molecular mechanism. Endocr Relat Cancer. 2009;16(4):1273–82. doi:10.1677/ERC-08-0325. Epub 2009 Jul 22. PubMed.
40. Rieker RJ, Aulmann S, Penzel R, Schnabel PA, Blaeker H, Esposito I, Morresi-Hauf A, Otto HF, Hecker E, Dienemann H, Schirmacher P, Mechtersheimer G. Chromosomal imbalances in sporadic neuroendocrine tumours of the thymus. Cancer Lett. 2005;223(1):169–74. Epub 2004 Dec 8. PubMed.
41. Teh BT, Zedenius J, Kytölä S, Skogseid B, Trotter J, Choplin H, Twigg S, Farnebo F, Giraud S, Cameron D, Robinson B, Calender A, Larsson C, Salmela P. Thymic carcinoids in multiple endocrine neoplasia type 1. Ann Surg. 1998;228(1):99–105. PubMed PMID: 9671073; PubMed Central PMCID: PMC1191434.
42. Arrigoni MG, Woolner LB, Bernatz PE. Atypical carcinoid tumors of the lung. J Thorac Cardiovasc Surg. 1972;64(3):413–21. PubMed PMID: 5054879.
43. Valli M, Fabris GA, Dewar A, Chikte S, Fisher C, Corrin B, Sheppard MN. Atypical carcinoid tumour of the thymus: a study of eight cases. Histopathology. 1994;24(4):371–5. PubMed PMID: 8045526.
44. Öberg K, Hellman P, Ferolla P, Papotti M, ESMO Guidelines Working Group. Neuroendocrine bronchial and thymic tumors: ESMO Clinical Practice Guidelines for diagnosis, treatment and follow-up. Ann Oncol. 2012;23(Suppl 7):vii120–3. PubMed PMID: 22997444
45. Ekeblad S, Sundin A, Janson ET, Welin S, Granberg D, Kindmark H, Dunder K, Kozlovacki G, Orlefors H, Sigurd M, Oberg K, Eriksson B, Skogseid B. Temozolomide as monotherapy is effective in treatment of advanced malignant neuroendocrine tumors. Clin Cancer Res. 2007;13(10):2986–91. PubMed PMID: 17505000.
46. Hamada S, Masago K, Mio T, Hirota S, Mishima M. Good clinical response to imatinib mesylate in atypical thymic carcinoid with KIT overexpression. J Clin Oncol. 2011;29(1):e9–10. doi:10.1200/JCO.2010.30.2455. PubMed PMID: 20876428, Epub 2010 Sep 27.
47. Warren WH, Gould VE. Long-term follow-up of classical bronchial carcinoid tumors. Clinicopathologic observations. Scand J Thorac Cardiovasc Surg. 1990;24(2):125–30. PubMed PMID: 2166332.
48. Oberg K, Jelic S, ESMO Guidelines Working Group. Neuroendocrine bronchial and thymic tumors: ESMO clinical recommendation for diagnosis, treatment and follow-up. Ann Oncol. 2009;20(Suppl 4):147–9. doi:10.1093/annonc/mdp157.Review. PubMed PMID: 19454438
49. Cardillo G, Treggiari S, Paul MA, Carleo F, De Massimi AR, Remotti D, Graziano P, Martelli M. Primary neuroendocrine tumours of the thymus: a clinicopathologic and prognostic study in 19 patients. Eur J Cardiothorac Surg. 2010;37(4):814–8. doi:10.1016/j.ejcts.2009.10.026. PubMed PMID: 19954997, Epub 2009 Dec 1.
50. Rindi G, Klöppel G, Alhman H, Caplin M, Couvelard A, de Herder WW, Erikssson B, Falchetti A, Falconi M, Komminoth P, Körner M, Lopes JM, McNicol AM, Nilsson O, Perren A, Scarpa A, Scoazec JY, Wiedenmann B, all other Frascati Consensus Conference participants; European Neuroendocrine Tumor Society (ENETS). TNM staging of foregut (neuro)endocrine tumors: a consensus proposal including a grading system. Virchows Arch. 2006;449(4):395–401. Epub 2006 Sep 12. PubMed PMID: 16967267; PubMed Central PMCID: PMC1888719

51. Fukai I, Masaoka A, Fujii Y, Yamakawa Y, Yokoyama T, Murase T, Eimoto T. Thymic neuroendocrine tumor (thymic carcinoid): a clinicopathologic study in 15 patients. Ann Thorac Surg. 1999;67(1):208–11. PubMed PMID: 10086551.
52. de Montpréville VT, Macchiarini P, Dulmet E. Thymic neuroendocrine carcinoma (carcinoid): a clinicopathologic study of fourteen cases. J Thorac Cardiovasc Surg. 1996;111(1):134–41. PubMed PMID: 8551758.
53. Wick MR, Scott RE, Li CY, Carney JA. Carcinoid tumor of the thymus: a clinicopathologic report of seven cases with a review of the literature. Mayo Clin Proc. 1980;55(4):246–54. PubMed PMID: 6153740.
54. Economopoulos GC, Lewis Jr JW, Lee MW, Silverman NA. Carcinoid tumors of the thymus. Ann Thorac Surg. 1990;50(1):58–61. PubMed PMID: 2196019, Review.
55. Travis WD, Rush W, Flieder DB, Falk R, Fleming MV, Gal AA, Koss MN. Survival analysis of 200 pulmonary neuroendocrine tumors with clarification of criteria for atypical carcinoid and its separation from typical carcinoid. Am J Surg Pathol. 1998;22(8):934–44. PubMed PMID: 9706973.
56. Righi L, Volante M, Rapa I, Scagliotti GV, Papotti M. Neuro-endocrine tumours of the lung. A review of relevant pathological and molecular data. Virchows Arch. 2007;451 Suppl 1:S51–9. Epub 2007 Aug 8. Review. PubMed PMID: 17684766.
57. Travis WD, Giroux DJ, Chansky K, Crowley J, Asamura H, Brambilla E, Jett J, Kennedy C, Rami-Porta R, Rusch VW, Goldstraw P, International Staging Committee and Participating Institutions. The IASLC Lung Cancer Staging Project: proposals for the inclusion of broncho-pulmonary carcinoid tumors in the forthcoming(seventh) edition of the TNM Classification for Lung Cancer. J Thorac Oncol. 2008;3(11):1213–23. doi:10.1097/JTO.0b013e31818b06e3. PubMed PMID: 18978555.
58. Asamura H, Kameya T, Matsuno Y, Noguchi M, Tada H, Ishikawa Y, Yokose T, Jiang SX, Inoue T, Nakagawa K, Tajima K, Nagai K. Neuroendocrine neoplasms of the lung: a prognostic spectrum. J Clin Oncol. 2006;24(1):70–6. PubMed PMID:16382115.

Neuroendocrine Tumors of the Lung

Farah Khalil

Introduction

Extensive research over the last several years has investigated the reproducible molecular alterations in lung cancers. The marked success in identifying specific molecular cohorts of patients has contributed to a new paradigm of classification of these tumors [1]. Based on the molecular and morphological type of tumor, the appropriately selected patients show better prognosis with targeted therapy as compared to conventional chemotherapy [2]. Great strides have been made in identifying the molecular alterations observed in the most common subtype of lung cancer, adenocarcinoma, which has led to improvement in therapy and prognosis of the patients [3, 4]. Neuroendocrine tumors (NETs) form a distinctive group of neoplasms, ranging in malignancy and aggression [5]. Lung is the second most common site for NET formation after the gastrointestinal tract, and these tumors account for approximately 25 % of primary lung neoplasms [6, 7]. The most common lung NETs are small cell lung cancer (SCLC), which comprise 20 % of all lung neoplasms [6]. Diagnosis of NETs, description of the predictive molecular markers in NET tumors with background on the role in tumorigenesis, and evidence for their value as productive markers will be discussed in this chapter.

F. Khalil, MD
Department of Anatomic Pathology, University of South Florida, Tampa, Florida, USA

H. Lee Moffitt Cancer Center and Research Institute, Tampa, Florida, USA
e-mail: farah.khalil@moffitt.org

A. Nasir, D. Coppola (eds.), *Neuroendocrine Tumors: Review of Pathology, Molecular and Therapeutic Advances*, DOI 10.1007/978-1-4939-3426-3_9

Historical Aspects of Lung Neuroendocrine Tumors

Siegfried Oberndorfer was one of the first to use the term carcinoid to describe lung NET tumors [8]; however, the described neoplasms were known for close to a century prior to his characterization of carcinoids. In 1904, a case described as "multiple primary carcinomata" by Bunting from Johns Hopkins referenced other possible descriptions as far back as the eighteenth century [9]. Similar tumors in the appendix are described by Gossett and Masson in 1914 who made an analogy to that described by Oberndorfer [8, 10].

Gmelich et al. identified the presence of Kulchitsky cells and bronchioles and associated the occurrence of these neoplasms in the lung to the cells [11]. About the same time, Hausman and Weimann published an interesting case of NET with lymph node metastasis and alluded to the fact that these tumors have low malignant potential [12].

The study of 100 cases of oat cell carcinoma was performed by Azzopardi in which he described the tumor morphology as that with rosettes, ribbons, streams, and ductules [13]. Kato et al. described a similar study of 138 cases of oat cell carcinoma [14]. Although neuroendocrine in nature, photographic evidence indicates that both Azzopardi and Kato's study cases correspond to the low- or intermediate-grade neuroendocrine tumors of today.

Pathogenesis of Lung Neuroendocrine Tumors

During the earliest stages of embryological lung development, the bronchial Kulchitsky cells are the first cells to form and differentiate in the epithelium [15]. Derived from the endoderm, they are found in the immature fetal epithelium and are part of the diffuse NE system, thus currently known as the pulmonary NE cells [16–18]. These pulmonary NE cells comprise a very minor component of the bronchial epithelial cells and are usually seen as solitary cells within the ciliated respiratory epithelium [19, 20]. Sometimes they form small nodules called neuroepithelial bodies (NEBs) [21]. Their function is to act as local modulators of lung growth and differentiation during embryological development with the expression of neuron-specific enolase and serotonin initially followed by gastrin-releasing peptide. In adult life, the pulmonary NE cells act as airway chemoreceptors by secreting serotonin in hypoxia and diverting blood flow to better ventilated areas of the lung resulting from vasoconstriction in the poorly ventilated areas [19, 20, 22].

Gene expression profiling supports that SCLC arises from normal bronchial epithelial cells [16, 22] and acquires NE characteristics. Sutherland et al. [23] introduced p53 and Rb mutations in different pulmonary cells in transgenic mice which showed that central SCLC arose from PNECs; however, peripheral SCLC arose from the alveolar type 2 cells. SCLC also occurs in combination with NSCLCs, making it a possibility for all of the NCLCs and NSCLCs to arise from pluripotent precursor stem cells. Linnoila et al. [24] have shown evidence that PNECs, alveolar type 2 cells, Clara cells, and respiratory ciliated cells are derived from a common cell which expresses AHS1/ASCL1 (achaete-scute complex homolog 1). Experiments with mouse cell lines have also shown that lung tumors have heterogeneity and adenocarcinoma can arise from SCLC [25] after Ras oncogene expression. There has been debate over clustering SCLC with LCNEC, because they have been observed to occur in a combination. Gene expression profiling has supported this notion [16, 26]; however, Nasgashio et al. [27] observed lower ASH1 intensity in LCNEC and suggested that it is more closely related to non-NETs. The few studies performed on CTs indicate that they also arise from PNECs and alveolar type 2 cells.

Precursor Lesions

The precursor lesions for pulmonary carcinoid tumors show histological resemblance to CT [28, 29]. These precursor lesions can be seen in two orientations: as 2–5 mm small extraluminal nodules called tumorlets and as minute linear proliferations of PNECs or NEBs, referred to as diffuse idiopathic pulmonary NE cell hyperplasia (DIPNECH) [16]. Tumorlets were originally described as benign lesions; however, they have shown to behave like CTs, with metastasis to the lymph nodes and distant sites [30–32]. DIPNECH is always seen in patients with tumorlets and CTs leading to the belief that the hyperplastic foci are the precursors to nodule formation [33]. All three are positive for p53 and Ki-67 [34], whereas reactive NEC hyperplasia does not show this expression.

Terminology and Current Classification of Lung Neuroendocrine Tumors

The pathologic terminology that has been used to describe neuroendocrine tumors had been perplexing over the last decades. Kulchitsky cell carcinoma, bronchial adenoma, carcinoid tumor, atypical carcinoid tumor, cutaneous Merkel cell carcinoma, medullary thyroid carcinoma, islet cell tumor, and oat cell carcinoma have been used for the epithelial group of neuroendocrine tumors. Terms used for a separate group of nonepithelial or neural tumors have included paraganglioma, pheochromocytoma, chemodectoma, neuroblastoma, retinoblastoma, glomus jugulare tumor, and pineoblastoma [35–39]. Lung NET is known to arise from bronchial Kulchitsky cells, but differs in terms of histopathology. Each category of NET has different grades (low, intermediate, high) depending on the presence of nuclear pleomorphism, necrosis, and rate of mitosis, and is also characterized based on the TNM staging system [40]. This section will expound upon the histological and other determining characteristics of each type of NET.

Carcinoid Tumor (Grade 1 Neuroendocrine Carcinoma)

Carcinoid tumor (CT) was previously also known as "classical carcinoid" or "typical carcinoid"; these low-grade NECs demonstrate typical neuroendocrine features which are histologically easy to recognize. Centrally located tumors (Fig. 1a) are typically 2–4 cm and both cellular and vascular and show nested, trabecular, pseudoglandular/rosette, insular, or solid sheetlike growth pattern, with delicate fibrovascular stroma (Fig. 1b, c). They lack internal hemorrhage and necrosis and contain abundant cytoplasm, but it may be granular or oncocytic. The nuclear chromatin is finer compared to the higher grade tumors, and the proliferation index is low (up to two mitoses per ten high-power fields). Peripherally located tumors usually show a spindle cell growth pattern (Fig. 2a, b); however, in cases where the growth pattern resembles the central tumors, the histological recognition is easier. There may be evidence of fibrosis or stromal hyalinization, calcification, and ossification [41]. CTs smaller than 5 mm are designated as "carcinoid tumorlets" based on the observation that these are usually incidentally found and carry almost a negligible chance of metastasis [40].

Immunohistochemical markers that can be used to identify carcinoid NET in differential diagnosis include CD56, chromogranin A, neuron-specific enolase, serotonin, synaptophysin, and ACTH [42]. Furthermore, proliferation rates determined by Ki-67 staining can be used to distinguish TC (Fig. 1d–g) from AC, with lower staining in TC (<5 %) and increased staining (5–20 %) in AC [43]. Although tissues of AC show higher rates of mitosis, it is uncommon for the neoplasm to be metastatic.

Atypical Carcinoid (Grade 2 Neuroendocrine Carcinoma)

Atypical carcinoid tumors (AC) are very similar to CTs with respect to the growth pattern and cell morphology; however, the mitotic activity is limited to fewer than 10 mitoses in 2 mm^2. AC may have punctuate necrosis and some degree of nuclear pleomorphism [41]. AC cells have a characteristic eosinophilic cytoplasm with finely granular chromatin, and nucleoli are only seen in AC cells [43].

Clinical Symptoms and Treatment of CT and AC

Cases of bronchial carcinoids are TC 75–90 % of the time and 10–25 % AC. TCs are slightly more common in females and children, pulmonary neoplasm being the most common up until late adolescence [40]. Indeed, carcinoid NETs have an earlier age of onset than SCLC and LCNC, the average age of diagnosis being 45–55 years [43]. TCs are more likely to be in stage I during diagnosis (>80 % of the time),

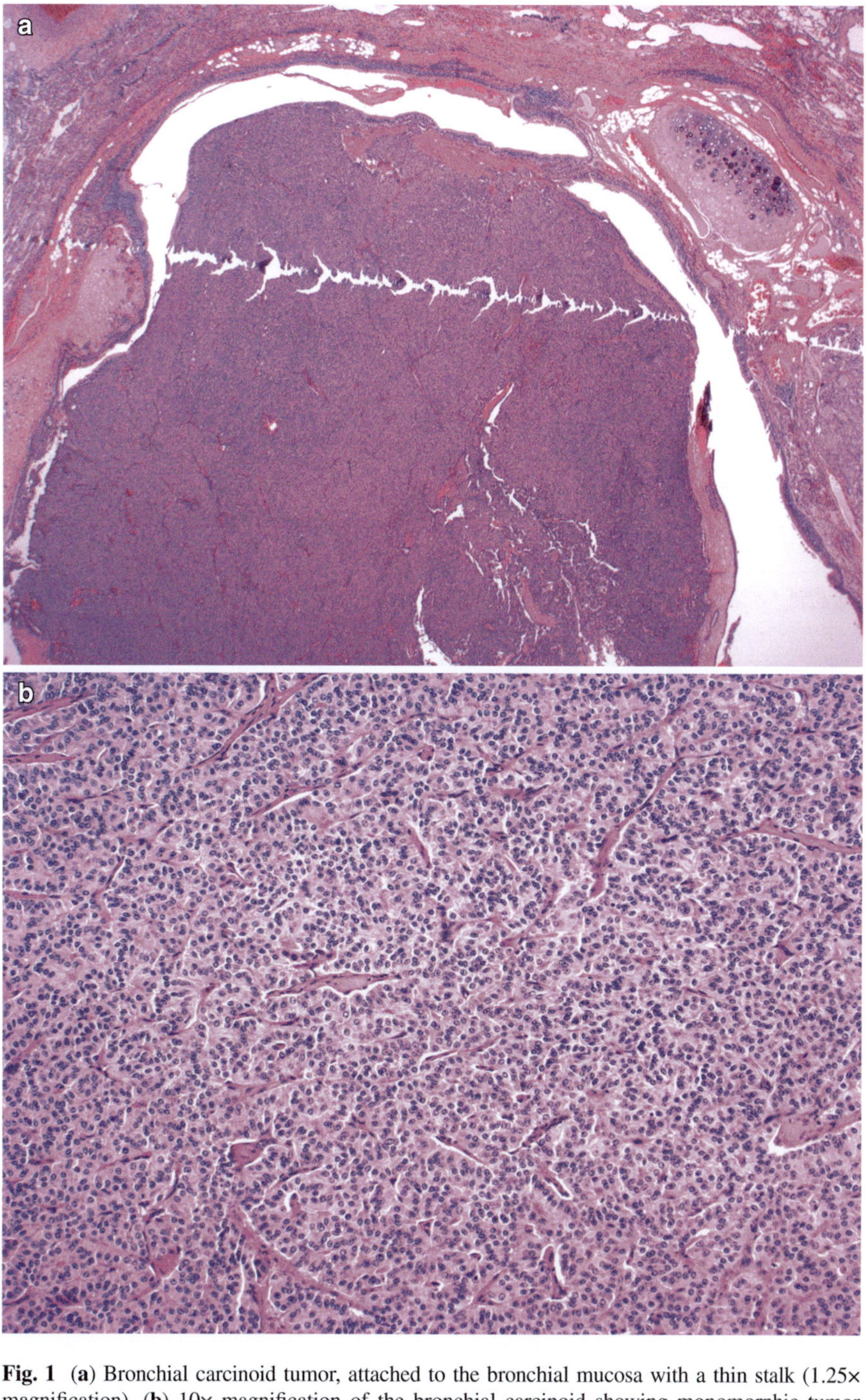

Fig. 1 (**a**) Bronchial carcinoid tumor, attached to the bronchial mucosa with a thin stalk (1.25× magnification). (**b**) 10× magnification of the bronchial carcinoid showing monomorphic tumor cells. (**c**) 20× magnification of the bronchial carcinoid with minimal stroma, no necrosis/apoptosis, and salt-and-pepper nuclear chromatin. (**d**) Carcinoid tumor (CT) with crisp reactivity for CD56. (**e**) CT positive for synaptophysin. (**f**) CT positive for chromogranin. (**g**) CT showing low Ki-67 index

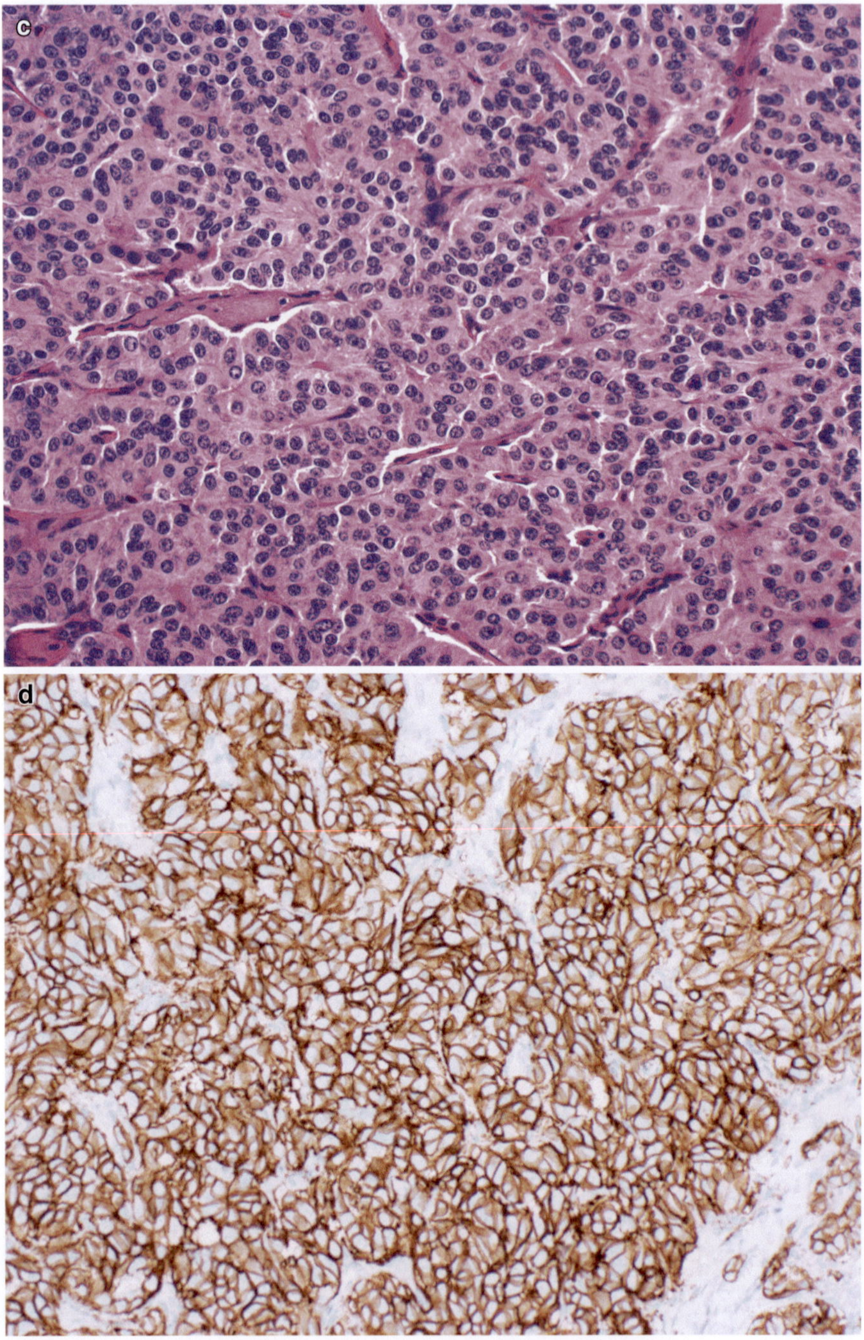

Fig. 1 (continued)

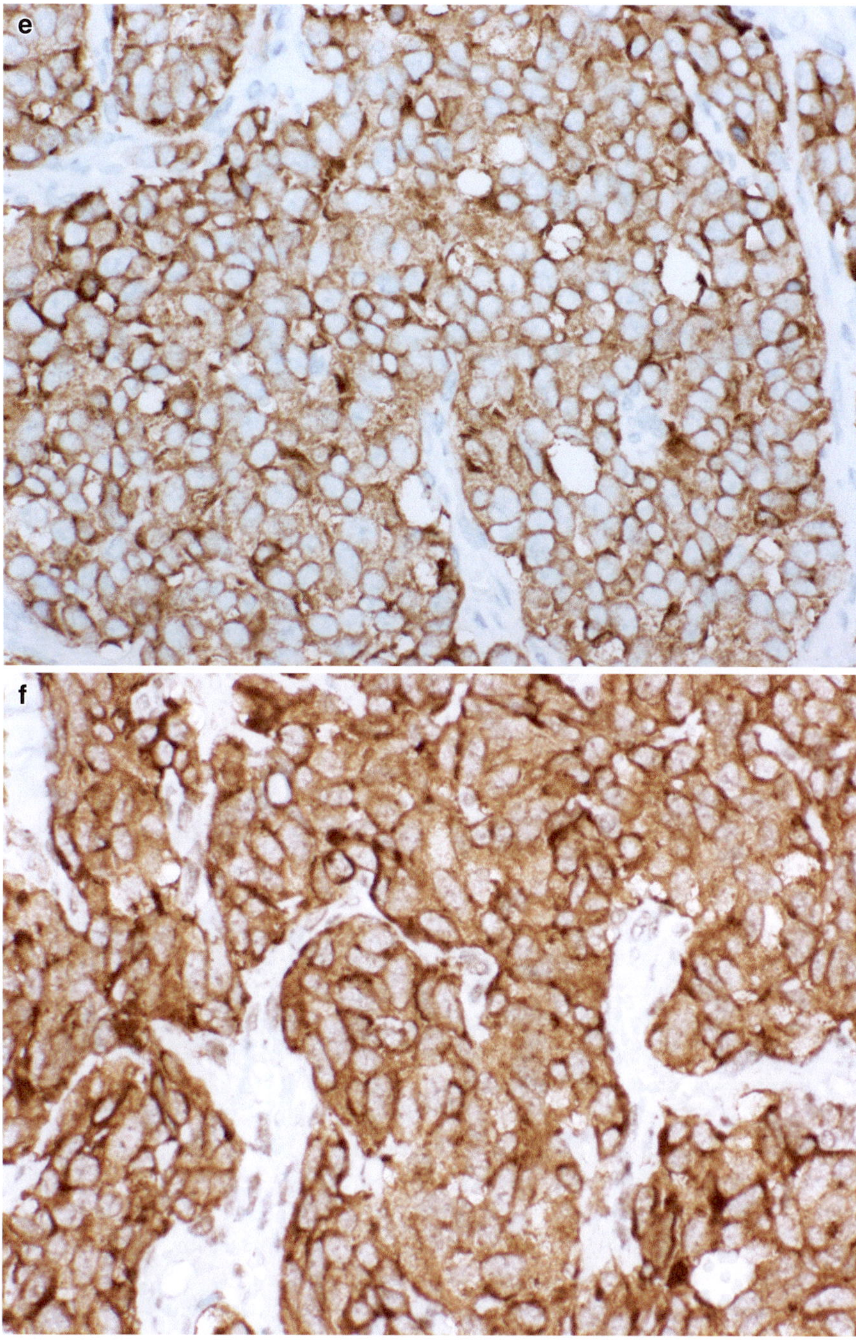

Fig. 1 (continued)

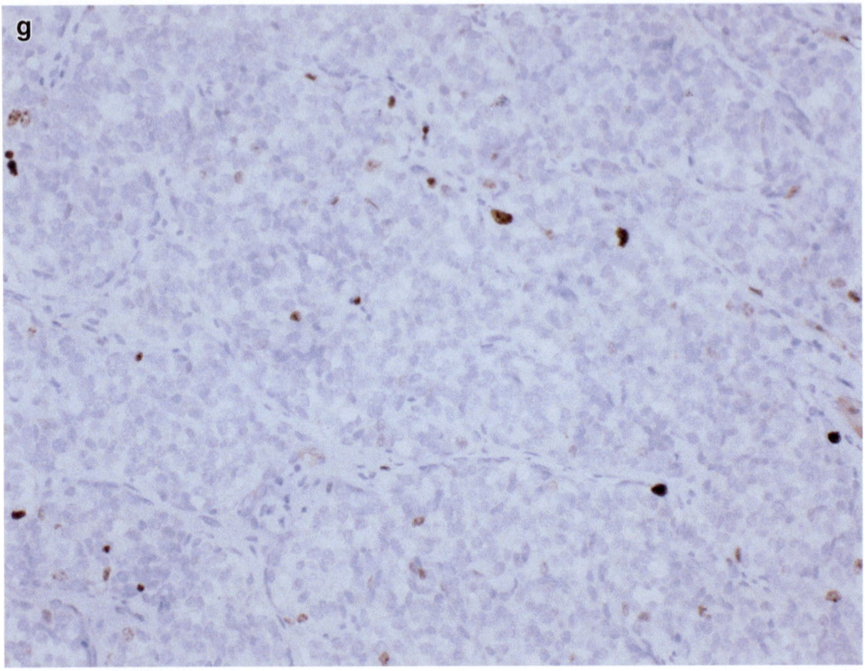

Fig. 1 (continued)

whereas ACs are more aggressive and are less likely to be diagnosed at stage I (up to 50 %). Furthermore, metastasis to regional lymph nodes is also more common in the more aggressive AC than TC. Distant site metastasis is a relatively rare feature in grade 1 NETs of the lung [40].

Patients with carcinoid tumors present with bronchial symptoms, including coughing, wheezing, and other obstructive symptoms [40]. In addition, due to the high angiogenic characteristic of lung carcinoid neoplasms, hemoptysis is another common presenting feature [44]. Metastatic progression of AC and TC leads to the presentation of carcinoid syndrome symptoms (2–7 % of patients) including wheezing, diarrhea, symptoms of valvular heart disease, cutaneous flushing, and occasionally a unique cutaneous manifestation, as well as Crushing's syndrome [40, 45, 46]. Interestingly, most cases of carcinoid NETs are discovered by routine investigation before symptoms become apparent [40].

Surgery is the procedure of choice for carcinoid NET because of its slow-growing nature and the ability to remove the neoplasm while preserving lung function. Complete surgical resection of carcinoid NET, even in cases of lymph node metastasis, shows favorable rates of prognosis; the lung parenchyma should be preserved in cases of TC [47, 48]. However, in cases of AC, radical surgery should be chosen because of the higher rates of lymph node involvement [48]; lymph node dissection is an important factor for good prognosis in cases of carcinoid NET [49]. Lymph

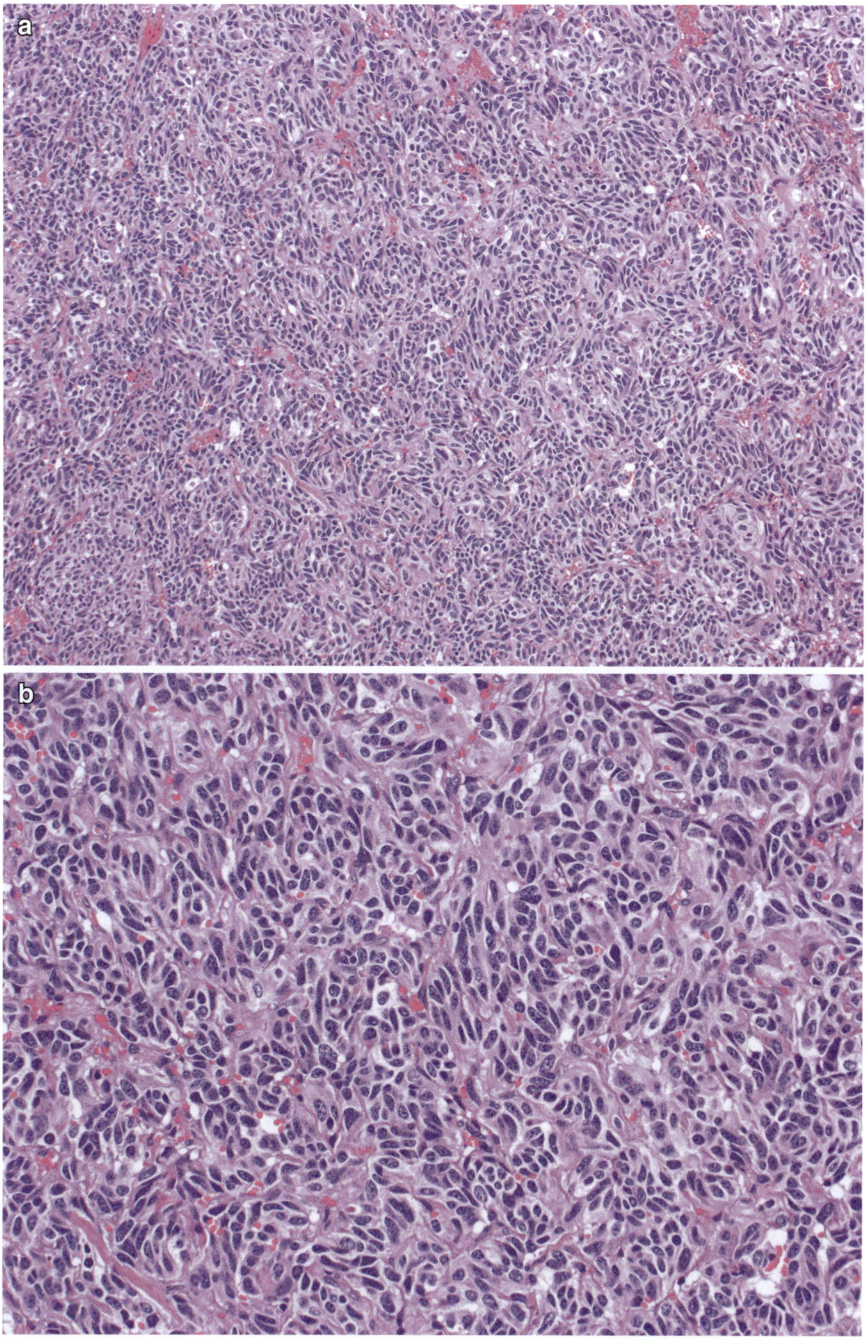

Fig. 2 (**a**) Peripheral carcinoid tumor with spindle cell features. (**b**) 20× magnification of the peripheral carcinoid tumor showing monomorphic neuroendocrine tumor cells

node involvement, metastasis, and histology of neoplasm are main prognostic factors for carcinoid NETs, and prognostic rates after surgery have been found to be 97 and 78 % for TC and AC, respectively [42, 49, 50]. Despite surgical resection being an effective treatment against carcinoid NET, adjuvant therapies have also been studied to improve the prognosis of the disease. Radiotherapy may be used after surgical resection to remove any remaining neoplasm that was not removed by surgical means [42]. Sun et al. showed that fluorouracil with streptozocin improved survival rates in patients with AC when compared to doxorubicin-based treatments, but overall results were not very convincing [51]. Other chemotherapy treatments investigated in studies of carcinoid NET include temozolomide and somatostatin analogs among other treatments without convincing results [42]. Somatostatin receptor (SSTR) analogs such as octreotide have shown effectiveness in relieving symptoms associated with carcinoid symptoms in patients with carcinoid NET [42, 52]. Targeted therapy of VEGF in carcinoid tumors by sunitinib malate (tyrosine kinase receptor inhibitor) evaluated in two-cohort phase II clinical study in AC patients versus pancreatic NET showed an indeterminate activity against AC [53]. Treatments with bevacizumab (BEV) showed a reduction of tumor blood flow and longer progression-free survival (PFS) in carcinoid patients; however, larger studies are warranted to adequately ascertain its effectiveness [42]. Such therapies may not be indicated due to the high success rates that are seen with surgical resection of carcinoid neoplasms; however, this is a growing field of scholarship and may lead to better treatments in the future. However, the importance of routine screening and examination cannot be undervalued, as most cases of carcinoid NETs are incidentally diagnosed without any presentation of symptoms.

Small Cell Lung Cancer (SCLC/Grade 3 Neuroendocrine Carcinoma, Small Cell Type)

SCLC is one of the most common lung neoplasms and is commonly seen in smokers and the elderly. Although the incidences of SCLC have been steadily decreasing in the United States due to changes in smoking patterns in the population, its prevalence is higher in countries with a high percentage of smokers [54]. SCLC is a highly malignant neoplasm which is histologically identified as having small tumor cell size, a high nuclear-cytoplasmic ratio, and absent or deformed nuclei (Fig. 3a, b). The cell sizes of SCLC are smaller than that of LCNC by using the size of three resting lymphocytes as the cutoff size. In addition, the absence of nucleoli is characteristic of SCLC [55]. The delicate cells are easily damaged during preparation and exhibit the Azzopardi phenomenon as basophilic DNA material outlining vessel walls, which is typical for pulmonary neoplasms when looking for SCLC diagnosis. In addition, cells are arranged in a stratified formation and may exhibit pseudorosette patterns [41] and exhibit a high mitotic rate (>70/10 HPF). The nuclei are prone to damage during slide preparation, complicating histological investigation, when lymphocytes are present in the vicinity [41, 56].

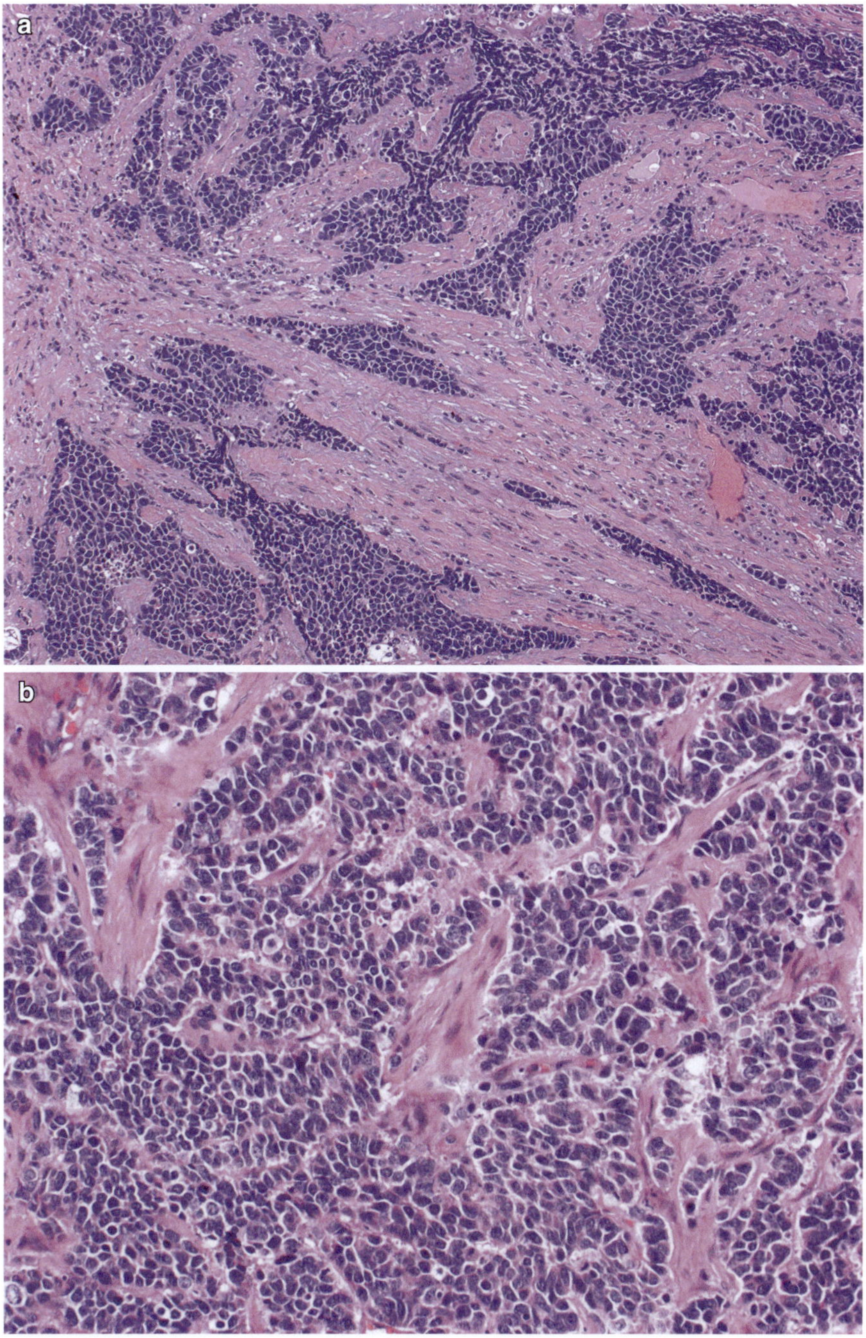

Fig. 3 (**a**) Low magnification of small cell lung cancer (SCLC), showing small tumor cells with minimal cytoplasm and nuclear molding. (**b**) SCLC cells with neuroendocrine nuclear features

Up to 90 % of SCLC are positive for at least one NE marker such as nuclear cell adhesion molecule, chromogranin A, and synaptophysin [55]. The MIB-1 marker can also be used as a marker for low-grade SCLC. As in other neoplasms, SCLC exhibits the inhibition of tumor suppression genes, the activation of oncogenes, and exaggerated growth pathways [54]. Almost all cases of SCLC exhibit the deletion of tumor suppressor gene FHIT from chromosome 3p and increase in MAD1 expression, which is involved in assembly of mitotic apparatus, suggesting a proliferative nature of the neoplasm [57, 58]. Indeed, Ki-67 proliferative marker is positively stained in tissues of SCLC, confirming that SCLC is a highly proliferative neoplasm. Furthermore, SCLC patients exhibit loss of RB1 tumor suppressor gene; however, there may not necessarily be increases in expression of KRAS and EGFR [54].

Clinical Symptoms and Treatment of SCLC

Due to the bronchial nature of NET, patients with SCLC commonly present with symptoms of pulmonary obstruction similar to that of carcinoid patients, including coughing, wheezing, and dyspnea; hemoptysis is also common due to the increase in vascularization of the neoplasm. The aggressive and metastatic nature of SCLC neoplasms means that pain, fatigue, and neurological symptoms are also common due to the potential intrathoracic spread [54]. Uncommon symptoms of SCLC include changes in blood glycemic and calcium levels as well as dermatomyositis [54]. It is not uncommon to find the development of immunological complications in SCLC. These include the development of Lambert-Eaton syndrome in which autoantibodies are produced against voltage-gated calcium channels of the neuromuscular junction similar to those in the neoplasm. It is also common that Lambert-Eaton syndrome does not develop in patients, but these patients still express autoantibodies against the same voltage-gated calcium channels [59, 60].

Patients are not usually treated by surgical resection of SCLC because they usually present at a late stage. The neoplasm is highly responsive to chemotherapy, and multiple cycles of etoposide with cisplatin or carboplatin is the initial chemotherapy of choice [55]; however, the effectiveness of the combination versus etoposide alone has been debated [54]. Six trials of 1476 Asian and White patients with extensive-stage SCLC treated with irinotecan and platinum investigated by meta-analysis revealed better survival rates with the latter than with etoposide in combination with cisplatin. There were toxic side effects to irinotecan and platinum such as nausea and diarrhea as opposed to severe anemia, neutropenia, and thrombocytopenia with etoposide and cisplatin which may have had an ethnicity-based pattern, but this has not yet been investigated [54]. Another study showed that amrubicin alone or with platinum has been shown to be a better alternative to irinotecan [54, 61]. Unfortunately, unlike carcinoid NET, it is not unusual for patients to relapse because of the highly proliferative nature of tumor stem cells that may not have been damaged by chemotherapy [55]. A number of different therapeutic options have been investigated to reduce relapse following SCLC resection. One such treatment option is radiotherapy; it was found that radiotherapy following three cycles of etoposide and cisplatin resulted in preliminary positive responses against extensive-stage SCLC [54]. Molecular targeting has also been investigated as another adjuvant therapy, as a number of molecular receptor targets have been identified in tissue studies of SCLC. Receptor tyrosine kinase, specifically c-Kit receptor, is positively expressed in up to 70 % of SCLC cases and presents a potential route of therapeutic intervention of SCLC [55, 62]. Indeed, imatinib mesylate, an inhibitor of c-Kit, was shown to inhibit growth of SCLC cells *in vitro* [63]. The Bcl-2 antiapoptotic protein family has been found to be overexpressed in SCLC and is a potential route of therapeutic intervention through use of ABT-737, AT-101, and obatoclax [54]. Clinical trials involving molecular targets have not been extensively conducted but present a unique route for future therapeutics to help reduce the morbidity of this aggressive and malignant neoplasm.

Large Cell Neuroendocrine Carcinoma (LCNC/Grade 3 Neuroendocrine Carcinoma, Large Cell Type)

LCNC are described as high-grade lung cancers and have some neuroendocrine characteristics [64]. As the name implies, they are distinguished by having a larger cell size when comparing them to other NET, but this is not the only LCNC specific characteristic [41]. Although LCNCs are of higher grade, they do not show better developed NE cell cytology. Histological characteristics of LCNC include the presence of occasional nucleoli, cytoplasm with a high nuclear-cytoplasmic ratio, polygonal shape, necrosis, and larger cell size [41] (Fig. 4a–e). Although many characteristics of LCNC overlap with SCLC, such as the similar telomerase activity [65], retrospective studies show that histological samples of LCNC better overlap with large cell carcinoma than SCLC [66].

There are a number of markers used for the immunohistochemical identification of LCNC apart from NET markers (nuclear cell adhesion molecule, chromogranin A, and synaptophysin). In many instances, genetic markers are used to rule out certain types of cancers during differential diagnosis. Bcl-2 and Ki-67 can be used as effective markers of LCNC when large cell carcinoma is also part of the differential diagnosis; these markers were expressed in significantly higher rates by LCNC than large cell carcinoma [67, 68]. Furthermore, cytological features of basaloid carcinoma and basaloid squamous carcinoma show similar features to LCNC but do not express NE markers [41]. CDX-2 has also been identified as a reliable marker for LCNC, as corroborated with RT-qPCR and immunohistological data [69]. Given the morphological similarities of LCNC and SCLC, there are a number of genetic characteristics that can be used to differentiate the two when cell size alone is not sufficient. Immunohistochemical markers specific for LCNC and not SCLC include CK7, CK18, E-cadherin, and B-catenin [67, 70]. Comparative genomic hybridization has also found differences in the chromosomal expression of 2q, 3p, 3q, 4q, 6p, 6q, 10q, 16q, and 17p between the two types of NET [67, 71, 72].

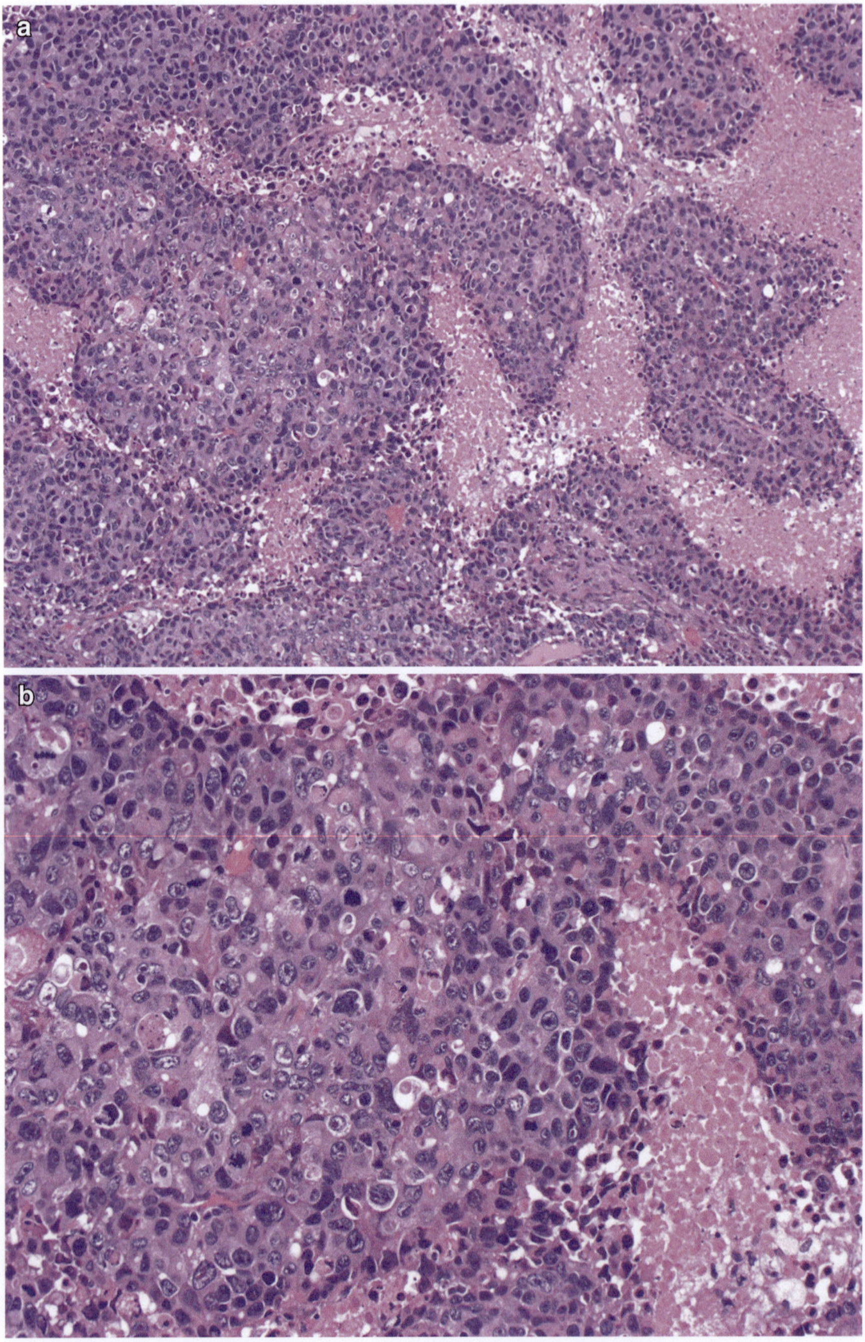

Fig. 4 (**a**) Large cell neuroendocrine carcinoma (LCNEC) with geographic areas of necrosis. (**b**) LCNEC highly pleomorphic cells with ample cytoplasm. (**c**) LCNEC showing reactivity for CD56. (**d**) LCNEC with reactivity for synaptophysin. (**e**) LCNEC showing high Ki-67 index

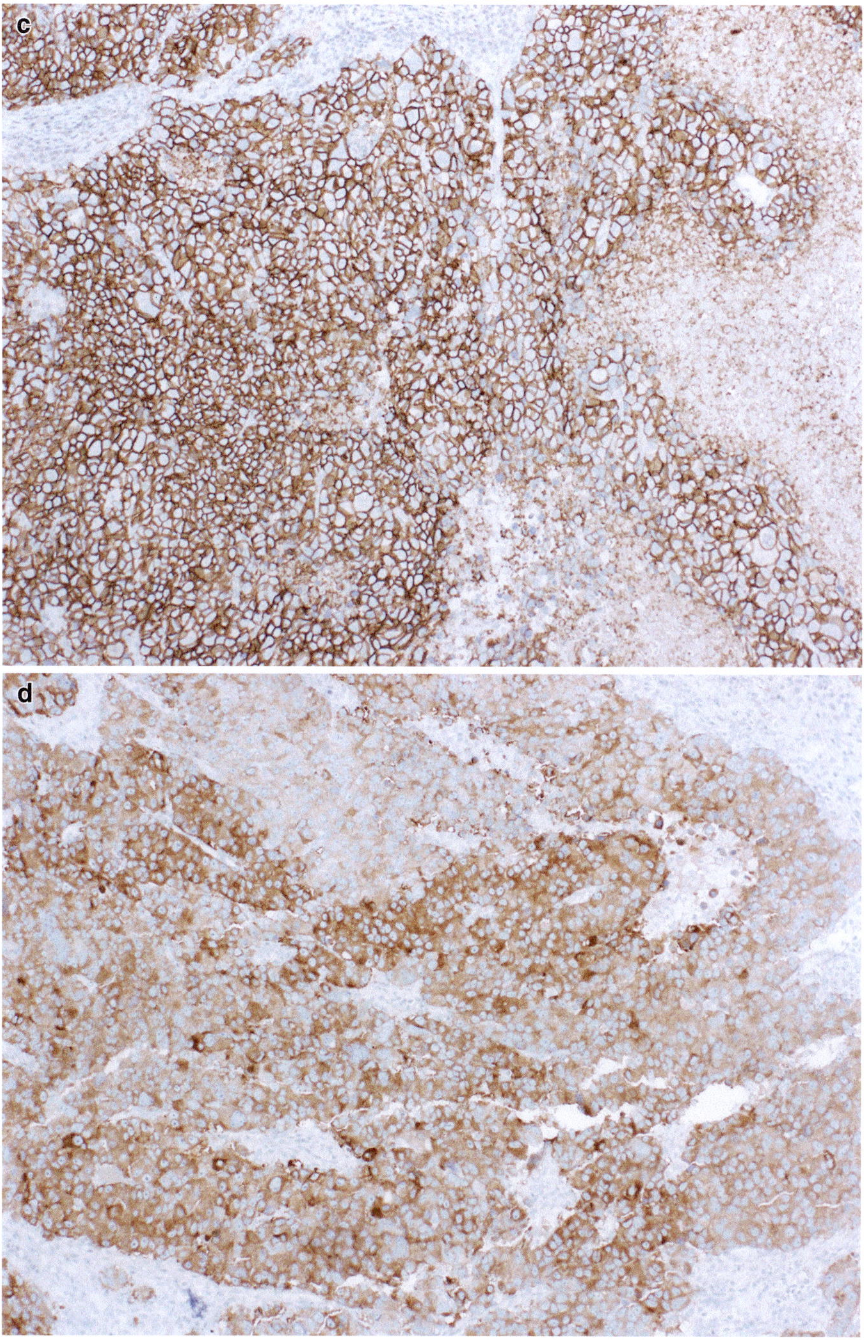

Fig. 4 (continued)

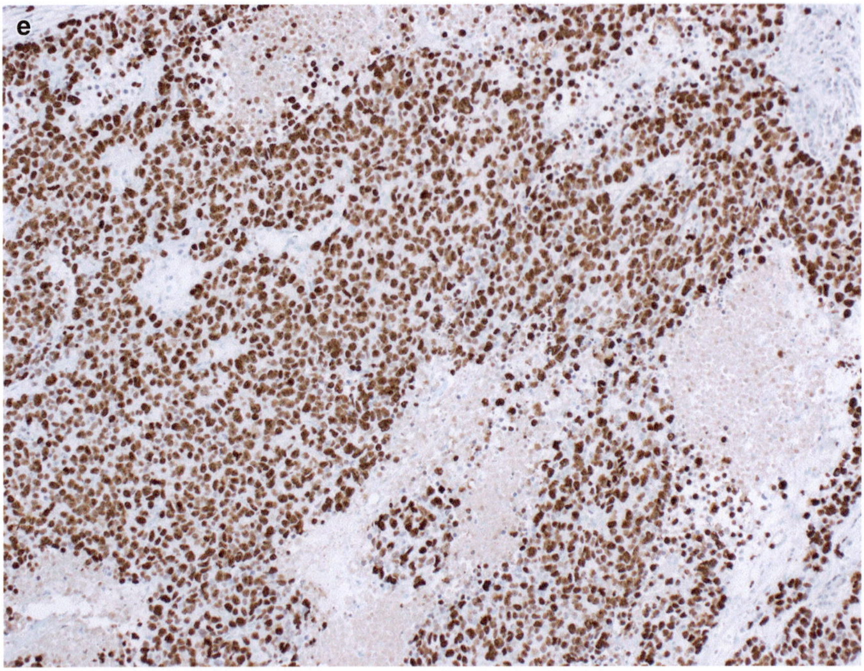

Fig. 4 (continued)

Clinical Symptoms and Treatment of LCNC

LCNC is a relatively aggressive NET and is usually characterized following surgical resection, which gives the disease an overall low prognosis. LCNC shows an aggressive nature with a 5-year survival rate of 54.5 % and metastasis of residual tumor after resection, indicating that surgery alone may not be an adequate treatment option [67, 73]. Indeed, adjuvant therapy against LCNC was found to be effective in postoperative settings by Iyoda et al. [74]. Retrospective and prospective studies of LCNC patients showed that patients treated with CDDP + VP-16 adjuvant chemotherapy had better prognosis than those treated with just surgical resection [67]. Tanaka et al. found that perioperative chemotherapy may be better for the prognosis of LCNC patients if the neoplasm is not immunoreactive to synaptophysin, chromogranin A, and neural cell adhesion molecule [75]. Furthermore, platinum-based adjuvant chemotherapy was found to be an effective therapy after LCNC resection by Sarkaria et al. [76]. In patients with LCNC positive for EGFR mutation, EGFR receptor tyrosine kinase inhibitors such as gefitinib have been shown to be an effective treatment [77, 78]; however, not all LCNC patients have EGFR mutations, and this presents a unique opportunity for personalized medicine to be implemented in their treatment [67]. Additionally, Iyoda et al. found that anti-VEGF, anti-c-KIT, and anti-HER2 treatments may also be effective against LCNC [79]. Other potential targeted therapies against LCNC include nedaplatin plus irinotecan and amrubicin therapies [67].

Molecular Pathways in Lung Neuroendocrine Tumors

Progress has been made in understanding the molecular pathogenesis of cancer over the past two decades. Identification of genes that help suppress tumor growth and the identification of genes that activate tumor cell growth are common in many different types of cancer including lung cancer. Lung cancer cells often show deletions at multiple chromosome sites, and several tumor suppressor genes are located at these regions which can cause loss of heterozygosity. There are a small number of tumor suppressor genes inactivated (loss of heterozygosity) in lung cancer, which include p53, RB, p16, FHIT, and PPP2R1B. Loss of heterozygosity can occur by chromosome breakage, deletions, nucleotide changes, amplification, and hypermethylation. These causes have been identified in lung cancer, preneoplastic tissue, and even in normal lung epithelium of nonsmokers [80]. In neuroendocrine tumors, a stepwise progression occurs from hyperplasia, low-grade tumor, and finally to high-grade tumors.

Chromosomal Changes

Chromosome analysis of lung tumor cells has shown multiple nonrandom breaks of chromosomes 1, 3, 7, 15, and 17 [81]. These breaks can cause loss of heterozygosity in tumor suppressor genes which cause tumor development. Lung cancer cells often show deletions at multiple chromosomal regions, and deletion mapping has found more than 30 regions in 21 different chromosomes as candidates for tumor suppressor loci [82].

Deletion of chromosome 3p is known to be one of the first chromosomal alterations in lung cancer, particularly NETs, and is highly associated with smoking. SCLC and LCNEt almost universally show allelic loss of 3p, which precedes deletion of 5q, 9p, and 17p.

Genetic analysis of NETs shows a stepwise loss of heterozygosity (LOH) first in chromosome 3p21.3 (site of RASSF1A, a member of the Ras association domain family, and FUS1), 3p14.2 (FHIT, a fragile histidine triad gene), followed by 9p21 (p16), 8p, 17p13 (p53), and finally 5q which are all tumor suppressor genes [83]. The loss of heterozygosity is one of the earliest molecular changes found in greater than 90 % of SCLC of slightly abnormal and even normal-appearing epithelium of smokers [80]. In the future, surgical margins may be examined by molecular analysis to identify patients most likely to benefit from adjuvant therapy [84].

Microsatellites are repeated sequence motifs of one to six base pairs found in the regulatory regions of genes and influence gene expression and transcriptional activity. Microsatellite alterations are found in 35 % of SCLCs and correlate with a younger age of incidence and more advanced stage at diagnosis [83].

Normal somatic cells have decreasing amounts of telomerase that eventually leads to cell death unlike tumor cells and germ cells that have increased telomerase that extend the telomeres and cell immortality. How telomerase is re-expressed in lung cancer is unknown, but this may be used as a marker and a target for therapy. Telomerase activity and telomere replications are increased in almost 100 % of SCLC.

Tumor Suppressor Genes

The p53 gene is located on chromosome 17. The p53 protein binds to DNA which stimulates another gene to produce proteins p21 and GADD45. P21 binds with cdk2, a cell division-stimulating protein, and inhibits the cell from passing through to the next stage of cell division. P21 controls G1/S cell cycle advancement, and GADD45 controls the G2/M cycle; both stop the replication of DNA if it is damaged [85]. BAX, PERP, and other proteins can activate p53 and cause apoptosis. MDM2, a proteasome, degrades p53 and keeps the levels low by autoregulatory feedback. Higashiyama et al. (1997) found that MDM2 is overexpressed in 25 % of NSCLCs [80]. Mutant p53 cannot bind DNA or is ineffective, so no p21 or GADD45 is made to stop cell division; therefore, the cell divides uncontrollably creating cancer. The p53 and Rb genes are the most common tumor suppressor genes affected in lung carcinoma and are inactivated by mutations, chromosomal deletions, gamma radiation, UV radiation, and carcinogens like tobacco smoke. Tobacco smoke often causes a p53 mutation, with G to T transversions, and hypermethylation of the promoter regions of p53 gene. Benzoapyrene, a tobacco smoke metabolite, damages three specific loci on the p53 gene. These three loci are known to be abnormal in approximately 50 % of primary lung cancer and 75 of SCLC [83]. P53 mutations can be found in lung tumors of nonsmokers but at a significantly lower rate than that of smokers [86].

The retinoblastoma gene is found on chromosome 13 which encodes a protein that also stops the cell cycle. The Rb protein prevents cells from entering S phase of the cell cycle. The Rb protein binds to a transcription factor E2F. E2F is not able to bind to the promoters of proto-oncogenes c-myc and c-fos. Transcription of c-myc and c-fos is needed for mitosis, so blocking the transcription factor needed to turn on these genes prevents cell division. In summary, if there is a mutation in the Rb gene, no suppressor protein is made to bind with EF2, and EF2 is free to start transcription of genes c-myc and c-fos that creates uncontrolled mitosis and tumorigenesis. Mutations in the RB protein have been found in 90 % of SCLC (Gazzeri et al. 1998). Mutations of the RB and $P16^{INK4A}$ are rarely found in the same lung tumor; however, $P16^{INK4A}$, cyclin D1, and cdk4 are usually seen in NSCLC, whereas RB gene inactivation is usually seen in SCLCs. Other members of the RB family, p107 and pR2/p130, are found mutated rarely in NSCLCs and SCLCs [80].

The RAS genes encode a GTPase protein that signals growth and survival after the membrane-bound RAS tyrosine kinase receptors are activated. The GTP is hydrolyzed to GDP and starts the RAS signaling. If there are RAS mutations, sometimes GTP hydrolysis is decreased or nonfunctional and there is an increase or constant signaling that causes uncontrolled cell growth [80]. The RAS genes (HRAS, KRAS, and NRAS) are transformed into oncogenes by a point mutation with a G-T transversion caused by bulky DNA adducts present in tobacco smoke like benzopyrene diethlyoxide and nitrosamides [87]. The mutations of the RAS gene are highly associated with smoking and found in 20–30 % of lung adenocarcinomas and in 25–40 % of atypical alveolar hyperplasia [88]. These point mutations are most commonly found at codon 12 [87] followed by codons 13 and 61 and affect the KRAS gene 90 % of the time. Patients with tumors that have K-ras, N-ras, or H-ras mutations have a decreased survival [81, 87].

BCL-2 is an antiapoptotic protein and counteracts BAX, a proapoptotic protein that acts on p53 that stops the cell cycle. The proto-oncogene BCl-2 is overexpressed in 10 % of adenocarcinomas, 25–30 % of squamous cell carcinomas, and 75–95 % of SCLCs. BCL-2 expression in NSCLC is believed to be a favorable prognostic factor, while BCL-2 expression does not influence survival in SCLCs. High BCL-2 and low BAX expression are frequently found in SCLCs that are p53 deficient and are very sensitive to chemotherapy [80].

MYC protein is a basic helix-loop-helix transcription factor that regulates the expression of genes involved in DNA synthesis, RNA metabolism, and cell cycle regulation [80]. Overexpression of MYC is found in 5–10 % of non-small cell lung carcinomas but up to 36 % of SCLC and may indicate chemotherapy-resistant tumors. Activation of MYC genes c-myc, L-myc, and N-myc occurs by amplification or loss of transcriptional control and causes an uncontrolled cell growth and tumorigenesis.

The $p16^{INK4A}$ is a major step in controlling the G1/S cell cycle advancement. $P16^{INK4A}$ binds to cyclin-dependent protein kinase 4 (CDK4) which inhibits CDK4 to interact with cyclin D1. The cyclin D1-associated CDK4 phosphorylates RB, releasing the cell from RB-mediated cell cycle arrest. $P16^{INK4A}$, cyclin D1-CDK4-RB pathway, is usually altered, mutated, or hypermethylated in 30–50 % of NSCLC and rarely in SCLC [80].

The FHIT gene (family histidine triad) encodes a diadenosine 5′,5‴-P1,P3-triphosphate hydrolase involved in purine metabolism. The gene encompasses the common fragile site FRA3B on chromosome 3p14.2, where carcinogen-induced damage can lead to translocations and aberrant transcripts of this gene. The FHIT gene shows LOH in 40 % of NSCLCs and 80 % of SCLC even though the FHIT protein is found in only 50 % of all lung cancers. Other candidate tumor suppressor genes in the 3p region include RASSF1, SEMA3B, FUS1, and RARB [80].

Another pathway that suppressor genes are inactivated by is hypermethylation of the promoter regions resulting in transcriptional inactivation of one allele with the other allele lost by mutation [80]. Hypermethylation has been shown to lead to the silencing of mRNA expression [82]. This occurs in SCLC but can also be detected in early preneoplastic lesions of smokers. Methylated promoter rejoins of genes TIMP-3, P16, p14, CDH13 (H-cadherin), DAPK, and GSTP1 and the genes of the chromosome 3p region have been reported [80]. Hypermethylated spots on chromosomal regions 4q, 10q, and 17p are present in SCLC, but so far no candidate tumor suppressor genes have been found in these regions [80].

Proliferation Markers

Lung cancer cells can express receptors for growth-promoting and inhibitory factors and are often associated with poor prognosis [80].

Gastrin-releasing or other bombesin-like peptides (GRP/BN) can stimulate the growth of both normal and malignant lung cells. Increase in GRP levels occurs in fetal lung development and differentiation [81, 82]. Most SCLCs express gastrin-releasing or other bombesin-like peptide (GRP/BN) receptors and GRPBN peptides although no mutations or amplifications of these genes have been found and the mechanism of this growth stimulatory pathway remains unknown. High levels of GRP-like activity have also been recorded in bronchial lavages of smokers compared with nonsmokers [81]. The GRP receptor is located on the X chromosome but does not undergo X inactivation so that women have two genes but men have only have one gene. This may be one reason why women are more susceptible to lung cancer from smoking [83].

EGFR regulates proliferation, apoptosis, angiogenesis, and tumor invasion. EGFR is frequently overexpressed in 10 % of NSCLCs. EGFR mutations are increased in women and nonsmokers, and 80 % of these mutations involve in-frame deletions within exon 19 or the L858R mutant within exon 21 [89]. EGFR mutations can transform fibroblast and lung epithelial cells into atypical alveolar hyperplasia, then into bronchioloalveolar carcinoma, and finally into adenocarcinomas in transgenic mice [90]. Clinical trials of the EGFR tyrosine kinase inhibitor, erlotinib, a monoclonal antibody against EGFR, are used for the treatment of previously untreated advanced lung adenocarcinoma.

IGF-1 and IGF-2 are tyrosine kinase receptors that bypass EGFR to activate downstream signaling pathways like KRAS [91]. IGF-1 and IGF-2 also induce self-regulation in NSCLC and SCLC. c-Kit receptor and hormone are highly expressed and cause growth in SCLC but much less in NSCLC and are an important negative prognostic factor [83].

VGRF induces neovascularization and is secreted by tumor cells and stromal tumor cells. VEGF expression is associated with loss of p53 function. VEGF is expressed in 50 % of NSCLCs and is associated with increased microvascular density in tumors and poor prognosis. IL-8 is also a strong angiogenic factor and is part of the CXC chemokine family and is expressed in 50 % of NSCLCs.

PD-ECFGs are expressed in 30–40 % of adenocarcinomas. Metalloproteinases (MMP) and their inhibitors are major causes of metastasis and promotion of tumor-related angiogenesis. MMP expression in NSCLC and SCLC is not well studied and an undetermined prognostic significance.

E-cadherin-catenin is important for maintaining normal tissue architecture. Lung cancers have reduced expression of laminins and integrins which is associated with disrupted tumor cells and extracellular matrix. This disrupted tumor cells and extracellular matrix lead to fragmentation of the basement membrane and invasion into the surrounding stroma. E-cadherin-catenin complex loss is seen in lung cancer invasion and metastasis and is associated with poor prognosis.

Cyfra 21–1 is a serum marker uniquely found in high levels in NSCLCs like adenocarcinoma and squamous cell carcinoma, and low levels were found in patients with nonmalignant pulmonary diseases and patients with small cell lung cancer [92].

Retinoic acid induces early cancer cells to stop proliferating, but advanced cancer cells lose responsiveness to retinoids. In an MD Anderson trial, 13-cis retinoic acid was used to reduce the development of a new primary cancer in people previously treated for head and neck cancer. Most head and neck cancers and lung cancer are caused by cigarette smoke, and if the first cancer is controlled, the patients have a very high risk of developing a second primary cancer of the upper aerodigestive tract. In the MD Anderson trial, none of the patients who received retinoic acid developed lung cancer, whereas four of the patients receiving placebo did three. In contrast to the rate of new primary cancers, the rate of head and neck primary cancer relapse was not affected by the treatment of retinoic acid [81].

Future Perspectives

Fifty percent of all newly diagnosed lung cancers in the United States occur in patients who had stopped smoking in the last 5 years. If we can detect some of these genetic alterations in preneoplastic respiratory epithelial lesions before cancer develops, early intervention and chemoprevention in such high-risk individuals could greatly increase survival rates. Patients with increased baseline risk may be appropriate candidates for screening with procedures such as bronchoscopy to obtain epithelial cells to detect amplifications, mutations, or deletions of genes involved in signal transduction, regulation of gene expression, or cellular proliferation and may result in clinically useful detection of early cancer. Interventional approaches that interfere with tumor growth and invasion may keep cells from undergoing malignant transformation [81].

Never smokers are people who have smoked less than 100 cigarettes in their lifetime. In Asia 60–80 % of women with lung cancer never smoked [93]. In the United States, 19 % of lung cancer in women occurs in never smokers, compared to

53 % in the rest of the world [94]. Small cell lung cancer and squamous cell carcinoma are associated with heavy smokers, while adenocarcinoma is more associated with never smokers, light smokers, and former smokers [93].

In summary, early detection of high-grade lung NETs in smokers may help in increasing the survival rate. The different chromosomal, molecular tumor suppressors, oncogene, and proliferation markers may be the key to identifying early lung cancer.

Abbreviations

AC	Atypical carcinoid
LCNC	Large cell neuroendocrine carcinoma
NET	Neuroendocrine tumor
NSCLC	Non-small cell lung cancer
SCLC	Small cell lung cancer
TC	Typical carcinoid

References

1. Travis WD, Brambilla E, Noguchi M, et al. International Association for the Study of Lung Cancer/American Thoracic Society/European Respiratory Society International multidisciplinary classification of lung adenocarcinoma. J Thorac Oncol. 2011;6(2):244–85.
2. Schiller JH, Harrington D, Belani CP, Eastern Cooperative Oncology Group, et al. Comparison of four chemotherapy regimens for advanced non-small-cell lung cancer. N Engl J Med. 2002;346(2):92–8.
3. Emery IF, Battelli C, Auclair PL, et al. Response to gefitinib and erlotinib in non-small cell lung cancer: a retrospective study. BMC Cancer. 2009;9:333.
4. Modjtahedi H, Essapen S. Epidermal growth factor receptor inhibitors in cancer treatment: advances, challenges and opportunities. Anticancer Drugs. 2009;20(10):851–5.
5. Chong S, et al. Neuroendocrine tumors of the lung: clinical, pathologic, and imaging findings. Radiographics. 2006;26(1):41–57.
6. Gustafsson BI, Kidd M, Modlin IM. Neuroendocrine tumors of the diffuse neuroendocrine system. Curr Opin Oncol. 2008;20(1):1–12.
7. Rekhtman N. Neuroendocrine tumors of the lung: an update. Arch Pathol Lab Med. 2010;134(11):1628–38.
8. Oberndorfer S. Karzinoide Tumoren des Dunndarms. Frankfurter Zeischrift Pathol. 41: 1907;1:425–429.
9. Bunting CH. Multiple primary carcinomata of the ileum. Johns Hopkins Hosp Bull. 1904;165:389–94. 7.
10. Gosset A, Masson P. Tumeurs endocrines de l'appendice. Presse Med. 1914;25:237–40.
11. Gmelich JT, Bensch KG, Liebow AA. Cells of Kultschitzky type in bronchioles and their relation to the origin of peripheral carcinoid tumor. Lab Invest. 1967;17:88–98.
12. Hausman DH, Weimann R. Pulmonary tumorlet with hilar lymph node metastasis. Cancer. 1967;20:1515–9.
13. Azzopardi JG. Oat cell carcinoma of the bronchus. J Pathol Bacteriol. 1959;78:513–9.
14. Kato Y, Ferguson TB, Bennett DE, et al. Oat cell carcinoma of the lung: a review of 138 cases. Cancer. 1969;23:517–24.

15. Warburton D, Schwarz M, Tefft D, Flores-Delgado G, Anderson KD, Cardoso WV. The molecular basis of lung morphogenesis. Mech Dev. 2000;92(1):55–81.
16. Travis WD, Brambilla E, Müller-Hermelink HK, Harris CC, editors. Tumors of the lung, pleura, thymus and heart. Lyon: IARC Press; 2004.
17. Ito T, Udaka N, Okudela K, Yazawa T, Kitamura H. Mechanisms of neuroendocrine differentiation in pulmonary neuroendocrine cells and small cell carcinoma. Endocr Pathol. 2003;14(2):133–9.
18. Sidhu GS. The endodermal origin of digestive and respiratory tract APUDcells. Histopathologic evidence and a review of the literature. Am J Pathol. 1979;96:5–20.
19. Linnoila RI. Functional facets of the pulmonary neuroendocrine system. Lab Invest. 2006;86(5):425–44.
20. Boers JE, den Brok JL, Koudstaal J, Arends JW, Thunnissen FB. Number and proliferation of neuroendocrine cells in normal human airway epithelium. Am J Respir Crit Care Med. 1996;154:758–63.
21. Gustafsson BI, Kidd M, Chan A, Malfertheiner MV, Modlin IM. Bronchopulmonary neuroendocrine tumors. Cancer. 2008;113:5–21.
22. Cutz E, Jackson A. Neuroepithelial bodies as airway oxygen sensors. Respir Physiol. 1999;115:201–14.
23. Sutherland KD, Proost N, Brouns I, Adriaensen D, Song JY, Berns A. Cell of origin of small cell lung cancer: inactivation of Trp53 and rb1 in distinct cell types of adult mouse lung. Cancer Cell. 2011;19:754–64.
24. Linnoila IR, Li Y. Neuroendocrine transcription factor ASCL1 defines multiple progenitors in the lung during the development and repair. J Thorac Oncol. 2011;6:S372–3.
25. Calbo J, van Montfort E, Proost N, van Drunen E, Beverloo HB, Meuwissen R, Berns A. A functional role for tumor cell heterogeneity in a mouse model of small cell lung cancer. Cancer Cell. 2011;19:244–56.
26. Jones MH, Virtanen C, Honjoh D, Miyoshi T, Satoh Y, Okumura S, Nakagawa K, Nomura H, Ishikawa Y. Two prognostically significant subtypes of high-grade lung neuroendocrine tumours independent of small-cell and large cell neuroendocrine carcinomas identified by gene expression profiles. Lancet. 2004;363:775–81.
27. Nasgashio R, Sato Y, Matsumoto T, Kageyama T, Hattori M, Iyoda A, Satoh Y, Ryuge S, Masuda N, Jiang SX, Saegusa M. The balance between the expressions of hASH1 and HES1 differs between large cell neuroendocrine carcinoma and small cell carcinoma of the lung. Lung Cancer. 2011;74:405–10.
28. Finkelstein SD, Hasegawa T, Colby T, Yousem SA. 11q13 allelic imbalance discriminates pulmonary carcinoids from tumorlets. A microdissection-based genotyping approach useful in clinical practice. Am J Pathol. 1999;155:633–40.
29. Lantuejoul S, Salameire D, Salon C, Brambilla E. Pulmonary preneoplasia sequential molecular carcinogenetic events. Histopathology. 2009;54:43–54.
30. Arioglu E, Doppman J, Gomes M, Kleiner D, Mauro D, Barlow C, Papanicolaou DA. Cushing's syndrome caused by corticotropin secretion by pulmonary tumorlets. N Engl J Med. 1998;339:883–6.
31. Liu SM, Wu HH, Wu CJ, Kuo CL, Mo LR. Adrenocorticotropin-producing pulmonary tumorlets with lymph node metastasis. Pathol Int. 2003;53:883–6.
32. D'Agati VD, Perzin KH. Carcinoid tumorlets of the lung with metastasis to a peribronchial lymph node. Report of a case and review of the literature. Cancer. 1985;55:2472–6.
33. Davies SJ, Gosney JR, Hansell DM, Wells AU, du Bois RM, Burke MM, Sheppard MN, Nicholson AG. Diffuse idiopathic pulmonary neuroendocrine cell hyperplasia: an under-recognised spectrum of disease. Thorax. 2007;62:248–52.
34. Gosney JR, Williams IJ, Dodson AR, Foster CS. Morphology and antigen expression profile of pulmonary neuroendocrine cells in reactive proliferations and diffuse idiopathic pulmonary neuroendocrine cell hyperplasia (DIPNECH). Histopathology. 2011;59:751–62.
35. Lloyd RV. Endocrine pathology. New York: Springer; 1990. p. 1–15.
36. Lee JE, Evans DB. Advances in the diagnosis and treatment of gastrointestinal neuroendocrine tumors. Cancer Treat Res. 1997;90:227–38.

37. Warner RR. Gut neuroendocrine tumors. Curr Ther Endocrinol Metab. 1997;6:606–14.
38. Mendelshon G. Diagnosis and pathology of endocrine diseases. Philadelphia: JB Lippincott; 1998. p. 1–205.
39. Argani P, Erlandson RA, Rosai J. Thymic neuroblastoma in adults: report of three cases with special emphasis on its association with the syndrome of inappropriate secretion of antidiuretic hormone. Am J Clin Pathol. 1997;108:537–43.
40. Jacobs MA, et al. Neuroendocrine tumors: beyond the abdomen. J Comput Assist Tomogr. 2014;38(6):898–914.
41. den Bakker M, Thunnissen F. Neuroendocrine tumours—challenges in the diagnosis and classification of pulmonary neuroendocrine tumours. J Clin Pathol. 2013;66(10):862–9. jclinpath-2012-201310.
42. Noel-Savina E, Descourt R. Focus on treatment of lung carcinoid tumor. Onco Targets Ther. 2013;6:1533.
43. Travis W. Advances in neuroendocrine lung tumors. Ann Oncol. 2010;21 suppl 7:vii65–71.
44. Jeung M-Y, et al. Bronchial carcinoid tumors of the thorax: spectrum of radiologic findings. Radiographics. 2002;22(2):351–65.
45. Phan AT, et al. NANETS consensus guideline for the diagnosis and management of neuroendocrine tumors: well-differentiated neuroendocrine tumors of the thorax (includes lung and thymus). Pancreas. 2010;39(6):784–98.
46. McElaney B, McAdams H. Chest case of the day. Metastatic bronchial carcinoid. Am J Roentgenol. 1995;165(1):186–7.
47. Bölükbas S, Schirren J. Parenchyma-sparing bronchial sleeve resections in trauma, benign and malign diseases. Thorac Cardiovasc Surg. 2010;58(01):32–7.
48. Ducrocq X, et al. Operative risk and prognostic factors of typical bronchial carcinoid tumors. Ann Thorac Surg. 1998;65(5):1410–4.
49. García-Yuste M, et al. Typical and atypical carcinoid tumours: analysis of the experience of the Spanish Multi-centric Study of Neuroendocrine Tumours of the Lung. Eur J Cardiothorac Surg. 2007;31(2):192–7.
50. Machuca TN, et al. Surgical treatment of bronchial carcinoid tumors: a single-center experience. Lung Cancer. 2010;70(2):158–62.
51. Sun W, et al. Phase II/III study of doxorubicin with fluorouracil compared with streptozocin with fluorouracil or dacarbazine in the treatment of advanced carcinoid tumors: Eastern Cooperative Oncology Group Study E1281. J Clin Oncol. 2005;23(22):4897–904.
52. Öberg K, et al. Neuroendocrine bronchial and thymic tumours: ESMO clinical practice guidelines for diagnosis, treatment and follow-up. Ann Oncol. 2010;21 suppl 5:v220–2.
53. Kulke MH, et al. Activity of sunitinib in patients with advanced neuroendocrine tumors. J Clin Oncol. 2008;26(20):3403–10.
54. van Meerbeeck JP, Fennell DA, De Ruysscher DK. Small-cell lung cancer. The Lancet. 2011;378(9804):1741–55.
55. Swarts DR, Ramaekers F, Speel E-JM. Molecular and cellular biology of neuroendocrine lung tumors: evidence for separate biological entities. Biochimica et Biophysica Acta (BBA)-Reviews on Cancer. 2012;1826(2):255–71.
56. Kaufmann O, Dietel M. Expression of thyroid transcription factor-1 in pulmonary and extrapulmonary small cell carcinomas and other neuroendocrine carcinomas of various primary sites. Histopathology. 2000;36(5):415–20.
57. Franklin W, Chanin T, Gonzalez A. Molecular and cellular pathology of lung cancer. In: Lung cancer: principles and practice. 3rd ed. Philadelphia: Lippincott Williams & Williams; 2005. p. 245Á248.
58. Coe BP, et al. Gain of a region on 7p22. 3, containing MAD1L1, is the most frequent event in small-cell lung cancer cell lines. Genes Chromosomes Cancer. 2006;45(1):11–9.
59. Darnell RB, Posner JB. Paraneoplastic syndromes involving the nervous system. N Engl J Med. 2003;349(16):1543–54.

60. Payne M, et al. Prospective study into the incidence of Lambert Eaton myasthenic syndrome in small cell lung cancer. J Thorac Oncol. 2010;5(1):34–8.
61. Inoue A, et al. A phase II study of amrubicin combined with carboplatin for elderly patients with small-cell lung cancer: North Japan Lung Cancer Study Group Trial 0405. Ann Oncol. 2010;21(4):800–3.
62. López-Martin A, et al. Prognostic value of KIT expression in small cell lung cancer. Lung Cancer. 2007;56(3):405–13.
63. Krystal GW, et al. The selective tyrosine kinase inhibitor STI571 inhibits small cell lung cancer growth. Clin Cancer Res. 2000;6(8):3319–26.
64. Moran CA, et al. Neuroendocrine carcinomas of the lung a critical analysis. Am J Clin Pathol. 2009;131(2):206–21.
65. Zaffaroni N, et al. Differential expression of telomerase activity in neuroendocrine lung tumours: correlation with gene product immunophenotyping. J Pathol. 2003;201(1):127–33.
66. Varlotto JM, et al. Should large cell neuroendocrine lung carcinoma be classified and treated as a small cell lung cancer or with other large cell carcinomas? J Thorac Oncol. 2011;6(6):1050–8.
67. Iyoda A, et al. Pulmonary large cell neuroendocrine carcinoma demonstrates high proliferative activity. Ann Thorac Surg. 2004;77(6):1891–5.
68. Iyoda A, et al. Treatment options for patients with large cell neuroendocrine carcinoma of the lung. Gen Thorac Cardiovasc Surg. 2014;62(6):351–6.
69. Bari MF. Biomarkers for the classification of high grade neuroendocrine lung cancers. Great Britain: University of Warwick; 2012.
70. Nitadori J, et al. Immunohistochemical differential diagnosis between large cell neuroendocrine carcinoma and small cell carcinoma by tissue microarray analysis with a large antibody panel. Am J Clin Pathol. 2006;125(5):682–92.
71. Peng WX, et al. Array-based comparative genomic hybridization analysis of high-grade neuroendocrine tumors of the lung. Cancer Sci. 2005;96(10):661–7.
72. Ullmann R, et al. Chromosomal aberrations in a series of large-cell neuroendocrine carcinomas: unexpected divergence from small-cell carcinoma of the lung. Hum Pathol. 2001;32(10):1059–63.
73. Iyoda A, et al. Postoperative recurrence and the role of adjuvant chemotherapy in patients with pulmonary large-cell neuroendocrine carcinoma. J Thorac Cardiovasc Surg. 2009;138(2):446–53.
74. Iyoda A, et al. Adjuvant chemotherapy for large cell carcinoma with neuroendocrine features. Cancer. 2001;92(5):1108–12.
75. Tanaka Y, et al. Immunohistochemical studies of pulmonary large cell neuroendocrine carcinoma: a possible association between staining patterns with neuroendocrine markers and tumor response to chemotherapy. J Thorac Cardiovasc Surg. 2013;145(3):839–46.
76. Sarkaria IS, et al. Neoadjuvant and adjuvant chemotherapy in resected pulmonary large cell neuroendocrine carcinomas: a single institution experience. Ann Thorac Surg. 2011;92(4):1180–7.
77. De Pas TM, et al. Large-cell neuroendocrine carcinoma of the lung harboring EGFR mutation and responding to gefitinib. J Clin Oncol. 2011;29(34):e819–22.
78. Kozuki T, et al. Complexity in the treatment of pulmonary large cell neuroendocrine carcinoma. J Cancer Res Clin Oncol. 2005;131(3):147–51.
79. Iyoda A, et al. Expression profiling and identification of potential molecular targets for therapy in pulmonary large-cell neuroendocrine carcinoma. Exp Ther Med. 2011;2(6):1041–5.
80. Meuwissen R, Berns A. Mouse models for human lung cancer. Genes Dev. 2005;19(6):643–64.
81. Mulshine JL, et al. Initiators and promoters of lung cancer. Chest. 1993;103(1 Suppl):4S–11.
82. Kohno T, Yokota J. How many tumor suppressor genes are involved in human lung carcinogenesis? Carcinogenesis. 1999;20(8):1403–10.
83. Forgacs E, et al. Molecular genetic abnormalities in the pathogenesis of human lung cancer. Pathol Oncol Res. 2001;7(1):6–13.
84. Herbst RS, Heymach JV, Lippman SM. Lung cancer. N Engl J Med. 2008;359(13):1367–80.

85. Wakamatsu N, et al. Overview of the molecular carcinogenesis of mouse lung tumor models of human lung cancer. Toxicol Pathol. 2007;35(1):75–80.
86. Husgafvel-Pursiainen K, et al. p53 mutations and exposure to environmental tobacco smoke in a multicenter study on lung cancer. Cancer Res. 2000;60(11):2906–11.
87. Johnson BE, Kelley MJ. Overview of genetic and molecular events in the pathogenesis of lung cancer. Chest. 1993;103(1 Suppl):1S–3.
88. Humphrey PA, Dehner LP, Pfeifer JD. The Washington manual of surgical pathology. Philadelphia: Lippincott Williams & Wilkins; 2008.
89. Ciardiello F, Tortora G. EGFR antagonists in cancer treatment. N Engl J Med. 2008;358(11):1160–74.
90. Ji H, et al. The impact of human EGFR kinase domain mutations on lung tumorigenesis and in vivo sensitivity to EGFR-targeted therapies. Cancer Cell. 2006;9(6):485–95.
91. Pao W, et al. KRAS mutations and primary resistance of lung adenocarcinomas to gefitinib or erlotinib. PLoS Med. 2005;2(1), e17.
92. Oremek GM, et al. [Cyfra 21-1--a new tumor marker of the cytokeratin series in differential diagnosis of lung diseases]. Med Klin (Munich). 1995;90(1):23–6.
93. Sun S, Schiller JH, Gazdar AF. Lung cancer in never smokers – a different disease. Nat Rev Cancer. 2007;7(10):778–90.
94. Wakelee HA, et al. Lung cancer incidence in never smokers. J Clin Oncol. 2007;25(5):472–8.

Breast Carcinomas with Neuroendocrine Features (Neuroendocrine Carcinomas of the Breast)

Marilin Rosa, Ujalla Sheikh, and Aejaz Nasir

Introduction

Primary breast carcinoma with neuroendocrine features is an uncommon malignancy that constitutes approximately 1 % of all breast cancers and mostly affects elderly patients [1, 2]. According to the most recent World Health Organization (WHO) classification, it affects almost exclusively the female population between the sixth and seventh decades [1, 3]. The presence of neuroendocrine differentiation in primary breast carcinomas has been debated for years. In 1977, Cubilla and Woodruff [4] described for the first time tumors in the breast resembling carcinoid tumors from other organs. They described eight patients with tumors demonstrating argyrophil granules and showing membrane-bound "neurosecretory" granules on electron microscopy. Because some of the tumors had an associated in situ component, they suggested that they were most probably of breast origin. Afterward, sporadic case reports and small case series of neuroendocrine breast carcinomas appeared in the literature.

Over the years, several authors have investigated and try to prove the presence of "normal" endocrine cells and primary breast endocrine carcinomas with mixed and not reproducible results. It is now of consensus that breast tumors with neuroendocrine features do not arise from preexisting breast endocrine cells or neuroendocrine precursor lesions because a benign endocrine component or atypical

M. Rosa, MD (✉)
Department of Anatomic Pathology and Comprehensive Breast Program,
H. Lee Moffitt Cancer Center, Tampa, FL, USA
e-mail: Marilin.Rosa@moffitt.org

U. Sheikh, MD • A. Nasir, MD, MPhil, FCAP (✉)
Diagnostic & Experimental Pathology (Tailored Therapeutics), Lilly
Research Laboratories, Eli Lilly & Co., Indianapolis, IN, USA
e-mail: nasirae@lilly.com

A. Nasir, D. Coppola (eds.), *Neuroendocrine Tumors: Review of Pathology, Molecular and Therapeutic Advances*, DOI 10.1007/978-1-4939-3426-3_10

endocrine lesion has not been conclusively demonstrated in the breast glandular tree [5–7].

For years, the diagnostic terminology of breast carcinomas with neuroendocrine features has also been a matter of debate and confusion. Different terminologies have been used and variable diagnostic criteria applied. When first described by Cubilla and Woodruff, they used the term "carcinoid tumor of the breast" [4]. This term has been used by some over the years, but is considered inappropriate because these breast tumors are true carcinomas [8]. In addition, methods of detecting neuroendocrine differentiation have evolved. Initially, histochemical methods and electron microscopy were the standard. Later, IHC replaced these methods and is now routinely used for this purpose. However, since no guidelines regarding what constituted positivity were available, the variability and inconsistency in diagnosis continued.

Histopathology

In 2003, the World Health Organization (WHO) classifications of tumors accepted for the first time the existence of primary breast neuroendocrine tumors [9]. At the time, breast neuroendocrine tumors were defined as tumors having morphological features similar to neuroendocrine tumors of the GI tract and lung and expressing neuroendocrine markers in more than 50 % of the tumor cells. In the most recent WHO classification of breast tumors published in 2012, these criteria were modified because it was acknowledged that the 50 % cutoff for diagnosis was arbitrary [3, 10]. Currently, three categories of tumors with neuroendocrine features are accepted: [1] neuroendocrine tumor, well differentiated (NET-WD); [2] neuroendocrine carcinoma, poorly differentiated/small cell carcinoma of the breast (NEC-PD/SCCB); [3] and invasive breast carcinoma with neuroendocrine differentiation (NEBC). At present, to establish the diagnosis of neuroendocrine carcinoma, it is required that the tumor has morphological features similar to neuroendocrine carcinomas of the lung and GI tract. In addition, other special- and no-special-type invasive carcinomas with proven neuroendocrine differentiation using IHC, regardless of the percentage of positive cells, are included in this group. Using these criteria, it is estimated that carcinomas with neuroendocrine differentiation of the breast constitute less than 1 % of breast carcinomas.

Neuroendocrine Tumor, Well Differentiated (NET-WD)

These tumors (true carcinomas) can be recognized as having neuroendocrine features on HE alone, although IHC is usually used for confirmation [6]. They resemble neuroendocrine tumors of the GI tract and lung and are morphologically low or intermediate grade (grade I and II). Histologically, they are formed by ill-circumscribed, solid nests or trabeculae of cells with plasmacytoid, spindle, and less commonly clear cell features (Fig. 1a, b) [3, 6, 8, 10]. Nuclear palisading toward the stroma and

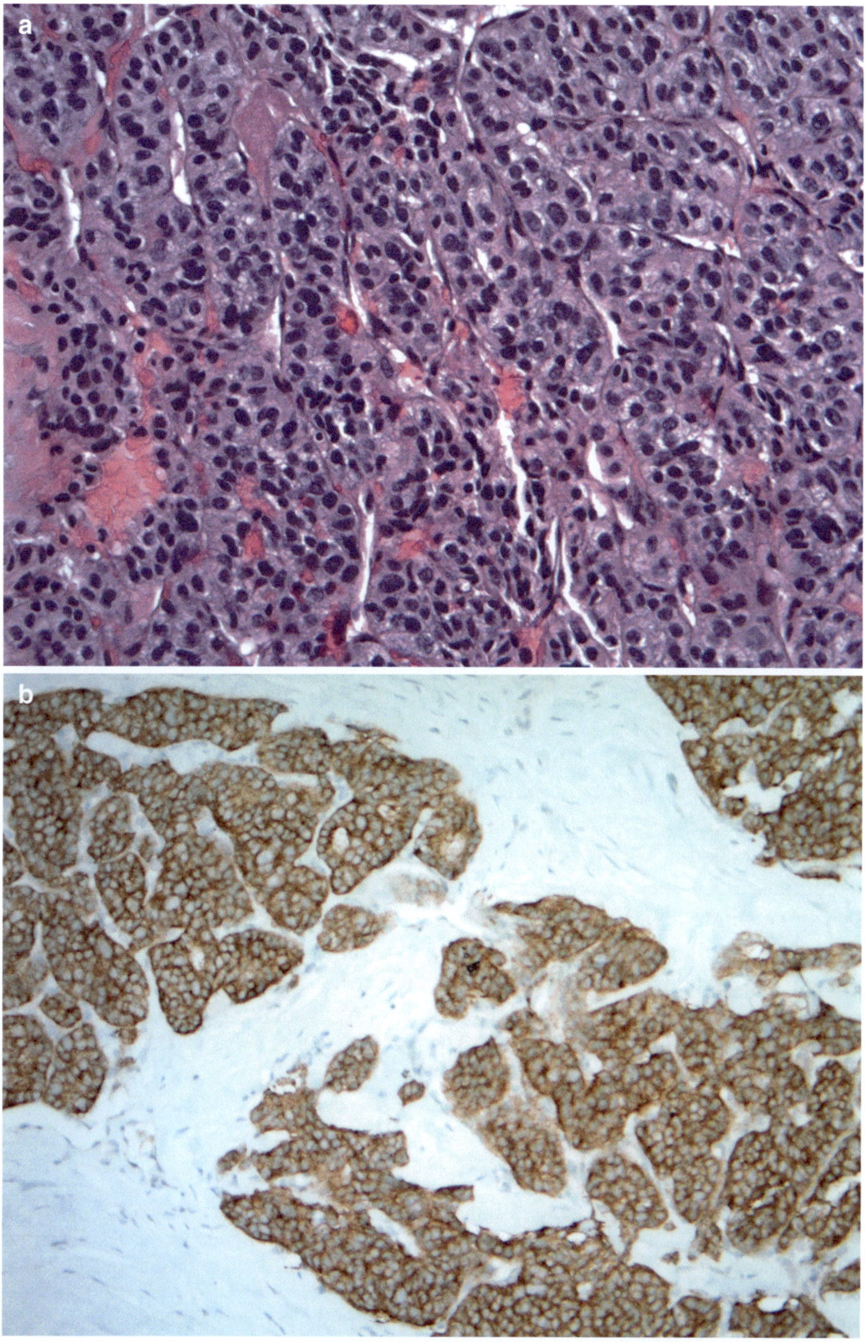

Fig. 1 (**a**) Well-differentiated neuroendocrine carcinoma of the breast displaying a trabecular growth pattern, closely resembling neuroendocrine tumors from other organs. The cells have abundant granular cytoplasm and round to oval nuclei (H&E, ×200). (**b**) Immunohistochemistry with chromogranin is diffusely positive, confirming neuroendocrine differentiation (×100)

pseudorosettes are usually seen, but true tubular or glandular formation is rare [3, 6]. Cytologically, NET-WD consists of a uniform tumor cell population with abundant eosinophilic cytoplasm and nuclei with stippled ("salt and pepper") chromatin; the tumor cells range from oval to spindle and plasmacytoid, separated by delicate fibrous stroma [11–14]. An in situ component may or may not be present.

Neuroendocrine Carcinoma, Poorly Differentiated/Small Cell Carcinoma of the Breast (NEC-PD/SCCB)

Primary small cell carcinoma of the breast is rare and only occasionally reported. It appeared for the first time in the literature in 1983 when Wade et al. [15] reported a patient with small cell carcinoma in the breast that also had disseminated disease with axillary, hepatic, and bone metastases. In this case, the clinical presentation makes the diagnosis of SCCB uncertain.

SCCB is morphologically and immunohistochemically indistinguishable from lung small cell carcinoma and therefore can only be diagnosed when an extramammary primary has been ruled out or if an in situ component is present. Histologically, the tumors have infiltrative borders and high-grade features. These include hyperchromatic tumor cells with scant cytoplasm, absent or inconspicuous nuclei, numerous mitoses, apoptosis, associated tumor necrosis, and molding and crushing artifact (Fig. 2a–c) [3, 5, 16–18]. Lymphovascular invasion is frequently observed [3, 5]. Growth pattern can be solid, trabecular, alveolar, or single cell infiltration [5]. Some authors have reported a dimorphic histologic pattern, where the small cell carcinoma pattern merges with other morphological patterns such as invasive lobular, tubulolobular, squamous, or ductal carcinoma [5, 17, 19, 20]. Cytologically, SCCB is composed of hyperchromatic cells with scant cytoplasm, arranged in small clusters or as single cells. Nuclear molding and crushing artifacts are key diagnostic features in cytology (Fig. 2d). Salt and pepper chromatin is better observed with Papanicolaou stain [18]. IHC with neuroendocrine markers confirms neuroendocrine differentiation; however, it is not essential for rendering the diagnosis, if the morphological features are classic [5].

Fig. 2 (**a**) Core needle biopsy of a breast mass revealing fragments of a high-grade tumor composed of malignant cells with scant cytoplasm, hyperchromatic, pleomorphic nuclei, numerous mitoses, and apoptotic bodies. These features are diagnostic of small cell carcinoma (H&E, ×200). (**b**) Higher magnification of the same case demonstrates high pleomorphism, mitoses, apoptosis, smudged chromatin, and nuclear molding (H&E, ×400). (**c**) Immunohistochemistry for the myoepithelial marker SMM (smooth muscle myosin) highlights the presence of an in situ component in a case of primary breast small cell carcinoma (×200). (**d**) Cytologic features of small cell carcinoma characterized by cells with scant or devoid of cytoplasm, hyperchromasia, and molding (Diff-Quik stain, ×400)

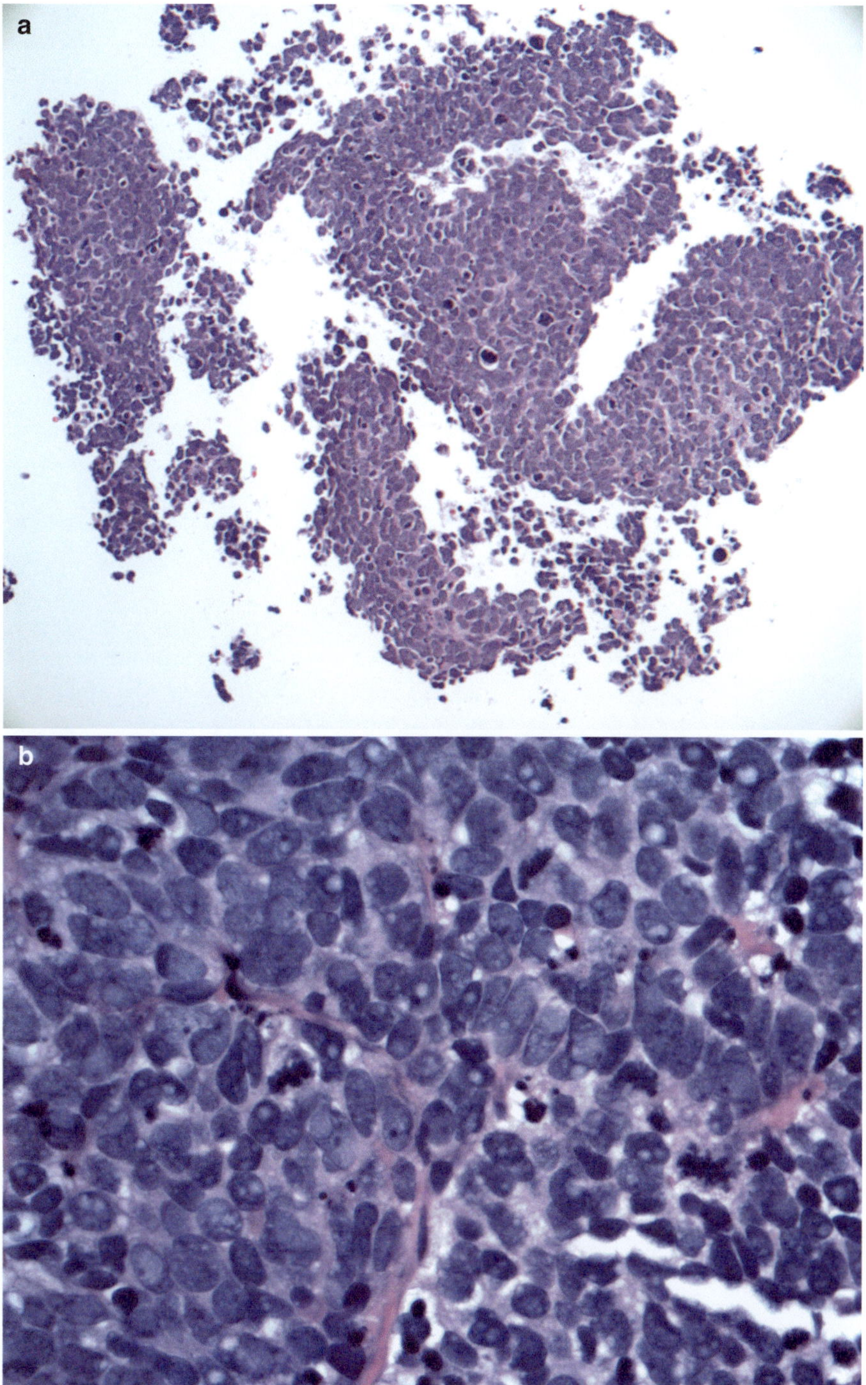
a
b

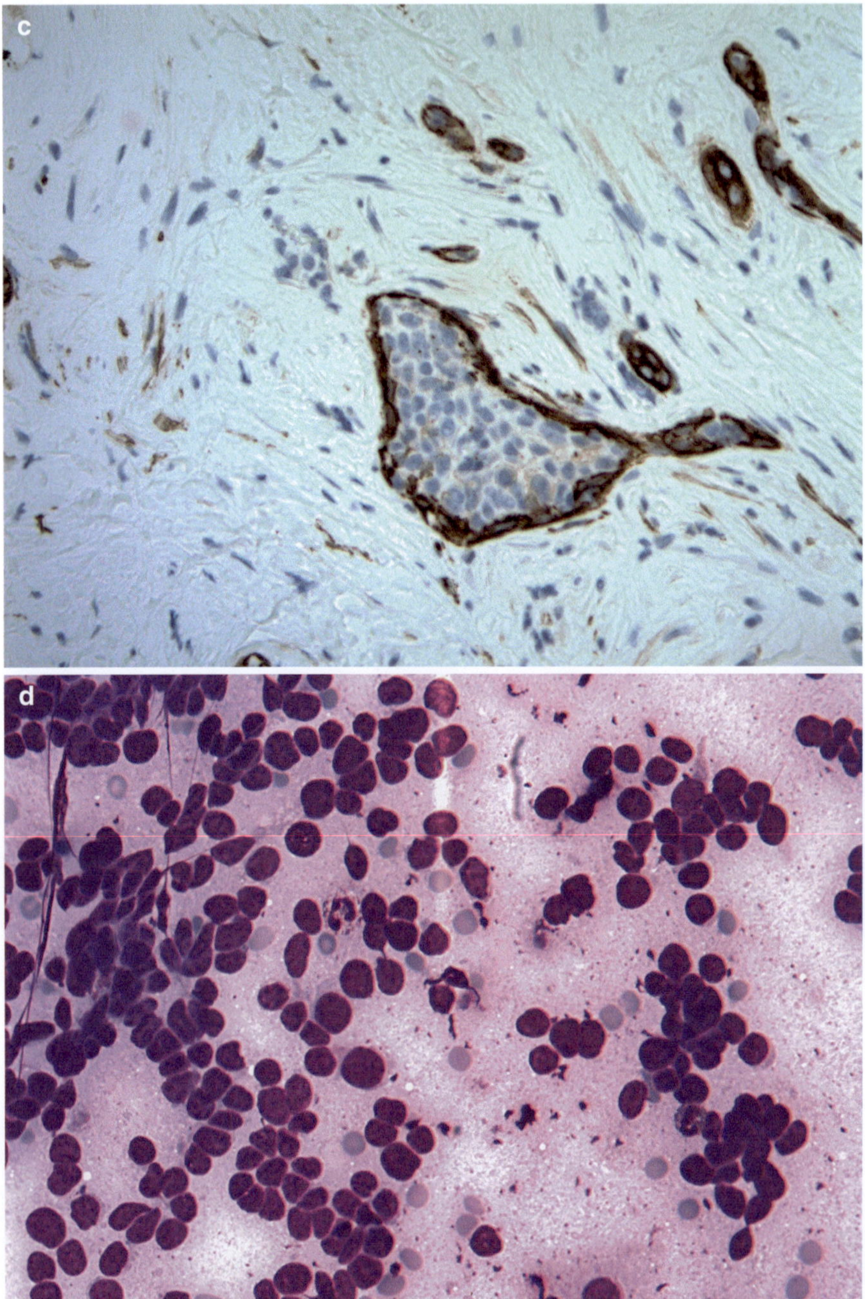

Fig. 2 (continued)

Invasive Breast Carcinoma with Neuroendocrine Differentiation (NEBC)

Invasive breast carcinomas with neuroendocrine differentiation are a heterogeneous group of tumors with variable morphology and accompanied neuroendocrine differentiation [10]. In contrast with the two previously described groups (well-differentiated neuroendocrine tumor and SCCB), NEBC does not necessarily show morphological features of neuroendocrine tumors in other organs; instead, neuroendocrine differentiation is identified using special histochemical stains or preferably IHC. IHC with neuroendocrine markers is not routinely used in the diagnostic work-up of invasive breast carcinomas; therefore, the true incidence of neuroendocrine differentiation in breast tumors is unknown. While it varies in the literature, it has been reported that neuroendocrine differentiation using IHC markers can be detected in up to 30 % of invasive no-special- and special-type breast carcinomas [3]. Many histologic types of invasive breast carcinomas can have neuroendocrine differentiation [8]. This includes ductal, lobular, and special-type carcinomas, but mainly the cellular variant of mucinous carcinoma and solid papillary carcinomas [3, 21]. Thorough sampling in order to identify at least focal areas suggesting neuroendocrine differentiation is the key to recognizing the possibility of NEBC, and immunohistochemical staining for neuroendocrine markers is necessary for confirmation of this rare diagnosis [14].

Mucinous carcinomas with neuroendocrine differentiation are usually of low-grade histology and have an indolent behavior [22]. The same as pure mucinous carcinomas, they usually affect older patients and are positive for estrogen (ERs) and progesterone receptors (PRs) and negative for Her-2 oncoprotein. When positive, neuroendocrine marker staining is usually focal (Fig. 3a, b) [22, 23]. Solid papillary carcinomas (SPC) are uncommon low-grade tumors that most often affect elderly women. Morphologically, they are composed of round, well-defined nodules composed of ductal cells separated by fibrovascular cores [21]. SPC are considered in situ tumors and approximately half of the cases are associated with invasive carcinoma [24]. The invasive component may have a pure or mixed mucinous, neuroendocrine-like, invasive ductal, rarely lobular, or tubular pattern. In general, the invasive carcinoma component is morphologically similar to the adjacent SPC [24, 25]. Solid papillary carcinomas and its associated invasive carcinoma are usually positive for ER and PR and negative for Her-2. Proliferation index is low. Additionally, tumor cells are variably positive for neuroendocrine markers (Fig. 4a, b) [21, 25].

Ductal carcinoma in situ (DCIS) seen in association with invasive carcinomas with neuroendocrine differentiation is usually of neuroendocrine and solid types [5]. Neuroendocrine ductal carcinoma in situ (NE-DCIS) is a distinct variant of DCIS that can also occur without an associated invasive component. Histologically, the NE-DCIS has a solid or papillary growth pattern. The neoplastic cells have monotonous appearance and small to medium size according to the tumor grade with

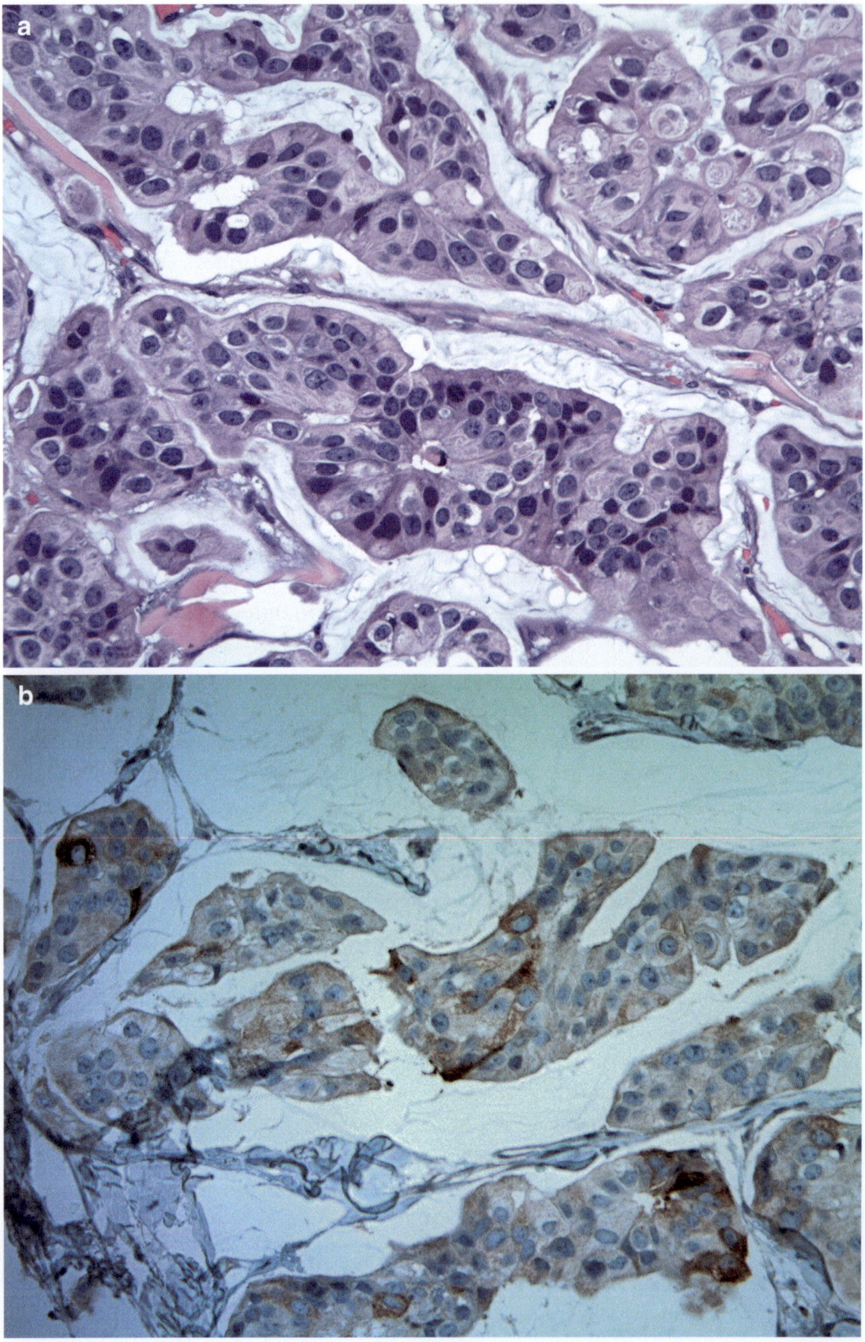

Fig. 3 (**a**) Mucinous carcinoma (type B) shows more cellularity and higher degree of pleomorphism than expected in mucinous carcinomas (H&E, ×200). (**b**) The tumor is focally positive for neuroendocrine marker synaptophysin (×200)

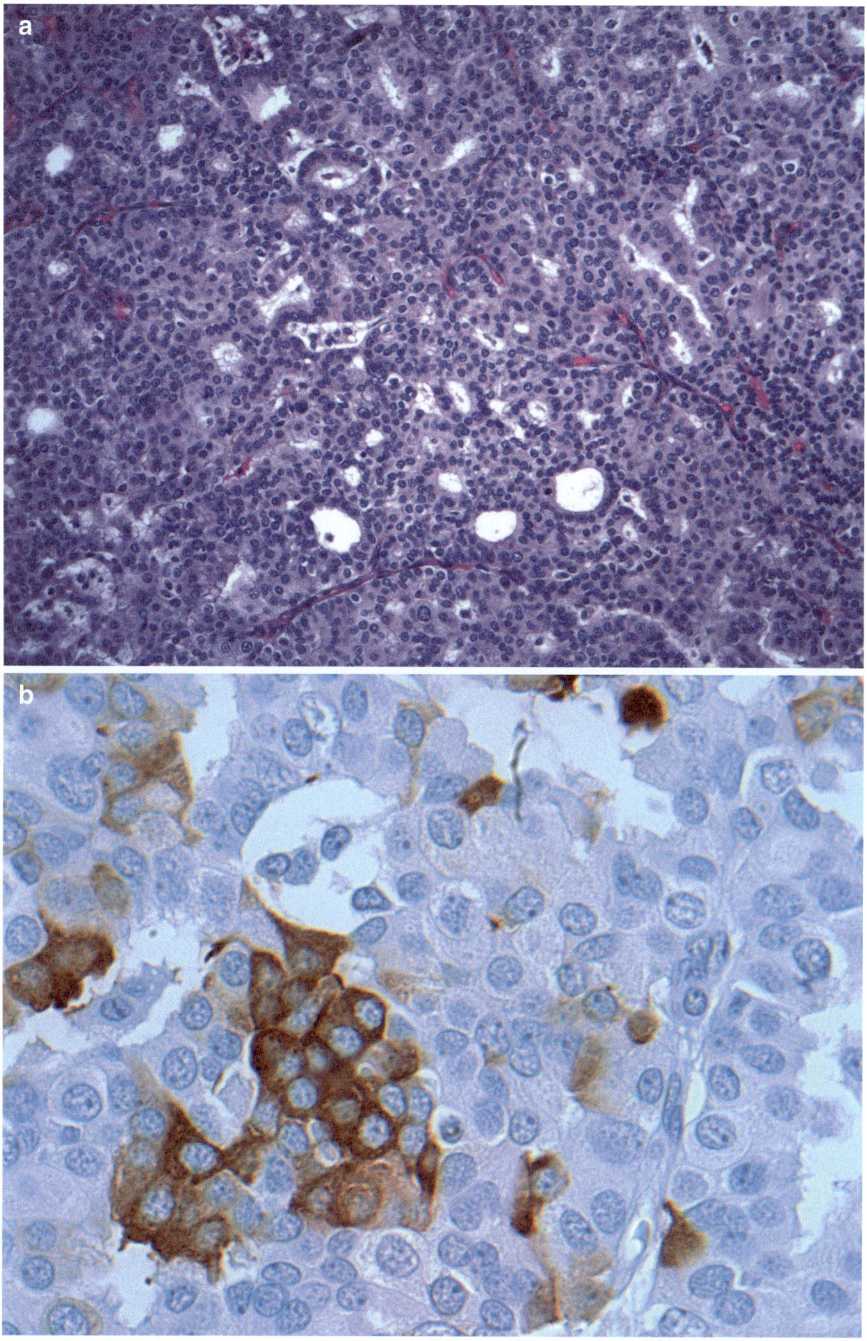

Fig. 4 (**a**) Solid papillary carcinoma of the breast composed of monotonous cells with a low to intermediate nuclear grade. The cells grow in a solid pattern with intermingled fibrovascular network and no apparent papillary structures. In this case, the cells have endocrine appearance with eosinophilic, granular cytoplasm. Focal pseudorosette and tubular formation are present (H&E, ×100). (**b**) Focal positivity with neuroendocrine marker synaptophysin is seen (×630)

columnar, ovoid, or spindle cell morphology [8, 26]. NE-DCIS is usually positive for ER and PR and negative for Her-2 [27].

Preoperative diagnosis of NEBC by fine needle aspiration cytology (FNAC) is possible, though not without difficulty [28]. In general, features are those of ductal, mucinous, or papillary carcinomas. May-Grünwald-Giemsa or Diff-Quik may show moderate cellularity and low cohesiveness, with polygonal to plasmacytoid tumor cells, with abundant cytoplasm, oval nuclei, and small nucleoli. More frequently, however, NEBC is diagnosed based on its histologic features using tissue biopsy [28–32].

Clinical Features and Prognosis

Breast carcinomas with neuroendocrine features most commonly affect postmenopausal women [1]. They usually present as a palpable mass in the central and retroareolar region of the breast [8]. In contrast, SCCB does not show any specific breast distribution predilection [5, 8]. Some patients with SCCB reported a rapidly growing mass [5, 18]. Interestingly, in contrast to non-neuroendocrine DCIS, a significant number of patients with NE-DCIS present with bloody nipple discharge [33], and mammographically detectable microcalcifications are uncommon in NE-DCIS [8]. Other than these subtle characteristics, there are no other clinical or radiological features specific to breast carcinomas with neuroendocrine features [3]. In fact, mammographic findings are substantially similar to other types of breast carcinomas [1].

The prognosis of breast carcinomas with neuroendocrine features depends on the tumor type, tumor grade, and stage at presentation. As expected, SCCB has the worse prognosis in this group; however, even SCCB can respond to treatment if detected early [5]. Metastases most commonly involve the axillary lymph nodes, bone, liver, and lung, among others [8]. Proliferation rate measured by Ki-67 immunohistochemistry may be useful in providing prognosis information [34].

Although there is lack of consensus, the presence of neuroendocrine differentiation in breast carcinomas is believed to lack clinical significance. Some authors have reported a better prognosis, while others believe neuroendocrine differentiation is associated with aggressive disease [8, 23, 35–38]. Mucinous differentiation, low-grade features, and positivity for estrogen and progesterone receptors are considered favorable prognostic factors [12, 39–42].

In a retrospective analysis of 96 patients with NEBC, tumors were grouped into those with expression of a neuroendocrine marker in >50 % of neoplastic cells and those with a minor neuroendocrine component [1]; NEBC cases showed a better prognosis as compared to breast carcinomas with a minor neuroendocrine component and to conventional invasive ductal or lobular cancers. In another study of 74 cases of invasive NEBC of the breast (per 2003 WHO criteria), excluding small cell carcinoma and low-grade solid papillary carcinoma with a predominant in situ component, these cancers were found to have worse clinical outcome compared with age- and stage-matched controls of invasive ductal carcinoma, not otherwise specified (IDC, NOS) [37]. In addition, these investigators found that these tumors did not respond as well to chemotherapy, hormonal therapy, or radiation therapy when treated using conventional therapies for IDC, NOS. An important clinical challenge is that apart from the relatively small numbers of primary NEC of the breast reported in literature, patient follow-up data is scarce. Therefore, at the present time, definitive conclusions about clinical implications of primary NEC of the breast cannot be reached [10]. The difficulties in determining the clinical significance of neuroendocrine differentiation in breast carcinomas are in part due to the rarity of the disease, the lack of diagnostic uniformity and the variability in testing methodology, and IHC stains used. It is noticeable how the diagnostic terminology varies across the published series that include patient follow-up, making hard to extrapolate prognosis and survival characteristics to the currently accepted WHO tumor classification. Although this may change in the future, at present, the routine use of IHC to detect neuroendocrine differentiation in tumors that do not show morphological neuroendocrine features is not necessary. Judicious use of neuroendocrine immunohistochemical markers in cases displaying morphological features suggestive of neuroendocrine differentiation should be encouraged because these stains are needed for diagnostic purposes and will also help establish the true incidence of these tumors.

Immunohistochemistry and Differential Diagnosis

Neuroendocrine markers including chromogranin proteins, synaptophysin, neuron-specific enolase (NSE), CD-56, and Leu 7 (CD-57) are commonly used to evaluate neuroendocrine differentiation in breast carcinomas [3, 5, 8, 16]. While no consensus currently exists regarding markers of election, chromogranin A and synaptophysin appear to be the most sensitive. In our experience, CD-56 has also demonstrated to be of value, although it is less specific. As mentioned before, no specific percentage of positive tumor cells is needed to establish the diagnosis. The expression of high molecular weight cytokeratins favors the diagnosis of non- neuroendocrine carcinoma [7].

Some breast carcinomas are capable of producing a variety of hormonal products normally not secreted by the breast such as human placental lactogen (hPl), adrenocorticotropic hormone, and norepinephrine. Human chorionic gonadotropin (hCG) can be detected in blood in about 12–33 % of patients with breast carcinoma; yet, many of these tumors do not show histologic evidence of choriocarcinomatous differentiation. One classical example of this tumor is the primary breast carcinoma with choriocarcinomatous differentiation [43]. The routine use of IHC to detect peptide hormone expression in cases of breast carcinomas with neuroendocrine features is not necessary unless morphological features of these specific tumors are present or there is clinical evidence of elevated serum hormonal levels. The main differential diagnosis of carcinomas with choriocarcinomatous differentiation is metastatic choriocarcinoma to the breast. However, this is a rare event; most of the patients are pregnant, have been previously pregnant, or have a known history of hydatiform mole or choriocarcinoma [43, 44]. The presence of in situ ductal carcinoma as well as a negative gynecologic history is crucial for a correct diagnosis [44, 45].

Metastasis to the breast from extramammary neuroendocrine tumors should be always considered. The presence of an associated in situ component is consistent with breast primary. It should be kept in mind that metastatic neuroendocrine tumors can appear very similar to lobular carcinomas, especially in small biopsies (Fig. 5). Also, the nesting pattern of some metastatic neuroendocrine tumors can mimic ductal carcinoma in situ. Primary breast small cell carcinoma must be differentiated from metastatic small cell carcinoma. Lung primary should always be excluded clinically. The use of thyroid transcription factor 1 (TTF-1) is not effective because nonpulmonary neuroendocrine tumors can express this marker [46]. Other possibilities to consider in this scenario are direct involvement of the breast by Merkel cell carcinoma from the overlaying skin, lymphoma (either primary or as a manifestation of systemic disease), carcinoid tumor, and melanoma [18]. Clinical history and radiologic findings as well as immunohistochemical stains are necessary to establish a

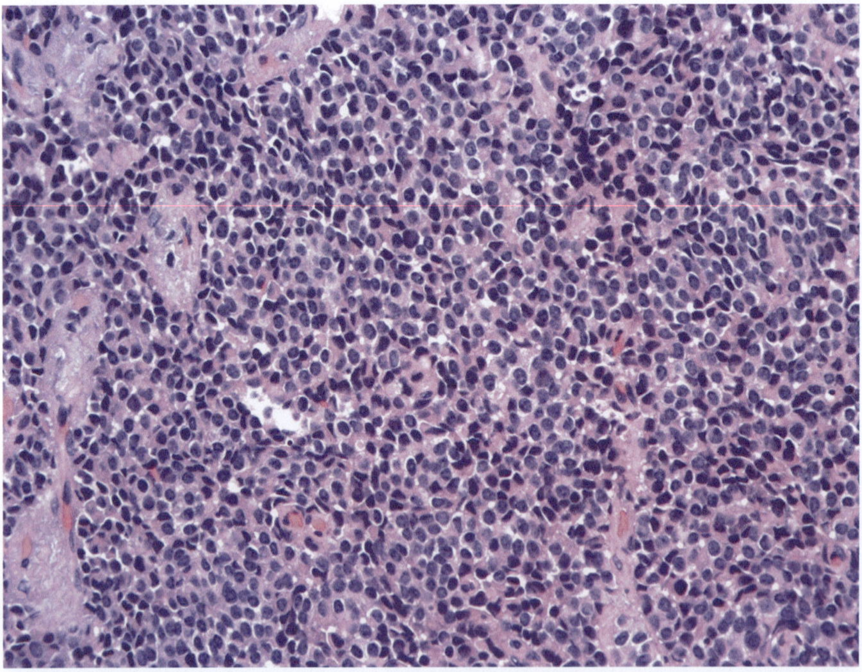

Fig. 5 Metastatic carcinoid tumor from small bowel looks remarkably similar to invasive primary lobular carcinoma in this core needle biopsy. Without the proper history, this case could be easily misdiagnosed (H&E, ×200)

correct diagnosis. Based on morphological features, a panel of immunostains that includes at least three cytokeratins, in addition to CK-20 (shows characteristic perinuclear dot-like staining in Merkel cell carcinoma), leukocyte common antigen (LCA), neuroendocrine markers, S-100 protein, Melan-A, and human melanoma black 45 (HMB-45), should be used. Of note, no single immunostain is unique to the breast. The most commonly used gross cystic disease fluid protein 15 (GCDFP-15) and mammaglobin are of limited value. GCDFP-15 is relatively specific for the breast, but it lacks sensitivity and shows a patchy staining which may be problematic mainly on biopsies. Mammaglobin is more sensitive than GCDFP-15, but it lacks specificity. Also, they may show some positivity on extramammary carcinomas [47]. GATA-3 (GATA3 binding protein) has been proven to be more sensitive than GCDFP-15, especially in ER-positive tumors (Fig. 6a–d) [48]. However, the expression of these markers has not been systematically studied in carcinomas with neuroendocrine differentiation. Therefore, their sensitivity in this setting is unclear.

It has been reported that CK-7 and caudal-type homeobox-2 (CDX-2) are useful when GI primary is being considered. Breast NEC are positive for CK-7 and negative for CDX-2, while GI primaries show an opposite expression pattern (Figs. 7a, b, and 8a, b). CDX-2 positivity favors GI origin [49]. Primary breast carcinomas with neuroendocrine features are variably positive for ER and PR. Well-differentiated tumors are usually diffusely positive, whereas SCCB tends to be positive in up to 50 % of cases [3, 8, 16, 18]. ER and PR are also often included in the diagnostic work-up because although extramammary tumors may be positive for these markers, expression is usually focal and weak [8]. Up to 45 % of cases are positive for androgen receptor [7]. Calcitonin to rule out metastasis from thyroid medullary carcinoma can also be used in the right clinical scenario [5].

With rare exceptions [37, 50], breast carcinomas with neuroendocrine features are negative for Her-2. Reported tumors have also expressed e-cadherin, bcl-2, and sometimes CD-117 and CD-99 [5, 8]. However, these markers are not useful to establish tumor origin.

Molecular and Genetic Features

Only a few studies have analyzed the molecular alterations in breast carcinomas with neuroendocrine features. It has been demonstrated that SPC and mucinous carcinomas showing neuroendocrine differentiation belong to the luminal A molecular subgroup [3]. In a genome-wide oligonucleotide-based microarray study using unsupervised hierarchical clustering analysis, NEBCs and mucinous (mucinous A or paucicellular and mucinous B or hypercellular) carcinomas were found to have a distinct expression profile, compared to molecular subtype-matched IDC, NOS [51]. In their study, mucinous carcinomas consistently displayed a luminal A expression profile, while neuroendocrine carcinomas were assigned to the luminal A or B. In the case of NEBC, compared with the same grade IDC (luminal A phenotype), genes

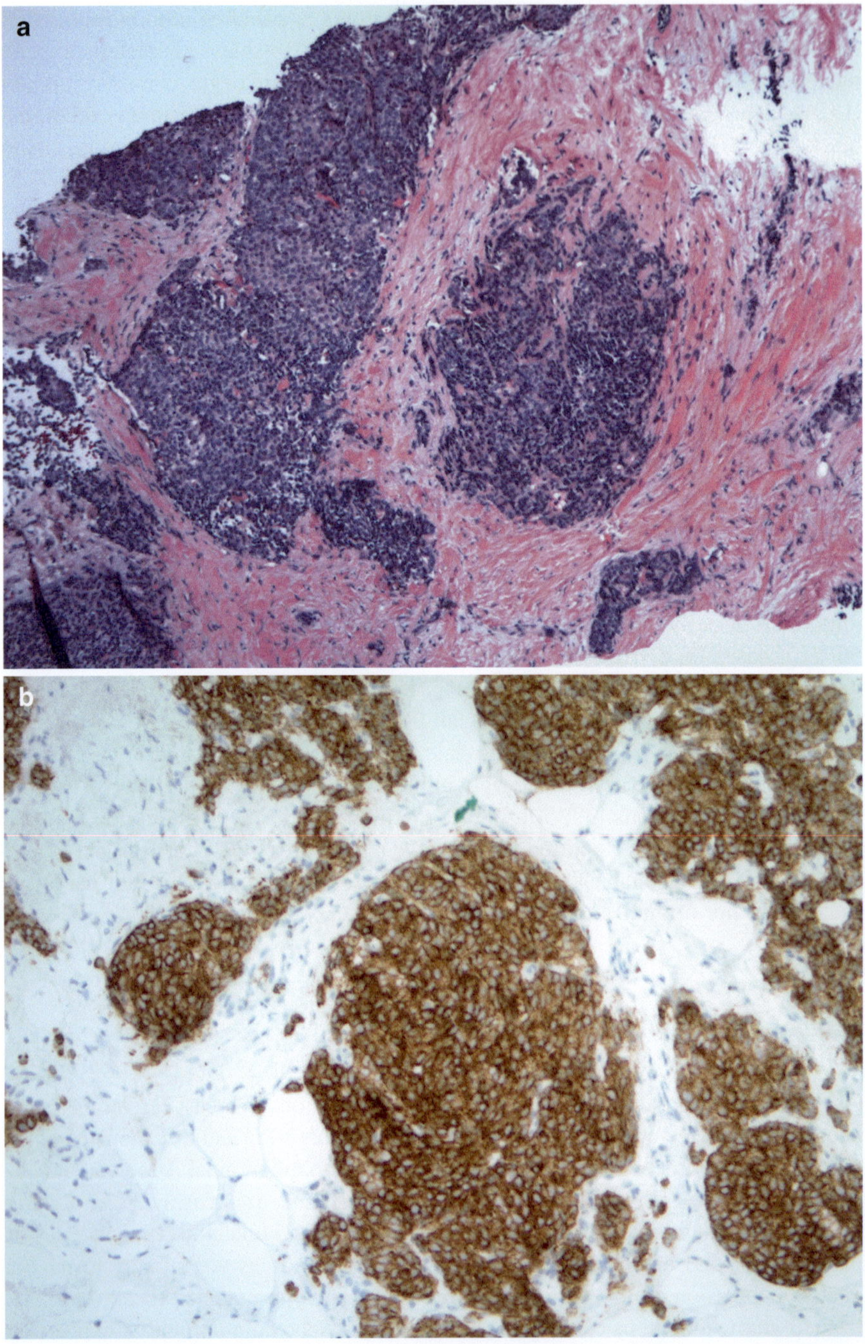

Fig. 6 (**a**) Poorly differentiated invasive ductal carcinoma of the breast displays infiltrative growth pattern with no tubular/glandular formation (H&E, ×50). (**b**) The tumor shows diffused positivity with neuroendocrine markers synaptophysin and chromogranin (synaptophysin stain ×100). To establish the origin of the tumor, a panel of immunostains was performed. Tumor cells were positive for GCDFP-15 (**c**) and GATA-3 (**d**), supporting the diagnosis of primary invasive carcinoma with neuroendocrine differentiation (×100)

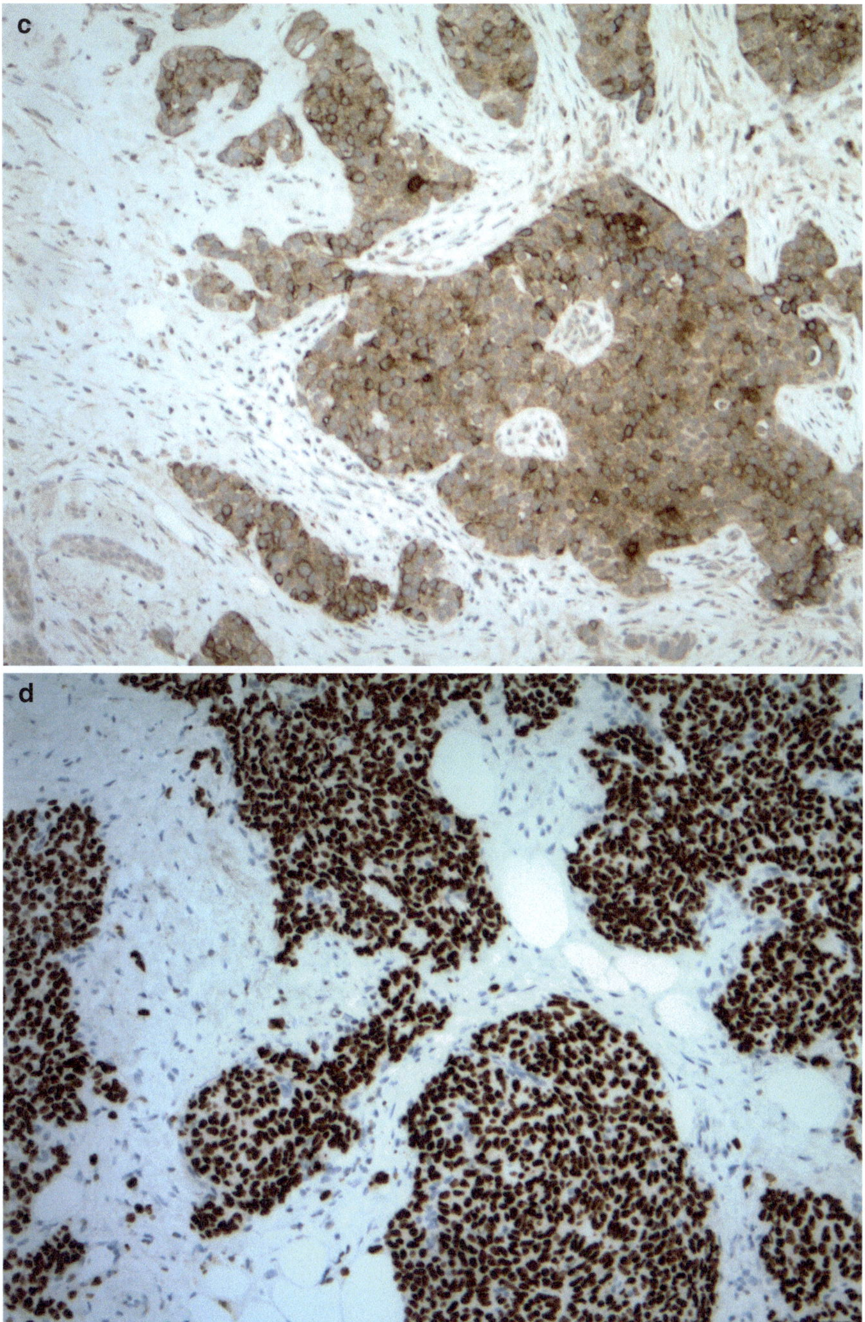

Fig.6 (continued)

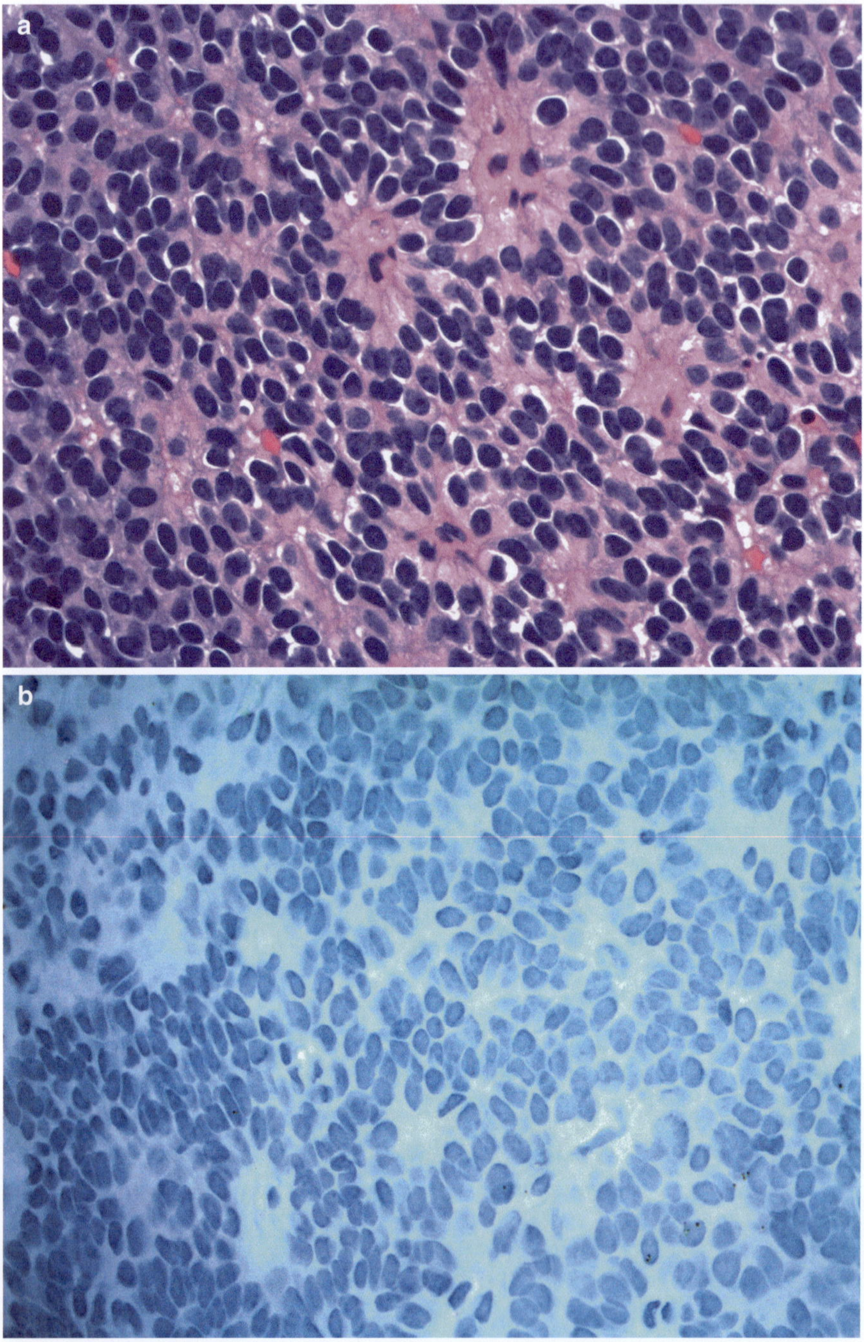

Fig. 7 (**a**) Another case of metastatic GI carcinoid to the breast shows more apparent neuroendocrine features and pseudorosettes (H&E, ×400). (**b**) Metastatic carcinoid is negative for cytokeratin 7 (×400)

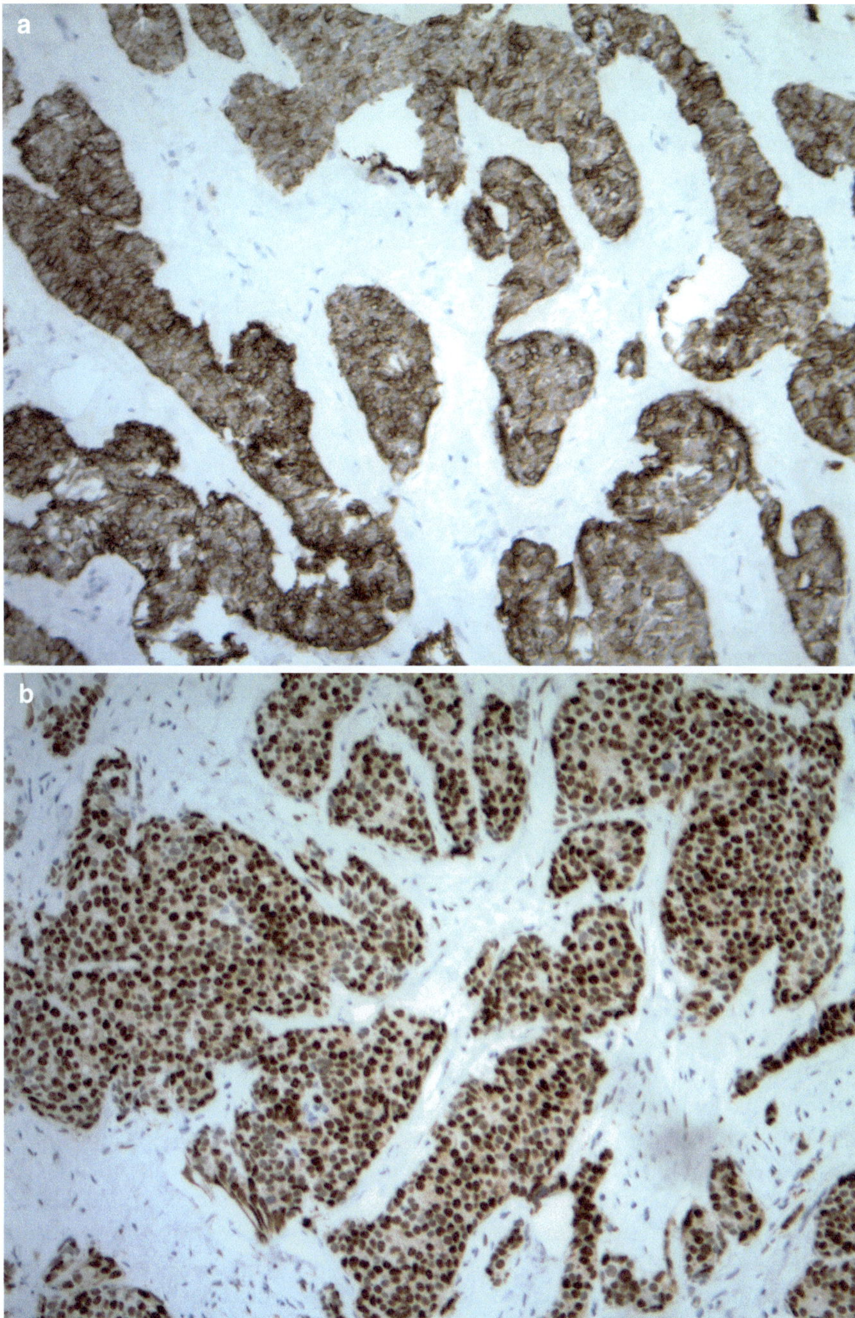

Fig. 8 A case of primary neuroendocrine breast carcinoma metastatic to the liver is positive for cytokeratin 7 (**a**) and estrogen receptor (**b**) (×100)

coding for the chromogranins, synaptophysin, CD-56, bombesin, metalloproteases, and collagenases were found to be amplified [51]. Similarly, the genes coding for FOXA1, XBP1, and ERBB4 were upregulated; these genes determine the expression of estrogen receptors, progesterone, and, in 45 % of cases, androgen. In the contrary, gene networks involved in cell migration, invasion, proliferation, and the expression of high molecular weight cytokeratins are downregulated.

In another study, Wachter et al. [52] investigated the frequency of neuroendocrine differentiation per molecular subtypes of no-special-type breast carcinoma. They found neuroendocrine differentiation in 20 % of luminal B carcinomas, using the 50 % cutoff established by the WHO in 2003 [9]. They did not find neuroendocrine expression in any of the other molecular groups (luminal A, Her-2 amplified, and triple negative).

Hoang et al. [53] described numerous molecular alterations in two cases of small cell breast carcinomas. Complex karyotypes, defined as three or more chromosomal aberrations including both numerical and structural aberrations per cell [54], are associated with aggressive cancers and those with poor clinical outcomes [55]. A recent study [1] carried out cytogenetic characterization of mammary NEC using both conventional G-banding and spectral karyotype and identified complex karyotypes and clonal chromosomal aberrations, including gain of chromosome 7, loss of chromosome 15, and aberrations involving chromosomes 1, 3, 6q, and 17q. These investigators also found mammary NEC to share some cytogenetic abnormalities (trisomies 7 and 12) with other neuroendocrine tumors in the lung and gastrointestinal tract, suggesting trisomies 7 and 12 as potential common molecular aberrations in neuroendocrine tumors. More comprehensive histomorphologic and molecular studies are necessary to understand this rare variant of human breast cancer.

Treatment

Treatment in general does not differ from other forms of breast carcinomas, and there is no standard treatment protocol for breast NEC. Treatment selection depends upon tumor stage and ER, PR, and Her-2 status [8]. Radical surgery with axillary lymph node dissection and neoadjuvant chemotherapy followed by breast conservation have all been used. Various chemotherapy regimens include FAC (fluorouracil, doxorubicin, cyclophosphamide), CMF (cyclophosphamide, methotrexate, fluorouracil), CAE (cyclophosphamide, doxorubicin, etoposide), and CP (cisplatin, etoposide) as single agents or in combination [18, 39, 56]. As a consequence of the absence of a standard treatment protocol, a large variety of chemotherapy protocols have been employed in treating this disease, as seen in our cases (FEC regimen, Taxol, and anastrozole). In SCCB, available data suggest that chemotherapy should be similar to the pulmonary counterpart [57]. Studies involving large cohorts of these cases are needed to further standardize and customize therapeutic approaches to individual patients.

Summary and Conclusions

Although clinicopathologic and molecular understanding of breast carcinomas with neuroendocrine features is still an evolving, controversial topic, there is increasing evidence that mammary NEC may represent a distinct subtype of breast carcinoma with somewhat different prognosis compared to other conventional breast cancer subtypes. In order to fully recognize biologic and clinical relevance of NEC as a separate entity (or otherwise), large well-designed clinicopathologic and molecular studies at protein, RNA, and DNA levels will be required to rationalize future recommendations on correct diagnosis, prognostication, treatment, and surveillance of patients with these rare subtypes of breast carcinoma.

It is of critical importance that anatomic pathologists adhere to accepted diagnostic criteria uniformly and reproducibly, so that clinical and translational research studies can rely on accurate data on incidence of these breast cancer subtypes. It is quite obvious that the future figures on incidence of breast carcinoma with neuroendocrine features will depend on the criteria used. An argument in support of the most recent recommendation by the WHO would be that by using any neuroendocrine marker positivity cutoff (rather than the previous 50 % immunoreactive tumor cells), it will be possible to identify cases with smaller proportions of neuroendocrine differentiation, allowing inclusion of a broader range of cases. The counterargument against this approach will be that by using such a low cutoff, future clinical or molecular analyses may provide misleading data on "lack of significance" of neuroendocrine differentiation in primary human breast cancer and exclude potential opportunity to recognize different biologic or clinical significance of more stringently defined criteria. It is recommended that pathologists communicate the strengths and limitations of current knowledge to their clinical colleagues, so that until sufficiently large data become available, oncologists and pathologists can work as a team to provide the most benefit to these patients. In the meanwhile, careful collection of multicenter data and appropriate analyses may help providing insightful biologic, clinical, and therapeutic leads to better serve the patients with these unusual forms of breast cancer.

Abbreviations

CDX-2	Caudal-type homeobox-2
DCIS	Ductal carcinoma in situ
ER	Estrogen receptor
FNAC	Fine needle aspiration cytology
GATA-3	GATA3 binding protein
GCDFP-15	Gross cystic disease fluid protein 15
GI	Gastrointestinal

H&E	Hematoxylin and eosin
hCG	Human chorionic gonadotropin
HMB-45	Human melanoma black 45
hPl	Human placental lactogen
IDC	Invasive ductal carcinoma
IHC	Immunohistochemical/immunohistochemistry
LCA	Leukocyte common antigen
NEBC	Invasive breast carcinoma with neuroendocrine differentiation
NEC	Breast carcinomas with neuroendocrine features
NEC-PD/SCCB	Neuroendocrine carcinoma, poorly differentiated/ small cell carcinoma of the breast
NE-DCIS	Neuroendocrine ductal carcinoma in situ
NET-WD	Neuroendocrine tumor, well differentiated
NOS	Not otherwise specified
NSE	Neuron-specific enolase
PR	Progesterone receptor
SPC	Solid papillary carcinomas
TTF-1	Thyroid transcription factor 1
WHO	World Health Organization

References

1. Rovera F, Lavazza M, La Rosa S, Fachinetti A, Chiappa C, Marelli M, et al. Neuroendocrine breast cancer: retrospective analysis of 96 patients and review of literature. Int J Surg. 2013;11 Suppl 1:S79–83. Epub 2014/01/02.
2. Xiang DB, Wei B, Abraham SC, Huo L, Albarracin CT, Zhang H, et al. Molecular cytogenetic characterization of mammary neuroendocrine carcinoma. Hum Pathol. 2014;45(9):1951–6. Epub 2014/07/31.
3. Bussolati G, Badve S. Carcinomas with neuroendocrine features. In: Lakhani SR, Ellis IO, Schnitt SJ, Tan PH, Van de Vijver MJ, editors. WHO classification of tumors of the breast. 4th ed. Lyon: International Agency for Research on Cancer; 2012. p. 62–3.
4. Cubilla AL, Woodruff JM. Primary carcinoid tumor of breast: a report of eight patients. Am J Surg Pathol. 1977;1:283–92.
5. Shin SJ, DeLellis RA, Ying L, Rosen PP. Small cell carcinoma of the breast: a clinicopathologic and immunohistochemical study of nine patients. Am J Surg Pathol. 2000;24(9):1231–8. Epub 2000/09/08.
6. Asioli S, Foschini MP, Masetti R, Eusebi V. Working formulation of neuroendocrine tumors of the skin and breast. Endocr Pathol. 2014;25(2):141–50. Epub 2014/04/15.
7. Righi L, Sapino A, Marchio C, Papotti M, Bussolati G. Neuroendocrine differentiation in breast cancer: established facts and unresolved problems. Semin Diagn Pathol. 2010;27(1):69–76. Epub 2010/03/24.
8. Brogi E. Mammary carcinomas with endocrine features. In: Hoda SA, Brogi E, Koerner FC, Rosen PP, editors. Rosen's breast pathology. 4th ed. Philadelphia: Lippincott Williams & Wilkins; 2014. p. 667–78.
9. Ellis IO, Schnitt SJ, Sastre-Garau X. Invasive breast carcinoma. In: Tavassoli FA, Devillee P, editors. Tumors of the breast and female genital organs. Lyon: IARC Press; 2003. p. 32–4.

10. Tan PH, Schnitt SJ, van de Vijver MJ, Ellis IO, Lakhani SR. Papillary and neuroendocrine breast lesions: the WHO stance. Histopathology. 2015;66(6):761–70. Epub 2014/05/23.
11. Kawasaki T, Nakamura S, Sakamoto G, Kondo T, Tsunoda-Shimizu H, Ishii Y, et al. Neuroendocrine ductal carcinoma in situ of the breast: cytological features in 32 cases. Cytopathology. 2011;22(1):43–9. Epub 2010/03/20.
12. Richter-Ehrenstein C, Arndt J, Buckendahl AC, Eucker J, Weichert W, Kasajima A, et al. Solid neuroendocrine carcinomas of the breast: metastases or primary tumors? Breast Cancer Res Treat. 2010;124(2):413–7. Epub 2010/09/28.
13. Singh S, Aggarwal G, Kataria SP, Kalra R, Duhan A, Sen R. Primary neuroendocrine carcinoma of breast. J Cytol. 2011;28(2):91–2. Epub 2011/06/30.
14. Tang F, Wei B, Tian Z, Gilcrease MZ, Huo L, Albarracin CT, et al. Invasive mammary carcinoma with neuroendocrine differentiation: histological features and diagnostic challenges. Histopathology. 2011;59(1):106–15. Epub 2011/06/15.
15. Wade Jr PM, Mills SE, Read M, Cloud W, Lambert 3rd MJ, Smith RE. Small cell neuroendocrine (oat cell) carcinoma of the breast. Cancer. 1983;52(1):121–5. Epub 1983/07/01.
16. Koerner FC. Small cell carcinoma. In: Hoda SA, Brogi E, Koerner FC, Rosen PP, editors. Rosen's breast pathology. 4th ed. Philadelphia: Lippincott Williams & Wilkins; 2014. p. 679–87.
17. Kitakata H, Yasumoto K, Sudo Y, Minato H, Takahashi Y. A case of primary small cell carcinoma of the breast. Breast Cancer. 2007;14(4):414–9. Epub 2007/11/08.
18. Latif N, Rosa M, Samian L, Rana F. An unusual case of primary small cell neuroendocrine carcinoma of the breast. Breast J. 2010;16(6):647–51. Epub 2010/11/13.
19. Fukunaga M, Ushigome S. Small cell (oat cell) carcinoma of the breast. Pathol Int. 1998;48(9):744–8. Epub 1998/10/20.
20. Papotti M, Gherardi G, Eusebi V, Pagani A, Bussolati G. Primary oat cell (neuroendocrine) carcinoma of the breast. Report of four cases. Virchows Arch A Pathol Anat Histopathol. 1992;420(1):103–8. Epub 1992/01/01.
21. Saremian J, Rosa M. Solid papillary carcinoma of the breast: a pathologically and clinically distinct breast tumor. Arch Pathol Lab Med. 2012;136(10):1308–11. Epub 2012/10/02.
22. Charfi S, Ayed CB, Mnif H, Ellouze S, Chaabane K, Feki J, et al. Mammary neuroendocrine carcinoma with mucinous differentiation: a clinicopathological study of 15 cases. Breast Dis. 2013;34(2):87–93. Epub 2013/09/06.
23. Tse GM, Ma TK, Chu WC, Lam WW, Poon CS, Chan WC. Neuroendocrine differentiation in pure type mammary mucinous carcinoma is associated with favorable histologic and immunohistochemical parameters. Mod Pathol. 2004;17(5):568–72. Epub 2004/03/06.
24. Nassar H, Qureshi H, Adsay NV, Visscher D. Clinicopathologic analysis of solid papillary carcinoma of the breast and associated invasive carcinomas. Am J Surg Pathol. 2006;30(4):501–7. Epub 2006/04/21.
25. Maluf HM, Koerner FC. Solid papillary carcinoma of the breast. A form of intraductal carcinoma with endocrine differentiation frequently associated with mucinous carcinoma. Am J Surg Pathol. 1995;19(11):1237–44. Epub 1995/11/01.
26. Honami H, Sotome K, Sakamoto G, Iri H, Tanaka Y, Fukamachi S, et al. Synchronous bilateral neuroendocrine ductal carcinoma in situ. Breast Cancer. 2014;21(4):508–13. Epub 2011/07/08.
27. Tsang WY, Chan JK. Endocrine ductal carcinoma in situ (E-DCIS) of the breast: a form of low-grade DCIS with distinctive clinicopathologic and biologic characteristics. Am J Surg Pathol. 1996;20(8):921–43. Epub 1996/08/01.
28. Sapino A, Papotti M, Pietribiasi F, Bussolati G. Diagnostic cytological features of neuroendocrine differentiated carcinoma of the breast. Virchows Arch. 1998;433(3):217–22. Epub 1998/10/13.
29. Fujimoto Y, Yagyu R, Murase K, Kawajiri H, Ohtani H, Arimoto Y, et al. A case of solid neuroendocrine carcinoma of the breast in a 40-year-old woman. Breast Cancer. 2007;14(2):250–3. Epub 2007/05/09.
30. Gupta RK, Holloway LJ, Wakefield SJ. Needle aspiration cytology, immunocytochemistry, and electron microscopic study in a case of carcinoid of the male breast. Diagn Cytopathol. 1993;9(4):461–4. Epub 1993/08/01.

31. Ni K, Bibbo M. Fine needle aspiration of mammary carcinoma with features of a carcinoid tumor. A case report with immunohistochemical and ultrastructural studies. Acta Cytol. 1994;38(1):73–8. Epub 1994/01/01.
32. Wee A, Nilsson B, Chong SM, Raju GC. Bilateral carcinoid tumor of the breast. Report of a case with diagnosis by fine needle aspiration cytology. Acta Cytol. 1992;36(1):55–9. Epub 1992/01/01.
33. Kawasaki T, Mochizuki K, Yamauchi H, Yagata H, Kondo T, Tsunoda H, et al. High prevalence of neuroendocrine carcinoma in breast lesions detected by the clinical symptom of bloody nipple discharge. Breast. 2012;21(5):652–6. Epub 2012/03/09.
34. Tian Z, Wei B, Tang F, Wei W, Gilcrease MZ, Huo L, et al. Prognostic significance of tumor grading and staging in mammary carcinomas with neuroendocrine differentiation. Hum Pathol. 2011;42(8):1169–77. Epub 2011/02/22.
35. Kwon SY, Bae YK, Gu MJ, Choi JE, Kang SH, Lee SJ, et al. Neuroendocrine differentiation correlates with hormone receptor expression and decreased survival in patients with invasive breast carcinoma. Histopathology. 2014;64(5):647–59. Epub 2013/10/15.
36. Wang J, Wei B, Albarracin CT, Hu J, Abraham SC, Wu Y. Invasive neuroendocrine carcinoma of the breast: a population-based study from the surveillance, epidemiology and end results (SEER) database. BMC Cancer. 2014;14:147. Epub 2014/03/05.
37. Wei B, Ding T, Xing Y, Wei W, Tian Z, Tang F, et al. Invasive neuroendocrine carcinoma of the breast: a distinctive subtype of aggressive mammary carcinoma. Cancer. 2010;116(19):4463–73. Epub 2010/06/24.
38. Zhang Y, Chen Z, Bao Y, Du Z, Li Q, Zhao Y, et al. Invasive neuroendocrine carcinoma of the breast: a prognostic research of 107 Chinese patients. Neoplasma. 2013;60(2):215–22. Epub 2012/12/25.
39. Lopez-Bonet E, Alonso-Ruano M, Barraza G, Vazquez-Martin A, Bernado L, Menendez JA. Solid neuroendocrine breast carcinomas: incidence, clinico-pathological features and immunohistochemical profiling. Oncol Rep. 2008;20(6):1369–74. Epub 2008/11/21.
40. Rovera F, Masciocchi P, Coglitore A, La Rosa S, Dionigi G, Marelli M, et al. Neuroendocrine carcinomas of the breast. Int J Surg. 2008;6 Suppl 1:S113–5. Epub 2009/01/27.
41. Stita W, Trabelsi A, Gharbi O, Mokni M, Korbi S. Primary solid neuroendocrine carcinoma of the breast. Can J Surg. 2009;52(6):E289–90. Epub 2009/12/17.
42. Zekioglu O, Erhan Y, Ciris M, Bayramoglu H. Neuroendocrine differentiated carcinomas of the breast: a distinct entity. Breast. 2003;12(4):251–7. Epub 2003/12/09.
43. Mohammadi A, Rosa M. Carcinoma of the breast with choriocarcinomatous features. Arch Pathol Lab Med. 2011;135(9):1097–100. Epub 2011/09/01.
44. Resetkova E, Sahin A, Ayala AG, Sneige N. Breast carcinoma with choriocarcinomatous features. Ann Diagn Pathol. 2004;8(2):74–9. Epub 2004/04/03.
45. Erhan Y, Ozdemir N, Zekioglu O, Nart D, Ciris M. Breast carcinomas with choriocarcinomatous features: case reports and review of the literature. Breast J. 2002;8(4):244–8. Epub 2002/07/09.
46. Kaufmann O, Dietel M. Expression of thyroid transcription factor-1 in pulmonary and extrapulmonary small cell carcinomas and other neuroendocrine carcinomas of various primary sites. Histopathology. 2000;36(5):415–20. Epub 2000/05/03.
47. Khazai L, Rosa M. Use of immunohistochemical stains in epithelial lesions of the breast. Cancer Control. 2015;22(2):220–5. Epub 2015/06/13.
48. Miettinen M, McCue PA, Sarlomo-Rikala M, Rys J, Czapiewski P, Wazny K, et al. GATA3: a multispecific but potentially useful marker in surgical pathology: a systematic analysis of 2500 epithelial and nonepithelial tumors. Am J Surg Pathol. 2014;38(1):13–22. Epub 2013/10/23.
49. Perry KD, Reynolds C, Rosen DG, Edgerton ME, Albarracin C T, Gilcrease MZ, et al. Metastatic neuroendocrine tumour in the breast: a potential mimic of in-situ and invasive mammary carcinoma. Histopathology. 2011;59(4):619–30. Epub 2011/10/22.
50. Yamamoto J, Ohshima K, Nabeshima K, Ikeda S, Iwasaki H, Kikuchi M. Comparative study of primary mammary small cell carcinoma, carcinoma with endocrine features and invasive ductal carcinoma. Oncol Rep. 2004;11(4):825–31. Epub 2004/03/11.

51. Weigelt B, Geyer FC, Horlings HM, Kreike B, Halfwerk H, Reis-Filho JS. Mucinous and neuroendocrine breast carcinomas are transcriptionally distinct from invasive ductal carcinomas of no special type. Mod Pathol. 2009;22(11):1401–14. Epub 2009/07/28.
52. Wachter DL, Hartmann A, Beckmann MW, Fasching PA, Hein A, Bayer CM, et al. Expression of neuroendocrine markers in different molecular subtypes of breast carcinoma. Biomed Res Int. 2014;2014:408459. Epub 2014/04/05.
53. Hoang MP, Maitra A, Gazdar AF, Albores-Saavedra J. Primary mammary small-cell carcinoma: a molecular analysis of 2 cases. Hum Pathol. 2001;32(7):753–7. Epub 2001/08/04.
54. Gohring G, Michalova K, Beverloo HB, Betts D, Harbott J, Haas OA, et al. Complex karyotype newly defined: the strongest prognostic factor in advanced childhood myelodysplastic syndrome. Blood. 2010;116(19):3766–9. Epub 2010/08/31.
55. Chen CC, Yang CF, Lee KD, You JY, Yu YB, Ho CH, et al. Complex karyotypes confer a poor survival in adult acute myeloid leukemia with unfavorable cytogenetic abnormalities. Cancer Genet Cytogenet. 2007;174(2):138–46. Epub 2007/04/25.
56. Buttar A, Mittal K, Khan A, Bathini V. Effective role of hormonal therapy in metastatic primary neuroendocrine breast carcinoma. Clin Breast Cancer. 2011;11(5):342–5. Epub 2011/07/07.
57. El Hassani LK, Bensouda Y, M'Rabti H, Boutayeb S, Kamouni M, Gamra L, et al. Primary neuroendocrine carcinoma of the breast, which chemotherapy? Indian J Cancer. 2009;46(4):352–4. Epub 2009/09/15.

Neuroendocrine Tumors of the Esophagus

Shabnam Seydafkan and Domenico Coppola

Introduction

Neuroendocrine cells are normally present in the esophageal mucosa and are present in larger number in the mucosal glands of the distal esophagus, hence the predominant distribution of esophageal neuroendocrine tumors in the lower third of the esophagus [1, 2]. Neuroendocrine cells may have different degrees of cellular proliferation (Table 1).

Gastrointestinal neuroendocrine neoplasms (GI-NENs) arise from neuroendocrine cells of mucosa and submucosa of the gastrointestinal tract [4].

The most commonly seen pattern of neuroendocrine differentiation in GI neoplasms is the presence of scattered tumor cells with neuroendocrine differentiation in a typical adenocarcinoma. This phenomenon is very well known, and a subset of GI adenocarcinomas and poorly differentiated carcinomas of stomach and colon express focal chromogranin (CG), indicative of neuroendocrine differentiation. In colonic adenocarcinomas, neuroendocrine differentiation does not affect the prognosis, in contrast to gastric adenocarcinomas where the presence of neuroendocrine differentiation may be associated with a slightly better prognosis [5].

Neuroendocrine tumors (NETs), on the other hand, are epithelial neoplasms composed of cells with either a well-developed neuroendocrine phenotype or with poorly developed but still recognizable and prominent neuroendocrine features. GI tumors with diffuse neuroendocrine differentiation usually are classified as differentiated neuroendocrine tumors, of grade 1 or 2 depending on the mitotic activity, or as poorly differentiated neuroendocrine carcinomas (NEC) (grade 3) [5, 6]. The term neuroendocrine tumor comprehends a spectrum of different neoplasms that originate from various neuroendo-

S. Seydafkan, MD • D. Coppola, MD (✉)
Department of Anatomic Pathology, Moffitt Cancer Center, Tampa, FL, USA
e-mail: domenico.coppola@moffitt.org

A. Nasir, D. Coppola (eds.), *Neuroendocrine Tumors: Review of Pathology, Molecular and Therapeutic Advances*, DOI 10.1007/978-1-4939-3426-3_11

Table 1 Spectrum of gastrointestinal neuroendocrine lesions [3]

Endocrine cell hyperplasia
Microcarcinoid
Carcinoid tumors
Mixed endocrine/exocrine tumors
Poorly differentiated neuroendocrine carcinoma (small cell carcinomas)

crine cells [cells of the amine precursor uptake and decarboxylation (APUD) system] and are classically defined by silver stains as either argyrophilic or argentaffinic [7, 8].

Gastrointestinal neuroendocrine tumors can also arise in the setting of two genetic syndromes: multiple endocrine neoplasia type 1 (MEN1) and neurofibromatosis type 1. The genetic defect in MEN1 is localized in chromosome 11q136 and consists of a mutation or a deletion in the tumor suppressor gene, MEN1, that codes for a nuclear protein called menin. However, most reported cases of esophageal NET are sporadic [9, 10].

Gastrointestinal NETs are classified into foregut, midgut, or hindgut.

Foregut NETs include those arising in the esophagus, stomach, pancreas, and duodenum. Foregut NETs have a broad range of benign to metastatic clinical behavior. Stomach is the most common foregut location for NETs and esophagus is the rarest site [6].

Neuroendocrine Neoplasms of the Esophagus

Neuroendocrine system is not well developed in the esophagus; thus, esophageal neuroendocrine neoplasm (NENs) tumors are extremely rare (Table 2) [10], and less than 500 cases have been reported in literature since 1952 when McKeown reported the first case.

According to the English literature, esophageal NETs occur more frequently in males of age ranging from 60 to 70 years. The most common presenting symptom is dysphagia [9]. Cases of typical carcinoid syndrome in NET of esophagus and extremely rare cases of syndrome of inappropriate secretion of antidiuretic hormone (SIADH) in the context of esophageal small cell NEC variant have also been reported [10, 13].

Foregut NENs are generally argyrophilic, and the esophagus, particularly near the esophagogastric junction, contains many argyrophilic cells.

Esophageal NET is found either as an incidental finding associated with BE and adenocarcinoma or as a single large polypoid or nodular tumor. It is hypothesized that esophageal NENs, Barrett's mucosa, and adenocarcinomas have common stem cell origin.

Neuroendocrine argyrophilic cells are present in 65–90 % of cases of metaplastic Barrett's mucosa (BE), in approximately 30 % of lower esophageal adenocarcinomas, and in cases of esophageal small cell carcinoma.

In esophageal adenocarcinomas, scattered CG-positive tumor cells may be generally found in the lower portion of the crypt, at the periphery of neoplastic glands, and away from luminal surfaces, especially in intestinal-type adenocarcinoma. This pattern of distribution is similar to that seen in nonneoplastic GI mucosa. However,

Table 2 Incidence of carcinoid tumors in esophagus [3]

Incidence per 100,000 population (Europe and the USA): [11] 3/100,000
Percentage of all GI carcinoid tumors: <0.4–0.5 %
Percentage of tumors arising at esophagus: <1 % of esophageal neoplasms (may be ~7.6 % in Japan and China [11])
SCNEC (small cell neuroendocrine carcinoma): 1.0–2.8 % of all esophageal cancers [12]

in dysplastic Barrett's mucosa, the CG-positive cells often extend higher up in the crypt as compared to the nondysplastic mucosa. The presence or absence of neuroendocrine cells and their pattern of distribution is not a diagnostic criterion for dysplasia in BE, as CG-positive cells are present in both dysplastic and nondysplastic mucosa.

In BE, neuroendocrine differentiation is preserved in low- and high-grade dysplasia but is usually lost in esophageal adenocarcinoma.

The presence of scattered neuroendocrine cells does not affect patient outcome, and the significance of neuroendocrine differentiation in esophageal adenocarcinomas is not clear [3, 14].

Most cases of esophageal NENs are poorly differentiated endocrine carcinoma (NEC) and mixed adenoneuroendocrine carcinoma.

If the tumor shows mixed phenotype and contains both adenocarcinoma and neuroendocrine cells, it is classified as "mixed adenoneuroendocrine carcinoma (MANEC). Importantly, for a tumor to be classified as MANEC each components must represent at least 30 % of the entire tumor." Localized areas of carcinoid or neuroendocrine carcinoma neighboring an adenocarcinoma or adenoma are classified as intimately intermixed, "collision" tumors. Neuroendocrine tumors colliding with papillary adenocarcinoma and squamous cell carcinoma have also been reported in esophagus. Amphicrine tumors are rare tumors showing neuroendocrine and glandular differentiation within the same cell [5]. By definition, the presence of scattered neuroendocrine positivity pattern does not make a tumor mixed type or neuroendocrine tumor [15].

Classification

As elsewhere in the foregut, 2010 WHO classification system divides NENs of esophagus into low- to intermediate-grade (grade 1–2) neuroendocrine tumors (NETs) and high-grade (grade 3) neuroendocrine carcinomas (NECs, large or small cell type), according to their histopathologic characterization by mitotic activity per ten high-power fields and/or by proliferation index (Ki-67). The histologic features alone do not usually predict malignancy, and the distinction between a benign and a malignant neuroendocrine tumor usually relies on the presence or absence of metastases. Thus, it is recommended to include results of immunohistochemical staining, lymphovascular invasion, perineural invasion, and lymph node metastasis in pathology reports when assessing a NET of the esophageal or of any other site.

When a tumor invades beyond the submucosa or if metastatic spread is present, the lesion is considered potentially aggressive. The prognosis of esophageal NETs is dependent on the mitotic rate and the presence or absence of lymph node metastasis. If the lesion is limited to the mucosa or submucosa but invades vessels or it is larger than 1 cm, it is considered to be of uncertain malignant potential.

Most high-grade NECs arising in the squamous lined parts (esophagus and anal canal) are small cell type (78 %), whereas most occurring in the glandular mucosa are large cell (53 %) or mixed (82 %) subtype; associated adenocarcinomas are more common in large cell (61 %) or mixed (36 %) type than in small cell type (26 %) [16].

Small Cell Neuroendocrine Carcinoma of Esophagus

McKeown reported the first case of small cell carcinoma of the esophagus in 1952. Small cell neuroendocrine carcinomas usually show aggressive behavior and can occur anywhere in the gastrointestinal tract, but the esophagus is the most common site of small cell carcinoma in the gastrointestinal tract [17]. Small cell cancers of the gastrointestinal tract are histologically indistinguishable from its counterpart in the lung and tend to metastasize early. However, SCNEC of esophagus may have a much more aggressive clinical course and has a poor prognosis despite combination radio-chemotherapies. SCNEC of esophagus are usually ulcerative, more than 1.0 cm in diameter, and present with early involvement of the esophageal wall and/or metastasis to regional lymph nodes [18, 19].

Gross

Esophageal carcinoid tumors usually arise distally in lower third of either the native esophageal tissue or in areas of Barrett esophagus, regions where neuroendocrine cells are more numerous. They tend to be single, large infiltrative lesions, measuring 4–7 cm and deep within the esophageal wall. Smaller lesions may appear polypoid. The overlying squamous epithelium shows patchy erosions [10], or it is covered with shiny reddish normal-appearing squamous mucosa [3, 20].

Histologic Features

Gastrointestinal carcinoid tumors show five histologic patterns [2]:

1. Solid, nodular, and narrow cords
2. Trabecular anastomosing patterns
3. Tubules and glands or rosette-like patterns

4. Poorly differentiated (atypical patterns)
5. Mixed tumors

Esophageal NET usually shows anastomosing ribbons, solid nests, trabeculae, acini, or rosette patterns. Mixed patterns with more typical solid nests may also be seen. Some tumors resemble more to that of appendicular goblet cell carcinoids. There are also atypical esophageal carcinoid tumors present which display diverse patterns, including organoid, trabecular, and sheet-like. The cells in NETs are usually round or polygonal but may be oval or cylindrical and have large, irregular, hyperchromatic nuclei with prominent nucleoli and up to four mitoses per ten high-power fields (HPF). There is discrete cell necrosis present as well. Tumors in early stages usually show little or no mitotic activity.

Molecular Pathways

Pathways regulating chromatin remodeling and epigenetic modification rather than genetic changes may play a key role in regulating NET growth. Inactivation of MEN gene, which codes for protein menin (part of a histone methyltransferase complex), is a well-documented genetic alteration in neuroendocrine tumors of the gastrointestinal tract which further supports the role for epigenetic. This genetic alteration is location-specific phenomena: MEN1 somatic mutations occur most frequently in foregut neuroendocrine tumors 18q loss of heterozygosity (LOH) almost exclusively in midgut and hindgut neuroendocrine tumors [21, 22].

The genomics of NETs has been extensively studied and has been resulted in suggestion of further mutations and expression anomalies in genes and pathways, for example, PI3K/Akt/mTOR, DAXX/ATRX, TSC2, IL1RN, and *CYP1B1* [23]. PCR-based analysis of 51 marker genes in the blood also has proposed genes, which their expression is altered and shown to have mRNAs in peripheral blood of NET cases at the time of diagnosis (Figs. 1, 2, and 3) [25]. Such circulating transcription products can be used not only as a sensitive and specific marker to diagnose NET more reliably than commonly used markers but also can be targeted to develop therapeutic agents [27].

The Fox Chase Cancer Center (FCCC) experience of molecular profiling of neuroendocrine tumors has indicated that unlike high-grade NETs in which tumor-specific mutations are common, it is only seen in minority of low-grade tumors.

Mutations and resulting instability in neuroendocrine tumorigenesis, which may occur as gain or more commonly losses, can happen at the level of alleles or at the chromosomal level (aneuploidy). Loss of chromosome 18 with site-specific propensity has been commonly reported in NETs, and 13 % of nonileal carcinoid tumors show genetic polymorphisms in chr18q22. In addition to chromosome 18, loss of part or all of chromosome 21 has been reported to significantly associate with nonileal site and larger size of NETs. The next most frequent reported chromosomal imbalances among well-differentiated NETs included loss of chromosome 13 or 13q, chromosome 16 or 16q, and amplification of chromosome 20 or 20p.

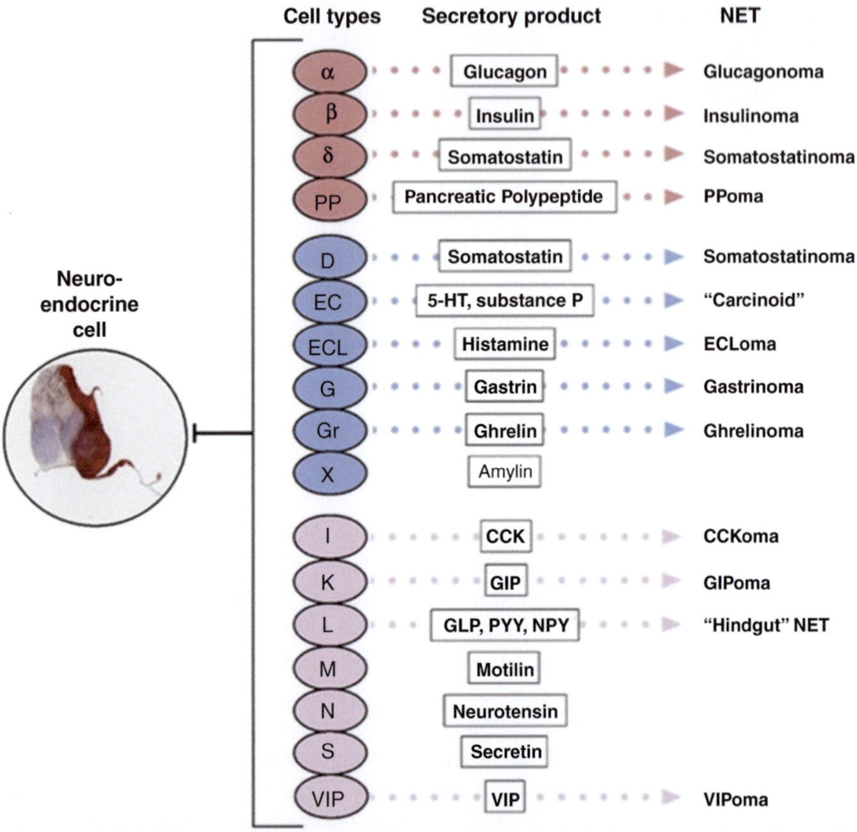

Fig. 1 Gastrointestinal and pancreatic neuroendocrine cell types, secretory products, and associated neoplasms. *CCK* cholecystokinin, *GIP* gastric inhibitory peptide, *GLP-1* glucagon-like peptide1, *NPY* neuropeptide Y (tyrosine), *PP* pancreatic polypeptide, *PYY* polypeptide YY (tyrosine, tyrosine) (Image courtesy of Hauso et al., Kidd et al. [24])

Bcl-2

Overexpression of Bcl-2, an antiapoptotic protein, has been detected in large number of NECs and 100 % in the small cell subtype but not very commonly in NETs. Overexpression of Bcl-2 is significantly associated with higher mitotic rate.

Heparanase

A newly suggested marker of invasiveness in NETs, heparanase, has roles in degradation of extracellular matrix and with the enzymatic activity allows NETs to damage their extracellular matrix and to invade through endothelium. Higher heparanase expression is correlated with higher grade and stage of tumor and a tendency for

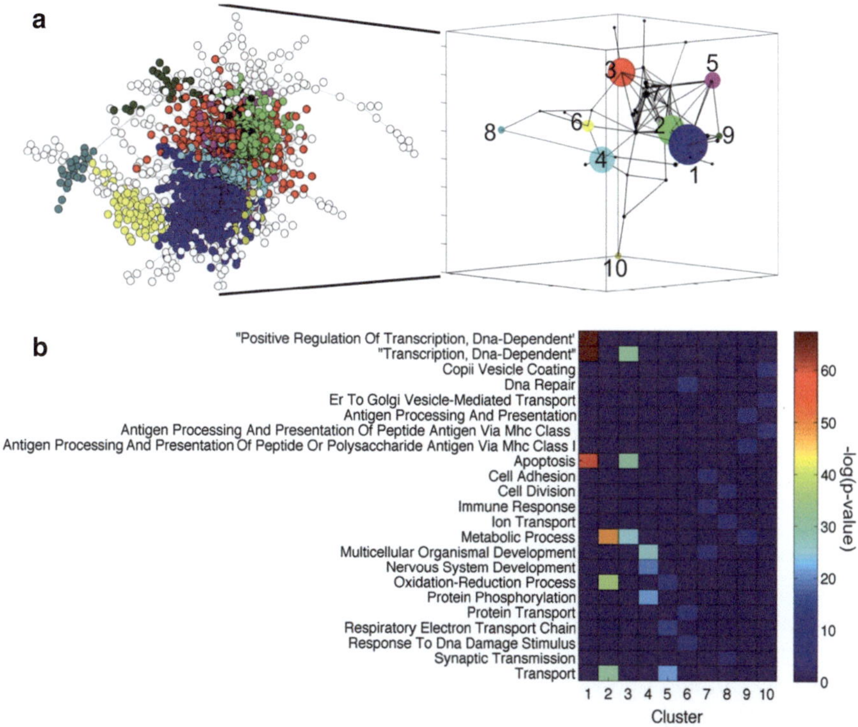

Fig. 2 GEP-NEN gene co-expression network. (**a**) Visualization of the GEP-NEN gene co-expression network (2545 genes, 30,249 edges). Each node represents a gene, while a link represents a GEP-NEN-specific co-expression. Nodes that localized to the same network community are marked in the same color. The community structure of the GEP-NEN network is further visualized in the three-dimensional inset, whereby each node represents a community while edges are drawn between communities that contain co-expressed genes. Larger nodes indicate bigger gene communities. (**b**) Heatmap visualizing enrichment for overrepresented gene ontology (GO) biological process (BP) terms assigned to the ten largest clusters (>20 genes). Heatmap colors represent the significance of the enrichment [25]

metastasis. Heparanase upregulation is associated with lymphangiogenesis and resulting dissemination in contrast to heparanase deletion, which results in endothelial cell aggregation and inhibiting the tumor from further spread [27].

p53 and Rb

High degree of abnormal immunolabeling of p53 and Rb has been discovered in high-grade neuroendocrine carcinomas but not in well-differentiated variant. The tumor suppressor p53 plays a critical role in maintaining genomic stability and tumor prevention and is tightly regulated by a number of proteins, including the critical negative regulators MDM2, MDM4, and WIP1. Extra gene copies of these proteins have been reported in Pancreatic NET, which may lead to an attenuated p53 function.

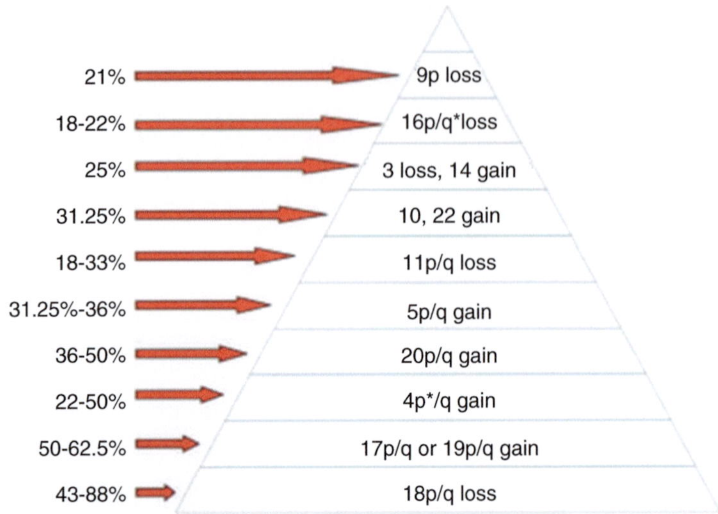

Fig. 3 GI carcinoid chromosomal aberrations [26]

Cyclin-dependent protein kinases (CDK) 4 and 6 are involved in phosphorylation of the retinoblastoma (Rb) tumor suppressor gene. Loss of Rb function results in unchecked transcriptional activation that can occur either by loss of Rb protein itself via RB1 gene mutations or by aberrations in other regulatory elements of the Rb pathway that increase phosphorylation of the Rb protein. Loss of Rb protein via RB1 gene mutation is frequently observed in poorly differentiated and high-grade NETs [21, 28].

Ataxia Telangiectasia Mutated (ATM) Gene

Ataxia telangiectasia mutated (ATM) gene is a regulator of cell cycle and down-regulation of ATM has been proposed as a promoter for metastasis. ATM is negatively correlated with metastatic behavior in 85 % of metastatic cases. The higher levels of ATM mRNA are associated with lower Ki-67 indices [27].

Other signaling pathways are involved in the tumor growth and include but not limited to inhibitory or activating G protein-coupled receptors, receptor tyrosine kinases, ligands, and intracellular targets such as the mammalian target of rapamycin (mTOR) [29].

Angiogenesis

NETs are vascular tumors and have a high expression of proangiogenic molecules, such as the angiogenic cytokine VEGF (vascular endothelial growth factor). c-Met is among the genes involved in the invasiveness and metastatic behavior of tumor cells. Inhibition of c-Met reduces the invasive and metastatic capabilities caused by VEGF-pathway inhibition [21].

mTOR Pathway

Mammalian target of rapamycin (mTOR) is a Ser/Thr protein kinase complex and is activated via phosphorylation through feedback regulatory loops and is a main regulator of different cell functions including growth, proliferation, and protein synthesis. Activation of the MTOR pathway may play a central role in the pathogenesis of NET, and strong MTOR expression is associated with higher proliferative index [22]. There are enough clues on the involvement of mTOR pathway in sporadic diseases and vast majority of well-differentiated NETs. mTOR activation in highly aggressive tumors is suggested as well [30]. mTOR forms two protein complexes known as mTORC1 and mTORC2, which have different activation loops and roles but with correlated function in pathogenesis of NETs. mTOR pathway components can be readily measured using immunohistochemical techniques [21, 22, 29].

Somatostatin Receptor Signaling

Somatostatin acts through a family of 5G protein-coupled receptors termed sst1–sst5 to exert a variety of functions, including inhibition of endocrine and exocrine secretions and tumor cell growth [21].

KIT and PDGFRA

In all the investigated cases of small cell NEC of esophagus, expression of KIT and PDGFRA (platelet-derived growth factor receptor, alpha polypeptide proteins) has been noticed as in its lung counterpart. There has not been any mutation of KIT (exons 9, 11, 13, and 17) and PDGFRA (exons 12 and 18) genes associated in any of the investigated cases [26, 31, 32].

Diagnosis

The diagnosis of esophageal NENs is confirmed by immunohistochemistry. Esophageal NETs express chromogranin (CgA) and synaptophysin (Syn) strongly, confirming the endocrine nature of the neoplastic cells. Neuron-specific enolase (NSE) has been used as general common biomarker. Less frequently, expression of serotonin, glucagon, or pancreatic polypeptide has been reported [33]. Poorly differentiated esophageal NECs commonly demonstrate no or very weak CgA positivity. Syn can be detected in all NETs. Other neuroendocrine markers including protein cell product 9.5, CD56, E-cadherin, and p53 have been used in the study of NETs but are not considered to have diagnostic value.

Carcinoids from the foregut are generally positive for CD56, while those from the hindgut are usually negative [27].

Similarly to the majority of pulmonary small cell carcinomas, esophageal small cell carcinomas frequently express TTF-1 (33–71 %) [34].

Based on one study by Yun et al. [35] showed the following immunohistochemistry profile, Syn, 95.2 %; CD56, 76.2 %; TTF-1, 71.4 %; NSE, 61.9 %; CgA, 61.9 %; CK, 57.1 %; EMA, 61.9 %; and S100, 19.0 %, whereas primary high-grade neuroendocrine carcinoma of the esophagus neoplastic cells is immunoreactive to synaptophysin (100 %), CD56 (93 %), chromogranin A (67 %), p63 (55 %), TTF1 (71 %), CK8/18 (90 %), CD117 (86 %), HER2 (16 %), and p16 (84 %) antibodies [36].

Treatment

Optimal management of early foregut NETs is controversial and generally a personalized approach based on the clinical characteristics, pathologic diagnosis, grade, and staging of each individual case is recommended.

In many phases of NET management, surgery is mainstay of treatment; however, multidisciplinary management has been shown to have superior results over surgery or radiotherapy alone. The treatment of choice for a localized limited NET is usually surgery. Esophagogastrectomy is a commonly used approach.

If NETs are diagnosed at early stages during the screening endoscopy due to low frequency of lymph node involvement or distant metastasis, they can usually be managed with endoscopic treatment. Small polypoid esophageal carcinoid tumors may be removed by polypectomy if the lesions are not deeply invasive. Deeply invasive esophageal carcinoid tumors have a poor prognosis even in the absence of metastases and require surgical resection.

Well-differentiated neuroendocrine carcinomas have an excellent prognosis and may even be cured with limited resection [10].

Treatment of SCNET of esophagus follows the treatment approach for small cell cancers of lung, but even with low stage disease, there is usually rapid dissemination within a year of diagnosis. With a multidisciplinary approach of chemotherapy combined with radiation therapy, patients with small cell neuroendocrine carcinoma of the esophagus may be able to achieve long-term survival without devastating surgery [12].

A multivariate analysis of esophageal small cell NEC by Shia et al. [37] identified the following three factors as adverse predictors on 2-year disease-specific survival: the absence of an associated adenocarcinoma component, the presence of synaptophysin staining, and high disease stage [12, 38].

General Management Approach

1. Tumor size <1 cm, clear margin, and no LN metastasis (usually are rarely metastatic thus good candidate for endoscopic approach): endoscopic resection
2. Tumor size >1 cm: surgical resection only or combined chemotherapy
3. Regional and distant metastasis: palliative chemotherapy [6, 10, 20]

Note: Chemotherapy has little value in the treatment of advanced esophageal NETs with aggressive clinical course.

Abbreviations

CG	Chromogranin
GEP-NETs	Gastroenteropancreatic neuroendocrine tumors
GI-NENs	Gastrointestinal neuroendocrine neoplasms
INETs	Ileal neuroendocrine tumors
MANEC	Mixed adenoneuroendocrine carcinoma
NEC	Neuroendocrine carcinoma
NEN	Neuroendocrine neoplasm
NET	Neuroendocrine tumor
NSE	Neuron-specific enolase
SCNEC	Small cell neuroendocrine carcinoma
Syn	Synaptophysin

References

1. Bennouna J, Bardet E, Deguiral P, Douillard JY. Small cell carcinoma of the esophagus: analysis of 10 cases and review of the published data. Am J Clin Oncol. 2000;23:455–9.
2. Attar BM, Levendoglu H, Rhee H. Small cell carcinoma of the esophagus. Report of three cases and review of the literature. Dig Dis Sci. 1990;35:145–52.
3. Fenoglio-Preiser CM. Gastrointestinal neuroendocrine/neuroectodermal tumors. Am J Clin Pathol. 2001;115(Suppl):S79–93.
4. Hirabayashi K, Zamboni G, Nishi T, Tanaka A, Kajiwara H, Nakamura N. Histopathology of gastrointestinal neuroendocrine neoplasms. Front Oncol. 2013;3:2.
5. Hamilton K, Chiappori A, Olson S, Sawyers J, Johnson D, Washington K. Prevalence and prognostic significance of neuroendocrine cells in esophageal adenocarcinoma. Mod Pathol. 2000;13:475–81.
6. Park MI. Endoscopic treatment for early foregut neuroendocrine tumors. Clin Endosc. 2013;46:450–5.
7. Nawroz IM. Malignant carcinoid tumour of oesophagus. Histopathology. 1987;11:879–80.
8. Ready AR, Soul JO, Newman J, Matthews HR. Malignant carcinoid tumour of the oesophagus. Thorax. 1989;44:594–6.
9. Estrozi B, Bacchi CE. Neuroendocrine tumors involving the gastroenteropancreatic tract: a clinicopathological evaluation of 773 cases. Clinics. 2011;66:1671–5.

10. Lee CG, Lim YJ, Park SJ, Jang BI, Choi SR, Kim JK, Kim YT, Cho JY, Yang CH, Chun HJ, Song SY. Neuroendocrine tumor study g. The clinical features and treatment modality of esophageal neuroendocrine tumors: a multicenter study in Korea. BMC Cancer. 2014;14:569.
11. Yekeler E, Koca T, Vural S. A rare cause of the cough: primary small cell carcinoma of esophagus-case report. Case Rep Med. 2012;2012:870783.
12. Funakoshi S, Hashiguchi A, Teramoto K, Miyata N, Kurita S, Adachi M, Hamamoto Y, Higuchi H, Takaishi H, Hibi T. Second-line chemotherapy for refractory small cell neuroendocrine carcinoma of the esophagus that relapsed after complete remission with irinotecan plus cisplatin therapy: case report and review of the literature. Oncol Lett. 2013;5:117–22.
13. Ando T, Hosokawa A, Yamawaki H, Hasumoto Y, Kajiura S, Itaya Y, Ueda A, Suzuki N, Nishikawa J, Fujinami H, Miyazaki T, Ogawa K, Sugiyama T. Esophageal small-cell carcinoma with syndrome of inappropriate secretion of antidiuretic hormone. Intern Med. 2011;50:1099–103.
14. Jankowski JA, Wright NA, Meltzer SJ, Triadafilopoulos G, Geboes K, Casson AG, Kerr D, Young LS. Molecular evolution of the metaplasia-dysplasia-adenocarcinoma sequence in the esophagus. Am J Pathol. 1999;154:965–73.
15. Yang L, Sun X, Zou Y, Meng X. Small cell type neuroendocrine carcinoma colliding with squamous cell carcinoma at esophagus. Int J Clin Exp Pathol. 2014;7:1792–5.
16. Gumprich T, Johnen G, Hummel T, Jaworska M, Schmitz I, Muller KM. A rare case of a neuroendocrine carcinoma of the esophagus. Intermediate between a well-differentiated neuroendocrine carcinoma and a low-differentiated neuroendocrine carcinoma. Pathologe. 2004;25:229–34.
17. Maru DM, Khurana H, Rashid A, Correa AM, Anandasabapathy S, Krishnan S, Komaki R, Ajani JA, Swisher SG, Hofstetter WL. Retrospective study of clinicopathologic features and prognosis of high-grade neuroendocrine carcinoma of the esophagus. Am J Surg Pathol. 2008;32:1404–11.
18. Al Mansoor S, Ziske C, Schmidt-Wolf IG. Primary small cell carcinoma of the esophagus: patient data metaanalysis and review of the literature. Ger Med Sci. 2013;11:Doc12.
19. Brenner B, Shah MA, Gonen M, Klimstra DS, Shia J, Kelsen DP. Small-cell carcinoma of the gastrointestinal tract: a retrospective study of 64 cases. Br J Cancer. 2004;90:1720–6.
20. Yagi M, Abe Y, Sasaki Y, Nomura E, Sato T, Iwano D, Yoshizawa K, Sakuta K, Kanno N, Nishise S, Ueno Y. Esophageal carcinoid tumor treated by endoscopic resection. Dig Endosc. 2015;27:527–30.
21. Oberg K, Casanovas O, Castano JP, Chung D, Delle Fave G, Denefle P, Harris P, Khan MS, Kulke MH, Scarpa A, Tang LH, Wiedenmann B. Molecular pathogenesis of neuroendocrine tumors: implications for current and future therapeutic approaches. Clin Cancer Res. 2013;19:2842–9.
22. Qian ZR, Ter-Minassian M, Chan JA, Imamura Y, Hooshmand SM, Kuchiba A, Morikawa T, Brais LK, Daskalova A, Heafield R, Lin X, Christiani DC, Fuchs CS, Ogino S, Kulke MH. Prognostic significance of MTOR pathway component expression in neuroendocrine tumors. J Clin Oncol. 2013;31:3418–25.
23. Capdevila J, Meeker A, Garcia-Carbonero R, Pietras K, Astudillo A, Casanovas O, Scarpa A. Molecular biology of neuroendocrine tumors: from pathways to biomarkers and targets. Cancer Metastasis Rev. 2014;33:345–51.
24. Kidd M, Modlin IM, Bodei L, Drozdov I. Decoding the molecular and mutational ambiguities of gastroenteropancreatic neuroendocrine neoplasm pathobiology. Gastroenterol Hepatol. 2015;1:131–53.
25. Modlin IM, Drozdov I, Kidd M. The identification of gut neuroendocrine tumor disease by multiple synchronous transcript analysis in blood. PLoS One. 2013;8:e63364.
26. Zikusoka MN, Kidd M, Eick G, Latich I, Modlin IM. The molecular genetics of gastroenteropancreatic neuroendocrine tumors. Cancer. 2005;104:2292–309.
27. Lewis MA, Yao JC. Molecular pathology and genetics of gastrointestinal neuroendocrine tumours. Curr Opin Endocrinol Diabetes Obes. 2014;21:22–7.

28. Yachida S, Vakiani E, White CM, Zhong Y, Saunders T, Morgan R, de Wilde RF, Maitra A, Hicks J, Demarzo AM, Shi C, Sharma R, Laheru D, Edil BH, Wolfgang CL, Schulick RD, Hruban RH, Tang LH, Klimstra DS, Iacobuzio-Donahue CA. Small cell and large cell neuroendocrine carcinomas of the pancreas are genetically similar and distinct from well-differentiated pancreatic neuroendocrine tumors. Am J Surg Pathol. 2012;36:173–84.
29. Pavel M. Translation of molecular pathways into clinical trials of neuroendocrine tumors. Neuroendocrinology. 2013;97:99–112.
30. Cingarlini S, Bonomi M, Corbo V, Scarpa A, Tortora G. Profiling MTOR pathway in neuroendocrine tumors. Target Oncol. 2012;7:183–8.
31. Terada T. Small cell neuroendocrine carcinoma of the esophagus: report of 6 cases with immunohistochemical and molecular genetic analysis of KIT and PDGFRA. Int J Clin Exp Pathol. 2013;6:485–91.
32. Terada T. Esophageal small cell carcinoma without neuroendocrine features but with KIT and PDGFRA expression: kit as a useful marker of this type of tumor. J Gastrointest Cancer. 2014;45 Suppl 1:132–5.
33. Wong HH, Chu P. Immunohistochemical features of the gastrointestinal tract tumors. J Gastrointest Oncol. 2012;3:262–84.
34. Yamamoto J, Ohshima K, Ikeda S, Iwashita A, Kikuchi M. Primary esophageal small cell carcinoma with concomitant invasive squamous cell carcinoma or carcinoma in situ. Hum Pathol. 2003;34:1108–15.
35. Yun JP, Zhang MF, Hou JH, Tian QH, Fu J, Liang XM, Wu QL, Rong TH. Primary small cell carcinoma of the esophagus: clinicopathological and immunohistochemical features of 21 cases. BMC Cancer. 2007;7:38.
36. Huang Q, Wu H, Nie L, Shi J, Lebenthal A, Chen J, Sun Q, Yang J, Huang L, Ye Q. Primary high-grade neuroendocrine carcinoma of the esophagus: a clinicopathologic and immunohistochemical study of 42 resection cases. Am J Surg Pathol. 2013;37:467–83.
37. Shia J, Tang LH, Weiser MR, Brenner B, Adsay NV, Stelow EB, Saltz LB, Qin J, Landmann R, Leonard GD, Dhall D, Temple L, Guillem JG, Paty PB, Kelsen D, Wong WD, Klimstra DS. Is nonsmall cell type high-grade neuroendocrine carcinoma of the tubular gastrointestinal tract a distinct disease entity? Am J Surg Pathol. 2008;32:719–31.
38. Gollard R, Ellis C, VanderHarten C. Small cell/neuroendocrine tumors of the esophagus: presentation of two cases and review of the literature. Tumori. 2010;96:780–3.

Neuroendocrine Neoplasms of the Stomach

Evita Henderson-Jackson, Ujalla Sheikh, Jalil Muhammad, Domenico Coppola, and Aejaz Nasir

Introduction

Neuroendocrine neoplasms of the stomach include neuroendocrine tumors (NETs) and neuroendocrine carcinomas (NECAs). The gastric neuroendocrine tumors (G-NETs) or gastric carcinoids (GCs) arise in enterochromaffin-like (ECL) cells in the stomach cells that play a role in the regulation of gastric acid production. These tumors are increasingly diagnosed at endoscopy and account for 0.6–2 % of all gastric polyps identified [1–4]. Gastric NETs represent almost a quarter of all gastroenteropancreatic neuroendocrine tumors (GEP-NETs) [5] with an incidence of 0.002–0.1 per 100,000 population per year [6–8]. In Japan the incidence of G-NETs is higher representing 30 % of all gastrointestinal NETs. This may be due to the high incidence of chronic atrophic gastritis as well as intensive endoscopy screening [9]. The majority of G-NETs are incidentally diagnosed by histologic examination of "simple" gastric polyps identified at endoscopy, which is the dominant diagnostic, therapeutic, and surveillance modality for G-NETs. Originally, there were three types of GCs (G-NETs) described by Rindi et al.: type I and type II related to hypergastrinemia and type II which occurs sporadically and independent of gastrin [10]. Subsequently, type IV has been identified as high-grade poorly differentiated neuroendocrine carcinoma (NECA), which is also sporadic malignancy. There are

E. Henderson-Jackson, MD • U. Sheikh, MD • D. Coppola, MD
Department of Anatomic Pathology, Moffitt Cancer Center, Tampa, FL, USA

J. Muhammad
George Mason University, Falls Church, VA, USA

A. Nasir, MD, MPhil, FCAP (✉)
Diagnostic & Experimental Pathology (Tailored Therapeutics),
Lilly Research laboratories, Eli Lilly & Co.,
893 South Delaware St., Building 98C/2C, Room 2391, Indianapolis, IN, USA
e-mail: nasirae@lilly.com

A. Nasir, D. Coppola (eds.), *Neuroendocrine Tumors: Review of Pathology, Molecular and Therapeutic Advances*, DOI 10.1007/978-1-4939-3426-3_12

important epidemiological, pathophysiological, endoscopic, and histologic differences between each type that affects prognosis, management, and follow-up [11].

Epidemiology

According to SEER database in the United States, the incidence of gastric NETs has increased from 2.2 % between 1950 and 1969 to 6.0 % between 2000 and 2007 [3, 4]. This increase in incidence can be explained by factors like increased access to endoscopy (including repeated procedures and surveillance programs), more widespread biopsies of "simple" gastric polyps, improved immunohistologic assessment, and greater understanding of G-NETs [12, 13]. However, the overall incidence of diagnosed G-NETs remains low at 0.2 cases per 100, 000 population with a significantly higher prevalence resulting from a favorable prognosis [5]. Women are increasingly diagnosed with G-NETs, rising from 55 % in 1970 to 66 % in 2010, reflecting a changing gender distribution [14, 15]. This may relate to the increased use of endoscopy to diagnose "incidental"-type I G-NETs that are more prevalent in women.

Etiology and Pathogenesis of Gastric NETs

Physiologically, the hormone gastrin acts on ECL cells to regulate gastric acid production [16]. On ingestion of a meal, G cells in the gastric antrum secrete gastrin that then binds to cholecystokinin-2 receptors on ECL cells in the gastric body and fundus. ECL cells release histamine to stimulate gastric parietal cells to produce hydrochloric acid. As part of a negative feedback loop in acid conditions, antral D cells secrete the hormone somatostatin that acts on G cells to inhibit the production of gastrin [17]. Pathologically, lack of gastric acid production (achlorhydria), as in chronic atrophic gastritis, results in hyperplasia of antral G cells to augment gastrin secretion. Hypergastrinemia causes compensatory hyperplasia and proliferation of ECL cells through growth factors in order to increase acid production [18, 19] and, working with other cofactors, can also mediate the development of G-NETs from ECL cells [20]. Both type I and II G-NETs mainly develop through the morphologic sequence of "hyperplasia–dysplasia–neoplasia" [21, 22]. There is no hypergastrinemia or abnormal gastric acidity in type III or type IV G-NETs, both of which occur as sporadic neoplasms.

Diagnostic Approach

Approach to diagnosis and prognostication of gastric NETs is multidisciplinary and includes the following modalities.

Endoscopy

Careful inspection of the mucosa for multiple small lesions is advised, as type I and type II G-NETs are commonly multifocal. The size of the largest lesion should be recorded as type I G-NETs <1 cm, which do not require additional assessment or resection. Type I G-NETs >1 cm require assessment with endoscopic ultrasound (EUS) and imaging for locally invasive, nodal, and metastatic disease prior to resection.

Gastric Biopsies

Biopsies should be taken from the suspected G-NET lesion plus two non-lesional biopsies from gastric antrum and four biopsies from the gastric body/fundus to help identify the G-NET type by assessing for the presence of atrophic gastritis and intestinal metaplasia [11, 23].

An assessment of *H. pylori* status should be made as infection is associated with atrophic gastritis in type I G-NETs as well as sporadic type III G-NETs [24]. pH testing of gastric fluid may offer clarification when there is uncertainty over the G-NET type; type I has a higher pH (>4), and type II has a lower pH (<2) than normal.

Biochemical Investigations

Fasting serum gastrin levels are elevated in type I and 2 G-NETs but not in type III G-NETs. Levels are also elevated in patients treated with acid suppression therapy. Levels >1000 pg/mL with a pH <2 are diagnostic of Zollinger-Ellison syndrome (ZES), although the majority of cases do not reach these levels. CgA (chromogranin A) is secreted by ECL cells, particularly under the influence of gastrin, and is the most useful serum diagnostic marker for NETs with high sensitivity and correlation with tumor burden and liver metastases [25–27]. However, CgA can be raised in patients on proton pump inhibitor (PPI) therapy as well as in the presence of chronic atrophic gastritis alone.

Imaging

The investigation of G-NETs is dependent on the histologic type and the associated risk of locally advanced or metastatic disease. The role of more specialized investigations, like EUS and somatostatin receptor scintigraphy, again depends on histologic type [28]. Positive somatostatin receptor imaging with indium-111-labeled pentetreotide (OctreoScan) may help with tailoring therapy. The role of fluorodeoxyglucose (FDG)–positron emission tomography (PET) remains unclear in G1 or G2 tumors, but is of greater utility in metabolically active G3 NECAs.

Histopathologic Classification

Most gastric NETs are well-differentiated, nonfunctioning enterochromaffin-like cell carcinoids (ECL cell NETs), arising in gastric body and fundus. The diagnosis of G-NETs is confirmed by histopathologic examination of the tissue specimen. All gastric NETs are identifiable at histology by their characteristic histomorphologic features and immunohistochemical staining for the neuroendocrine markers like CgA and synaptophysin (Syn) [29, 30]. Recently, the term "neuroendocrine tumor" (NET) has been adopted by the World Health Organization (WHO) to define "carcinoids" [31], and the new classification schemes provided by the European Neuroendocrine Tumor Society (ENETS) have been accepted for site-specific grading and staging [31, 32].

Broadly, gastric NETs are divided into well-differentiated and poorly differentiated categories. They have also been subclassified into four distinct types: (1) type I, associated with chronic atrophic gastritis/pernicious anemia (70–80 %); (2) type II, associated with MENI and ZES (5 %); (3) type III, sporadic (15–20 %); and (4) type IV, poorly differentiated NECAs, which are rare [33–35] (Table 1).

Gross

Type I NETs are frequently multiple, less than 1.5 cm (97 %), tan nodules or polyps in the gastric mucosa or submucosa that involve muscularis propria in a minority of cases. Type II gastric NETs result in gastric wall thickening due to severe hypertrophic hypersecretory gastropathy or multiple mucosal or submucosal tumors, <1.5 cm in 75 % of cases. Type III NETs are >2 cm (33 %) solitary, sometime ulcerated, tumors that can cause significant hemorrhage. They arise in the background of histologically normal gastric mucosa with frequent infiltration of muscularis propria (76 %) and serosa (58 %) [35]. Type IV (NECAs) may form large infiltrative gastric tumor mass with frequent lymph node and liver metastases [36]. Mixed adenoneuroendocrine carcinoma (MANEC) grossly resembles conventional gastric carcinomas [31].

Microscopic

Microscopically, well-differentiated gastric NETs demonstrate characteristic nesting, trabecular, or gyriform patterns with relatively uniform neoplastic cells with granular cytoplasm (Fig. 1a). Immunoexpression of neuroendocrine markers, such as chromogranin and synaptophysin, is strong and diffuse [32].

Table 1 Subtypes of gastric NETs

Criteria	Type I	Type II	Type III	Type IV
Frequency	70–80 % of cases	5 %	15–20 % of cases	Rare
Focality	Multifocal	Multifocal	Solitary	Solitary
Size	0.5–1.0 cm	1.5 cm or less	Variable	Large
Location within the stomach	Corpus (body)	Corpus (body)	Anywhere	Anywhere
Clinical associations	Hypergastrinemic states; chronic atrophic gastritis enterochromaffin-like cell (ECL) hyperplasia, pernicious anemia	Multiple endocrine neoplasia (MEN) type I, with hypergastrinemia or Zollinger-Ellison syndrome (ZES)	Sporadic	Sporadic
Clinical behavior	Usually benign	30 % metastasize	71 % >2 cm with muscularis propria and vascular invasion, lymph node metastases	High-grade carcinoma Metastases common; poor prognosis
Demographic profile	70–80 % females, 50–60 years of age	Males = females, mean age 50	More common in males, mean age 55	More common in males

ECL Cell NETs

Most gastric NETs consist predominantly of ECL cells (ECL cell carcinoids), stain for vesicular monoamine transporter 2 (VMAT2), and contain vesicular secretory granules [10, 37, 38]. ECL cell carcinoids can also contain minor component of serotonin, ghrelin, gastrin, somatostatin, pancreatic polypeptide (PP), or alpha-human chorionic gonadotropin staining neoplastic cells [10, 39]. Majority of type I and type II and a minority of type III ECL cell NETs consist of small aggregates of uniform neoplastic cells with regular, monomorphic nuclei, inapparent nucleoli, and rather abundant, fairly eosinophilic cytoplasm. Mitoses are almost absent, and angioinvasion is infrequent [40]. These neoplasms will be consistent with the histologic grade G1 in the current grading system [41]. Type III sporadic ECL cell NETs often display more aggressive histology with solid or trabecular pattern of round, spindled, or polyhedral neoplastic cells, large vesicular nuclei, prominent eosinophilic nucleoli, scarce necrosis, and considerable mitotic activity, including atypical mitoses (mean mitotic count 9/10 HPF) and high Ki67 index (mean about 1000/10 HPFs), consistent with histologic grade G2 [41]. Type III NETs frequently show angiolymphatic invasion and are deeply invasive with local spread and/or distant metastases [40].

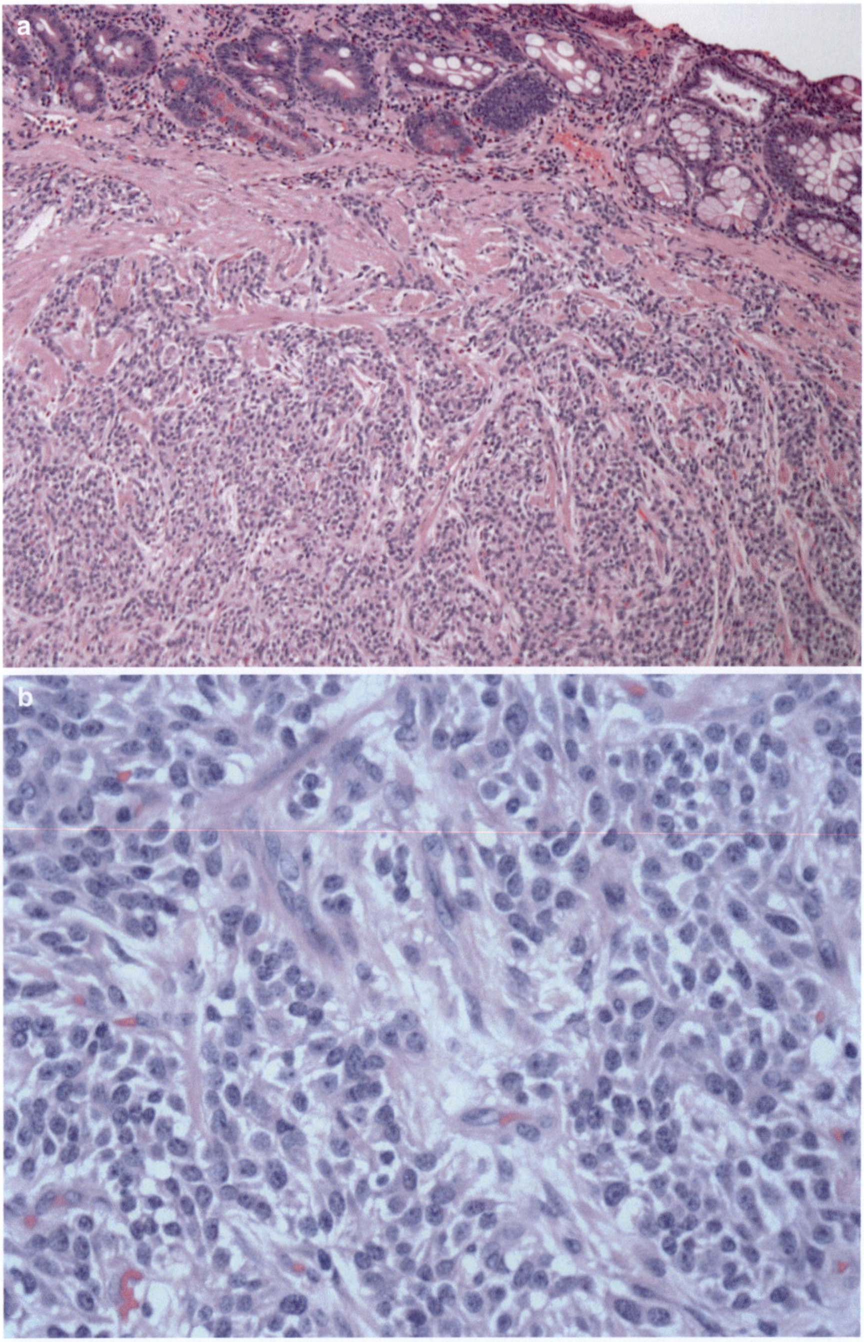

Fig. 1 Type I gastric NET, well-differentiated (G1) featuring nested pattern of uniform neoplastic cells, in a background of chronic atrophic gastritis with intestinal metaplasia (**a**). Tumor cell nuclei are uniform without any obvious mitoses (**b**). Ki-67 index is low (**c**)

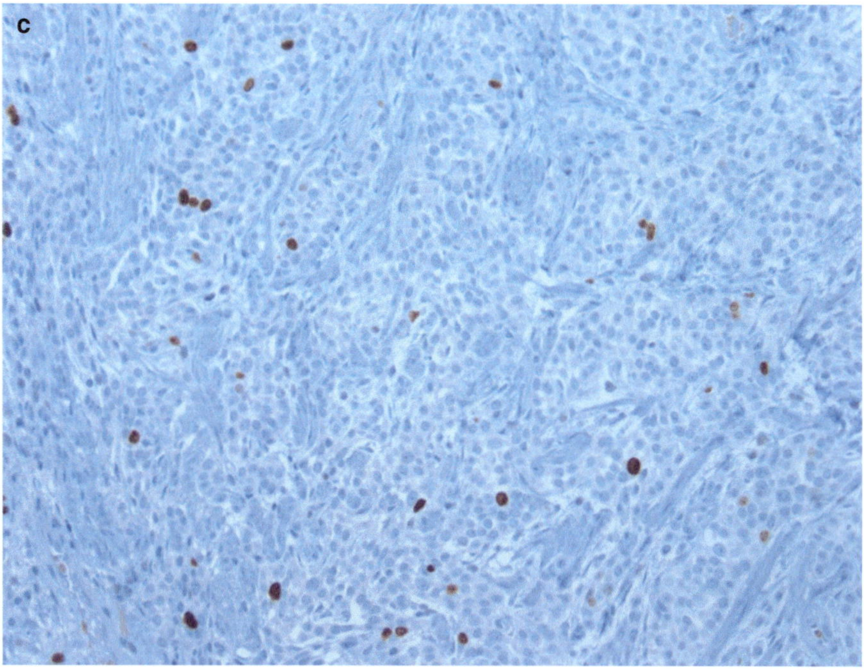

Fig. 1 (continued)

ECL Cell Serotonin-Producing NETs

Histologically similar to ileal NETs, these are very rare in the stomach [10, 42]. Apart from CgA and Syn, tumor cells are also immunoreactive for serotonin.

Gastrin-Producing NETs (Gastrinomas)

These are very rare in the stomach [43]. They tend to form small mucosal–submucosal nodules near the pylorus or in the duodenum and show thin trabecular gyriform or solid pattern of uniform neoplastic cells (Fig. 2a, b) with predominant immunoreactivity for gastrin (Fig. 2c) [31].

Gastric Neuroendocrine Carcinomas (Poorly Differentiated, Small-Cell, Large-Cell NECAs)

These make up 6–16 % of gastric NETs [31] with male predominance. Microscopically, they consist of large poorly formed trabeculae, nests, or sheets of anaplastic, variable-sized, round, or polyhedral to spindle cells that stain for general

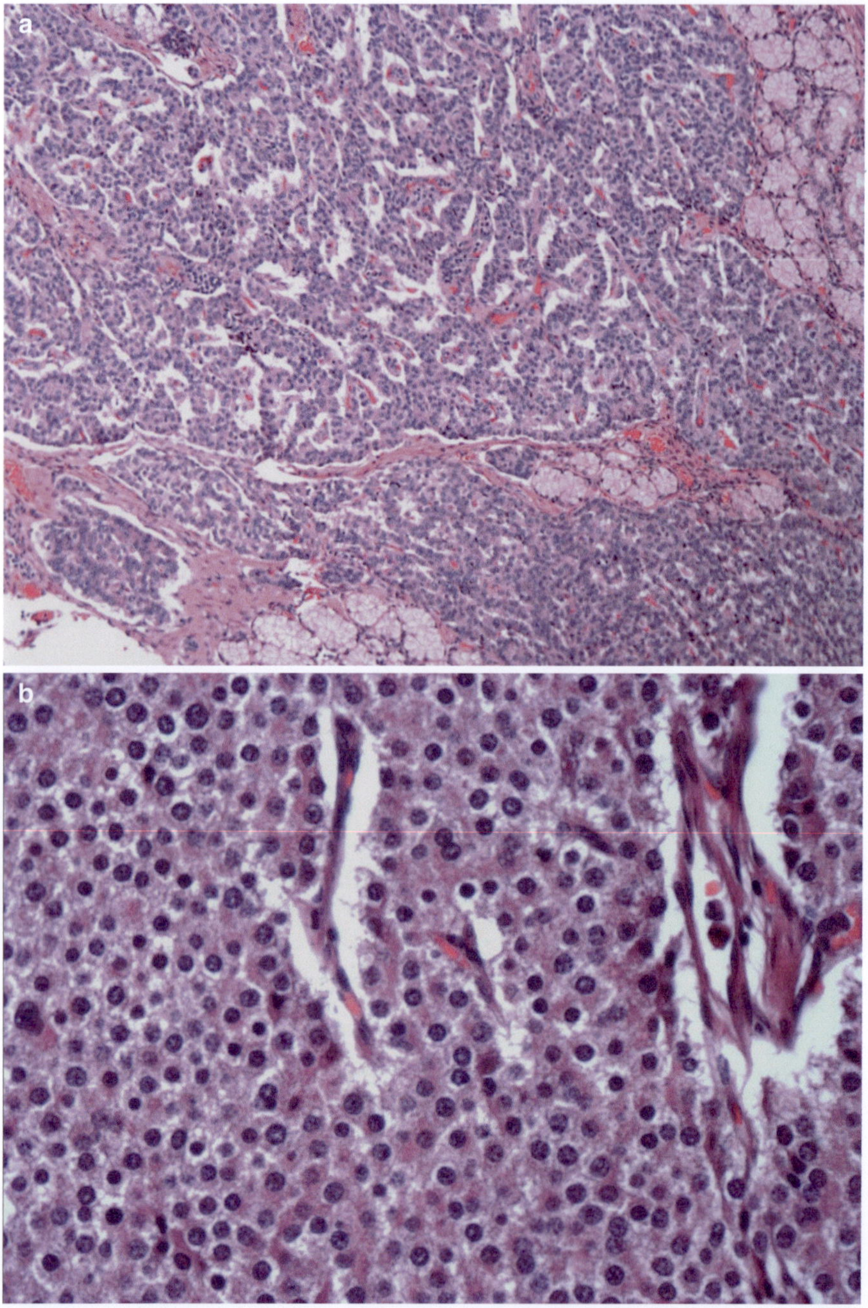

Fig. 2 Gastrin-producing NET (gastrinoma) arising in duodenal wall, featuring trabecular growth pattern (**a**) and uniform round neoplastic cells (**b**) and distinct tumor cell immunostaining for gastrin (**c**)

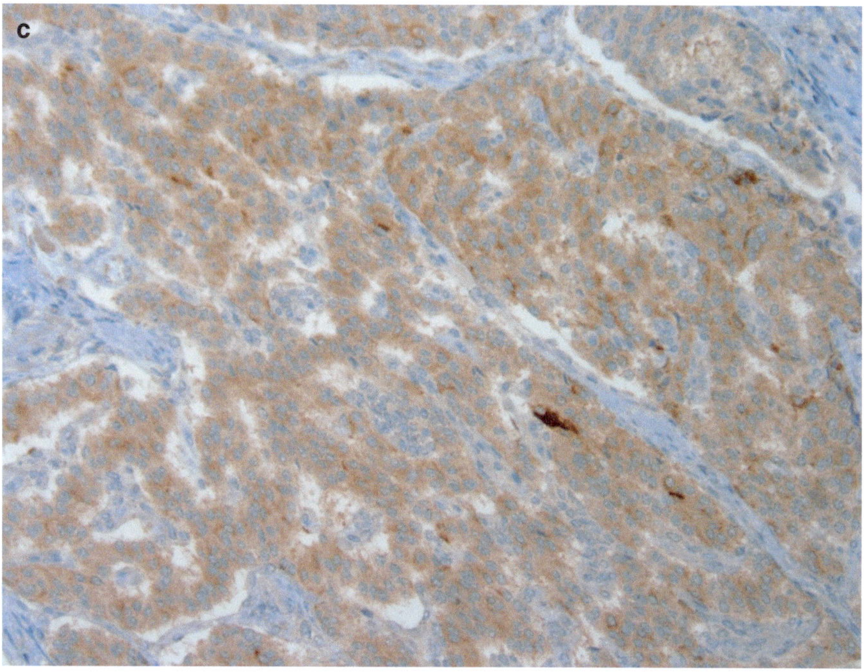

Fig. 2 (continued)

neuroendocrine markers like, CGA, Syn, CD56, PGP9.5, and NSE (Fig. 3a, b) [10, 32, 40, 44, 45]. Often, these are high-grade malignancies with high mitotic rate (>20 mitoses/10HPF) and very high Ki67 index (Fig. 3c), consistent with histologic grade G3 in the current guidelines [41]. Based on cell size and nuclear structure, these are further grouped into small-cell NECAs with fine nuclear chromatin and large-cell neuroendocrine carcinomas (LCNECAs) with more vesicular nuclei and prominent nucleoli [31]. Gastric epithelial malignancies with histologic features suspicious of neuroendocrine differentiation and with an NE marker expression in >50 and 1 % to approximately 50 % tumor cells by expressing chromogranin A and/or synaptophysin have been defined as LCNECAs and adenocarcinoma with neuroendocrine differentiation (ACNED), respectively [44]. LCNECAs demonstrate less predominant NE morphology than carcinoids and may show solid, tubular, and scirrhous growth patterns.

Gastric MANECs

Mixed adenoneuroendocrine carcinoma (MANEC) of the stomach is an invasive carcinoma with exocrine and endocrine components, one of which is more than 30 % [31].

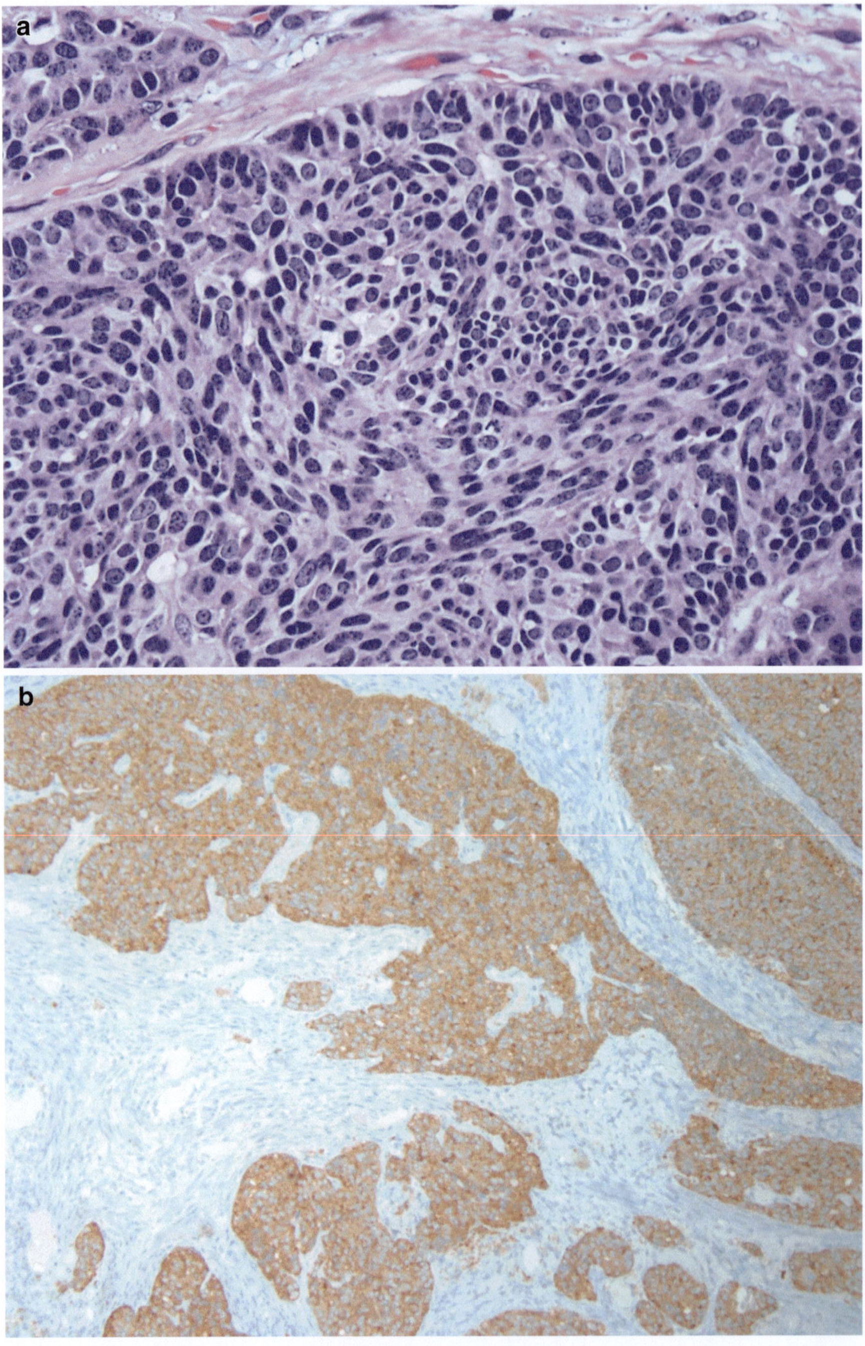

Fig. 3 Poorly differentiated neuroendocrine carcinoma (G3) arising within the stomach, composed of large, poorly formed nests/sheets of round, polyhedral to spindle-shaped cells (**a**), and immunoreactive for synaptophysin (**b**). Ki-67 index is high (**c**)

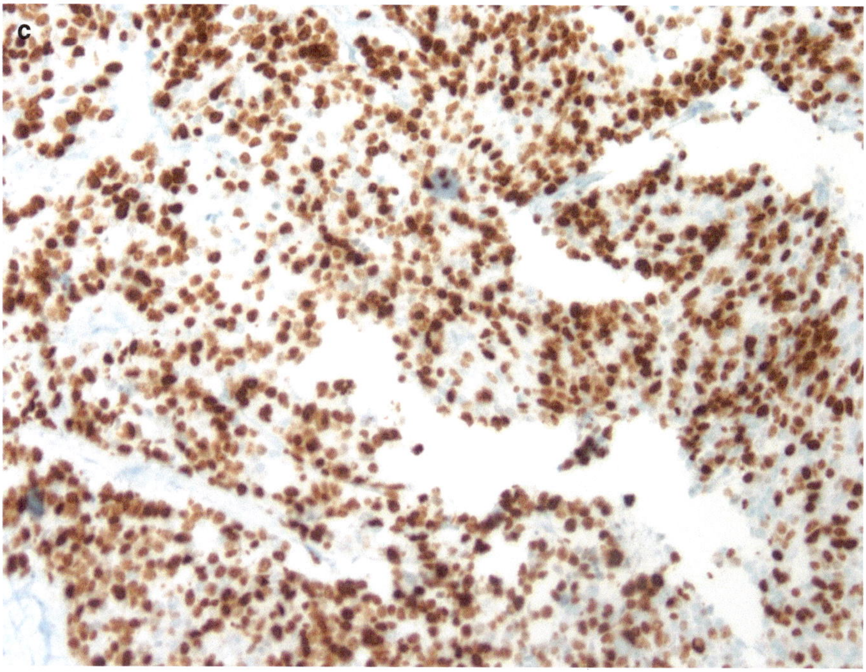

Fig. 3 (continued)

Histologic Grading

The histologic grading of G-NETs is based on differentiation. The mitotic count in 10 high-power fields HPF (1 HPF = 2 mm^2) and the Ki67 index are used to determine the grade of G-NETs. The 2010 WHO histologic classification utilizes the Ki67 index to grade G-NETs as part of gastroenteropancreatic (GEP) NETs [31]. Well-differentiated G-NETs have a low (G1) grade with a Ki67 index of ≤2 % or intermediate grade (G2) with Ki67 index of 3–20 %. Poorly differentiated NECAs have a high grade (G3) with a Ki67 index of >20 % (Table 2) [41]. Some of the challenges with Ki67 index are intra- and interobserver variability and inconsistency in differentiating G1 and G2 tumors [46]. Some investigators have suggested a Ki67 cutoff of 5 % to differentiate between G1 and G2 and in predicting survival and recurrence in other NETs [47, 48].

Prognosis of Gastric NETs

The most critical factor for prognostication is the type of G-NET; other variables that predict malignancy in G-NETs include size, invasion, and grade [40]. Most type I, autoimmune chronic atrophic gastritis (A-CAG)-associated gastric NETs, have excellent prognosis like the majority of type II MEN1-ZES-associated gastric

Table 2 Grading classification for neuroendocrine tumors of the stomach, duodenum, and pancreas by Rindi et al. [41]

Grade	Mitotic count per 10 HPF	Ki67 proliferative index
1	<2	≤2
2	2–20	3–20
3	>20	>20

Grading requires mitotic count in at least 50 HPFs and Ki67 index using the MIB antibody as a percentage of 500–2000 cells counted in areas of strongest nuclear labeling

NETs [10, 35]. Invasion of muscularis propria or beyond, size >1 cm, angioinvasion, presence of endocrine syndrome, high mitotic activity (grade G2), and sporadic occurrence are associated with aggressive behavior in ECL cell NETs [10, 35, 40, 49]. Prognosis of gastric NECAs is uniformly poor [40, 50], including for LCNECAs, which tend to be significantly more aggressive than conventional gastric adenocarcinomas [44]. Most patients present with deeply invasive, advanced-stage disease and short survival [31].

Type I Gastric NETs

Pathogenesis: Hypergastrinemia, Chronic Atrophic Gastritis, and Achlorhydria

Several conditions associated with achlorhydria (chronic atrophic gastritis, vagotomy, and chronic acid suppression therapy) result in hypergastrinemia [17], although not all are associated with increased prevalence of G-NETs [51]. Both enterochromaffin-like cell dysplasia and severe ECL cell hyperplasia are associated with increased risk of G-NET development in type A chronic atrophic gastritis with hypergastrinemia/G-cell hyperplasia [52].

Experimental studies in rats have shown development of type I gastric NETs following prolonged H2-receptor antagonist therapy [53]. In humans, chronic proton pump inhibitor (PPI) therapy is associated with ECL cell hyperplasia, which is seen in 10–30 % of patients who are infected with *Helicobacter pylori* [54]. These infected patients have a greater prevalence of atrophic gastritis and markedly higher gastrin levels. In animal models, *H. pylori* lipopolysaccharides and peptidoglycans have been shown to cause proliferation of ECL cells [55].

Diagnosis

Type I G-NETs represent 74–78 % of all G-NETs and are more common in women [10, 33]. They are associated with pernicious anemia and autoimmune chronic atrophic gastritis. However, only 5 % of patients with chronic atrophic gastritis develop type I G-NET with 2.4 % at the time of diagnosis and a low annual incidence (0.4 %) [23, 33, 56]. They are nonfunctioning tumors and become symptomatic when they ulcerate and can result in bleeding and anemia. The associated atrophic gastritis can cause both B12 and iron deficiency and dyspepsia from slow gastric emptying [57]. The diagnosis should be considered on endoscopy for gastric polyps in patients with atrophic gastritis and/or B12 and iron deficiency.

Type I G-NETs are often found in the gastric fundus and are mostly polypoid (78 %), small (size 5–8 mm), and multicentric [58, 59]. Characteristic features include an irregularly shaped erythematous depression or central ulcer [60]. Almost a quarter of type I G-NETs are microcarcinoids that are diagnosed at histology or through narrowband imaging and high-resolution magnification endoscopy [61–63]. Gastric pH is elevated (>4) because of a lack of parietal cells secreting acid. Elevated serum CgA is more specific (55–85 %) than elevated serum gastrin (35–55 %) in type I G-NETs as hypergastrinemia is also present in chronic atrophic gastritis without G-NET [58, 64].

Most type I G-NETs are G1 tumors (82.7 %) with a low Ki67 (Fig. 1a–c) that present with stage I (73.9 %) disease limited to the mucosa or submucosa [58, 65]. They rarely invade the muscularis propria or metastasize to local lymph nodes if <1 cm. Patients diagnosed with type I G-NET have an excellent prognosis, even with metastatic disease, and have normal life expectancy and no associated mortality [24, 58, 65, 66]. Type I G-NETs are recurring tumors (median time 24 months), due to persistent antral-mediated hypergastrinemia, with 3 % developing poorly differentiated G3 NECAs [21].

Rarely composite carcinoid–adenocarcinoma lesions are found in lesions >2 cm and represent two pathophysiological processes associated with atrophic gastritis: G-NET development from ECL cell hyperplasia and adenocarcinoma development from *H. pylori*-associated intestinal metaplasia [67–72]. Nonlesional gastric biopsies may reveal gastric mucosal atrophy, which may be severe [59]. Gastric pH testing (>4) can support the diagnosis of type I G-NETs in cases where gastric atrophy is not obvious. Associated autoimmune conditions like pernicious anemia, diabetes mellitus, Hashimoto's thyroiditis, and primary biliary cirrhosis should be considered and appropriately investigated. H. pylori status should be also assessed because of its association with intestinal metaplasia and gastric adenocarcinoma.

For lesions ≤1 cm, there is no indication for further assessment as they are invariably confined to the mucosa or submucosa. For lesions >1 cm, EUS is useful to assess for invasion beyond the submucosa prior to resection [59, 73]. For lesions >2 cm, CT or MRI is recommended to assess for invasion and nodal disease. Functional imaging with OctreoScan is unlikely to reveal any additional lesions above conventional imaging in early resectable disease [58]. Somatostatin receptor imaging positivity may indicate a role for somatostatin analogues (SSAs) in advanced, unresectable, or residual G-NETs [74].

Treatment

The majority of type I G-NETs are managed by endoscopy. Lesions <1 cm should undergo annual endoscopic surveillance as they have a low risk of invasion or metastasis. Lesions >1 cm should be resected, as there is a small risk of lymph node metastases. Endoscopic mucosal resection (EMR) is indicated if EUS demonstrates the lesion to be localized to the mucosa or submucosa. Endoscopic submucosal dissection (ESD) can be performed for larger lesions and/or those not are amenable to EMR [75–78]. Endoscopic resection of nonmetastatic localized lesions <2 cm with ≤6 lesions has been demonstrated to be as effective as surgical resection. For more advanced lesions >1 cm, with EUS-assessed involvement of the muscularis propria and/or local lymph nodes, surgical resection is indicated. Gastric antrectomy for type I G-NET is an option for patients with multifocal (>6 lesions, 3–4 lesions >1 cm or 1 lesion >2 cm), invasive, or recurrent disease. Antrectomy removes G cells-mediated hypergastrinemia that leads to regression of G-NET lesions in over 90 % of cases [33, 58, 79].

Somatostatin analogues (SSAs) act on G cells to suppress gastrin secretion that drives ECL cell hyperplasia and may also exert a direct antiproliferative effect on ECL cells via somatostatin receptors (SSTRs). SSAs may have a role in reducing tumor burden and progression in type I G-NETs, especially if multiple [80, 81], and may cause reduction or normalization in gastrin and CgA levels. The majority of patients will have complete regression of lesions or a reduction in tumor size at follow-up endoscopy, though lesions soon recur after cessation of SSA therapy. Netazepide (Trio Medicines Ltd, England) is a new orally active selective antagonist of the gastrin/CCK-2 receptor that has been shown to reduce gastric acid secretion [82, 83], normalize plasma CgA, and cause regression of type 1 G-NETs with a reduction in the number and size of the largest lesions at 12 weeks' posttreatment [84, 85]. Endoscopic surveillance is recommended annually for unresected lesions <1 cm and for recurrent G-NETs. Since chronic atrophic gastritis is an independent risk factor for gastric adenocarcinoma, surveillance is required.

Type II Gastric NETs

Pathogenesis: Gastrinoma, Hypergastrinemia, and Peptic Ulcers

Autonomous gastrin secretion from a gastrinoma (Zollinger-Ellison syndrome – ZES), in the presence of normal parietal cell function, results in hypergastrinemia [17] that leads to marked gastric acidity and associated peptic ulcers. Gastrinomas are located in the wall of the duodenum in 50–88 % of sporadic ZES patients and 70–100 % of ZES patients associated with MEN1 [86]. ECL cell changes are invariably seen in both sporadic and MEN1-related cases of ZES [87, 89–91]. Advanced hyperplasia and G-NETs are seen in 53 % and 23 %, respectively, of cases with MEN1/ZES cases.

Risk factors for developing G-NETs in patients with MEN1/ZES include elevated fasting serum gastrin (>490 pg/mL), gastric nodules (present in 44 % of patients), severe ECL cell changes, and long disease duration (>7 years) [89]. Type II G-NETs associated with ZES invariably show loss of heterozygosity (LOH) at the MEN1 gene locus 11q13 [92, 93].

Diagnosis

These are the least common (<5 %) type of all gastric NETs and result from hypergastrinemia caused by gastrinomas, almost invariably in patients with multiple endocrine neoplasia type I (MEN1) syndrome although some arise sporadically [94–96]. About 30 % of patients with MEN1 develop G-NETs and up to 50 % if ZES is present [97, 98]. The majority of patients have symptoms of peptic ulcers refractory to treatment as a result of increased gastric secretion [92]. However, the G-NET lesion itself rarely causes symptoms.

Endoscopy

Type II G-NETs are usually multiple small (<1 cm) polypoid tumors that may involve the gastric fundus or antrum. Peptic ulcers may also be present.

Type II G-NETs are usually well differentiated (G1 or G2), though invasion beyond the submucosa and metastases to abdominal lymph nodes and liver are more common than in type I [10]. The prognosis is good with a mortality rate of less than 10 %. In contrast to type I G-NET, the background gastric mucosa may show chemical gastritis or ulcers, rather than atrophy, because of increased gastric acidity (pH <2). Measuring random or overnight gastric pH may help substantiate this diagnosis. Serum gastrin levels are elevated and may be more than 1000 pg/mL [92]. Serum CgA levels are elevated in all patients, often showing marked elevation. MEN1 gene mutations can be identified in 25 % of cases with ZES. Screening for parathyroid and pituitary tumors associated with MEN1 is recommended [92].

Imaging

EUS, CT, MRI, and scintigraphy can be helpful to detect locally advanced and metastatic disease and also the site of gastrinoma [92]. Selective angiography with calcium stimulation may be necessary to identify small tumors that are not visible on cross-sectional imaging or EUS [99]. PET CT with 68 Ga-DOTA-NOC may localize occult gastrinomas [100].

Treatment

All type II G-NETs should be resected due to high probability of lymph node involvement and metastases, endoscopic resection for localized disease, and surgery for invasive or metastatic disease. Gastrinoma should be localized and resected. Annual endoscopic surveillance is advocated for recurrence, particularly if ZES persists from an in situ gastrinoma. Acid hypersecretion in ZES should be controlled to prevent complications [88], using high-dose PPIs or long-acting SSAs.

Type III Gastric NETs

Pathogenesis: Sporadic Gastric NETs with Normal Gastrin Levels

These tumors occur sporadically without evidence of predisposing factors, like chronic atrophic gastritis or gastrinoma causing hypergastrinemia. There is no ECL hyperplasia in the gastric body mucosa, in contrast to type I and II G-NETs [33]. Although these tumors do not develop in MEN1 patients, there is LOH at the MEN1 gene locus 11q13 in 25–50 % of type III G-NETs [93].

Diagnosis

Type III G-NETs form 15–20 % of gastric NETs and have the worst prognosis with the highest rate of distant metastases [101]. They occur sporadically, unrelated to gastrin, and are more frequently observed in men over the age of 50 years [7, 10, 21, 35, 40]. Patients may present with pain, weight loss, gastrointestinal hemorrhage, and iron deficiency anemia. They may be associated with an atypical form of carcinoid syndrome due to high levels of histamine released from ECL cells that may cause itching, cutaneous wheals, and bronchospasm [102].

They are commonly associated with *H. pylori*-related gastritis [24]. There is no associated gastric atrophy or significant peptic ulcers that are commonly seen with type I or II G-NET, respectively.

Type III G-NETs can vary in histologic grade and differentiation, although G3 tumors (gastric NEC) are more common. The well-differentiated group shows slow disease progression, while poorly differentiated group shows rapid disease progression. Invasion beyond the submucosa is common, and metastases are found in 50–100 % patients [10, 103]. The prognosis is poor with a mortality rate of 22–30 % [24]. Concurrent gastric adenocarcinoma can be present in 5–10 % of these cases [30, 72, 104]. In contrast to other G-NETs, the gastric pH is normal, and there is poor correlation with serum gastrin and CgA levels.

Type III gastric NETs behave like gastric adenocarcinomas and should be similarly investigated and staged with CT [17]. OctreoScan is usually negative in poorly differentiated high-grade tumors (G3 NEC) but occasionally highlights the extent of disease [17].

Treatment

All type III G-NETs, irrespective of grade and stage, should be treated with partial or total gastrectomy with local lymph node resection, followed by postoperative surveillance as for gastric adenocarcinoma. In patients with metastatic disease at presentation, systemic therapy is often the first-line therapy. In a recent study, EMR and ESD of well-differentiated type III G-NETs, <2 cm, limited to the submucosa have shown efficacy [105], although long-term follow-up is still awaited. The treatment of metastatic liver disease from NETs is multimodal, including surgical, locoregional, and systemic treatment modalities [106, 107]. SSAs may have a role as an antiproliferative agent in advanced but low proliferative (G1) G-NETs that are OctreoScan positive [108–111] or in patients with functioning tumors causing carcinoid syndrome as an antisecretory agent [107, 112].

Systemic chemotherapy is indicated in G3 NECA with etoposide and cisplatin, particularly if OctreoScan is negative [113]. Peptide receptor radionuclide therapy (PRRT) with 90 Y- and/or 177 Lu-labeled SSA has a role in patients with a positive OctreoScan and advanced extrahepatic disease [114, 115].

Type IV Gastric NETs (NECAs)

A distinct subset (type IV) of G-NETs comprises poorly differentiated G3 neuroendocrine carcinomas (NECAs) that invariably present with metastases [7, 33]. This may be a clinically important subtype both in terms of prognosis and patient management, in contrast to G1/G2 gastric NETs. Aggressive surgery and chemotherapy (cisplatin plus irinotecan) should be considered for these high-grade malignancies [33, 50, 113].

Molecular Advances in Gastric NETs

Gastric NETs may occur in association with multiple endocrine neoplasia type I (MEN1) and neurofibromatosis type I (NF1) [116–119]. Molecular genetic pathways have not been fully investigated in sporadic type III G-NETs.

MEN1

MEN1 is caused by alterations of the MEN1 tumor suppressor gene located at chromosome 11q13. It encodes a 610 amino acid nuclear protein known as "menin," whose suppressor function involves direct binding to JunD and inhibition of JunD-activated transcription [67, 120]. Most well-differentiated gastric NETs associated with MEN1 appear to be of foregut origin [117]. Loss of heterozygosity (LOH) at 11q13 in type II gastric NETs has been found in 9 out of 10 patients with MEN1 [95, 121–123]. In multiple NETs from the same stomach, the deletion size in the wild-type allele differed from one neoplasm to another, suggesting a multiclonal origin [123, 124]. MEN1 mutation is rarely observed in cases of sporadic gastric NETs [125–127].

NF1

NF1 is an autosomal dominant genetic disorder caused by an alteration of the NF1 gene at chromosome 17q11 [93]. LOH at the NF1 locus has been demonstrated in a gastric NET from an NF1 patient [128].

Chromosomal Abnormalities

Many chromosomal imbalances have been identified by comparative genome hybridization (CGH) analysis in sporadic gastric NETs. Gains involving chromosomes 5, 14, 17 (especially 17q), and 19 and losses involving chromosomes 11 (especially 11q) and 18 appear to be the most common [129–131]. Beta-catenin (CTNNB1) is the most frequent mutated gene in gastric NETs. In one report, beta-catenin exon 3 mutations were found in 27 (37.5 %) of 72 cases [132].

Other Genetic Abnormalities

These include mutations of the REG1A gene involved in ECL cell cycle control in type I gastric NETs [133] and X chromosomal marker loss, with common minimal deletion region restricted to Xq25 and Xq26 in gastric NETs and NECs [134–136]. Recently, the association of gastric NETs and primary hyperparathyroidism has been proposed as a familial syndrome independent from MEN1, but this hypothesis requires further genetic confirmation [137]. Similar to NECs at other sites of the gastrointestinal tract, gastric NECs demonstrate multiple chromosomal alterations involving cell cycle regulatory genes, including TP53, FHIT (fragile histidine triad gene) (3p), DCC (deleted in colorectal carcinoma) and SMAD4/DPC4 (deleted in pancreatic cancer locus 4) (18q), and MEN1, with a higher frequency of allelic imbalances than NETs [136, 138].

Gene Expression Signatures

Gene expression profiling comparing metastatic versus nonmetastatic NETs revealed that the ataxia telangiectasia mutated (ATM) gene was negatively correlated with metastatic behavior [139]. Absence of immunoexpression of ATM protein (seen in over 85 % of the metastatic samples) was associated with decreased overall survival (OS) in comparison to patients with ATM positivity [139]. Therefore, downregulation of ATM may promote metastases in case of G-NETs.

Clinical and pathologic data are important to manage patients with gastric NETs. However, genetic alterations may aid in evaluating tumor behavior and may provide rationale to personalize treatment decisions further.

Multidisciplinary Approach Toward Gastric NETs

Despite rising incidence of G-NETs in recent years, the majority of clinicians will rarely come across such patients in their routine practice. Therefore, management of these patients will be best accomplished in a multidisciplinary setting by neuroendocrine oncologists, pathologists, gastroenterologists, surgeons, radiologists, and nuclear medicine experts. It is critical that a dedicated pathology team with subspecialty expertise or interest in NETs reviews all cases to ensure accurate subtyping and grading of each case, since these assessments have direct impact on patient management decisions. Studies from centers with experience in managing NET patients have shown significant improvement in patient [140].

Proton Pump Inhibitors and Gastric NETs

Gastric NETs have been reported in patients taking PPI therapy with associated ECL cell hyperplasia without chronic atrophic gastritis. Acid suppression therapy can lead to hypergastrinemia that acts as a trophic factor for ECL cells [51, 141, 142]. Recently, PPI use has been associated with a poorly differentiated neuroendocrine carcinoma [143]. Stopping PPI therapy led to the regression of ECL hyperplasia and even regression of a well-differentiated gastric NET [144]. The role of PPI therapy on rising incidence of G-NETs is still controversial and needs further investigation [145, 146].

Future Directions

Currently, there is no clinically validated single or panel of markers that can impact histologic or molecular subtyping or risk stratification of gastric NETs [147]. An improved understanding of the molecular pathogenesis of G-NETs will facilitate the development of clinically relevant biomarkers. Current advances in functional imaging may allow more accurate staging and more personalized patient management. SSTR imaging with 68Ga-DOTATATE PET is more sensitive than OctreoScan to identify additional lesions in well-differentiated NETs [148]. The role of netazepide in managing type I G-NET needs further evaluation in randomized controlled trials to determine its clinical efficacy and define patient selection criteria.

Abbreviations

ACNED	Adenocarcinoma with neuroendocrine differentiation
ATM	Ataxia telangiectasia mutated
ECL	Enterochromaffin-like cells
EMR	Endoscopic mucosal resection
ESD	Endoscopic submucosal dissection
EUS	Endoscopic ultrasound
GCs	Gastric carcinoids
GEP-NET	Gastroenteropancreatic neuroendocrine tumors
G-NETs	Gastric neuroendocrine tumors
LCNECAs	Large-cell neuroendocrine carcinoma
LOH	Loss of heterozygosity
MANEC	Mixed adenoneuroendocrine carcinoma
MEN	Multiple endocrine neoplasms
NECAs	Neuroendocrine carcinomas
NF	Neurofibromatosis
PPI	Proton pump inhibitor
PRRT	Peptide receptor radionuclide therapy
SSAs	Somatostatin analogues
SSTRs	Somatostatin receptors
VMATS 2	Vesicular monoamine transporter 2
ZES	Zollinger-Ellison syndrome
ZES	Zollinger-Ellison syndrome

References

1. Modlin IM, Latich I, Zikusoka M, Kidd M, Eick G, Chan AK. Gastrointestinal carcinoids: the evolution of diagnostic strategies. J Clin Gastroenterol. 2006;40(7):572–82.
2. Modlin IM, Lye KD, Kidd M. A 50-year analysis of 562 gastric carcinoids: small tumor or larger problem? Am J Gastroenterol. 2004;99(1):23–32.
3. Lawrence B, Gustafsson BI, Chan A, Svejda B, Kidd M, Modlin IM. The epidemiology of gastroenteropancreatic neuroendocrine tumors. Endocrinol Metab Clin North Am. 2011;40(1):1–18, vii.
4. Lawrence B, Kidd M, Svejda B, Modlin I. A clinical perspective on gastric neuroendocrine neoplasia. Curr Gastroenterol Rep. 2011;13(1):101–9.
5. Niederle MB, Hackl M, Kaserer K, Niederle B. Gastroenteropancreatic neuroendocrine tumours: the current incidence and staging based on the WHO and European Neuroendocrine Tumour Society classification: an analysis based on prospectively collected parameters. Endocr Relat Cancer. 2010;17(4):909–18.
6. Godwin 2nd JD. Carcinoid tumors. An analysis of 2,837 cases. Cancer. 1975;36(2):560–9.
7. Modlin IM, Lye KD, Kidd M. Carcinoid tumors of the stomach. Surg Oncol. 2003;12(2):153–72.
8. Modlin IM, Kidd M, Latich I, Zikusoka MN, Shapiro MD. Current status of gastrointestinal carcinoids. Gastroenterology. 2005;128(6):1717–51.
9. Morishita Y, Tanaka T, Kato K, Kawamori T, Amano K, Funato T, et al. Gastric collision tumor (carcinoid and adenocarcinoma) with gastritis cystica profunda. Arch Pathol Lab Med. 1991;115(10):1006–10.
10. Rindi G, Luinetti O, Cornaggia M, Capella C, Solcia E. Three subtypes of gastric argyrophil carcinoid and the gastric neuroendocrine carcinoma: a clinicopathologic study. Gastroenterology. 1993;104(4):994–1006.
11. Delle Fave G, Kwekkeboom DJ, Van Cutsem E, Rindi G, Kos-Kudla B, Knigge U, et al. ENETS Consensus Guidelines for the management of patients with gastroduodenal neoplasms. Neuroendocrinology. 2012;95(2):74–87.
12. Ellis L, Shale MJ, Coleman MP. Carcinoid tumors of the gastrointestinal tract: trends in incidence in England since 1971. Am J Gastroenterol. 2010;105(12):2563–9.
13. Lehy T, Roucayrol AM, Mignon M. Histomorphological characteristics of gastric mucosa in patients with Zollinger-Ellison syndrome or autoimmune gastric atrophy: role of gastrin and atrophying gastritis. Microsc Res Tech. 2000;48(6):327–38.
14. Gencosmanoglu R, Sen-Oran E, Kurtkaya-Yapicier O, Avsar E, Sav A, Tozun N. Gastric polypoid lesions: analysis of 150 endoscopic polypectomy specimens from 91 patients. World J Gastroenterol. 2003;9(10):2236–9.
15. Scherubl H, Cadiot G, Jensen RT, Rosch T, Stolzel U, Kloppel G. Neuroendocrine tumors of the stomach (gastric carcinoids) are on the rise: small tumors, small problems? Endoscopy. 2010;42(8):664–71.
16. Dockray GJ. Clinical endocrinology and metabolism. Gastrin. Best Pract Res Clin Endocrinol Metab. 2004;18(4):555–68.
17. Basuroy R, Srirajaskanthan R, Prachalias A, Quaglia A, Ramage JK. Review article: the investigation and management of gastric neuroendocrine tumours. Aliment Pharmacol Ther. 2014;39(10):1071–84.
18. Fanelli MF, Chinen LT, Begnami MD, Costa Jr WL, Fregnami JH, Soares FA, et al. The influence of transforming growth factor-alpha, cyclooxygenase-2, matrix metalloproteinase (MMP)-7, MMP-9 and CXCR4 proteins involved in epithelial-mesenchymal transition on overall survival of patients with gastric cancer. Histopathology. 2012;61(2):153–61.
19. Sanui A, Yotsumoto F, Tsujioka H, Fukami T, Horiuchi S, Shirota K, et al. HB-EGF inhibition in combination with various anticancer agents enhances its antitumor effects in gastric cancer. Anticancer Res. 2010;30(8):3143–9.

20. Pritchard DM, Berry D, Przemeck SM, Campbell F, Edwards SW, Varro A. Gastrin increases mcl-1 expression in type I gastric carcinoid tumors and a gastric epithelial cell line that expresses the CCK-2 receptor. Am J Physiol Gastrointest Liver Physiol. 2008;295(4):G798–805.
21. Bordi C. Gastric carcinoids. Ital J Gastroenterol Hepatol. 1999;31 Suppl 2:S94–7.
22. Solcia E, Bordi C, Creutzfeldt W, Dayal Y, Dayan AD, Falkmer S, et al. Histopathological classification of nonantral gastric endocrine growths in man. Digestion. 1988;41(4): 185–200.
23. Annibale B, Azzoni C, Corleto VD, di Giulio E, Caruana P, D'Ambra G, et al. Atrophic body gastritis patients with enterochromaffin-like cell dysplasia are at increased risk for the development of type I gastric carcinoid. Eur J Gastroenterol Hepatol. 2001;13(12):1449–56.
24. Rappel S, Altendorf-Hofmann A, Stolte M. Prognosis of gastric carcinoid tumours. Digestion. 1995;56(6):455–62.
25. Manfe AZ, Norberto L, Marchesini M, Lumachi F. Usefulness of chromogranin A, neuron-specific enolase and 5-hydroxyindolacetic acid measurements in patients with malignant carcinoids. In Vivo. 2011;25(6):1027–9.
26. Nikou GC, Lygidakis NJ, Toubanakis C, Pavlatos S, Tseleni-Balafouta S, Giannatou E, et al. Current diagnosis and treatment of gastrointestinal carcinoids in a series of 101 patients: the significance of serum chromogranin-A, somatostatin receptor scintigraphy and somatostatin analogues. Hepatogastroenterology. 2005;52(63):731–41.
27. Zatelli MC, Torta M, Leon A, Ambrosio MR, Gion M, Tomassetti P, et al. Chromogranin A as a marker of neuroendocrine neoplasia: an Italian Multicenter Study. Endocr Relat Cancer. 2007;14(2):473–82.
28. Gibril F, Reynolds JC, Lubensky IA, Roy PK, Peghini PL, Doppman JL, et al. Ability of somatostatin receptor scintigraphy to identify patients with gastric carcinoids: a prospective study. J Nucl Med. 2000;41(10):1646–56.
29. Bordi C. Gastric carcinoids: an immunohistochemical and clinicopathologic study of 104 patients. Cancer. 1995;75(1):129–30.
30. Bordi C, Yu JY, Baggi MT, Davoli C, Pilato FP, Baruzzi G, et al. Gastric carcinoids and their precursor lesions. A histologic and immunohistochemical study of 23 cases. Cancer. 1991;67(3):663–72.
31. Solcia E, Arnold R, Capella C, Klimstra DS, Kloppel G, Komminoth P, et al. Nomenclature and classification of neuroendocrine neoplasms of the digestive system. In: Bosman FT, Carneiro F, Hruban RH, Theise ND, editors. WHO classification of tumours of the digestive system. 4th ed. IARC: Lyon; 2010.
32. Kulke MH, Anthony LB, Bushnell DL, de Herder WW, Goldsmith SJ, Klimstra DS, et al. NANETS treatment guidelines: well-differentiated neuroendocrine tumors of the stomach and pancreas. Pancreas. 2010;39(6):735–52.
33. Borch K, Ahren B, Ahlman H, Falkmer S, Granerus G, Grimelius L. Gastric carcinoids: biologic behavior and prognosis after differentiated treatment in relation to type. Ann Surg. 2005;242(1):64–73.
34. Annibale B, Lahner E, Negrini R, Baccini F, Bordi C, Monarca B, et al. Lack of specific association between gastric autoimmunity hallmarks and clinical presentations of atrophic body gastritis. World J Gastroenterol. 2005;11(34):5351–7.
35. Rindi G, Bordi C, Rappel S, La Rosa S, Stolte M, Solcia E. Gastric carcinoids and neuroendocrine carcinomas: pathogenesis, pathology, and behavior. World J Surg. 1996;20(2):168–72.
36. Chejfec G, Gould VE. Malignant gastric neuroendogrinomas. Ultrastructural and biochemical characterization of their secretory activity. Hum Pathol. 1977;8(4):433–40.
37. Capella C, Polak JM, Timson CM, Frigerio B, Solcia E. Gastric carcinoids of argyrophil ECL cells. Ultrastruct Pathol. 1980;1(3):411–8.
38. Rindi G, Paolotti D, Fiocca R, Wiedenmann B, Henry JP, Solcia E. Vesicular monoamine transporter 2 as a marker of gastric enterochromaffin-like cell tumors. Virchows Arch. 2000;436(3):217–23.

39. Papotti M, Cassoni P, Volante M, Deghenghi R, Muccioli G, Ghigo E. Ghrelin-producing endocrine tumors of the stomach and intestine. J Clin Endocrinol Metab. 2001;86(10):5052–9.
40. Rindi G, Azzoni C, La Rosa S, Klersy C, Paolotti D, Rappel S, et al. ECL cell tumor and poorly differentiated endocrine carcinoma of the stomach: prognostic evaluation by pathological analysis. Gastroenterology. 1999;116(3):532–42.
41. Rindi G, Kloppel G, Alhman H, Caplin M, Couvelard A, de Herder WW, et al. TNM staging of foregut (neuro)endocrine tumors: a consensus proposal including a grading system. Virchows Arch. 2006;449(4):395–401.
42. Christodoulopoulos JB, Klotz AP. Carcinoid syndrome with primary carcinoid tumor of the stomach. Gastroenterology. 1961;40:429–40.
43. Kloppel G, Clemens A. The biological relevance of gastric neuroendocrine tumors. Yale J Biol Med. 1996;69(1):69–74.
44. Jiang SX, Mikami T, Umezawa A, Saegusa M, Kameya T, Okayasu I. Gastric large cell neuroendocrine carcinomas: a distinct clinicopathologic entity. Am J Surg Pathol. 2006;30(8):945–53.
45. Shia J, Tang LH, Weiser MR, Brenner B, Adsay NV, Stelow EB, et al. Is nonsmall cell type high-grade neuroendocrine carcinoma of the tubular gastrointestinal tract a distinct disease entity? Am J Surg Pathol. 2008;32(5):719–31.
46. Tang LH, Gonen M, Hedvat C, Modlin IM, Klimstra DS. Objective quantification of the Ki67 proliferative index in neuroendocrine tumors of the gastroenteropancreatic system: a comparison of digital image analysis with manual methods. Am J Surg Pathol. 2012;36(12):1761–70.
47. Khan MS, Luong TV, Watkins J, Toumpanakis C, Caplin ME, Meyer T. A comparison of Ki-67 and mitotic count as prognostic markers for metastatic pancreatic and midgut neuroendocrine neoplasms. Br J Cancer. 2013;108(9):1838–45.
48. Boninsegna L, Panzuto F, Partelli S, Capelli P, Delle Fave G, Bettini R, et al. Malignant pancreatic neuroendocrine tumour: lymph node ratio and Ki67 are predictors of recurrence after curative resections. Eur J Cancer. 2012;48(11):1608–15.
49. Norton JA, Melcher ML, Gibril F, Jensen RT. Gastric carcinoid tumors in multiple endocrine neoplasia-1 patients with Zollinger-Ellison syndrome can be symptomatic, demonstrate aggressive growth, and require surgical treatment. Surgery. 2004;136(6):1267–74.
50. Matsui K, Jin XM, Kitagawa M, Miwa A. Clinicopathologic features of neuroendocrine carcinomas of the stomach: appraisal of small cell and large cell variants. Arch Pathol Lab Med. 1998;122(11):1010–7.
51. Schenk BE, Kuipers EJ, Klinkenberg-Knol EC, Bloemena E, Nelis GF, Festen HP, et al. Hypergastrinaemia during long-term omeprazole therapy: influences of vagal nerve function, gastric emptying and Helicobacter pylori infection. Aliment Pharmacol Ther. 1998;12(7):605–12.
52. Vanoli A, La Rosa S, Luinetti O, Klersy C, Manca R, Alvisi C, et al. Histologic changes in type A chronic atrophic gastritis indicating increased risk of neuroendocrine tumor development: the predictive role of dysplastic and severely hyperplastic enterochromaffin-like cell lesions. Hum Pathol. 2013;44(9):1827–37.
53. Larsson H, Carlsson E, Hakanson R, Mattsson H, Nilsson G, Seensalu R, et al. Time-course of development and reversal of gastric endocrine cell hyperplasia after inhibition of acid secretion. Studies with omeprazole and ranitidine in intact and antrectomized rats. Gastroenterology. 1988;95(6):1477–86.
54. Klinkenberg-Knol EC, Nelis F, Dent J, Snel P, Mitchell B, Prichard P, et al. Long-term omeprazole treatment in resistant gastroesophageal reflux disease: efficacy, safety, and influence on gastric mucosa. Gastroenterology. 2000;118(4):661–9.
55. Kidd M, Miu K, Tang LH, Perez-Perez GI, Blaser MJ, Sandor A, et al. Helicobacter pylori lipopolysaccharide stimulates histamine release and DNA synthesis in rat enterochromaffin-like cells. Gastroenterology. 1997;113(4):1110–7.
56. Vannella L, Sbrozzi-Vanni A, Lahner E, Bordi C, Pilozzi E, Corleto VD, et al. Development of type I gastric carcinoid in patients with chronic atrophic gastritis. Aliment Pharmacol Ther. 2011;33(12):1361–9.

57. Marignani M, Delle Fave G, Mecarocci S, Bordi C, Angeletti S, D'Ambra G, et al. High prevalence of atrophic body gastritis in patients with unexplained microcytic and macrocytic anemia: a prospective screening study. Am J Gastroenterol. 1999;94(3):766–72.
58. Thomas D, Tsolakis AV, Grozinsky-Glasberg S, Fraenkel M, Alexandraki K, Sougioultzis S, et al. Long-term follow-up of a large series of patients with type 1 gastric carcinoid tumors: data from a multicenter study. Eur J Endocrinol. 2013;168(2):185–93.
59. Merola E, Sbrozzi-Vanni A, Panzuto F, D'Ambra G, Di Giulio E, Pilozzi E, et al. Type I gastric carcinoids: a prospective study on endoscopic management and recurrence rate. Neuroendocrinology. 2012;95(3):207–13.
60. Nakamura S, Iida M, Yao T, Fujishima M. Endoscopic features of gastric carcinoids. Gastrointest Endosc. 1991;37(5):535–8.
61. Kitago M, Inada T, Igarashi S, Mizutani S, Ogata Y, Kubota T. Multiple gastric carcinoid tumors with type A gastritis concomitant with gastric cancer: a case report. Oncol Rep. 2001;8(2):343–6.
62. Reinecke P, Borchard F. Pattern of gastric endocrine cells in microcarcinoidosis – an immunohistochemical study of 14 gastric biopsies. Virchows Arch. 1996;428(4–5):237–41.
63. Singh R, Yao K, Anagnostopoulos G, Kaye P, Ragunath K. Microcarcinoid tumor diagnosed with high-resolution magnification endoscopy and narrow band imaging. Endoscopy. 2008;40 Suppl 2:E12.
64. Campana D, Nori F, Piscitelli L, Morselli-Labate AM, Pezzilli R, Corinaldesi R, et al. Chromogranin A: is it a useful marker of neuroendocrine tumors? J Clin Oncol. 2007;25(15):1967–73.
65. La Rosa S, Inzani F, Vanoli A, Klersy C, Dainese L, Rindi G, et al. Histologic characterization and improved prognostic evaluation of 209 gastric neuroendocrine neoplasms. Hum Pathol. 2011;42(10):1373–84.
66. Hosokawa O, Kaizaki Y, Hattori M, Douden K, Hayashi H, Morishita M, et al. Long-term follow up of patients with multiple gastric carcinoids associated with type A gastritis. Gastric Cancer. 2005;8(1):42–6.
67. Caruso ML, Pilato FP, D'Adda T, Baggi MT, Fucci L, Valentini AM, et al. Composite carcinoid-adenocarcinoma of the stomach associated with multiple gastric carcinoids and nonantral gastric atrophy. Cancer. 1989;64(7):1534–9.
68. Pasquinelli G, Santini D, Preda P, Cariani G, Bonora G, Martinelli GN. Composite gastric carcinoma and precursor lesions with amphicrine features in chronic atrophic gastritis. Ultrastruct Pathol. 1993;17(1):9–24.
69. Vannella L, Lahner E, Annibale B. Risk for gastric neoplasias in patients with chronic atrophic gastritis: a critical reappraisal. World J Gastroenterol. 2012;18(12):1279–85.
70. Mendelsohn G, de la Monte S, Dunn JL, Yardley JH. Gastric carcinoid tumors, endocrine cell hyperplasia, and associated intestinal metaplasia. Histologic, histochemical, and immunohistochemical findings. Cancer. 1987;60(5):1022–31.
71. Gladdy RA, Strong VE, Coit D, Allen PJ, Gerdes H, Shia J, et al. Defining surgical indications for type I gastric carcinoid tumor. Ann Surg Oncol. 2009;16(11):3154–60.
72. Kim BS, Oh ST, Yook JH, Kim KC, Kim MG, Jeong JW, et al. Typical carcinoids and neuroendocrine carcinomas of the stomach: differing clinical courses and prognoses. Am J Surg. 2010;200(3):328–33.
73. Varas MJ, Gornals JB, Pons C, Espinos JC, Abad R, Lorente FJ, et al. Usefulness of endoscopic ultrasonography (EUS) for selecting carcinoid tumors as candidates to endoscopic resection. Rev Esp Enferm Dig. 2010;102(10):577–82.
74. Grozinsky-Glasberg S, Thomas D, Strosberg JR, Pape UF, Felder S, Tsolakis AV, et al. Metastatic type 1 gastric carcinoid: a real threat or just a myth? World J Gastroenterol. 2013;19(46):8687–95.
75. Suzuki S, Ishii N, Uemura M, Deshpande GA, Matsuda M, Iizuka Y, et al. Endoscopic submucosal dissection (ESD) for gastrointestinal carcinoid tumors. Surg Endosc. 2012;26(3):759–63.

76. Oshima T, Okugawa T, Hori K, Kim Y, Tanaka J, Watari J, et al. Successful endoscopic submucosal dissection of gastric carcinoid in a patient with autoimmune gastritis and systemic lupus erythematosus. Intern Med. 2012;51(10):1211–3.
77. Hulagu S, Senturk O, Aygun C, Kocaman O, Celebi A, Konduk T, et al. Endoscopic submucosal dissection for premalignant lesions and noninvasive early gastrointestinal cancers. World J Gastroenterol. 2011;17(13):1701–9.
78. Li QL, Zhang YQ, Chen WF, Xu MD, Zhong YS, Ma LL, et al. Endoscopic submucosal dissection for foregut neuroendocrine tumors: an initial study. World J Gastroenterol. 2012;18(40):5799–806.
79. Ozao-Choy J, Buch K, Strauchen JA, Warner RR, Divino CM. Laparoscopic antrectomy for the treatment of type I gastric carcinoid tumors. J Surg Res. 2010;162(1):22–5.
80. Grozinsky-Glasberg S, Kaltsas G, Gur C, Gal E, Thomas D, Fichman S, et al. Long-acting somatostatin analogues are an effective treatment for type 1 gastric carcinoid tumours. Eur J Endocrinol. 2008;159(4):475–82.
81. Campana D, Nori F, Pezzilli R, Piscitelli L, Santini D, Brocchi E, et al. Gastric endocrine tumors type I: treatment with long-acting somatostatin analogs. Endocr Relat Cancer. 2008;15(1):337–42.
82. Boyce M, Warrington S, Black J. Netazepide, a gastrin/CCK2 receptor antagonist, causes dose-dependent, persistent inhibition of the responses to pentagastrin in healthy subjects. Br J Clin Pharmacol. 2013;76(5):689–98.
83. Boyce M, David O, Darwin K, Mitchell T, Johnston A, Warrington S. Single oral doses of netazepide (YF476), a gastrin receptor antagonist, cause dose-dependent, sustained increases in gastric pH compared with placebo and ranitidine in healthy subjects. Aliment Pharmacol Ther. 2012;36(2):181–9.
84. Fossmark R, Sordal O, Jianu CS, Qvigstad G, Nordrum IS, Boyce M, et al. Treatment of gastric carcinoids type 1 with the gastrin receptor antagonist netazepide (YF476) results in regression of tumours and normalisation of serum chromogranin A. Aliment Pharmacol Ther. 2012;36(11–12):1067–75.
85. Moore AR, Boyce M, Steele IA, Campbell F, Varro A, Pritchard DM. Netazepide, a gastrin receptor antagonist, normalises tumour biomarkers and causes regression of type 1 gastric neuroendocrine tumours in a nonrandomised trial of patients with chronic atrophic gastritis. PLoS One. 2013;8(10):e76462.
86. Kloppel G, Anlauf M. Gastrinoma – morphological aspects. Wien Klin Wochenschr. 2007;119(19–20):579–84.
87. Anlauf M, Garbrecht N, Henopp T, Schmitt A, Schlenger R, Raffel A, et al. Sporadic versus hereditary gastrinomas of the duodenum and pancreas: distinct clinico-pathological and epidemiological features. World J Gastroenterol. 2006;12(34):5440–6.
88. Jensen RT, Cadiot G, Brandi ML, de Herder WW, Kaltsas G, Komminoth P, et al. ENETS Consensus Guidelines for the management of patients with digestive neuroendocrine neoplasms: functional pancreatic endocrine tumor syndromes. Neuroendocrinology. 2012;95(2):98–119.
89. Berna MJ, Annibale B, Marignani M, Luong TV, Corleto V, Pace A, et al. A prospective study of gastric carcinoids and enterochromaffin-like cell changes in multiple endocrine neoplasia type 1 and Zollinger-Ellison syndrome: identification of risk factors. J Clin Endocrinol Metab. 2008;93(5):1582–91.
90. Delle Fave G, Marignani M, Moretti A, D'Ambra G, Martino G, Annibale B. Hypergastrinemia and enterochromaffin-like cell hyperplasia. Yale J Biol Med. 1998;71(3–4):291–301.
91. Delle Fave G, Marignani M, Corleto VD, Angeletti S, D'Ambra G, Ferraro G, et al. Progression of gastric enterochromaffin-like cells growth in Zollinger-Ellison syndrome and atrophic body gastritis patients. Dig Liver Dis. 2002;34(4):270–8.
92. Nikou GC, Toubanakis C, Nikolaou P, Giannatou E, Marinou K, Safioleas M, et al. Gastrinomas associated with MEN-1 syndrome: new insights for the diagnosis and management in a series of 11 patients. Hepatogastroenterology. 2005;52(66):1668–76.

93. Zikusoka MN, Kidd M, Eick G, Latich I, Modlin IM. The molecular genetics of gastroentero-pancreatic neuroendocrine tumors. Cancer. 2005;104(11):2292–309.
94. Lehy T, Cadiot G, Mignon M, Ruszniewski P, Bonfils S. Influence of multiple endocrine neoplasia type 1 on gastric endocrine cells in patients with the Zollinger-Ellison syndrome. Gut. 1992;33(9):1275–9.
95. Cadiot G, Laurent-Puig P, Thuille B, Lehy T, Mignon M, Olschwang S. Is the multiple endocrine neoplasia type 1 gene a suppressor for fundic argyrophil tumors in the Zollinger-Ellison syndrome? Gastroenterology. 1993;105(2):579–82.
96. Gibril F, Schumann M, Pace A, Jensen RT. Multiple endocrine neoplasia type 1 and Zollinger-Ellison syndrome: a prospective study of 107 cases and comparison with 1009 cases from the literature. Medicine (Baltimore). 2004;83(1):43–83.
97. Norton JA, Jensen RT. Resolved and unresolved controversies in the surgical management of patients with Zollinger-Ellison syndrome. Ann Surg. 2004;240(5):757–73.
98. Cadiot G, Vissuzaine C, Potet F, Mignon M. Fundic argyrophil carcinoid tumor in a patient with sporadic-type Zollinger-Ellison syndrome. Dig Dis Sci. 1995;40(6):1275–8.
99. Norton JA. Gastrinoma: advances in localization and treatment. Surg Oncol Clin N Am. 1998;7(4):845–61.
100. Naswa N, Sharma P, Soundararajan R, Karunanithi S, Nazar AH, Kumar R, et al. Diagnostic performance of somatostatin receptor PET/CT using 68Ga-DOTANOC in gastrinoma patients with negative or equivocal CT findings. Abdom Imaging. 2013;38(3):552–60.
101. Hassan MM, Phan A, Li D, Dagohoy CG, Leary C, Yao JC. Risk factors associated with neuroendocrine tumors: A U.S.-based case-control study. Int J Cancer. 2008;123(4):867–73.
102. Giordano JA. Gastric carcinoid syndrome diagnosed by endoscopy. Am J Gastroenterol. 1981;76(1):41–3.
103. Gough DB, Thompson GB, Crotty TB, Donohue JH, Kvols LK, Carney JA, et al. Diverse clinical and pathologic features of gastric carcinoid and the relevance of hypergastrinemia. World J Surg. 1994;18(4):473–9; discussion 9–80.
104. Adhikari D, Conte C, Eskreis D, Urmacher C, Ellen K. Combined adenocarcinoma and carcinoid tumor in atrophic gastritis. Ann Clin Lab Sci. 2002;32(4):422–7.
105. Kwon YH, Jeon SW, Kim GH, Kim JI, Chung IK, Jee SR, et al. Long-term follow up of endoscopic resection for type 3 gastric NET. World J Gastroenterol. 2013;19(46):8703–8.
106. Basuroy R, Srirajaskanthan R, Ramage JK. A multimodal approach to the management of neuroendocrine tumour liver metastases. Int J Hepatol. 2012;2012:819193.
107. Pavel M, Baudin E, Couvelard A, Krenning E, Oberg K, Steinmuller T, et al. ENETS Consensus Guidelines for the management of patients with liver and other distant metastases from neuroendocrine neoplasms of foregut, midgut, hindgut, and unknown primary. Neuroendocrinology. 2012;95(2):157–76.
108. Modlin IM, Pavel M, Kidd M, Gustafsson BI. Review article: somatostatin analogues in the treatment of gastroenteropancreatic neuroendocrine (carcinoid) tumours. Aliment Pharmacol Ther. 2010;31(2):169–88.
109. Arnold R, Rinke A, Klose KJ, Muller HH, Wied M, Zamzow K, et al. Octreotide versus octreotide plus interferon-alpha in endocrine gastroenteropancreatic tumors: a randomized trial. Clin Gastroenterol Hepatol. 2005;3(8):761–71.
110. Faiss S, Pape UF, Bohmig M, Dorffel Y, Mansmann U, Golder W, et al. Prospective, randomized, multicenter trial on the antiproliferative effect of lanreotide, interferon alfa, and their combination for therapy of metastatic neuroendocrine gastroenteropancreatic tumors – the International Lanreotide and Interferon Alfa Study Group. J Clin Oncol. 2003;21(14):2689–96.
111. Rinke A, Muller HH, Schade-Brittinger C, Klose KJ, Barth P, Wied M, et al. Placebo-controlled, double-blind, prospective, randomized study on the effect of octreotide LAR in the control of tumor growth in patients with metastatic neuroendocrine midgut tumors: a report from the PROMID Study Group. J Clin Oncol. 2009;27(28):4656–63.
112. Appetecchia M, Baldelli R. Somatostatin analogues in the treatment of gastroenteropancreatic neuroendocrine tumours, current aspects and new perspectives. J Exp Clin Cancer Res. 2010;29:19.

113. Okita NT, Kato K, Takahari D, Hirashima Y, Nakajima TE, Matsubara J, et al. Neuroendocrine tumors of the stomach: chemotherapy with cisplatin plus irinotecan is effective for gastric poorly-differentiated neuroendocrine carcinoma. Gastric Cancer. 2011;14(2):161–5.
114. Kwekkeboom DJ, Krenning EP, Lebtahi R, Komminoth P, Kos-Kudla B, de Herder WW, et al. ENETS Consensus Guidelines for the Standards of Care in Neuroendocrine Tumors: peptide receptor radionuclide therapy with radiolabeled somatostatin analogs. Neuroendocrinology. 2009;90(2):220–6.
115. Kwekkeboom DJ, de Herder WW, van Eijck CH, Kam BL, van Essen M, Teunissen JJ, et al. Peptide receptor radionuclide therapy in patients with gastroenteropancreatic neuroendocrine tumors. Semin Nucl Med. 2010;40(2):78–88.
116. Easton DF, Eeles RA. Genome-wide association studies in cancer. Hum Mol Genet. 2008;17(R2):R109–15.
117. Duh QY, Hybarger CP, Geist R, Gamsu G, Goodman PC, Gooding GA, et al. Carcinoids associated with multiple endocrine neoplasia syndromes. Am J Surg. 1987;154(1):142–8.
118. Levy AD, Patel N, Dow N, Abbott RM, Miettinen M, Sobin LH. From the archives of the AFIP: abdominal neoplasms in patients with neurofibromatosis type 1: radiologic-pathologic correlation. Radiographics. 2005;25(2):455–80.
119. Levy AD, Taylor LD, Abbott RM, Sobin LH. Duodenal carcinoids: imaging features with clinical-pathologic comparison. Radiology. 2005;237(3):967–72.
120. Agarwal SK, Guru SC, Heppner C, Erdos MR, Collins RM, Park SY, et al. Menin interacts with the AP1 transcription factor JunD and represses JunD-activated transcription. Cell. 1999;96(1):143–52.
121. Beckers A, Abs R, Reyniers E, De Boulle K, Stevenaert A, Heller FR, et al. Variable regions of chromosome 11 loss in different pathological tissues of a patient with the multiple endocrine neoplasia type I syndrome. J Clin Endocrinol Metab. 1994;79(5):1498–502.
122. Bordi C, D'Adda T, Azzoni C, Pilato FP, Caruana P. Hypergastrinemia and gastric enterochromaffin-like cells. Am J Surg Pathol. 1995;19 Suppl 1:S8–19.
123. Debelenko LV, Emmert-Buck MR, Zhuang Z, Epshteyn E, Moskaluk CA, Jensen RT, et al. The multiple endocrine neoplasia type I gene locus is involved in the pathogenesis of type II gastric carcinoids. Gastroenterology. 1997;113(3):773–81.
124. Debelenko LV, Zhuang Z, Emmert-Buck MR, Chandrasekharappa SC, Manickam P, Guru SC, et al. Allelic deletions on chromosome 11q13 in multiple endocrine neoplasia type 1-associated and sporadic gastrinomas and pancreatic endocrine tumors. Cancer Res. 1997;57(11):2238–43.
125. Fujii T, Kawai T, Saito K, Hishima T, Hayashi Y, Imura J, et al. MEN1 gene mutations in sporadic neuroendocrine tumors of foregut derivation. Pathol Int. 1999;49(11):968–73.
126. Gortz B, Roth J, Krahenmann A, de Krijger RR, Muletta-Feurer S, Rutimann K, et al. Mutations and allelic deletions of the MEN1 gene are associated with a subset of sporadic endocrine pancreatic and neuroendocrine tumors and not restricted to foregut neoplasms. Am J Pathol. 1999;154(2):429–36.
127. Toliat MR, Berger W, Ropers HH, Neuhaus P, Wiedenmann B. Mutations in the MEN I gene in sporadic neuroendocrine tumours of gastroenteropancreatic system. Lancet. 1997;350(9086):1223.
128. Stewart W, Traynor JP, Cooke A, Griffiths S, Onen NF, Balsitis M, et al. Gastric carcinoid: germline and somatic mutation of the neurofibromatosis type 1 gene. Fam Cancer. 2007;6(1):147–52.
129. Tonnies H, Toliat MR, Ramel C, Pape UF, Neitzel H, Berger W, et al. Analysis of sporadic neuroendocrine tumours of the enteropancreatic system by comparative genomic hybridisation. Gut. 2001;48(4):536–41.
130. Terris B, Meddeb M, Marchio A, Danglot G, Flejou JF, Belghiti J, et al. Comparative genomic hybridization analysis of sporadic neuroendocrine tumors of the digestive system. Genes Chromosomes Cancer. 1998;22(1):50–6.
131. Oberg K. Genetics and molecular pathology of neuroendocrine gastrointestinal and pancreatic tumors (gastroenteropancreatic neuroendocrine tumors). Curr Opin Endocrinol Diabetes Obes. 2009;16(1):72–8.

132. Fujimori M, Ikeda S, Shimizu Y, Okajima M, Asahara T. Accumulation of beta-catenin protein and mutations in exon 3 of beta-catenin gene in gastrointestinal carcinoid tumor. Cancer Res. 2001;61(18):6656–9.
133. Higham AD, Bishop LA, Dimaline R, Blackmore CG, Dobbins AC, Varro A, et al. Mutations of RegIalpha are associated with enterochromaffin-like cell tumor development in patients with hypergastrinemia. Gastroenterology. 1999;116(6):1310–8.
134. Azzoni C, Bottarelli L, Pizzi S, D'Adda T, Rindi G, Bordi C. Xq25 and Xq26 identify the common minimal deletion region in malignant gastroenteropancreatic endocrine carcinomas. Virchows Arch. 2006;448(2):119–26.
135. D'Adda T, Annibale B, Delle Fave G, Bordi C. Oxyntic endocrine cells of hypergastrinaemic patients. Differential response to antrectomy or octreotide. Gut. 1996;38(5):668–74.
136. Pizzi S, D'Adda T, Azzoni C, Rindi G, Grigolato P, Pasquali C, et al. Malignancy-associated allelic losses on the X-chromosome in foregut but not in midgut endocrine tumours. J Pathol. 2002;196(4):401–7.
137. Christopoulos C, Balatsos V, Rotas E, Karoumpalis I, Papavasileiou D, Kontogeorgos G, et al. The syndrome of gastric carcinoid and hyperparathyroidism: a family study and literature review. Eur J Endocrinol. 2009;160(4):689–94.
138. Furlan D, Cerutti R, Uccella S, La Rosa S, Rigoli E, Genasetti A, et al. Different molecular profiles characterize well-differentiated endocrine tumors and poorly differentiated endocrine carcinomas of the gastroenteropancreatic tract. Clin Cancer Res. 2004;10(3):947–57.
139. Lee J, Sung CO, Lee EJ, Do IG, Kim HC, Yoon SH, et al. Metastasis of neuroendocrine tumors are characterized by increased cell proliferation and reduced expression of the ATM gene. PLoS One. 2012;7(4):e34456.
140. Strosberg J, Gardner N, Kvols L. Survival and prognostic factor analysis of 146 metastatic neuroendocrine tumors of the mid-gut. Neuroendocrinology. 2009;89(4):471–6.
141. Kuipers EJ. Proton pump inhibitors and gastric neoplasia. Gut. 2006;55(9):1217–21.
142. Brunner G, Athmann C, Schneider A. Long-term, open-label trial: safety and efficacy of continuous maintenance treatment with pantoprazole for up to 15 years in severe acid-peptic disease. Aliment Pharmacol Ther. 2012;36(1):37–47.
143. Jianu CS, Lange OJ, Viset T, Qvigstad G, Martinsen TC, Fougner R, et al. Gastric neuroendocrine carcinoma after long-term use of proton pump inhibitor. Scand J Gastroenterol. 2012;47(1):64–7.
144. Jianu CS, Fossmark R, Viset T, Qvigstad G, Sordal O, Marvik R, et al. Gastric carcinoids after long-term use of a proton pump inhibitor. Aliment Pharmacol Ther. 2012;36(7):644–9.
145. McCarthy DM. Adverse effects of proton pump inhibitor drugs: clues and conclusions. Curr Opin Gastroenterol. 2010;26(6):624–31.
146. McCarthy DM. Commentary: a gastrin antagonist against carcinoids – implications for PPI-induced hypergastrinaemia. Aliment Pharmacol Ther. 2013;37(2):276–7.
147. Lewis MA, Yao JC. Molecular pathology and genetics of gastrointestinal neuroendocrine tumours. Curr Opin Endocrinol Diabetes Obes. 2014;21(1):22–7.
148. van Essen M, Sundin A, Krenning EP, Kwekkeboom DJ. Neuroendocrine tumours: the role of imaging for diagnosis and therapy. Nat Rev Endocrinol. 2014;10(2):102–14.

Neuroendocrine Neoplasms of the Pancreas

Michael Markow and Barbara Ann Centeno

Introduction

Neuroendocrine tumors of the pancreas are composed of cells with evidence of neuroendocrine differentiation based on immunophenotypic and ultrastructural findings. These historically were called islet cell tumors, based on the assumption that they were derived from the islets of Langerhans. The first reported description came from Nicholls in 1902. He reported his discovery at autopsy of a simple adenoma of the pancreas arising from the island of Langerhans [1]. Fabozzi described a malignant counterpart in 1903 [2]. It has since been recognized that these neoplasms arise from neuroendocrine cells residing in the pancreatic ductal epithelium [3]. The WHO 2004 classification system referred to these as pancreatic endocrine neoplasms [4]. In the WHO 2010 classification, the terminology was modified to neuroendocrine tumor [5]. This chapter will cover the clinical, pathological, and molecular features of functional and nonfunctional pancreatic neuroendocrine tumors and adult nesidioblastosis.

M. Markow, MD
PGY 4 in Pathology, Department of Pathology and Cell Biology, Morsani College of Medicine at the University of South Florida, Tampa, FL, USA
e-mail: mmarkow@health.usf.edu

B.A. Centeno, MD (✉)
Morsani College of Medicine at the University of South Florida, Tampa, FL, USA

Vice Chair of Clinical Services, Department of Anatomic Pathology, H. Lee Moffitt Cancer Center and Research Institute, Tampa, FL, USA
e-mail: Barbara.Centeno@moffitt.org

A. Nasir, D. Coppola (eds.), *Neuroendocrine Tumors: Review of Pathology, Molecular and Therapeutic Advances*, DOI 10.1007/978-1-4939-3426-3_13

Neuroendocrine Tumors

Clinical

PanNETs are the second most common pancreatic neoplasm but account for 5 % or less of all pancreatic malignancies, with an annual incidence of 1 in 100,000 [6]. Many are detected incidentally during imaging for another process. They are more common in adults, with an age distribution of 30–60 years (mean of 50 years). Those occurring in children or adolescents are usually associated with a genetic syndrome [6]. There is a slight male predominance.

The tumors occur throughout the pancreas without a predilection for any site. PanNETs that occur in the head of the pancreas are only rarely associated with jaundice.

PanNETs may arise in association with familial syndromes including von Hippel-Lindau (VHL), tuberous sclerosis complex (TSC), neurofibromatosis type 1, and multiple neuroendocrine neoplasia type 1 (MEN 1) (see Table 1). Neoplasms arising in association with MEN 1 and VHL are frequently multifocal and occur in a younger age group [7, 8]. MEN 1 syndrome patients develop multiple microadenomas (<0.5 cm), and dysplastic islets, but can also develop macrotumors (>0.5 cm). The PanNETs that develop in VHL patients are nonfunctional, and up to 60 % show clear cell cytoplasm due to the presence of intracytoplasmic lipids [8, 9]. This morphology is not pathognomonic of VHL as originally presumed, since it is seen in sporadic, nonfunctional tumors and tumors associated with MEN 1 [10].

PanNETs have traditionally been classified as functioning or nonfunctioning. The majority of PanNETs are sporadic and nonfunctioning [11]. They are found during screening of patients with a syndrome that predisposes them to PanNET, the work-up of patients presenting with nonspecific symptoms, or the work-up of patients presenting with widespread metastatic disease. Functioning PanNETs are less common. They often present secondarily to patient symptoms related to the peptide produced by the PanNET. See Table 2 for a list of the syndromes and associated symptoms.

Table 1 Genetic syndromes associated with PanNET

Syndrome	Gene involved	Clinical features	Frequency of PanNET
Multiple endocrine neoplasia, type 1	*MEN 1*	Hyperplasia/neoplasms in multiple endocrine organs	Almost 100 %
von Hippel-Lindau	*VHL*	A variety of neoplasms, including pheochromocytoma, paraganglioma, hemangioblastoma, renal cell carcinoma, PanNET, serous cystadenoma, etc.	11–17 %
Neurofibromatosis, type 1	*NF-1*	Café au lait, neurofibromas, freckling, bony dysplasia	Rare
Tuberous sclerosis	*TSC1* *TSC2*	Hamartomas in many organs	2 %

Table 2 Summary of Clinical Presentations in Nonfunctional and Functional PanNET

Type	Incidence	Hormone	Clinical presentation
Nonfunctioning	1–3	CgA, NSE, PP	Incidental or nonspecific (related to tumor mass)
Insulinoma	0.1–0.3	Insulin	Whipple's triad
Gastrinoma	0.5–1.5	Gastrin	Zollinger-Ellison syndrome
Glucagonoma	0.01–0.1	Glucagon	Glucagonoma syndrome
VIPoma	0.05–0.2	VIP	Verner-Morrison syndrome
Somatostatinoma	<0.1	Somatostatin	SSoma syndrome (rare, <10 %), incidental, nonspecific symptoms related to tumor mass
PPoma	Rare	PP	Nonspecific, tumor mass related
Polyfunctional	Rare	Multiple	Depends on the hormones being secreted

Abbreviations: *CgA* chromogranin A, *PP*pancreatic polypeptide, *VIPoma* VIP-secreting tumor, *VIP* vasoactive intestinal polypeptide

Imaging

The imaging findings of PanNETs apply to both functional and nonfunctional tumors. Typical PanNETs present as solid, circumscribed enhancing masses on computed tomography (CT) imaging studies. They may appear somewhat lobulated and rarely appear infiltrative. Nonfunctioning tumors often are larger and have more irregular borders. Tumors in the head of the pancreas do not commonly obstruct the bile duct, in contrast to ductal adenocarcinomas, which frequently do. By endoscopic ultrasound (EUS), lesions are usually round and circumscribed, homogenous, and hypoechoic. Multiple tumors may be seen, particularly in patients with familial syndromes.

Cystic degeneration is a relatively common finding, identified in up to 10–20 % of PanNETs by CT scan and EUS. A key imaging feature of a cystic PanNET is a thick cyst wall, which is present in most cases.

Octreotide scintigraphy utilizes octreotide, a radiolabeled somatostatin analog, which binds to somatostatin receptors, to identify PanNETs. The Octreoscan, which uses ^{111}In-pentetreotide, was one of the first such functional imaging methods. Octreoscan is used to localize primary tumors and metastases and to plan treatments and monitor therapy response. Unfortunately, it has low sensitivity for the detection of tumors measuring less than 1 cm.

An emerging technology is the use of somatostatin analogs labeled with gallium. The somatostatin analogs are linked to ^{68}Ga with the use of a chelate, most commonly 1,4,7,10-tetraazacyclododecane-1,4,7,10-tetraacetic acid (DOTA). There are three ^{68}Ga-DOTA-labeled somatostatin analogs currently in use: DOTA-NOC, DOTA-TATE, and DOTA-TOC. Advantages over the traditional Octreoscan are the following: faster image acquisition, improved spatial resolution, higher affinity for somatostatin receptors, and the ability to quantify activity. It appears that a combination of imaging techniques including EUS, MDCT, and ^{68}Ga-DOTA-TOC provides the most optimal diagnosis [12]. ^{68}Ga-DOTA PET/CT imaging techniques can be used to localize functional as well as nonfunctional tumors [13].

Laboratory Testing

Plasma chromogranin A (CgA) is the most useful marker for diagnosing and monitoring patients with neuroendocrine tumors, including pancreatic neuroendocrine tumors. Limitations of the use of CgA as a biomarker include treatment with proton pump inhibitors, chronic atrophic gastritis, impaired renal function, and inflammatory bowel disease. Serum pancreatic polypeptide levels are used less frequently due to lower sensitivity, but when used in combination with CgA can improve sensitivity to 93 %.
Elevated levels of specific hormones are identified with functional syndromes and will be described in those specific sections.

Functional Neuroendocrine Tumors

Functional or syndromic PanNETs are named after the functional hormone they secrete, although some may secrete multiple hormones [11]. The diagnostic criteria vary. Based on the clinical definition of function – functional, hormone-producing, clinically symptomatic tumors – approximately 85 % of pancreatic neuroendocrine tumors are nonfunctional. Functional PanNETs are rare. The most common is insulinoma, followed by gastrinomas, glucagonomas, VIPomas, somatostatinomas, PanNET causing carcinoid syndrome, and other rare syndromes [11]. The most common syndromes are summarized in Table 2.

Insulinoma

Insulinomas are insulin-secreting PanNETs. The detection of the insulinoma relies upon the classical symptomatic presentation of Whipple's triad: hypoglycemia with glucose less than 50 mg/dL, neuroglycopenia, and symptomatic relief following administration of glucose. To establish the diagnosis of hyperinsulinism related to insulinoma, the parameters of serum glucose, C-peptide, and proinsulin are measured following a 72-h fast. Together, the criteria of decreased serum glucose, elevated C-peptide, and elevated proinsulin are 99 % sensitive for distinguishing insulinomas from other pancreatic mass lesions [14]. Some authors have reported higher overall sensitivity and specificity rates using the insulin/glucose ratio in conjunction with glucose, C-peptide, and insulin levels [15].

The characterization of a mass lesion is required to distinguish insulinoma from a rare, diffuse pancreatic insulin-secreting lesion known as nesidioblastosis. Conventional multi-detector CT imaging has been reported to have 68.8–94.4 % sensitivity [14, 16] for the detection of mass lesions; cases in which the CT is negative but clinical suspicion remains high can be augmented with MRI, EUS (86.6–92.3 % sensitivity) [14, 17], ^{18}F-FDOPA PET imaging [18],

^{18}F-radiolabeled GLP-1 analog exendin-4 imaging [18], and dual-energy spectral CT [16], among other imaging modalities. For cases in which these imaging modalities are negative, and nesidioblastosis cannot be excluded from the differential diagnosis, intra-arterial [14] calcium stimulation with venous sampling (ASVS) remains an option (see Nesidioblastosis, Adult Type, "Clinical diagnostic criteria") [14].

Glucagonoma

Glucagon targets some of the same pathways as insulin, and therefore has the contrary effect of raising blood glucose, but also has efficacy in pathways that are not directly related to glucose metabolism. The clinical diagnostic triad consists of diabetes mellitus, excess serum glucagon, and a skin rash known as necrolytic migratory erythema (NME) [19]. Diabetes is a simple diagnosis with well-established criteria; however, it is a nonspecific finding. Glucagon elevation is fairly specific in the context of a mass lesion. NME is seen in 70 % of cases and has dermatological and histopathological features that are nonspecific. Features of NME are psoriasiform in nature and include papillary dermal hyperplasia with prominent vessels, superficial epidermal necrosis, epidermal hyperplasia, and parakeratosis. Other symptoms of glucagonoma include weight loss, anemia, diarrhea, stomatitis, and psychiatric disorders [20].

When clinical suspicion is aroused enough to impel the use of imaging to search for a mass lesion, a pancreatic mass is readily detected, and the appropriate neuroendocrine tumor work-up can successfully lead to the diagnosis. The imaging studies already described may be employed.

Glucagon may be hypersecreted by enlarged, misshapen pancreatic islets, much in cases where a mass lesion is absent, like insulin is in nesidioblastosis. Some authors consider this phenomenon to be a glucagon-secreting nesidioblastosis [21, 22], while others have called it *glucagon cell adenomatosis*. It presents with the same symptoms of glucagonomas, but without a discrete mass. Instead, the islets are diffusely enlarged with glomeruloid morphology [20, 23]. In contrast to the association of insulinomas with MEN 1, only one case of glucagon cell adenomatosis has been found to have the *MEN 1* (11q13) deletion [23]. The significance of this is unclear.

Gastrinoma

Clinical presentation of gastrinomas includes abdominal pain (with or without gastric ulceration), bleeding, and chronic diarrhea due to unregulated acid production in the stomach. Gastrinomas are famous for their association with Zollinger-Ellison syndrome and are also known to be associated with MEN 1. In both syndromes, gastrinomas tend to be multifocal; nonsyndromic gastrinomas are usually solitary. *ZES* and *MEN 1* mutations can be identified through molecular studies. Care must be exercised in evaluating functional neuroendocrine tumors biochemically, as gastrinomas can produce separate neuroendocrine hormones (e.g., insulin) in up to 50 % of cases and many may be characterized as polyfunctional pancreatic neuroendocrine tumors if the separate hormone causes distinct clinical symptoms (page 6) [24].

The diagnosis of gastrinoma can be determined using fasting serum gastrinoma (FSG) concentration, endoscopic imaging, conventional CT and MRI for pancreatic masses, and newer imaging and biochemical methods. Any hypochlorhydric state can lead to serum hypergastrinemia, but hypergastrinemia (>2000 pg/mL) in the presence of a mass is highly suggestive of gastrinoma (98 % sensitive) [25]. With chronic functional gastrinomas, the stomach develops characteristically thickened rugal folds in 92 % of cases, grossly reflecting parietal cell hyperplasia due to unopposed gastrin stimulation [24]. Chromogranin A and progastrin have been studied for use in gastrinoma diagnosis, with some initial success of α-aminated gastrin assays. Overall, the biochemical diagnosis of gastrinomas can be complicated by treatment with common proton pump inhibitors and by problems with manufactured reagents that have occurred recently [24]. A stimulation test for gastrinoma can be performed using the glucagon provocation test, which is positive if plasma gastrin levels increase by 200 pg/mL or rise to greater than 35 % above baseline [26]. Secretin, a hormone that stimulates G cells, has been used historically as a clinical gold standard for diagnosis. Due to expense, it is now used primarily for tumor localization in cases of small but functional gastrinomas. The selective arterial secretagogue injection (SASI) test measures plasma gastrin levels after selective injection of secretin in various tributary arteries to the pancreas.

Prognosis is strongly correlated with the presence or absence of metastasis; 10-year survival with no metastasis is 96 %, and 10-year survival with diffuse metastasis is 16 % [24].

Vasoactive Intestinal Peptide-Secreting Tumor (VIPoma)

Pancreatic VIPomas are rare, with only about 1 in 10,000,000 per year [11]. These usually present as larger tumors, greater than 3 cm, and the vast majority occur in the tail of the pancreas (75 %). A majority, 60–80 %, present with metastatic disease. The classical clinical presentation is that of Verner-Morrison syndrome, also known as WDHA [27]. The signs and symptoms include watery diarrhea, with dehydration, hypokalemia, achlorhydria, and metabolic acidosis. Symptoms related to hypokalemia and dehydration include lethargy, nausea, vomiting, muscle weakness, and muscle cramps. Other symptoms include vasodilation with flushing and hypotension, hypercalcemia, and hyperglycemia. Abdominal pain, if present, is mild at most [11].

Somatostatin-Secreting Pancreatic Neuroendocrine Tumor (Somatostatinoma)

Due to the physiologic role of somatostatin as a general inhibitor of neuroendocrine secretion, the clinical presentation is highly variable. The classical presentation of somatostatinoma includes the development of diabetes mellitus, gallbladder disease (due to cholestasis), diarrhea, weight loss, and steatorrhea [28]. However, preferential inhibition of insulin or other hormones may occur idiosyncratically, leading to primary presentation with hypoglycemia or hypochlorhydria [29]. Pancreatic somatostatinomas are far more likely than duodenal somatostatinomas (2 %) to present with symptoms, presumably due to circumvention of the first-pass effect [28, 30]. Gallbladder disease, the most distinguishing clinical feature of somatostatinomas from other pancreatic neuroendocrine tumors, is seen in 59 % of pancreatic somatostatinomas [30].

Due to vague symptoms and rarity of disease, somatostatinomas present with metastatic lesions 80 % of the time, and overall survival at 5 years is 60 %. In addition to the detection of a mass lesion in the pancreas, somatostatinomas can be identified serologically using immunoassays for somatostatin-like immunoreactivity (SLI) levels. Stimulation of SLI production using tolbutamide or arginine may have clinical utility but remains to be validated in large studies. Reference intervals are difficult to establish due to the paucity of cases; however, elevation of SLI levels to greater than 50 times mean values is accepted by some as diagnostic for somatostatinoma.

Pancreatic Polypeptide-Secreting Tumor (PPoma)

Pancreatic polypeptide-secreting tumors are extremely rare; only 24 pure PPomas have been described in the literature [25, 31]. They more often occur secondarily with other neuroendocrine tumors, often as a separate pauci-functional mass or discrete cell population within a mass that is secreting another major hormone. The physiologic role of pancreatic polypeptide is not fully elucidated, but similarly to somatostatin, it has a role in inhibiting other hormones. Therefore, abdominal pain is the most prominent of symptoms. Other signs and symptoms include diarrhea (including WDHA syndrome: watery diarrhea, hypokalemia, achlorhydria) [26], steatorrhea, and gallbladder contraction [25].

Clinically, PPomas may be detected by performing an assay for fasting serum PP concentrations (>300 pM) or by administering secretin to stimulate PP production (positive cutoff >5000 pM). Of the 24 pure PPomas reported in the literature, eight metastasized (33 %); prognosis is guarded, but it appears that metastatic rate is not dissimilar from nonfunctional pancreatic neuroendocrine tumors (38 %) [23].

Polyfunctional Pancreatic Endocrine Tumor

A polyfunctional PanNET is one that produces more than one hormone type and therefore is associated with more than one clinical syndrome. These are extremely rare and mostly have been documented in case reports [24, 32, 33, 35, 36]. These may respond to surgical debulking and treatment with peptide receptor radiotherapy [35].

Pathology

Gross

PanNETs typically appear as well-circumscribed, solitary masses. The cut surface is tan-brown and fleshy when the stromal component is minimal and sometimes more yellow, firm, and sclerotic when there is a stromal reaction. Some cases have a complete capsule. A percentage of these tumors present as predominantly cystic masses or as masses with cystic degeneration.

Histopathology

PanNET is typically a stroma-poor neoplasm, in contrast to ductal adenocarcinoma. The stroma may contain amyloid. There are no specific features associated with any of the functional types or that differentiate nonfunctional from functional types. Two exceptions exist. PanNET with psammomatous calcifications and gland formations is suggestive of somatostatin-secreting tumors. When dense sclerotic stroma is present, it suggests a serotonin-secreting tumor.

The cells are arranged in anastomosing cords, nests, and trabeculae (Fig. 1). They may form glandular structures, pseudorosettes, or tubuloacinar structures. These structures are surrounded by intervening vascular rich, thin stroma. The individual cells have rounded, monotonous nuclei with salt-and-pepper chromatin. The cytoplasm may be abundant and eccentric, imparting a plasmacytoid appearance.

A number of morphological variants have been described. The lipid-rich (also known as clear cell) variant is characterized by abundant foamy/microvesicular cytoplasm (Fig. 2). Some of these are associated with von Hippel-Lindau syndrome (VHL) [9] or MEN 1 [10]. An oncocytic variant, characterized by abundant, granular, eosinophilic cytoplasm and large prominent nucleoli, is also recognized. This variant has been found to be more aggressive in some studies [37]. Other morphological variants include a rhabdoid variant that may also have signet ring features [38], a small cell variant with an increased nuclear to cytoplasmic ratio, lacking the necrosis and mitotic activity typically seen in small cell carcinomas, and also a peliotic variant (Fig. 3) with pools of blood and dilated blood vessels.

PanNETs may show significant nuclear pleomorphism, called endocrine atypia, similar to that seen in other endocrine organs [39]. These degenerative, symplastic cells can be abundant and atypical, leading to a misdiagnosis of carcinoma.

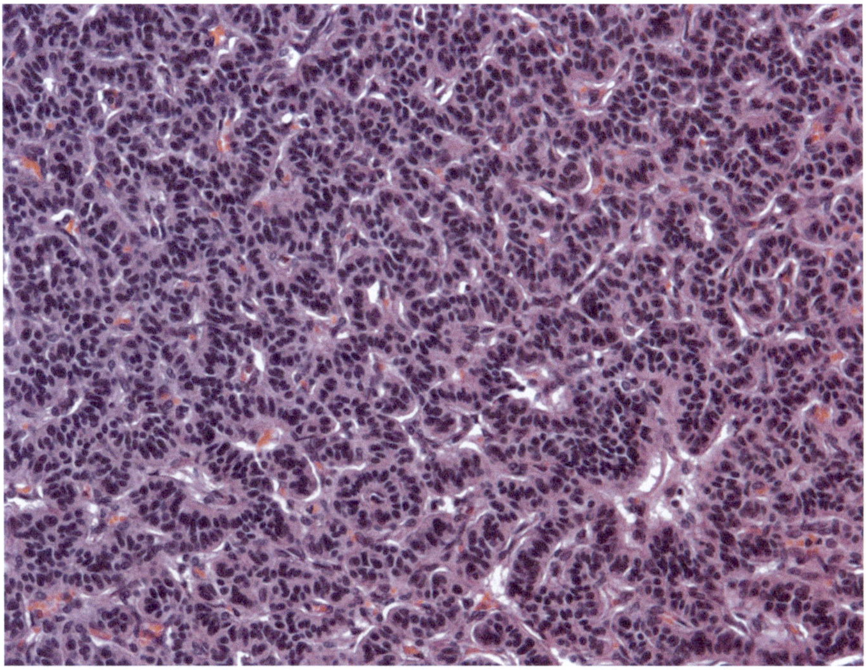

Fig. 1 Pancreatic neuroendocrine tumor growing in cords and trabeculae. The nuclei are round to oval with evenly dispersed chromatin. The cytoplasm is scant (hematoxylin and eosin, 200×)

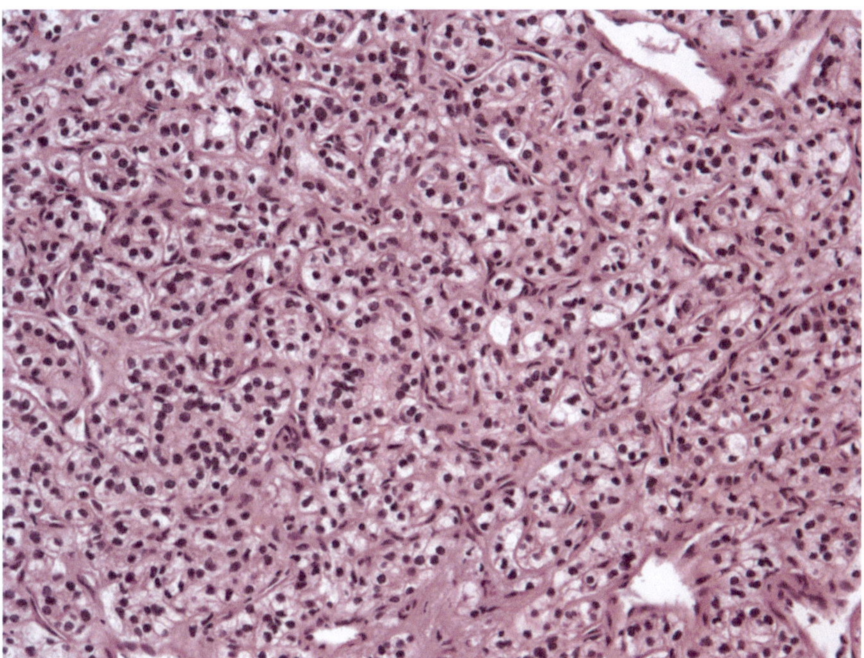

Fig. 2 Pancreatic neuroendocrine tumor with abundant clear cytoplasm (hematoxylin and eosin, 200×)

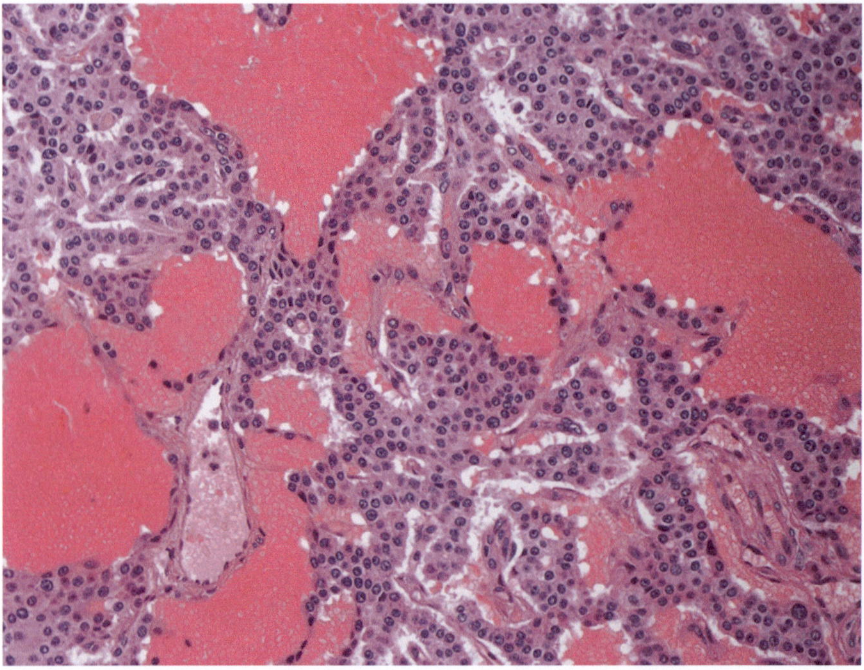

Fig. 3 Pancreatic neuroendocrine tumor showing a peliotic pattern. There are multiple dilated vascular spaces (hematoxylin and eosin, 200×)

Cytopathology

The low-power assessment of PanNET smears typically shows a cellular smear with a monomorphic cellular appearance (Fig. 4). The cells are arranged in loosely cohesive tissue fragments, which may have pseudorosettes, and as single cells. Due to the vascularity of these tumors, fibrovascular cores with loosely attached tumor cells may also be present. The cytoplasm varies from delicate, amphophilic scant cytoplasm to more abundant well-defined, granular cytoplasm with eccentric nuclei, imparting a plasmacytoid appearance [40, 41]. Cytoplasmic variations are seen in the oncocytic, rhabdoid, signet ring, lipid-rich, and clear cell variants [9, 42]. The lipid-rich variant commonly occurs in patients with von Hippel-Lindau syndrome [42]. The nuclei of all neuroendocrine tumor variants are usually round to oval, and the nuclear membranes remain smooth. The chromatin is finely granular with a "salt-and-pepper" appearance. The oncocytic variant retains the nuclear membrane configuration and chromatin pattern but also has prominent nucleoli. The pleomorphic variant of PanNET is the exception and shows anisonucleosis or "endocrine atypia" [42].

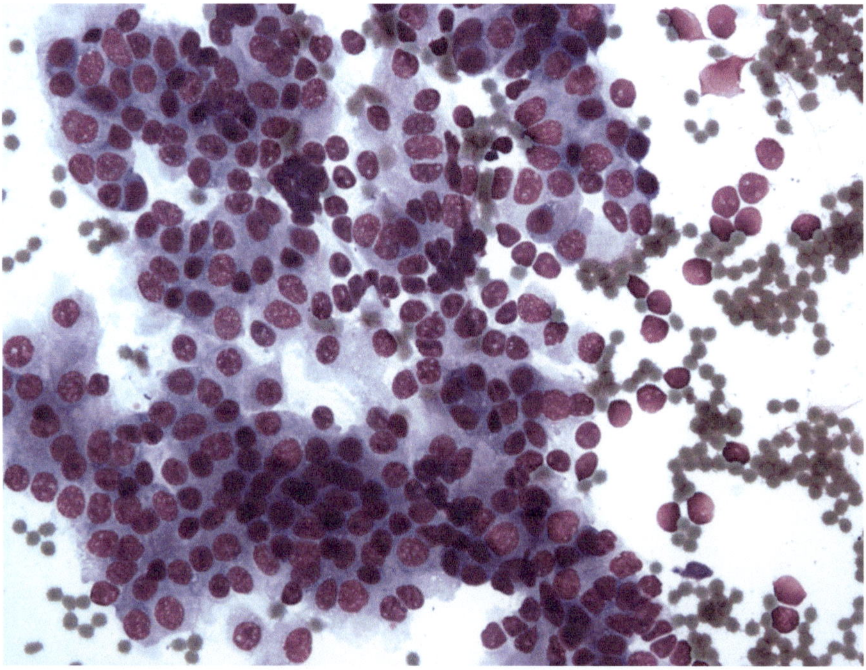

Fig. 4 Fine-needle aspirate smear demonstrating a monomorphic population of cells with round to oval uniform nuclei. The cytoplasm is variable in quantity and fragile. Stripped nuclei are seen in the background (Diff-Quik, 400×)

Ancillary Studies

Ki-67

The cell proliferation marker Ki-67 has gained substantial currency in the use of pancreatic neuroendocrine tumor prognosis. The Ki-67 index was incorporated in the 2010 WHO criteria for determining the histologic grade of pancreatic neuroendocrine tumors. Low grade is <3 %, intermediate is 3–20 %, and high grade is >20 % (Fig. 5a, b) [5]. It is used as an adjunct to mitotic index, which can have poor interobserver variability, and the highest possible grade is assigned according to either the Ki-67 or mitotic index criteria. The Ki-67 index is assessed by counting the areas of greatest proliferation, or so-called hot spots.

This new use of Ki-67 is controversial, as the scheme was incorporated into the WHO 2010 with very limited data to support it. Some advocate the alternative of using the Memorial Sloan-Kettering criteria (based on mitotic indices) or using a different proliferation marker like PHH3. Large head-to-head comparisons of repro-

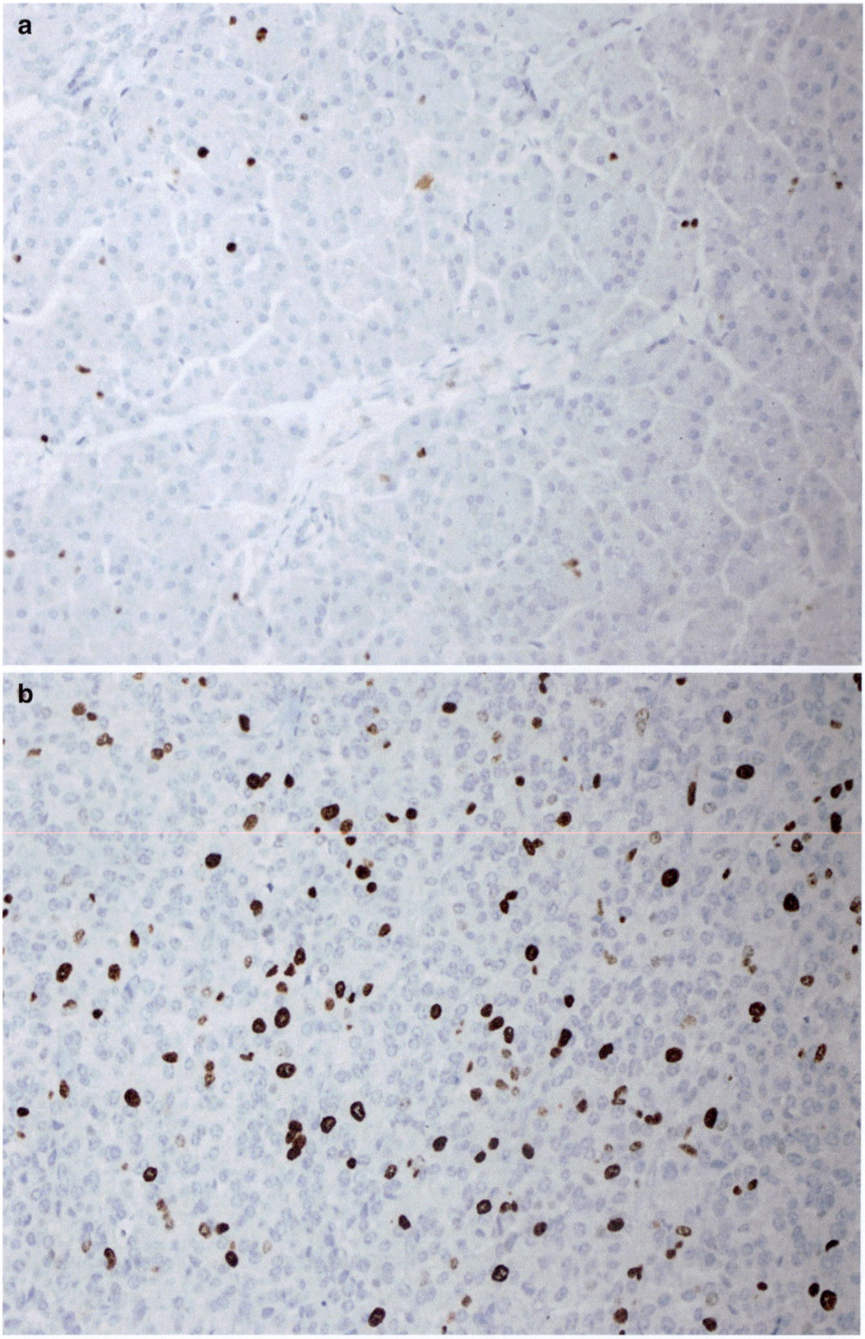

Fig. 5 Images of Ki-67 labeling (**a**) Pancreatic neuroendocrine tumor, grade 1, with a Ki-67 labeling index of 2 % (peroxidase, antiperoxidase, 200×). (**b**) Pancreatic neuroendocrine tumor, grade 2, with a Ki-67 labeling index of 15 % (peroxidase, antiperoxidase, 200×)

ducibility of these prognostic methods against Ki-67, using surgical resection specimens and under practical circumstances of hand counting, have not been performed. However, many studies have attempted to demonstrate the utility of Ki-67 and PHH3 in cell blocks from fine-needle aspirates, usually in conjunction with an automated cytometric counting system [43, 44].

Since the WHO 2010 reclassification, some data has come out to support the utility of Ki-67 in prognostication of pancreatic neuroendocrine tumors. It has use in upgrading grade 1 low-mitotic-count pancreatic neuroendocrine tumors to grade 2 based on an elevated Ki-67 index. PanNETs upgraded in this manner have been found to better correlate to tumor size and metastatic potential [45]. Still other studies have suggested making minor modifications to the WHO 2010 score, like altering the low-grade to intermediate-grade Ki-67 cutoff from 3 to 5 % [46]. A study comparing WHO 2010 Ki-67 index criteria to the WHO 2000/2004 showed that the Ki-67 index criteria are easier to use and more reproducible but that with this technique, there were no benign tumors since even G1 tumors metastasized. The WHO 2000/2004 was better at prognostication, most likely because this system included more parameters [47]. This study shows that the Ki-67 proliferation index alone is not sufficient to predict prognosis and needs to be combined with staging information at the time of resection.

Ultimately, Ki-67 index studies are hamstrung by the problem of site localization. It is widely recognized that different tissues have different mitotic or proliferation indices for assessing malignant potential. This becomes altogether more complicated in the GI tract, where the presence of a single or multiple sub-centimeter neoplasms prior to metastasis obscures discovery of the tissue of origin. Immunohistochemical markers for specific hormones are not helpful, as hormone-producing neuroendocrine tumors can arise in areas away from their native tissue, practically anywhere in the GI tract. Until it is possible to localize sites using immunohistochemical, molecular, or other methods, it will remain difficult to develop robust, site-specific criteria using the Ki-67 index. This is especially true in the pancreas, as its adjacency to multiple other GI organs can confuse radiographic localization of solitary neoplasms [48]. Another confounding problem with the use of the Ki-67 index is heterogeneity of Ki-67 expression within different parts of the same tumor.

PHH3

PHH3, or phosphohistone 3, is a marker of active mitosis (M phase). By contrast, Ki-67 is expressed during S, G2, and M phases. Theoretically, PHH3 should be a superior surrogate marker of mitotic activity, although this remains to be validated in large studies. PHH3 has been compared to the use of mitotic counts in pancreatic neuroendocrine tumors and found to have superior interobserver agreement (Fleiss' κ of 0.69 vs. 0.46) [49].

A comparison between PHH3 and Ki-67 suggests that Ki-67 should continue to remain the standard for now. This is due in part to the phenomenon of mitotic hot spots or aggregates of proliferating cells. The standard practice is to count Ki-67 expression across 500–2000 cells, and the preferred practice is to focus on the fields with the greatest numbers. The PHH3 antibodies used in immunoperoxidase reactions so far have stained less intensely than Ki-67, and PHH3 has therefore been less useful for detecting hot spots and led to underestimation of mitotic indices [43].

No large study has examined the use of PHH3 in the examination of metastatic potential or overall survival in pancreatic neuroendocrine tumors, although its use has shown promising results in other organ systems. Forthcoming validation of PHH3 as a prognostic marker for pancreatic neuroendocrine tumors may show substantial utility.

Molecular Alterations

Information about the genetic basis of this disease has been limited. DAXX/ ATRX, MEN 1, and mTOR pathway genes (*TSC2, PTEN, PIK3CA*) have recently been shown to be altered in sporadic pancreatic neuroendocrine tumors [50]. The genes most commonly affected in pancreatic ductal adenocarcinoma, including *KRAS*, *TGF-β* pathway (*TGFBR1, SMAD 3, SMAD 4*), *CDKN2A*, and *TP53*, were rarely altered, if at all [50]. These suggest an alternate oncogenetic pathway for PanNET.

DAXX/ATRX

Alpha thalassemia/mental retardation syndrome X-linked *(ATRX)* and death domain-associated protein (*DAXX)* are the two subunits of a transcription/remodeling complex. Mutation in one gene is mutually exclusive of mutations in the other. In the study by Jiao et al., 42.6 % of all PanNETs had loss in either ATRX or DAXX. Loss of immunolabeling for *DAXX* and *ATRX* correlated with mutation in the gene [50]. Subsequent studies detected mutations of *ATRX* or *DAXX* within 18 and 23 % of PanNETs by whole exome sequencing or FISH. PanNETs with mutations in *ATRX* or *DAXX* had a worse prognosis than *ATRX*- or *DAXX*-wild type tumors, including increased metastatic rate and decreased progression-free survival [51, 52].

Mutations of *ATRX* and *DAXX* lead to misplacement of histone H3.3 at pericentric and telomeric chromosome regions (at loci of DNA repeat sequencing), leading in turn to aberrant lengthening of telomeres. Failure to deposit H3.3 is an epigenetic phenomenon that leads to permanent somatic chromosome changes, possibly accounting for some of the additive cytogenetic abnormalities identified in sporadic pancreatic neuroendocrine tumors [53].

mTOR Pathway Genes

NF, TSC, and VHL are all associated with loss of suppression of the mTOR pathway. The mTOR pathway is a prominent regulator of cell growth, and its gain of function promotes oncogenesis.

Genes Associated with Familial Syndromes

Familial syndromes with increased pancreatic neuroendocrine tumors include multiple endocrine neoplasia (MEN) type 1, neurofibromatosis (NF) type 1, von Hippel-Lindau (VHL) syndrome, and tuberous sclerosis (TSC). MEN 1 is known to have multiple microcarcinomas of the neuroendocrine type, as well as multiple neuroendocrine tumors [54]. Loss-of-function mutations of the *MEN* gene are seen in 10–27 % of insulinomas and 39–45 % of gastrinomas. The pathways involved in PanNET development patients with a genetic predisposition are shown in Fig. 6. It is believed that genes on 11q distal to the *MEN* locus may harbor additional onco-suppressor exons.

Other Molecular Alterations and Cytogenetic Abnormalities

Sporadic pancreatic neuroendocrine tumors rarely have abnormalities in *TP53* and have various cytogenetic abnormalities, including 1 del, 11q del, 9q gain, 4 gain, 6q del, and 22q loss of heterozygosity (93 % of insulinomas). Deletions of *p16INK4a*

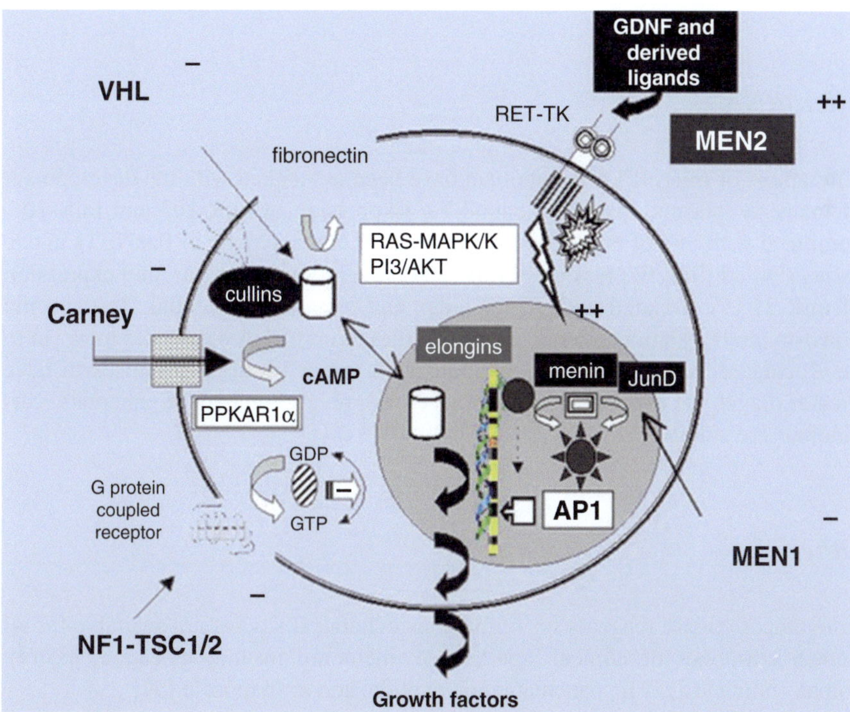

Fig. 6 This is a schematic summary of the pathways involved in genetic predisposition to neuroendocrine tumors (Reprinted with permission from [94])

and *p16/MTS1* are seen in gastrinomas. Cyclin D1 overexpression is seen in 43 % of pancreatic neuroendocrine tumors [55].

Palladin and RUNX1T1

Palladin is a nonproliferative prognostic immunohistochemical marker that is expressed in pancreatic neuroendocrine tumors. Physiologically, it has been demonstrated to play a role in regulating cell motility. It has been shown to have predictive value for liver metastasis. A study of 38 patients showed good immunohistochemical accuracy of palladin for predicting liver metastases. Using an Allred score cutoff of three of nine, palladin had a 100% sensitivity, 63% spcificity and overall positive predictive accuracy of 76% for predicting liver metastases in PanNET [56].

Another nonproliferative prognostic marker is *RUNX1T1* expression, discovered using gene expression profiling on frozen samples of PanNETs. Similar to the palladin protein, a study of RUNX1T1 expression loss in 37 patients using an Allred score of four of nine as the cutoff showed an 85 % sensitivity and 96 % specificity in predicting liver metastasis in tumors with a score of four or less [57]. RUNX1T1 is known to regulate neuronal differentiation in glial tissue; however, its function in the pancreas or pancreatic neuroendocrine cells is not yet elucidated [57].

MicroRNA

Alterations of microRNA metabolism have been associated with the development of many neoplasms, including PanNETs. Expression of miR-103 and miR-107, combined with loss of expression of miR-155, is characteristic of PanNETs in one series studied [58]. Expression of miR-204 is seen in insulinomas, and expression of miR-21 is correlated with Ki-67 index and metastatic potential. The specific downstream translational derangements of these microRNA sequences have yet to be elucidated. MicroRNA heat mapping with tumor profiling promises to have greater diagnostic and theragnostic efficacy as greater numbers of pancreatic carcinomas are studied [58].

Other

Immunoperoxidase reagents for immunohistochemical studies are available for all known hormones of clinical significance, including insulin, glucagon, gastrin, somatostatin (SLI), VIP, pancreatic polypeptide, and even motilin [59].

Nesidioblastosis, Adult Type

Background

Nesidioblastosis (also called congenital hyperinsulinism) is a controversial entity that is distinct from the insulinoma but is traditionally defined as proliferations of β cells which do not form discrete masses. Due to the rarity of nesidioblastosis, and the degree of overlap of clinical presentation between nesidioblastosis and insulinoma, no rigorously studied criteria have been developed to differentiate the two entities. The commonly accepted working definition is the exclusion of insulinoma using a combination of radiographic examination, bimanual surgical examination, and gross pathologic examination [60]. Microscopically, there are no absolute size criteria applied to differentiate nesidioblastosis and insulinoma; instead, nesidioblastosis and insulinomas have distinctly different pathological features, described below [61]. Meanwhile, the clinical criteria for the two entities are better defined. Although no specific marker exists to differentiate nesidioblastosis from insulinomas, there are clinical parameters that can be used to strongly support the diagnosis of nesidioblastosis [62]. For the diagnosis of nesidioblastosis, close clinicopathologic correlation is essential.

Nesidioblastosis comes in two main varieties, the diffuse type and focal type [60]. The focal type is characteristically seen only in infants; in fact, only one case has been reported in an adult [63]. Nesidioblastosis, focal type, is distinct from the insulinoma by not forming a discrete mass, and it is distinct from diffuse nesidioblastosis by forming patchy areas of irregular, hyperplasic islets that are increased in cellular density. These areas of islet hyperplasia are only sporadically affected, in contrast to the diffuse form in which islets are nearly equally affected throughout the pancreas [64]. We highlight the diagnostic criteria of nesidioblastosis, focal type, to offer evidence for its distinction as an entity from diffuse nesidioblastosis and insulinoma. Nesidioblastosis, focal type, has additional histopathological features that will not be described here. Further description of the clinical and histopathological features of diffuse nesidioblastosis can be seen below.

Prior to its subtyping, nesidioblastosis was first described as a phenomenon in children in 1938 [65] and first described in adults in 1975 [66]. Nesidioblastosis, diffuse type, is traditionally believed to be a rare entity; only 138 cases have been reported [60–63, 67–98]. Diffuse nesidioblastosis is responsible for 60 % of cases of neonatal nesidioblastosis and essentially 100 % of adult cases [60]. Although nesidioblastosis has been characterized as a β-cell proliferation, it has recently been reported to express glucagon in rare cases, although some believe this should be designated as a separate entity [81, 90]. Nesidioblastosis also can occur concomitantly with insulinomas [22, 76]; and nesidioblastosis, adult type, is associated with prior stomach surgery, especially gastric bypass surgery [69, 90–98]. The commonness of postprandial episodic hypoglycemia with hyperinsulinemia in postoperative gastric bypass patients, combined with the intrinsic difficulty of diagnosing nesidioblastosis, suggests an underdiagnosis of diffuse nesidioblastosis, adult type [98].

Pathogenesis and Molecular Biology

Nesidioblastosis was originally coined to reflect the phenomenon of endocrine cells appearing to displace ductal epithelial cells of the pancreas (*nesidio-*, islet; *blastos*, germ) [65]. Originally, pathologists believed that its etiology was embryogenic; therefore, some texts utilize the term nesidioblastosis to refer to the embryogenic displacement of epithelial cells by neuroendocrine cells. Others use the term nesidioblastosis only to describe the histological features, without any congenital connotation. Nesidioblastosis was believed to be a diffuse proliferation of neuroendocrine cells within glands (ectopic placement, as in heterotopic pancreas within upper alimentary tract) which was consistent with a congenital, presumed embryological, malformation. The identification of nesidioblastosis exclusively in the pediatric population during the first 37 years after its discovery likely contributed to the conception of nesidioblastosis as an embryologic or congenital disease [65, 66].

However, no convincing studies emerged to demonstrate an embryological pathogenesis for nesidioblastosis, and the recognition of adult-onset diffuse-type nesidioblastosis forced a reconsideration of pathogenesis. The growing evidence that a subset of postoperative gastric bypass patients are developing diffuse-type nesidioblastosis demonstrates that other factors must be at play.

What do we know now about the pathogenesis of nesidioblastosis? While the exact etiology remains unclear, and further studies are required to elucidate a working model to explain both pediatric- and adult-onset nesidioblastosis, we have determined some of the biochemical and molecular factors underlying the disease.

Familial cases of nesidioblastosis have been the underpinning of the challenge against an embryologic model of pathogenesis and include mutations in genes *ABCC8*, *KCNJ11*, *HADH1*, *GCK*, *GLUD1*, *SLC16A1*, *UCP2*, and *HNF4a* [89]. Of these mutations, authors focus on *GLUD1*, *GCK*, and *SLC16A1* as more likely to present in adults.

The *ABCC8* and *KCNJ11* genes, most common of the familial genes, are not typically found in adults with sporadic nesidioblastosis. Homozygous recessive genotypes for either gene, or heterozygosity of both genes, causes defects in ATP-driven K^+ channels on islet cells, leading to hyperplasia of islet cells. Impairment of K^+ receptors leads to constitutively active insulin secretion, of which cell hypertrophy and proliferation are downstream effects [60]. The effects of these two germline mutations can be modified by somatic mutations. Inheritance of paternal *ABCC8* or *KCNJ11* genes with a somatic loss of heterozygosity at the 11p15 region can likewise lead to hypertrophic islet cells and hyperplastic islets. Unsurprisingly, the therapeutic value of diazoxide, an agonist of the ATP-driven K+ channels, is limited in cases of nesidioblastosis with these mutations.

GCK mutations in glucokinase cause hyperinsulinism due to failure of the negative feedback loop in glycolysis. *GLUD1* mutation upregulates glutamate dehydrogenase, causing increased α-ketoglutarate and efficacy of insulin secretion that is stimulated by amino acids [99]. Together, mutations of *GCK* and *GLUD1* are generally responsive to medical therapy, and so their histopathology has been poorly studied due to absence of resection specimens [60]. Similarly to *GLUD1*, mutation of the gene *HADH1*, which encodes the protein SCHAD, is found in mice knockout studies to increase activity of glutamate dehydrogenase. Increased glutamate dehydrogenase activity is caused by the loss of functional inhibition by wild-type SCHAD glutamate dehydrogenase; the mutant is less capable of downregulating glutamate dehydrogenase. For this reason, both *GLUD1* and *HADH1* are associated with protein-induced hypoglycemia [99].

SLC16A1 encodes MCT1, which is a membrane-bound pyruvate transporter. Ostensibly, it removes excess pyruvate, allowing glycolysis to proceed faster. It is associated with anaerobic exercise-induced hypoglycemia. Ultimately, thorough work-up of nesidioblastosis may need to include testing for these genetic aberrances, as treatment efficacy varies demonstrably among nesidioblastosis cases with differing genetic mutations [99, 100].

Studies attempting to implicate the *menin* gene of MEN 1 failed to demonstrate a germline mutation in known cases of nesidioblastosis [61].

In studies surrounding the mechanism of gastric bypass surgery causing nesidioblastosis, glucagon-like protein 1 (GLP-1) has been identified as an inducer of cell proliferation in islets, with subsequent insulin overproduction and postprandial hypoglycemia. GLP-1 targets all islet cell types (including α and β cells) in rat models and also stimulates progenitor cell differentiation [100]. Meanwhile, GLP-1 is demonstrably elevated in gastric bypass patients after glucose intake [93, 101] and acts in a glucose-dependent manner [102]. GLP-1 is a logical candidate for causing β-cell hyperplasia "accidentally" while being endogenously produced to stimulate α-cell production, after bypass surgery, although its full effects remain to be elucidated. However, the GLP-1 hypothesis of nesidioblastosis development does not explain why β cells would predominate in number or function over α cells.

Increased levels of growth factor expression, including IGF1Rα, IGF2, and TGFRβ3, are also seen in nesidioblastosis. These factors stimulate β-cell proliferation and are also elevated in gastric bypass patients. The association is probably causal, but this remains to be demonstrated. The efficacy of growth factors as markers in individual cases of nesidioblastosis appears to be based on underlying subtype (diffuse vs. focal) [103].

Clinical Diagnostic Criteria

Nesidioblastosis is referred to more popularly in clinical circles as congenital hyperinsulinism (CH) due to the historical confusion, etiological uncertainty, and antiquated histological meaning of the term nesidioblastosis. However, the use of the term nesidioblastosis to describe the specific situation of adult-onset CH has gained traction due to the confusion of using "congenital" to describe an adult-onset disease with obvious environmental associations [60]. Given the confusion of terminology, clarification within the pathology report or during communication with clinicians can help facilitate understanding of the underlying diagnosis. Some also prefer use of the term persistent hyperinsulinemic hypoglycemia (PHH).

Clinically speaking, nesidioblastosis and insulinoma are both under the diagnostic category of organic hyperinsulinism or the overproduction of insulin regardless of blood glucose level. Therefore, in nesidioblastosis, fasting causes hypoglycemia as glucose is depleted over time, and the elevated insulin/glucagon ratio prohibits liberation of new glucose into the blood. The first diagnostic step is a 48- or 72-h fast. Serial measurements of serum insulin, proinsulin, and C-peptide are taken until the patient begins having symptoms of neuroglycopenia. If the above peptides remain elevated, then organic hyperinsulinism is the diagnosis, and the patient is evaluated for insulinoma or an endogenous insulin-producing mass. In the absence of a radiographically identifiable mass, the traditional approach has been to undertake a laparotomy with bimanual examination of the pancreas in an attempt to localize a smaller mass. Depending on clinical parameters, some have recommended stopping the bimanual evaluation in the absence of an identifiable mass and performing a spleen-sparing distal pancreatectomy.

A newer diagnostic modality has been developed, which is helpful for mass localization, and in the absence of mass localization, it is capable of demonstrating nesidioblastosis clinically without biopsy. The procedure is called intra-arterial calcium stimulation with venous sampling (ASVS). It begins with infusion of calcium gluconate serially into each of the arteries feeding the pancreas: pancreatic, hepatic, gastroduodenal, superior mesenteric, and splenic. Throughout, serial measurements of insulin content in the hepatic vein are taken before and after the introduction of calcium gluconate into the tributary arteries. In the event of a localized mass, only one or two of the arteries will have elevated insulin levels. In the event of nesidioblastosis, all of the arteries tested should cause elevations in insulin draining to the hepatic vein. ASVS is comparable to the histopathological gold standard, with 100 % sensitivity in cases studied [80].

Histopathology

The histopathological features of nesidioblastosis are quite distinct from insulinomas and other neuroendocrine neoplasms on histopathological sectioning. Cytopathological examination of the cells cannot distinguish among these entities.

Histologically, nesidioblastosis, diffuse type, appears as diffuse, scattered islets with no mass formation. Anlauf et al. proposed four major criteria as essential for diagnosis and four minor criteria as adjunctive for diagnosis [61].

Major Criteria:

Exclusion of an insulinoma by macroscopic, microscopic, and immunohistochemical examination

Multiple β cells with enlarged, hyperchromatic nuclei and abundant clear cytoplasm
Islets with normal spatial distribution of various cell types
No mitotic proliferative activity of endocrine cells

Minor Criteria:

Irregular shape and occasional enlargement of islets
Increased number of islets
Lobulated islet structure (histological nesidioblastosis)
Macronucleoli in β cells

Using the major criteria as the pathologic standard, the Anlauf et al. group obtained 100 % specificity and 88 % sensitivity [61]. Other authors endorse anisonucleosis of islet cells as the main determining factor for nesidioblastosis, in conjunction with the absence of an identifiable mass and with clinical symptoms. While little data is available to support these criteria, they are becoming more widely used. Least used is the older criteria of calculating β cells as a percentage of pancreatic mass or measuring islet diameters.

It is important to understand that prior to the adoption of the diffuse and focal types of nesidioblastosis, most descriptions (all of the minor criteria) were applied mostly to the focal type. The diffuse type is usually comparatively bland, with regularly shaped islets that have subtle anisonucleosis, subtle islet cell hypertrophy, and subtle islet hyperplasia. The major criterion of low proliferative activity for the diffuse type does not apply to the focal type; the focal type typically has a higher proliferative rate. There is no established cutoff for the Ki-67 index for either type.

Treatment

Treatment of nesidioblastosis can vary based on genetic subtype. Nesidioblastosis may be removed if focal, through either enucleation or distal pancreatectomy. Nesidioblastosis, diffuse type with *ABCC8* or *KCNJ11* mutations, can be treated with octreotide and diazoxide medical therapy, although total or subtotal pancreatectomy remains an option in refractory cases.

Abbreviations

ASVS	Arterial calcium stimulation with venous sampling
CgA	Chromogranin A
CH	Congenital hyperinsulinism
CT	Computed tomography

DOTA	1,4,7,10-tetraacetic acid
EUS	Endoscopic ultrasound
FISH	Fluorescence in situ hybridization
FSG	Fasting serum gastrinoma
GLP-1	Glucagon-like protein 1
MDCT	Multiple detector computed tomography
MEN 1	Multiple neuroendocrine neoplasia, type 1
NF	Neurofibromatosis
NME	Necrolytic migratory erythema
PanNET	Pancreatic neuroendocrine tumor
PET	Positron emission tomography
PHH	Persistent hyperinsulinemic hypoglycemia
PHH3	Phosphohistone 3
PP	Pancreatic polypeptide
PPoma	Pancreatic polypeptide-secreting tumor
SASI	Selective arterial secretagogue injection
SLI	Somatostatin-like immunoreactivity
TSC	Tuberous sclerosis complex
VHL	Von Hippel-Lindau
VIP	Vasoactive intestinal peptide
WHO	World Health Organization
ZES	Zollinger-Ellison syndrome

References

1. Nicholls AG. Simple Adenoma of the Pancreas arising from an Island of Langerhans. J Med Res. 1902;8(2):385–95.
2. Fabozzi S. Uber die Histogenese des primaren Krebses des Pankreas. Beitr Pathol Anat. 1903;34:199–212.
3. Apel RL, Asa SL. Endocrine tumors of the pancreas. Pathol Annu. 1995;30(Pt 1):305–49.
4. Kloppel G, Perren A, Heitz PU. The gastroenteropancreatic neuroendocrine cell system and its tumors: the WHO classification. Ann N Y Acad Sci. 2004;1014:13–27.
5. Klimstra DS, Modlin IR, Coppola D, Lloyd RV, Suster S. The pathologic classification of neuroendocrine tumors: a review of nomenclature, grading, and staging systems. Pancreas. 2010;39(6):707–12.
6. Shi C, Klimstra DS. Pancreatic neuroendocrine tumors: pathologic and molecular characteristics. Semin Diagn Pathol. 2014;31(6):498–511.
7. Anlauf M, Schlenger R, Perren A, Bauersfeld J, Koch CA, Dralle H, et al. Microadenomatosis of the endocrine pancreas in patients with and without the multiple endocrine neoplasia type 1 syndrome. Am J Surg Pathol. 2006;30(5):560–74.
8. Lubensky IA, Pack S, Ault D, Vortmeyer AO, Libutti SK, Choyke PL, et al. Multiple neuroendocrine tumors of the pancreas in von Hippel-Lindau disease patients: histopathological and molecular genetic analysis. Am J Pathol. 1998;153(1):223–31.
9. Hoang MP, Hruban RH, Albores-Saavedra J. Clear cell endocrine pancreatic tumor mimicking renal cell carcinoma: a distinctive neoplasm of von Hippel-Lindau disease. Am J Surg Pathol. 2001;25(5):602–9.

10. Fryer E, Serra S, Chetty R. Lipid-rich ("clear cell") neuroendocrine tumors of the pancreas in MEN I patients. Endocr Pathol. 2012;23(4):243–6.
11. Grozinsky-Glasberg S, Mazeh H, Gross DJ. Clinical features of pancreatic neuroendocrine tumors. J Hepatobiliary Pancreat Sci. 2015;22(8):578–85.
12. Versari A, Camellini L, Carlinfante G, Frasoldati A, Nicoli F, Grassi E, et al. Ga-68 DOTATOC PET, endoscopic ultrasonography, and multidetector CT in the diagnosis of duodenopancreatic neuroendocrine tumors: a single-centre retrospective study. Clin Nucl Med. 2010;35(5):321–8.
13. Ambrosini V, Morigi JJ, Nanni C, Castellucci P, Fanti S. Current status of PET imaging of neuroendocrine tumours ([18F]FDOPA, [68Ga]tracers, [11C]/[18F]-HTP). Q J Nucl Med Mol Imaging (Official Publication of the Italian Association of Nuclear Medicine). 2015;59(1):58–69.
14. Okabayashi T, Shima Y, Sumiyoshi T, Kozuki A, Ito S, Ogawa Y, et al. Diagnosis and management of insulinoma. World J Gastroenterol (WJG). 2013;19(6):829–37.
15. Ahn CH, Kim LK, Lee JE, Jung CH, Min SH, Park KS, et al. Clinical implications of various criteria for the biochemical diagnosis of insulinoma. Endocrinol Metab. 2014;29(4): 498–504.
16. Lin XZ, Wu ZY, Tao R, Guo Y, Li JY, Zhang J, et al. Dual energy spectral CT imaging of insulinoma-Value in preoperative diagnosis compared with conventional multi-detector CT. Eur J Radiol. 2012;81(10):2487–94.
17. Wu H, Liang S, Liu S, Pan Y, Cheng D, Zhang Y. 18F-radiolabeled GLP-1 analog exendin-4 for PET/CT imaging of insulinoma in small animals. Nucl Med Commun. 2013; 34(7):701–8.
18. Imperiale A, Sebag F, Vix M, Castinetti F, Kessler L, Moreau F, et al. 18F-FDOPA PET/CT imaging of insulinoma revisited. Eur J Nucl Med Mol Imaging. 2015;42(3):409–18.
19. Eldor R, Glaser B, Fraenkel M, Doviner V, Salmon A, Gross DJ. Glucagonoma and the glucagonoma syndrome – cumulative experience with an elusive endocrine tumour. Clin Endocrinol (Oxf). 2011;74(5):593–8.
20. Otto AI, Marschalko M, Zalatnai A, Toth M, Kovacs J, Harsing J, et al. Glucagon cell adenomatosis: a new entity associated with necrolytic migratory erythema and glucagonoma syndrome. J Am Acad Dermatol. 2011;65(2):458–9.
21. Kang H, Kim S, Lim TS, Lee HW, Choi H, Kang CM, et al. A case of alpha-cell nesidioblastosis and hyperplasia with multiple glucagon-producing endocrine cell tumor of the pancreas. Korean J Gastroenterol (Taehan Sohwagi Hakhoe chi). 2014;63(4):253–7.
22. Bright E, Garcea G, Ong SL, Madira W, Berry DP, Dennison AR. An unusual case of concurrent insulinoma and nesidioblastosis. JOP. 2008;9(5):649–53.
23. Henopp T, Anlauf M, Schmitt A, Schlenger R, Zalatnai A, Couvelard A, et al. Glucagon cell adenomatosis: a newly recognized disease of the endocrine pancreas. J Clin Endocrinol Metab. 2009;94(1):213–7.
24. Jensen RT, Niederle B, Mitry E, Ramage JK, Steinmuller T, Lewington V, et al. Gastrinoma (duodenal and pancreatic). Neuroendocrinology. 2006;84(3):173–82.
25. Imamura M, Nakamoto Y, Uose S, Komoto I, Awane M, Taki Y. Diagnosis of functioning pancreaticoduodenal neuroendocrine tumors. J Hepatobiliary Pancreat Sci. 2015; 22(8):602–9.
26. Shibata C, Kakyo M, Kinouchi M, Tanaka N, Miura K, Naitoh T, et al. Criteria for the glucagon provocative test in the diagnosis of gastrinoma. Surg Today. 2013;43(11):1281–5.
27. Amrilleva V, Slater EP, Waldmann J, Bonorden D, Fendrich V. A pancreatic polypeptide-producing pancreatic tumor causing WDHA syndrome. Case Rep Gastroenterol. 2008;2(2):238–43.
28. Ito T, Igarashi H, Jensen RT. Pancreatic neuroendocrine tumors: clinical features, diagnosis and medical treatment: advances. Best Pract Res. 2012;26(6):737–53.
29. He X, Wang J, Wu X, Kang L, Lan P. Pancreatic somatostatinoma manifested as severe hypoglycemia. J Gastrointestin Liver Dis. 2009;18(2):221–4.

30. Vinik A, Feliberti E, Perry RR. Somatostatinoma. In: De Groot LJ, Beck-Peccoz P, Chrousos G, Dungan K, Grossman A, Hershman JM, et al., editors. ENDOTEXT (www.endotext.org). South Dartmouth (MA): MDText.com, Inc.; 2000. 2013 Nov 28.
31. Kuo SC, Gananadha S, Scarlett CJ, Gill A, Smith RC. Sporadic pancreatic polypeptide secreting tumors (PPomas) of the pancreas. World J Surg. 2008;32(8):1815–22.
32. Ohneda A, Otsuki M, Fujiya H, Yaginuma N, Kokubo T, Ohtani H. A malignant insulinoma transformed into a glucagonoma syndrome. Diabetes. 1979;28(11):962–9.
33. Wynick D, Williams SJ, Bloom SR. Symptomatic secondary hormone syndromes in patients with established malignant pancreatic endocrine tumors. N Engl J Med. 1988; 319(10):605–7.
34. Maton PN, Gardner JD, Jensen RT. Cushing's syndrome in patients with the Zollinger-Ellison syndrome. N Engl J Med. 1986;315(1):1–5.
35. Nasir A, Gardner NM, Strosberg J, Ahmad N, Choi J, Malafa MP, et al. Multimodality management of a polyfunctional pancreatic endocrine carcinoma with markedly elevated serum vasoactive intestinal polypeptide and calcitonin levels. Pancreas. 2008;36(3):309–13.
36. Van Der Veer JS, Choufoer JC, Querido A, Van Der Heul RO, Hollander CF, Van Rijssel T. Metastasising islet-cell tumour of the pancreas associated with hypoglycemia and carcinoid syndrome. Lancet. 1964;2(7348):1416–9.
37. Volante M, La Rosa S, Castellano I, Finzi G, Capella C, Bussolati G. Clinico-pathological features of a series of 11 oncocytic endocrine tumours of the pancreas. Virchows Arch. 2006;448(5):545–51.
38. Perez-Montiel MD, Frankel WL, Suster S. Neuroendocrine carcinomas of the pancreas with 'Rhabdoid' features. Am J Surg Pathol. 2003;27(5):642–9.
39. Taniguchi K, Tomioka T, Komuta K, Ura K, Tsunoda T, Kanematsu T, et al. Pleomorphic nonfunctioning islet cell tumor of the pancreas. Int J Pancreatol. 1995;17(1):83–9.
40. Collins BT, Cramer HM. Fine-needle aspiration cytology of islet cell tumors. Diagn Cytopathol. 1996;15(1):37–45.
41. Collins BT, Saeed ZA. Fine needle aspiration biopsy of pancreatic endocrine neoplasms by endoscopic ultrasonographic guidance. Acta Cytol. 2001;45(5):905–7.
42. Reid MD, Balci S, Saka B, Adsay NV. Neuroendocrine tumors of the pancreas: current concepts and controversies. Endocr Pathol. 2014;25:65–79.
43. Fung A, Cohen C, Kavuri S, Lawson D, Gao X, Reid M. Phosphohistone H3 and Ki-67 labeling indices in cytologic specimens from well differentiated neuroendocrine tumors of the gastrointestinal tract and pancreas: a comparative analysis using automated image cytometry. Acta Cytol. 2013;57(5):501–8.
44. Weynand B, Borbath I, Bernard V, Sempoux C, Gigot JF, Hubert C, et al. Pancreatic neuroendocrine tumour grading on endoscopic ultrasound-guided fine needle aspiration: high reproducibility and inter-observer agreement of the Ki-67 labelling index. Cytopathology. 2014;25(6):389–95.
45. McCall CM, Shi C, Cornish TC, Klimstra DS, Tang LH, Basturk O, et al. Grading of well-differentiated pancreatic neuroendocrine tumors is improved by the inclusion of both Ki67 proliferative index and mitotic rate. Am J Surg Pathol. 2013;37(11):1671–7.
46. Khan MS, Luong TV, Watkins J, Toumpanakis C, Caplin ME, Meyer T. A comparison of Ki-67 and mitotic count as prognostic markers for metastatic pancreatic and midgut neuroendocrine neoplasms. Br J Cancer. 2013;108(9):1838–45.
47. Pasaoglu E, Dursun N, Ozyalvacli G, Hacihasanoglu E, Behzatoglu K, Calay O. Comparison of World Health Organization 2000/2004 and World Health Organization 2010 classifications for gastrointestinal and pancreatic neuroendocrine tumors. Ann Diagn Pathol. 2015;19(2):81–7.
48. Miller HC, Drymousis P, Flora R, Goldin R, Spalding D, Frilling A. Role of Ki-67 proliferation index in the assessment of patients with neuroendocrine neoplasias regarding the stage of disease. World J Surg. 2014;38(6):1353–61.
49. Voss SM, Riley MP, Lokhandwala PM, Wang M, Yang Z. Mitotic count by phosphohistone H3 immunohistochemical staining predicts survival and improves interobserver reproduc-

ibility in well-differentiated neuroendocrine tumors of the pancreas. Am J Surg Pathol. 2015;39(1):13–24.

50. Jiao Y, Shi C, Edil BH, de Wilde RF, Klimstra DS, Maitra A, et al. DAXX/ATRX, MEN1, and mTOR pathway genes are frequently altered in pancreatic neuroendocrine tumors. Science. 2011;331(6021):1199–203.
51. Pipinikas CP, Dibra H, Karpathakis A, Feber A, Novelli M, Oukrif D, et al. Epigenetic dysregulation and poorer prognosis in DAXX-deficient pancreatic neuroendocrine tumours. Endocr Relat Cancer. 2015;22(3):L13–8.
52. Marinoni I, Kurrer AS, Vassella E, Dettmer M, Rudolph T, Banz V, et al. Loss of DAXX and ATRX are associated with chromosome instability and reduced survival of patients with pancreatic neuroendocrine tumors. Gastroenterology. 2014;146(2):453–60.e5.
53. Voon HP, Hughes JR, Rode C, De La Rosa-Velazquez IA, Jenuwein T, Feil R, et al. ATRX plays a key role in maintaining silencing at interstitial heterochromatic loci and imprinted genes. Cell Rep. 2015;11(3):405–18.
54. Calender A. Dysregulation of genetic pathways in neuroendocrien tumors. In: Huret-Loup J, editor. Atals of genetics and cytogenetics in oncology and haemotology. http://AtlasGeneticsOncology.irg; 2001.
55. Chen M, Van Ness M, Guo Y, Gregg J. Molecular pathology of pancreatic neuroendocrine tumors. J Gastrointest Oncol. 2012;3(3):182–8.
56. Henderson-Jackson EB, Helm J, Strosberg J, Nasir NA, Yeatman TJ, Kvols LK, et al. Palladin is a marker of liver metastasis in primary pancreatic endocrine carcinomas. Anticancer Res. 2011;31(9):2957–62.
57. Nasir A, Helm J, Turner L, Chen DT, Strosberg J, Hafez N, et al. RUNX1T1: a novel predictor of liver metastasis in primary pancreatic endocrine neoplasms. Pancreas. 2011;40(4):627–33.
58. Roldo C, Missiaglia E, Hagan JP, Falconi M, Capelli P, Bersani S, et al. MicroRNA expression abnormalities in pancreatic endocrine and acinar tumors are associated with distinctive pathologic features and clinical behavior. J Clin Oncol. 2006;24(29):4677–84.
59. Fiasse R, Deprez P, Weynand B, De Clercq P, Wibin E, Pauwels S, et al. An unusual metastatic motilin-secreting neuroendocrine tumour with a 20-year survival. Pathological, biochemical and motility features. Digestion. 2001;64(4):255–60.
60. Kloppel G, Anlauf M, Raffel A, Perren A, Knoefel WT. Adult diffuse nesidioblastosis: genetically or environmentally induced? Hum Pathol. 2008;39(1):3–8.
61. Anlauf M, Wieben D, Perren A, Sipos B, Komminoth P, Raffel A, et al. Persistent hyperinsulinemic hypoglycemia in 15 adults with diffuse nesidioblastosis: diagnostic criteria, incidence, and characterization of beta-cell changes. Am J Surg Pathol. 2005;29(4):524–33.
62. Raffel A, Krausch MM, Anlauf M, Wieben D, Braunstein S, Kloppel G, et al. Diffuse nesidioblastosis as a cause of hyperinsulinemic hypoglycemia in adults: a diagnostic and therapeutic challenge. Surgery. 2007;141(2):179–84. discussion 85–6.
63. McElroy MK, Lowy AM, Weidner N. Case report: focal nesidioblastosis ("nesidioblastoma") in an adult. Hum Pathol. 2010;41(3):447–51.
64. Sempoux C, Guiot Y, Jaubert F, Rahier J. Focal and diffuse forms of congenital hyperinsulinism: the keys for differential diagnosis. Endocr Pathol. 2004;15(3):241–6.
65. Laidlaw GF. Nesidioblastoma, the islet tumor of the pancreas. Am J Pathol. 1938;14(2):125–34. 5.
66. Sandler R, Horwitz DL, Rubenstein AH, Kuzuya H. Hypoglycemia and endogenous hyperinsulinism complicating diabetes mellitus. Application of the C-peptide assay to diagnosis and therapy. Am J Med. 1975;59(5):730–6.
67. Starke A, Saddig C, Kirch B, Tschahargane C, Goretzki P. Islet hyperplasia in adults: challenge to preoperatively diagnose non-insulinoma pancreatogenic hypoglycemia syndrome. World J Surg. 2006;30(5):670–9.
68. Kim YW, Park YK, Park JH, Lee SM, Lee J, Ko SW, et al. Islet cell hyperplasia of the pancreas presenting as hyperinsulinemic hypoglycemia in an adult. Yonsei Med J. 2000;41(3):426–9.

69. Hong R, Choi DY, Lim SC. Hyperinsulinemic hypoglycemia due to diffuse nesidioblastosis in adults: a case report. World J Gastroenterol (WJG). 2008;14(1):140–2.
70. Witteles RM, Straus IF, Sugg SL, Koka MR, Costa EA, Kaplan EL. Adult-onset nesidioblastosis causing hypoglycemia: an important clinical entity and continuing treatment dilemma. Arch Surg. 2001;136(6):656–63.
71. Toyomasu Y, Fukuchi M, Yoshida T, Tajima K, Osawa H, Motegi M, et al. Treatment of hyperinsulinemic hypoglycemia due to diffuse nesidioblastosis in adults: a case report. Am Surg. 2009;75(4):331–4.
72. Won JG, Tseng HS, Yang AH, Tang KT, Jap TS, Lee CH, et al. Clinical features and morphological characterization of 10 patients with noninsulinoma pancreatogenous hypoglycaemia syndrome (NIPHS). Clin Endocrinol (Oxf). 2006;65(5):566–78.
73. Francesconi AB, Matos M, Lee JC, Wyld DK, Clouston AD, Macfarlane D. Nesidioblastosis as a cause of focal pancreatic 111In-pentetreotide uptake in a patient with putative VIPoma: another differential diagnosis. Ann Nucl Med. 2009;23(5):497–9.
74. Ahn J, Lee SE, Lee ES, Chung YJ, Oh YS, Shinn SH, et al. A case of nesidioblastosis causing hypoglycaemia after delivery. Diabetes Res Clin Pract. 2009;83(1):e5–7.
75. Ferrario C, Stoll D, Boubaker A, Matter M, Yan P, Puder JJ. Diffuse nesidioblastosis with hypoglycemia mimicking an insulinoma: a case report. J Med Case Reports. 2012;6:332.
76. Dissanayake AS, Jones V, Fernando DJ. Adult hyperinsulinaemic hypoglycaemia caused by coexisting nesidioblastosis and insulinoma. Eur J Intern Med. 2008;19(4):303.
77. Batra CM, Saluja SS, Bajaj R, Rajshekar U, Thakur V, Gupta V. Non-insulinoma pancreatogenous hypoglycemia syndrome. J Assoc Physicians India. 2011;59:256–8.
78. Kenney B, Tormey CA, Qin L, Sosa JA, Jain D, Neto A. Adult nesidioblastosis. Clinicopathologic correlation between pre-operative selective arterial calcium stimulation studies and post-operative pathologic findings. JOP. 2008;9(4):504–11.
79. Arao T, Okada Y, Hirose A, Tanaka Y. A rare case of adult-onset nesidioblastosis treated successfully with diazoxide. Endocr J. 2006;53(1):95–100.
80. Jabri AL, Bayard C. Nesidioblastosis associated with hyperinsulinemic hypoglycemia in adults: review of the literature. Eur J Intern Med. 2004;15(7):407–10.
81. Garcia-Santos EP, Manzanares-Campillo Mdel C, Padilla-Valverde D, Villarejo-Campos P, Gil-Rendo A, Munoz-Atienza V, et al. Nesidioblastosis. A case of hyperplasia of the islets of Langerhans in the adult. Pancreatology. 2013;13(5):544–8.
82. Koklu E, Ozkan KU, Sayar H, Koklu S, Keskin M. Treatment of hyperinsulinemic hypoglycemia because of diffuse nesidioblastosis with nifedipine after surgical therapies in a newborn. J Pediatr Endocrinol Metab (JPEM). 2013;26(11–12):1153–6.
83. Gupta RA, Patel RP, Nagral S. Adult onset nesidioblastosis treated by subtotal pancreatectomy. JOP. 2013;14(3):286–8.
84. Soares F, Providencia R, Pontes M. Nesidioblastosis: an undescribed cause of transient loss of conscience in young adults. Europace (European Pacing, Arrhythmias, and Cardiac Electrophysiology: Journal of the Working Groups on Cardiac Pacing, Arrhythmias, and Cardiac Cellular Electrophysiology of the European Society of Cardiology). 2013; 15(10):1506.
85. Limongelli P, Belli A, Cioffi L, Russo G, D'Agostino A, Fantini C, et al. Hepatobiliary and pancreatic: nesidioblastosis. J Gastroenterol Hepatol. 2012;27(9):1538.
86. Kibebew M, Bacha S, Feleke Y, Johnson O. Case reports of insulinoma and nesidioblastosis in Ethiopia. Ethiop Med J. 2010;48(1):73–9.
87. Wig JD, Nayak NC, Kumar S, Buxi TB, Nundy S, Mittal KC, et al. A 20-year-old man with recurrent abdominal pain and vomiting since the age of 5 years. Familial chronic pancreatitis with nesidioblastosis and hyperinsulinaemic hypoglycaemia. Natl Med J India. 2008;21(6):307–12.
88. Karawagh AM, Abdullah LS, Gasim AM, Abdelaziz MM. Noninsulinoma pancreatogenous hypoglycemia syndrome in a Saudi male. Saudi Med J. 2008;29(11):1654–7.
89. Kovacs E, Nemeth H, Pasztor E, Pfliegler G. Hyperinsulinemic hypoglycemia in adults. Case reports and a short review. Orv Hetil. 2008;149(35):1659–64.

90. Yu R, Nissen NN, Dhall D, Heaney AP. Nesidioblastosis and hyperplasia of alpha cells, microglucagonoma, and nonfunctioning islet cell tumor of the pancreas: review of the literature. Pancreas. 2008;36(4):428–31.
91. Rosman J, Bravo-Vera R, Sheikh A, Gouller A. Metastatic insulinoma in an adult patient with underlying nesidioblastosis. J Endocrinol Invest. 2007;30(6):521–4.
92. de Heide LJ, Glaudemans AW, Oomen PH, Apers JA, Totte ER, van Beek AP. Functional imaging in hyperinsulinemic hypoglycemia after gastric bypass surgery for morbid obesity. J Clin Endocrinol Metab. 2012;97(6):E963–7.
93. Myint KS, Greenfield JR, Farooqi IS, Henning E, Holst JJ, Finer N. Prolonged successful therapy for hyperinsulinaemic hypoglycaemia after gastric bypass: the pathophysiological role of GLP1 and its response to a somatostatin analogue. Eur J Endocrinol (European Federation of Endocrine Societies). 2012;166(5):951–5.
94. McLaughlin T, Peck M, Holst J, Deacon C. Reversible hyperinsulinemic hypoglycemia after gastric bypass: a consequence of altered nutrient delivery. J Clin Endocrinol Metab. 2010;95(4):1851–5.
95. Guseva N, Phillips D, Mordes JP. Successful treatment of persistent hyperinsulinemic hypoglycemia with nifedipine in an adult patient. Endocr Pract (Official Journal of the American College of Endocrinology and the American Association of Clinical Endocrinologists). 2010;16(1):107–11.
96. Abellan P, Camara R, Merino-Torres JF, Perez-Lazaro A, del Olmo MI, Ponce JL, et al. Severe hypoglycemia after gastric bypass surgery for morbid obesity. Diabetes Res Clin Pract. 2008;79(1):e7–9.
97. Alvarez GC, Faria EN, Beck M, Girardon DT, Machado AC. Laparoscopic spleen-preserving distal pancreatectomy as treatment for nesidioblastosis after gastric bypass surgery. Obes Surg. 2007;17(4):550–2.
98. Clancy TE, Moore Jr FD, Zinner MJ. Post-gastric bypass hyperinsulinism with nesidioblastosis: subtotal or total pancreatectomy may be needed to prevent recurrent hypoglycemia. J Gastrointest Surg. 2006;10(8):1116–9.
99. Service GJ, Thompson GB, Service FJ, Andrews JC, Collazo-Clavell ML, Lloyd RV. Hyperinsulinemic hypoglycemia with nesidioblastosis after gastric-bypass surgery. N Engl J Med. 2005;353(3):249–54.
100. Patti ME, McMahon G, Mun EC, Bitton A, Holst JJ, Goldsmith J, et al. Severe hypoglycaemia post-gastric bypass requiring partial pancreatectomy: evidence for inappropriate insulin secretion and pancreatic islet hyperplasia. Diabetologia. 2005;48(11):2236–40.
101. Palladino AA, Stanley CA. Nesidioblastosis no longer! It's all about genetics. J Clin Endocrinol Metab. 2011;96(3):617–9.
102. List JF, Habener JF. Glucagon-like peptide 1 agonists and the development and growth of pancreatic beta-cells. Am J Physiol Endocrinol Metab. 2004;286(6):E875–81.
103. Rumilla KM, Erickson LA, Service FJ, Vella A, Thompson GB, Grant CS, et al. Hyperinsulinemic hypoglycemia with nesidioblastosis: histologic features and growth factor expression. Mod Pathol. 2009;22(2):239–45.

Neuroendocrine Neoplasms of the Small Intestine

Shabnam Seydafkan and Domenico Coppola

General

There are more than 15 types of neuroendocrine cells located within the gastrointestinal mucosa and pancreas producing peptides and hormones including chromogranin A and B, synaptophysin, gastrin, serotonin, insulin, glucagon, PP, ACTH, VIP, somatostatin, etc. These secretions regulate several gastrointestinal activities including motility, digestion, and metabolism.

Neuroendocrine cells originate from the endocrine system and contain metabolic enzymes such as neuron-specific enolase (NSE) and secretory vesicles filled with amines and hormonal peptides. Most of these cells have the capability to express glycoproteins such as chromogranin and high levels of somatostatin cell surface receptors.

Neuroendocrine tumors (NETs) originating from these cells have secretory function including chromogranins and proteins involved in amine uptake, e.g., VMAT (vesicular monoamine transporter) [1], as well as vesicular trafficking and fusion, e.g., SNAP25 [2] (synaptosomal-associated protein, 25 kDa). Tumors developing from these neuroendocrine cells throughout the body keep the capacity to express the aforementioned products. The term "carcinoid tumor" had been previously used to name these neoplasms which are believed to have low malignant potential. However, recently, the term "carcinoid" was replaced by the WHO with "neuroendocrine tumors/carcinomas."

The WHO classification of neuroendocrine neoplasms of the digestive system released in 2010 reflects the views of the Working Group participating to the Consensus Conference at the International Agency for Research on Cancer (IARC), Lyon, 10

S. Seydafkan, MD • D. Coppola, MD (✉)
Department of Anatomic Pathology, Moffitt Cancer Center, Tampa, FL, USA
e-mail: domenico.coppola@moffitt.org

A. Nasir, D. Coppola (eds.), *Neuroendocrine Tumors: Review of Pathology, Molecular and Therapeutic Advances*, DOI 10.1007/978-1-4939-3426-3_14

December 2009. This classification categorizes all neuroendocrine neoplasms of the digestive system, including the small intestine, in the following distinct categories:

1. Neuroendocrine tumor (NET), grade 1 (carcinoid)
2. Neuroendocrine tumor (NET), grade 2
3. Neuroendocrine carcinoma (NEC), high grade (large or small cell type)
4. Mixed adenoneuroendocrine carcinoma (MANEC)
5. Hyperplastic and preneoplastic lesions
6. EC-cell serotonin-producing NET
7. Gangliocytic paraganglioma
8. Gastrinoma
9. L-cell glucagon-like peptide-producing NET
10. PP/PYY-producing NETs
11. Somatostatin-producing NET

Small intestine neuroendocrine neoplasms (SI-NENs) derive from enterochromaffin (EC) cells of the embryonic neural crest. Although rare in general, SI-NENs are the most common malignancy of the small bowel and represent about half of all small intestine neoplasms. Midgut NETs are the most common type of NEN in the gastrointestinal tract and arise in the lower jejunum, ileum, appendix, and cecum. The most common site of the GI-NET is ileum.

The annual incidence of SI-NET is about two cases per 1 000 000 persons, but the rate is increasing due to improved sensitivity of advanced endoscopic and radiologic imaging.

Males are affected more than female (M:F ratio, 1.5:1) and patients usually present during their fifth or sixth decade.

NETs show a broadly variable size, natural history, and survival. The size of NETs ranges from as small as 0.5 cm to more than 10 cm. They grow slowly (Ki67 proliferating index is often <2 %), unless of high grade. The median survival ranges from approximately 6 months, in aggressive high-grade tumors, to up to 20 years in grade 1 tumors. The overall 5-year survival is approximately 60 % [3].

Many cases remain asymptomatic and are diagnosed only later in the course of the disease, after the development of signs of bleeding, obstruction, mesenteric ischemia, or carcinoid syndrome. In most well-differentiated GI-NETs, there is usually metastatic spread to regional lymph nodes (LNs) and to the liver at the time of diagnosis.

The pathognomonic carcinoid syndrome is a rare finding present in only 10 % of cases. This syndrome is usually manifested after the development of liver metastasis. The most common presenting symptoms of intestinal NETs include intestinal obstruction, which is a result of tumor-induced fibrosis. Approximately 58 % of SI-NETs patients will present with metastatic disease. Many SI-NETs are far smaller than the size detectable from conventional imaging modalities. Therefore, less than 50 % of GI-NETs (small bowel, colorectal, and stomach) are seen on CT scan and an even lower percent of these tumors can be detected by Octreoscan.

Available biomarkers have low specificity in detecting these tumors making the diagnosis a challenge [4–16].

Gross Features

A GI-NET grossly appears as a tan mass with homogeneous surface. Hemorrhage and/or necrosis may be seen occasionally. Well-differentiated tumors usually show a well-circumscribed invasive edge while the malignant ones have an invasive infiltrative growth pattern. GI-NETs are slow-growing malignant tumors with metastatic potential and ileal NETs have the highest metastasis potential.

Microscopic Features

"Gastrointestinal NETS have different histologic patterns: (1) solid, nodular, and narrow cords; (2) trabeculae or ribbons with frequent anastomosing patterns; (3) tubules and glands forming rosette-like patterns; (4) poorly differentiated or atypical patterns; and (5) mixed tumors." The glandular subtype seems to have better prognosis when compared to the nested pattern. They often show peripheral palisading.

Most grade 1 GI-NETs have minimal cytoplasm, nuclear hyperchromasia, little or no cellular pleomorphism, little mitotic activity, and unclear cell borders. Their small, round to oval central nuclei have well-defined, regular nuclear membranes and a "salt-and-pepper" chromatin distribution. Eosinophilic cytoplasmic granules may be identified. Invasion of tumor cells in between the muscle fibers separates the muscle fibers apart but does not destroy them. There is prominent desmoplastic response to the invading tumor, which causes fibrosis and thickening of the bowel wall. Vascular sclerosis frequently is seen in large mesenteric vessels and can lead to ischemia. Elastosis and fibrosis can also involve tumor cell nest borders and lymph nodes resulting in fibrous adhesions [10, 17, 42]. Retroperitoneal fibrosis can occur during the development of neuroendocrine tumor [43].

Diagnosis

Duodenal

Duodenal NETs are more common within the first or second part of the duodenum and include gastrinoma, somatostatinoma, gangliocytic paraganglioma, and non-functioning NET. The most common duodenal NET is gastrinoma.

Gastrinoma can be sporadic or occur in association with multiple endocrine neoplasia 1/Zollinger-Ellison syndrome (MEN-1/ZES), whereas somatostatinomas are mostly associated with von Recklinghausen's disease (neurofibromatosis type 1) and usually occur in the ampullary/periampullary region. Mixed exocrine-endocrine tumors with both neuroendocrine and glandular differentiations (goblet cell carcinoids) are extremely rare in this region but they do exist [44].

Tumors that invade beyond the submucosa or present with lymph node or distant metastases usually have an aggressive behavior. Although distant metastasis is not very common (approximately 25 % in duodenal NETs), when present, it negatively affects the 5-year survival. Moreover, metastasis to lymph nodes may be seen in tumors less than 1 cm in diameter. For tumor less than 2 cm, confined to mucosa and/or submucosa of the bowel and without metastatic disease, endoscopic resection can be advised. If there is any evidence of lymph node involvement and/or if the tumor is larger than 2 cm, surgical resection should be performed [45].

Jejunoileal

Terminal ileum NETs are the most common type of GEP-NETs. Unlike the duodenal NETs, ileal NETs (INETs) are a primarily sporadic neoplasm (D'adda et al. 2002) [17]. INETs are more common in male population with the median age of diagnosis around 66 years. The growth of INETs is mainly dependent on angiogenesis and usually shows a very slow pattern of growth. However, there is a rare subtype of well-differentiated INETs with a more aggressive behavior and worse survival due to a downregulation in the expression of succinate dehydrogenase (SDHB) causing increased cellular proliferative activity (MIB1). The diagnosis of INET is late and usually, the patient has already advanced-stage disease. Regardless of the size of the primary tumor, liver and regional lymph node involvements are already present at diagnosis. INETs have nonspecific symptoms which range from abdominal pain, GI bleeding, to intermittent ischemia. In some cases, mesenteric fibrosis, nodal metastases, and desmoplastic reactions can cause bowel obstruction. The classic carcinoid syndrome is only seen in 20 % of cases, usually after liver metastasis. The liver metastasis is a strong predictor of survival and when present, the 5-year survival will significantly deteriorate. Ninety percent of INETs have an aggressive behavior since they deeply invade the bowel wall, the muscularis propria and beyond, or metastasize. Tumor grade and stage, according to WHO/AJCC/ENET criteria, are still the most important predictors of prognosis and to determine the appropriate therapeutic approach. Surgical resection is curative only in early stages of disease. However, the presence of liver metastasis does not preclude the need for surgery and it is still recommended for delaying the progression and to block local invasion.

European Neuroendocrine Tumour Society (ENETS) in 2012 has provided new guidelines to improve the quality of diagnosis and therapy for jejunoileal NETs with liver and distant metastasis [27, 45, 46].

Molecular Features

Gastrointestinal NETs overexpress p53 and have high cell proliferation rate, telomerase activation, Rb loss, p16 loss, and K-ras amplification [18].

Similar to other malignancies, angiogenesis and inflammation may have role in SI-NETs [11]. In addition, SI-NETs are regulated at a developmental level and the activation of hypoxic pathways, a regulator of malignant stem cell expression, and activation of genes involved in apoptosis and cell proliferation are responsible for tumorigenesis.

Expressions of core secretory regulatory elements, e.g., CPE, PCSK1, and secretogranins, including genes involved in depolarization, e.g., SCN3A, as well as transcription factors associated with neurodevelopment (NKX2-2, NeuroD1, INSM1) and glucose homeostasis (APLP1) have been involved in NET tumorigenesis recently. Genomic examination has shown that, in general, SI-NET tumors may consist of two different subtypes, serotonin-producing neoplasms, and serotonin/substance P/tachykinin lesions [16].

Genetic Profiling

Genes known to have an important role in the pathogenesis of neuroendocrine tumors include those involved in genetic syndromes such as MEN-1, RET, VHL, TSC1, and TSC2. MEN-1 mutation is the most common form of genetic predisposition to neuroendocrine tumors [19].

Recent studies have contributed an expanded gene expression profile linked to the development of SI-NET [5]. Novel genes proposed to play an important role in the pathogenesis of SI-NET include:

PNMA2, SPOCK1, SERPINA10, GRIA2, GRP112, OR51E1, CXCL14, NKX23, NAP1L1, MAGE-D2, MTA-1, and APLP [5, 16]. NAP1L1, NKX2-3, TGFβR2, CD302 [16], and overexpression of GPCR signaling regulators [19], cAMP synthetase, ADCY2, and protein kinase A (PRKAR1A).

In addition, SI-NETs express neural GPCRs that activate different CREB targets associated with cell proliferation and secretion and thus with transcripts associated with cell proliferation and secretion. BEX1, BICD1, CHGB, CPE, GABRB3, SCG2, ADCY2, and PRKAR1A have been shown to be upregulated in SI-NET [20]. The candidate metastasis-associated transcription factor, ST18, is also highly expressed. In contrast, studies have shown that the expression of some genes, previously known to be associated with neoplasia, e.g., CEBPA and SDHD, is decreased in SI-NETs [16]. Beside the usefulness of genetic profiling in detecting primary tumors, proteomic signature can be helpful in classifying SI-NETs, as well. In particular, four proteins have shown usefulness in the diagnosis of primary tumors: IGF1, IL1a, SHKBP1, and EGR3. IL1a, XIAP, STX2, and SKBP1 are significant in lymph node metastasis. IGF1, IL1a, IGFBP2, MAML3, and SHKBP1 have been suggested as liver metastasis proof [11].

CDX-2

CDX-2 is a homeobox gene product essential for intestinal development and differentiation. High CDX-2 expression is seen in all ileal and appendiceal WDNET while low levels were seen in WDNETs from stomach, duodenum, and rectum. Low levels of CDX-2 expression are seen in one third of nonfunctional pancreatic WDNET, as well. CDX-2 expression has been detected more commonly in metastatic disease, especially in metastatic ileal WDNETs. CDX-2 has also been shown to be expressed at high levels in intestinal NEC, suggesting a dysregulation in the expression of homeobox genes in NEC [21].

Chromosomal Abnormalities

Chromosomal-based alterations that may be associated with NEN include loss of 18q22-mer or SMAD4 loss of heterozygosity (LOH) [16].

Hemizygous loss of all or most of chromosome 18 is the most frequently observed genetic shift in SI-NETs followed by arm-level gains of chromosomes 4, 5, 14, and 20. Loss of heterozygosity on chromosome arms 9p and 16q has also been observed. The majority of tumors show loss of chromosome 18 while a subgroup of tumors have intact chromosome 18, but gain of chromosome 14. Gain of chromosome 14 is a predictor of poor survival.

Focal region of recurrent gain on 14q has been plotted to the locus of the gene encoding the antiapoptotic protein DAD1 and immunohistochemical staining has confirmed DAD1 protein expression in those tumor samples. However, no alterations in the tumor suppressor genes DPC4/SMAD4 and DCC, located on chromosome 18, are found in these tumors, indicating that other, currently unknown, genes are important for pathogenesis of SI-NET [22–26].

To date, only one gene with statistically significant recurrent somatic mutations and deletions in SI-NET cases has been identified: the cell cycle regulator CDKN1B, the cyclin-dependent kinase inhibitor gene, which encodes p27 protein. Small insertions and deletions within CDKN1B gene in some cases lead to frameshift mutations and hemizygous deletions involving CDKN1B. These observations suggest that the p21/p27/p57 family has an insufficient tumor suppressor activity in SI-NETs and implicates cell cycle dysregulation as the etiology of SI-NETs. Loss of P27 is associated with poor prognosis [25, 27].

There is a correlation between the loss of SDHB expression, increased Ki67 labeling index, and biological aggressiveness of advanced midgut neuroendocrine tumors [28].

TCEB3C (Elongin A3) is currently the only imprinted gene on chromosome 18 and it has been confirmed that TCEB3C (Elongin A3) has a role as a tumor suppressor gene in SI-NETs. TCEB3C gene expression is epigenetically regulated and it is specific in each tumor cell type. Its regulation involves both DNA and histone methylation [29].

Hypomethylation and Promoter Methylation

Hypomethylation and promoter methylation of tumor suppressor genes are associated with downregulation of tumor suppressor gene expression and DNA copy number alterations in SI-NETs. This is particularly true for SI-NET lymph node metastases.

Promoter methylation in SI-NETs has been observed in WIF1, RASSF1A, CXCL14, NKX2–NKX3, P16, LAMA1, and CDH1 genes. Other genes including APC, CDH3, HIC1, P14, SMAD2, and SMAD4 only had low levels of methylation.

WIF1 WIF1 is a Wnt antagonist that inhibits the interaction of Wnt with its receptor, and it is a heavily methylated gene, which is downregulated in ileal NET metastases as compared to the primary tumor.

RASSF1A RASSF1A regulates tubulin dynamics and localizes to centromeres and mitotic spindles during cell motility inhibition and cell-to-cell binding. RASSF1A contributes to cancer development by modulating cyclin D1 accumulation, inhibition of the JNK pathway 25, and pro-apoptotic activities achieved by binding to MST1 (Mammalian Sterile Twenty 1) and other apoptotic agents. RASSF1A hypermethylation has been shown in SI-NETs and has been associated with distant metastasis. Low RASSF1A expression is associated with shorter survival.

CXCL14 and NKX2–NKX3 Downregulated mRNA expression for CXCL14 and NKX2–NKX3 has been described in progressive SI-NETs.

P16 P16 promoter methylation has a limited role on cancer progression. However, downregulated P16 has been reported to be associated with less favorable patient outcome [30].

Cancer-Related Pathways

There are several cancer-related pathways involved in SI-NET pathogenesis, mainly including PI3K/Akt/mTOR signaling, the TGF-β pathway (through alterations in SMAD genes), the SRC oncogene, VEGF pathway, EGFR pathway, IGF-1R pathway, and histone deacetylase pathway (Figs. 1 and 2). Protein degradation

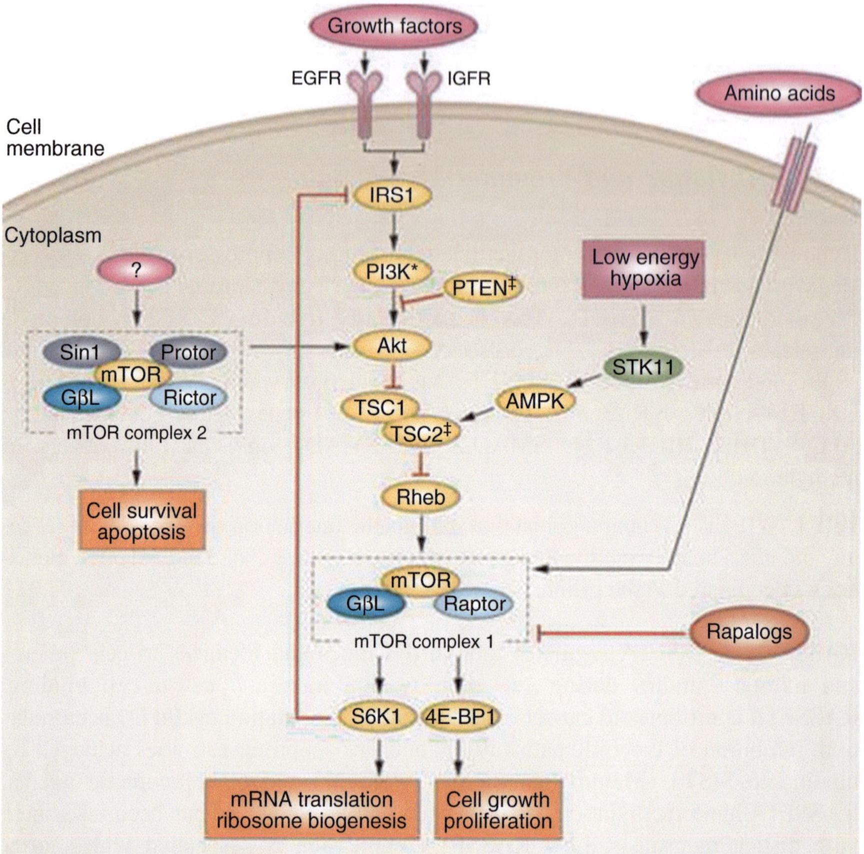

Fig. 1 mTOR signaling pathway [47]

pathways, c-kit, and PDGFR pathways have also been under investigation in an effort to recognize their role in NET development [3, 13, 31] (Fig. 3).

PI3K/Akt/mTOR Pathway

mTOR (the mammalian target of rapamycin, an intracellular serine-threonine kinase) expression and its phosphorylated downstream targets 4EBP1, S6K, and eIF4E are involved in pathogenesis of GEP-NET. mTOR expression and activity are higher in foregut than in midgut tumors and are even higher when distant metastases are present in foregut tumors. Strong mTOR activity is correlated with higher cell proliferative capacity and in patients with stage IV midgut tumors. Strong p-S6K expression can be associated with poor disease-specific survival [13, 32].

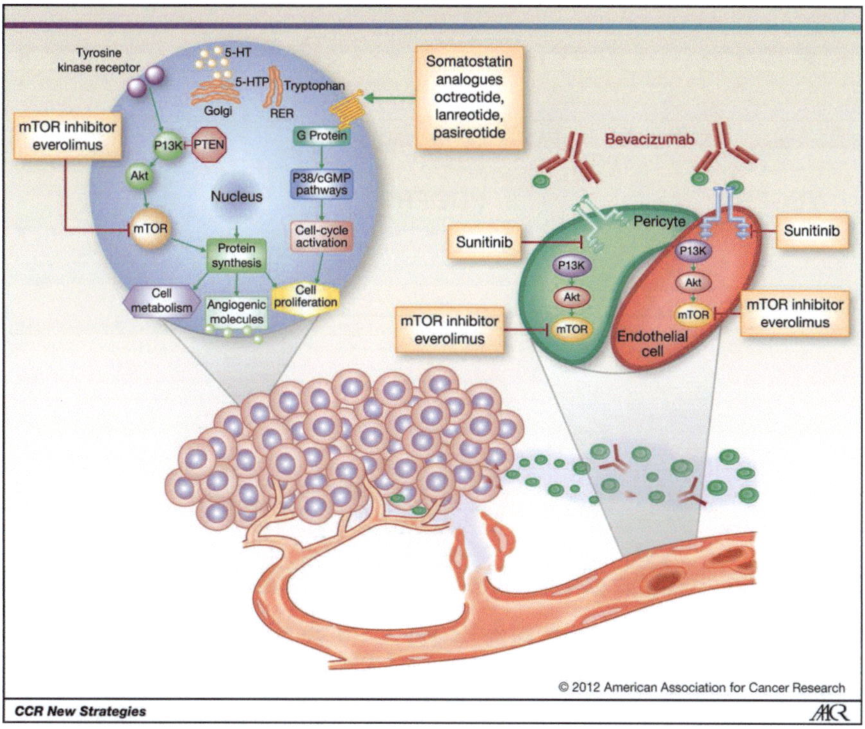

Fig. 2 mTOR (@ 2012 American Association for Cancer Research) [48]

In response to mTOR and Raf inhibitors, there is high compensatory activation of Akt and Erk signaling in NETs, and thus, downstream signaling of HSP90 can suppress both survival pathways [33].

TGF-β Pathway

Mutated or deleted SMAD genes have also been suggested as important regulators of growth in SI-NET through increased expression of TGF-β pathway. Gilbert et al. have shown high immunohistochemical levels of Hsp90, TGFBR1, IGF1R, and SSTR5 in SI-NETs [13, 34].

VEGF-R and IGF-R

There is an increased expression of VEGF-R and IGF-R in foregut and midgut carcinoids. Weak EGFR expression is observed in small-bowel NETs. IGF1/IGF1R system may play an important role, even in early stages of SI-NETs. IGF1

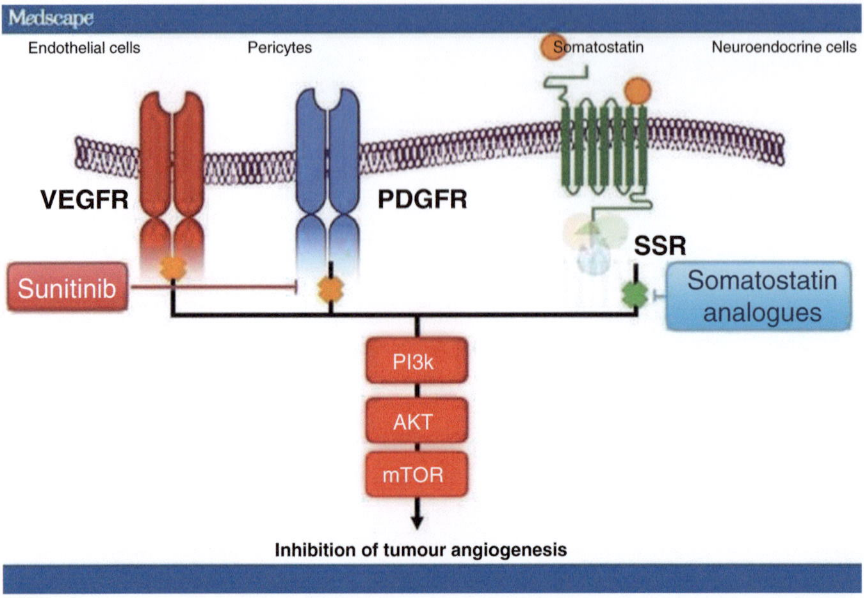

Fig. 3 Vascular endothelial growth factor receptor (*VEGF-R*) in endothelial cells and platelet-derived growth factor receptor (*PDGFR*) in pericytes resulting in the inhibition of angiogenesis in neuroendocrine tumors and somatostatin receptor involvement [50] (*Source*: Ther Adv Med Oncol ©2011 SAGA Publication Ltd)

expression levels can distinguish between normal and primary SI-NETs and it seems to represent a biomarker for SI-NET [11, 34, 35].

EpCAM Expression

Studies have shown EpCAM (epithelial cell adhesion molecule) expression in NETs. This finding is a demonstration of the epithelial features of these neural crest-derived tumors. NETs circulating tumor cells (CTC) have been detected especially in blood of patients with progressive and metastatic disease and may provide useful prognostic information given the variable survival rates of these patients [4].

Receptor and Membrane Proteins Changes in SI-NETs

Genes coding receptors and membrane proteins that may have a role and that are upregulated in SI-NETs include [36]:

BRS3 (bombesin-like receptor 3), GIPR, GPR98 (G-protein-coupled receptor 98), GPR113, GRM1 (metabotropic glutamate receptor 1), OPRK1 (k-opioid receptor), GPR113 (G-protein-coupled receptor 113), and GPR116 (G-protein-coupled receptor 116) [6].

In pancreatic cancer, the upregulation of GPR113 and OXTR is not as high as in SI-NET, and this difference in membrane gene profile may be a discriminator between the two diseases.

OPRK1: OPRK1 is overexpressed in SI-NET relative to normal tissue.

OXTR: Oxytocin receptor is highly expressed in SI-NET tumors relative to the small-bowel normal mucosa [37]. OXTR overexpression is present in both primary and metastasis of SI-NETs. OXTR may represent a target for future imaging and therapeutic interventions [6, 37].

G-Protein-Coupled Receptors

Transcriptional signaling in NETs involves the activation of cAMP/PKA/pCREB pathways with involvement of G-protein-coupled receptors. For SI-NETs cell line, somatostatin and dopamine are the most involved G-protein-coupled receptors defined [16, 20].

SRC Oncogene Pathway

Src is a proto-oncogene which through kinase activity transduces signals from the plasma membrane to control cell cycle and adhesion and motility [38]. Activated SRC stimulates MTOR activity in neuroendocrine cell and amplification of the SRC gene suggested to have role in carcinogenesis of neuroendocrine tumors [13].

Somatostatin Receptor (SSTR)

There are five SSTR subtypes in the somatostatin receptor family [39]. Somatostatin type 2 receptor (SSTR2) is the most extensively expressed receptor in GEP-NETs and is found in 80–95 % of cases. However, not all tumors express high levels of somatostatin receptor type 2 (SSTR2) [36].

Gastric Inhibitory Polypeptide Receptor (GIPR)

The gastric inhibitory polypeptide receptor (GIPR), also known as the glucose-dependent insulinotropic polypeptide receptor, is a G-protein-coupled receptor related to the glucagon receptor. GIPR is expressed in neuroendocrine tissues including pancreatic β cells [40]. Prabakaran *et al.* have shown that GIP increases proliferation and activation of the MAP kinase and mTOR pathways. GIPR is overexpressed in neuroendocrine tumors compared to normal tissue and hence suggesting the pro-malignant signaling mediated by this receptor involvement in NETs [6, 41].

Aldo-Keto Reductase Family One Member C3 (AKR1C3)

SI-NETs have the highest ratio of positive AKR1C3 among NE tumors and it could be a useful marker for the exclusion of the NE phenotype [42].

Biomarkers

Tumor cells with neuroendocrine differentiation show immunoreactivity for CgA and synaptophysin and are also often positive for carcinoembryonic antigen (CEA). Low-molecular-weight cytokeratin expression (CAM 5.2) is also common in these tumors [18].

When GEP-NET is suspected, the most commonly accepted approach would be the assessment of serum markers including chromogranin A, 24-h urinary 5-HIAA test, gastrin, histamine, serotonin, substance P, neuron-specific enolase, and neurokinin A levels. The serum biochemical markers are used not only as diagnostic test but also as prognostic indicators and for monitoring tumor response to treatment. Currently, CgA is the best tumor marker for well-differentiated NETs, whereas NSE is a better indicator for poorly differentiated NEC.

CgA and 5-HIAA levels are increased especially in metastatic tumors. PCR-based detection of CgA would be more sensitive than either H&E or CgA IHC for detecting lymph node metastases early on in SI-NETs.

Neurokinin A is a member of the tachykinin family found to be elevated in midgut neuroendocrine tumors. Neurokinin A is helpful in determining response to therapy in midgut neuroendocrine tumors. Elevated levels of neurokinin A failing to decrease after treatment are usually an indicator of worse survival. However, its reliability as a prognostic factor seeks further investigation.

Currently, it is difficult to detect WD-SI-NETs at early stages when metastases are not yet developed. New molecules have been proposed for the replacement of CgA for better detection, diagnosis, classification, and monitoring of these tumors. These molecules include IGFBP2, IGF1, SHKBP1, ETS1, IL1a, STX2, MAML3, EGR3, and XIAP.

Cytokeratin fragments (CKfr) have shown utility in patients with well-differentiated NET while both CKfr and progastrin-releasing peptide are good markers in patients with poorly differentiated NEC.

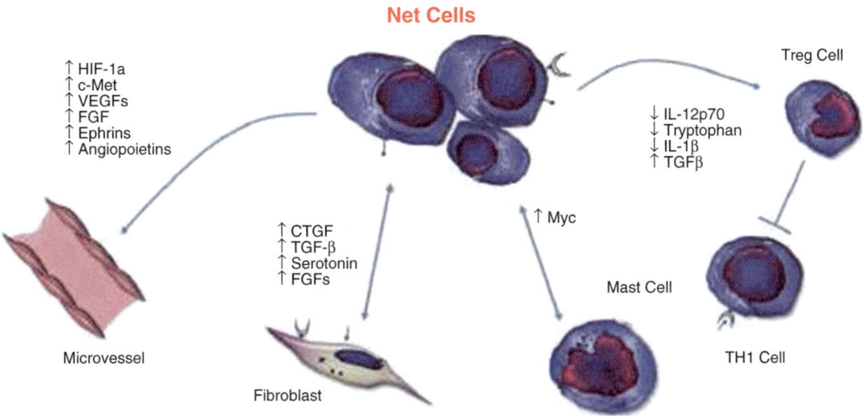

Fig. 4 Role of the microenvironment in the pathogenesis of neuroendocrine tumors (*NETs*). NET cells mutually interact with their microenvironment, prompting angiogenesis through cytokine secretion, inhibiting T-cell function by T-regulatory cell (*Treg*) dysregulation, prompting infiltration of mast cells via Myc upregulation, and driving fibroblast activation, which in turn enhances NET cell proliferation. *CTGF* connective tissue growth factor, *FGF* fibroblast growth factor, *HIF-1(α)* hypoxia-inducible factor alpha, IL interleukin, *TGF* transforming growth factor, *TH1* T-helper type 1 cell, *VEGF* vascular endothelial growth factor [49] (Information from Refs. [19, 22, 23])

Autoantibodies against the paraneoplastic MA antigen 2 and olfactory receptor 51E1 may be important in the detection of patient recurrences. Finally, *insulin-like growth factor 1 (IGF1)* has been previously described as a biomarker for SI-NETs (Fig. 4).

If the biochemical marker profile is suggestive of NET, the next clinical step would be to identify tumor location and assessment of mass lesion, fibrosis, and lymphadenopathy. 111Indium-labeled octreotide scan has 90 % sensitivity to detect tumor-related lesion and fibrosis [5, 7, 8, 11, 14, 43].

Prognosis

TNM staging and grading system is a reliable tool relevant to SI-NETs prognosis and can facilitate therapeutic approach [44, 45]. However, beside TNM system, other factors can be used to determine the overall disease prognosis. A better prognosis for midgut NETs usually can be expected with primary tumors <2.5 cm, in the absence of liver metastases and carcinoid symptoms, and a low Ki67 (Pape et al. 2008). In contrast, factors leading to bad prognosis include [5, 45] advanced age, LN involvement, presence of more than five liver metastases, lack of symptoms at the time of diagnosis, high levels of 5-HIAA, high levels of plasma chromogranin A or neuropeptide K, and the presence of carcinoid syndrome [5].

Treatment

Surgery is the only potential cure currently effective for SI-NETs. Treatment with cytotoxic, biological, and tumor-targeted radionucleotide agents can prolong survival and help to relieve symptoms [28]. NETs with high proliferative activity (Ki67 >20 %) are treated similar to lung small cell cancer with cisplatin-etoposide combination chemotherapy [28]. Surgery, radiofrequency ablation, and liver embolization all are included in current therapeutic approach for liver metastases [46].

Abbreviations

Cg	Chromogranin
GEP-NETs	Gastroenteropancreatic neuroendocrine tumors
INETs	Ileal neuroendocrine tumors
MANEC	Mixed adenoneuroendocrine carcinoma
NEC	Neuroendocrine carcinoma
NEN	Neuroendocrine neoplasm
NET	Neuroendocrine tumor
NSE	Neuron-specific enolase
SI-NENs	Small intestine neuroendocrine neoplasms
SI-NET	Small intestine neuroendocrine tumor
Syn	Synaptophysin

References

1. Jakobsen AM, et al. Differential expression of vesicular monoamine transporter (VMAT) 1 and 2 in gastrointestinal endocrine tumours. J Pathol. 2001;195(4):463–72.
2. Chieregatti E, Witkin JW, Baldini G. SNAP-25 and synaptotagmin 1 function in Ca2+–dependent reversible docking of granules to the plasma membrane. Traffic. 2002;3(7):496–511.
3. Modlin IM, et al. Blood transcript analysis and metastatic recurrent small bowel carcinoid management. BMC Cancer. 2014;14:564.
4. Khan MS, et al. Circulating tumor cells and EpCAM expression in neuroendocrine tumors. Clin Cancer Res. 2011;17(2):337–45.
5. Edfeldt K, et al. Different gene expression profiles in metastasizing midgut carcinoid tumors. Endocr Relat Cancer. 2011;18(4):479–89.
6. Carr JC, et al. Differentiation of small bowel and pancreatic neuroendocrine tumors by gene-expression profiling. Surgery. 2012;152(6):998–1007.
7. Simion NI, Muntean V, Fabian O. Current state of knowledge on neuroendocrine small bowel tumours: non-systematic review of the literature based on one case. BMJ Case Rep. 2013;2013.
8. Salyers WJ, et al. Neuroendocrine tumors of the gastrointestinal tract: case reports and literature review. World J Gastrointest Oncol. 2014;6(8):301–10.
9. Pfragner R, et al. Establishment and characterization of three novel cell lines – P-STS, L-STS, H-STS – derived from a human metastatic midgut carcinoid. Anticancer Res. 2009;29(6):1951–61.

10. Stoica-Mustafa E, et al. Pathological characteristics and clinical specifications in gastroentero-pancreatic neuroendocrine tumors: a study of 68 cases. Rom J Morphol Embryol. 2012;53(2):351–5.
11. Darmanis S, et al. Identification of candidate serum proteins for classifying well-differentiated small intestinal neuroendocrine tumors. PLoS One. 2013;8(11), e81712.
12. Walsh KM, et al. A pilot genome-wide association study shows genomic variants enriched in the non-tumor cells of patients with well-differentiated neuroendocrine tumors of the ileum. Endocr Relat Cancer. 2011;18(1):171–80.
13. Banck MS, et al. The genomic landscape of small intestine neuroendocrine tumors. J Clin Invest. 2013;123(6):2502–8.
14. Landry CS, et al. Biochemical prognostic indicators for pancreatic neuroendocrine tumors and small bowel neuroendocrine tumors. Gland Surg. 2014;3(4):215–8.
15. Peiffer S, Cathomas R, Villiger P. Bilocal recurrence of a neuroendocrine carcinoma of the small intestine: a case report. Int J Surg Case Rep. 2014;5(12):1117–9.
16. Kidd M, Modlin IM, Drozdov I. Gene network-based analysis identifies two potential subtypes of small intestinal neuroendocrine tumors. BMC Genomics. 2014;15:595.
17. D'Adda T, et al. Different patterns of 11q allelic losses in digestive endocrine tumors. Hum Pathol. 2002;33(3):322–9.
18. Fenoglio-Preiser CM. Gastrointestinal neuroendocrine/neuroectodermal tumors. Am J Clin Pathol. 2001;115(Suppl):S79–93.
19. Barakat MT, Meeran K, Bloom SR. Neuroendocrine tumours. Endocr Relat Cancer. 2004;11(1):1–18.
20. Drozdov I, et al. Gene network inference and biochemical assessment delineates GPCR pathways and CREB targets in small intestinal neuroendocrine neoplasia. PLoS One. 2011;6(8):e22457.
21. Barbareschi M, et al. CDX-2 homeobox gene product expression in neuroendocrine tumors: its role as a marker of intestinal neuroendocrine tumors. Am J Surg Pathol. 2004;28(9):1169–76.
22. Kulke MH, et al. High-resolution analysis of genetic alterations in small bowel carcinoid tumors reveals areas of recurrent amplification and loss. Genes Chromosomes Cancer. 2008;47(7):591–603.
23. Zhao J, et al. Genomic alterations in well-differentiated gastrointestinal and bronchial neuroendocrine tumors (carcinoids): marked differences indicating diversity in molecular pathogenesis. Am J Pathol. 2000;157(5):1431–8.
24. Kytola S, et al. Comparative genomic hybridization identifies loss of 18q22-qter as an early and specific event in tumorigenesis of midgut carcinoids. Am J Pathol. 2001;158(5):1803–8.
25. Francis JM, et al. Somatic mutation of CDKN1B in small intestine neuroendocrine tumors. Nat Genet. 2013;45(12):1483–6.
26. Andersson E, et al. High-resolution genomic profiling reveals gain of chromosome 14 as a predictor of poor outcome in ileal carcinoids. Endocr Relat Cancer. 2009;16(3):953–66.
27. Kim HS, et al. p27 loss is associated with poor prognosis in gastroenteropancreatic neuroendocrine tumors. Cancer Res Treat. 2014;46(4):383–92.
28. Milione M, et al. Succinate dehydrogenase B subunit immunohistochemical expression predicts aggressiveness in well differentiated neuroendocrine tumors of the ileum. Cancers (Basel). 2012;4(3):808–20.
29. Edfeldt K, et al. TCEB3C a putative tumor suppressor gene of small intestinal neuroendocrine tumors. Endocr Relat Cancer. 2014;21(2):275–84.
30. Fotouhi O, et al. Global hypomethylation and promoter methylation in small intestinal neuroendocrine tumors: an in vivo and in vitro study. Epigenetics. 2014;9(7):987–97.
31. Naraev BG, Strosberg JR, Halfdanarson TR. Current status and perspectives of targeted therapy in well-differentiated neuroendocrine tumors. Oncology. 2012;83(3):117–27.
32. Kasajima A, et al. mTOR expression and activity patterns in gastroenteropancreatic neuroendocrine tumours. Endocr Relat Cancer. 2011;18(1):181–92.
33. Zitzmann K, et al. Potent antitumor activity of the novel HSP90 inhibitors AUY922 and HSP990 in neuroendocrine carcinoid cells. Int J Oncol. 2013;43(6):1824–32.

34. Gilbert JA, et al. Molecular markers for novel therapies in neuroendocrine (carcinoid) tumors. Endocr Relat Cancer. 2010;17(3):623–36.
35. Bowen KA, et al. An analysis of trends and growth factor receptor expression of GI carcinoid tumors. J Gastrointest Surg. 2009;13(10):1773–80.
36. Sherman SK, et al. Gastric inhibitory polypeptide receptor (GIPR) is a promising target for imaging and therapy in neuroendocrine tumors. Surgery. 2013;154(6):1206–13; discussion 1214.
37. Murphy S, Carroll S. Importance of histological analysis of seroma fluid. Aesthetic Plast Surg. 2013;37(1):187–8.
38. Capurso G, et al. Molecular pathology and genetics of pancreatic endocrine tumours. J Mol Endocrinol. 2012;49(1):R37–50.
39. Kaemmerer D, et al. Molecular imaging with (6)(8)Ga-SSTR PET/CT and correlation to immunohistochemistry of somatostatin receptors in neuroendocrine tumours. Eur J Nucl Med Mol Imaging. 2011;38(9):1659–68.
40. Irwin N, Flatt PR. Therapeutic potential for GIP receptor agonists and antagonists. Best Pract Res Clin Endocrinol Metab. 2009;23(4):499–512.
41. Saxena R, et al. Genetic variation in GIPR influences the glucose and insulin responses to an oral glucose challenge. Nat Genet. 2010;42(2):142–8.
42. Chang TS, et al. Expression of aldo-keto reductase family 1 member C3 (AKR1C3) in neuroendocrine tumors & adenocarcinomas of pancreas, gastrointestinal tract, and lung. Int J Clin Exp Pathol. 2013;6(11):2419–29.
43. Lawrence B, et al. Comparison of PCR-based detection of chromogranin A mRNA with traditional histological lymph node staging of small intestinal neuroendocrine neoplasia. BMC Res Notes. 2012;5:318.
44. Jann H, et al. Neuroendocrine tumors of midgut and hindgut origin: tumor-node-metastasis classification determines clinical outcome. Cancer. 2011;117(15):3332–41.
45. Ahmed A, et al. Midgut neuroendocrine tumours with liver metastases: results of the UKINETS study. Endocr Relat Cancer. 2009;16(3):885–94.
46. Eriksson B, et al. Consensus guidelines for the management of patients with digestive neuroendocrine tumors--well-differentiated jejunal-ileal tumor/carcinoma. Neuroendocrinology. 2008;87(1):8–19.
47. de Wilde RF, Edil BH, Hruban RH, Maitra A. Well-differentiated pancreatic neuroendocrine tumors: from genetics to therapy. Nat Rev Gastroenterol Hepatol. 2012;9:199–208.
48. Dong M, Phan AT, Yao JC. New strategies for advanced neuroendocrine tumors in the era of targeted therapy. Clin Cancer Res. 2012;18:1830–6.
49. Cives M, Strosberg J. An update on gastroenteropancreatic neuroendocrine tumors. Oncology (Williston Park). 2014;28:749–56, 758.
50. Delbaldo C, Faivre S, Dreyer C, Raymond E. Sunitinib in advanced pancreatic neuroendocrine tumors: latest evidence and clinical potential. Ther Adv Med Oncol. 2012;4:9–18.

Neuroendocrine Neoplasms of the Appendix

Ujalla Sheikh, Evita Henderson-Jackson, Jalil Muhammad, Domenico Coppola, and Aejaz Nasir

According to the latest World Health Organization (WHO) classification [1], the neuroendocrine neoplasms of the appendix showing neuroendocrine differentiation include neuroendocrine tumors (NETs), neuroendocrine carcinomas (NECs), and mixed adenoneuroendocrine carcinomas (MANECs), including goblet cell carcinoids.

Neuroendocrine Tumors (NETs)

Neuroendocrine tumors are the most common primary malignant neoplasms of the appendix and are found in 0.3–0.9 % of patients undergoing appendectomy [2, 3]. Langhans first described a gut carcinoid tumor in 1867 [4]. The term "carcinoid" was introduced by Oberndorfer in 1907 for carcinoma-like lesions of the gastrointestinal tract, which showed a more benign behavior than conventional carcinomas. By definition, "carcinoid" is a neoplasm that arises in the neuroendocrine tissues of the GI tract and lung. Originally, carcinoids were grouped into foregut (respiratory tract, thymus, stomach, duodenum, and pancreas), midgut (small intestine, appendix, and right colon), and hindgut (transverse and descending colon, sigmoid, and rectum) tumors.

U. Sheikh, MD • E. Henderson-Jackson, MD • D. Coppola, MD
Department of Anatomic Pathology, Moffitt Cancer Center, Tampa, FL, USA

J. Muhammad
Department of Neuroscience, George Mason University, Falls Church, VA, USA

A. Nasir, MD, MPhil, FCAP (✉)
Diagnostic and Experimental Pathology (Tailored Therapeutics), Lilly Research Laboratories, Eli Lilly & Co., 893 South Delaware St., Building 98C/2C, Room 2391, Indianapolis, IN, USA
e-mail: nasirae@lilly.com

A. Nasir, D. Coppola (eds.), *Neuroendocrine Tumors: Review of Pathology, Molecular and Therapeutic Advances*, DOI 10.1007/978-1-4939-3426-3_15

Pathogenesis

In 1928 Masson identified the subepithelial "Kultschitzky" cells as the origin of appendiceal carcinoid tumors and demonstrated their endocrine and neural characteristics [5]. He also proposed that appendiceal carcinoids originated from subepithelial neuroendocrine cells (SNC), whereas other located NETs originated from epithelial neuroendocrine cells (ENC) [5].

Epidemiology

Primary appendiceal neoplasms are uncommon, comprising 0.4–1 % of all gastrointestinal malignancies [6]. In pediatric patients, the rate is 0.08–0.5 % [2, 7]. The overall incidence of carcinoid tumors in surgical specimens has been estimated to 1–2 cases per 1000 appendectomies [4]. Most frequently, the tumor is localized at the tip of the appendix and is diagnosed as an incidental finding in the appendectomy specimens [8]. Less frequently it may be found in the middle or the base. Frequently this tumor occurs in girls aged 12–13 years [4]. The incidence of appendiceal carcinoids peaks between 15 and 19 years of age in female patients and 20 and 29 years in men [9], while malignancies of the appendix are most frequent between the ages of 38 and 49 years [10–12].

Clinical Presentation

Most appendiceal NETs are clinically silent [4, 6]. When symptomatic, the clinical presentation of appendiceal carcinoids is similar to that of acute appendicitis, with intermittent abdominal pain or pain localized in the right lower abdominal quadrant. A carcinoid syndrome in association with a metastatic well-differentiated appendiceal NETs is exceedingly rare [13], except in the presence of widespread liver or retroperitoneal metastases [1, 14].

Diagnosis

Most appendiceal neoplasms are clinically silent [6], and the majority of appendiceal carcinoids are discovered during incidental histologic examination of the appendectomy specimen [15]. Obstruction of the tumor causes symptom of appendicitis, but histopathologic analysis confirms an obstructing factor in only 25 % of cases [16]. Even a symptomatic obstructive NET of an appendix will usually be identified during computed tomography scans or ultrasound as appendicitis [17].

Pathologic Findings

The tip of the organ is the preferred site of the appendiceal NETs that are mainly observed in women at an age of 40–50 years. Children may be also affected. The tumors are mostly between 1 and 2 cm in size and infiltrate the appendix wall. Occasionally, these tumors may involve and obstruct more proximal part of the appendix and may present as acute appendicitis.

EC Cell NETs

Majority of appendiceal NETs are EC cell NETs with uniform tumor cells arranged in solid nests, sometime with peripheral palisading [1]. Tumor cells are uniform with little or no pleomorphism or mitoses (Fig. 1) and Ki67 proliferative index of <2 % (Fig. 2), consistent with well-differentiated, histologic grade G1 NETs [18]. The tumor cells stain positive for CgA, Syn, CAM5.2 (Figs. 3, 4, and 5), CK8/CK19, CD56, and CDX2 and usually negative for CK7/CK20, CEA, and TTF-1 [18–20]. These tumors are also immunoreactive for serotonin and substance P and may contain S100-positive sustentacular cells [1]. Occasionally, clear cell pattern may predominate that may resemble goblet cell carcinoid (GCC).

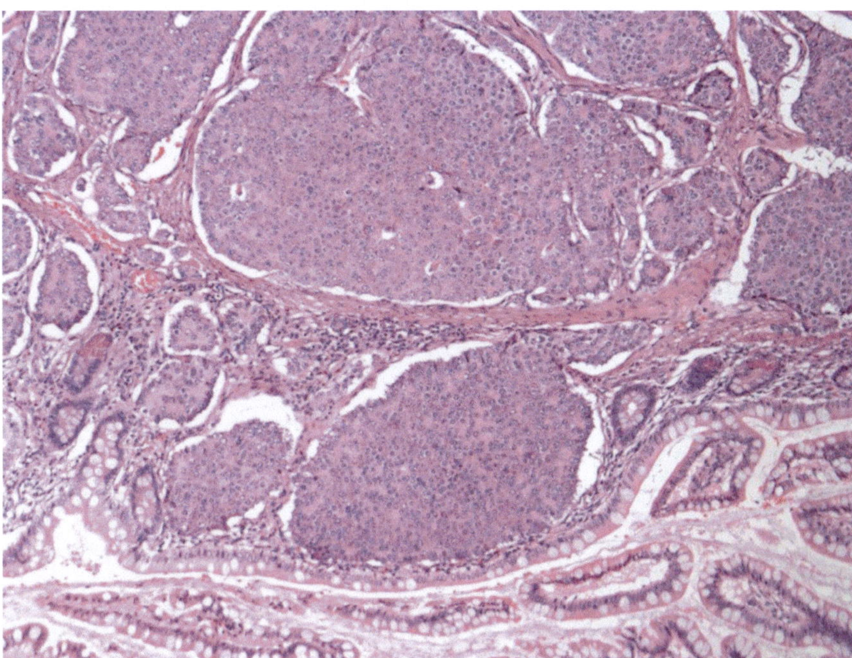

Fig. 1 Well-differentiated NET showing nested pattern of uniform neoplastic cells, infiltrating the wall of the appendix [H&E Original magnification 100×]

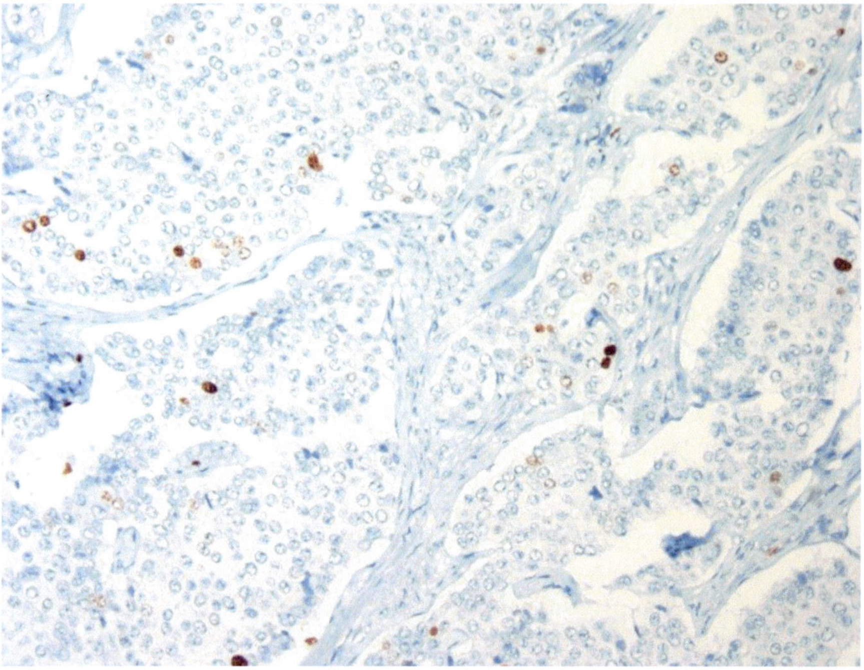

Fig. 2 Well-differentiated NET showing low Ki67 (<5 %) index [Ki67 IHC. Original magnification 200×]

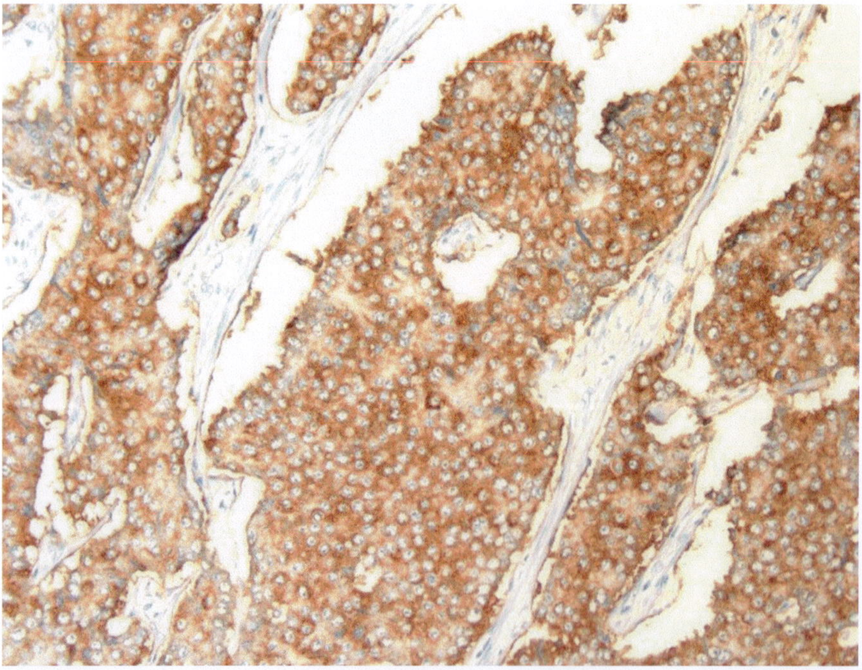

Fig. 3 Well-differentiated NET showing CgA-positive tumor cells [CgA IHC. Original magnification 200×]

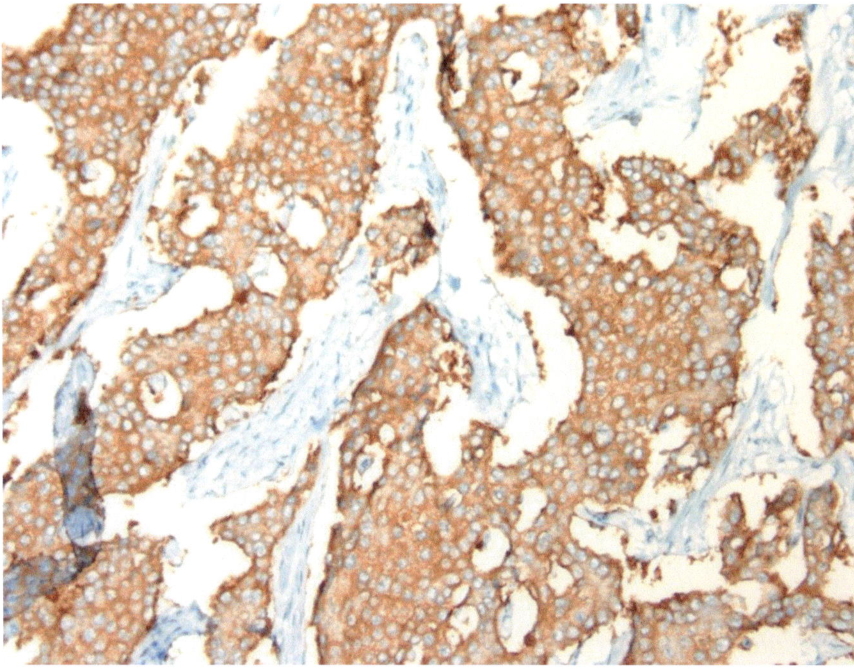

Fig. 4 Well-differentiated NET showing synaptophysin-positive tumor cells [Syn IHC. Original magnification 200×]

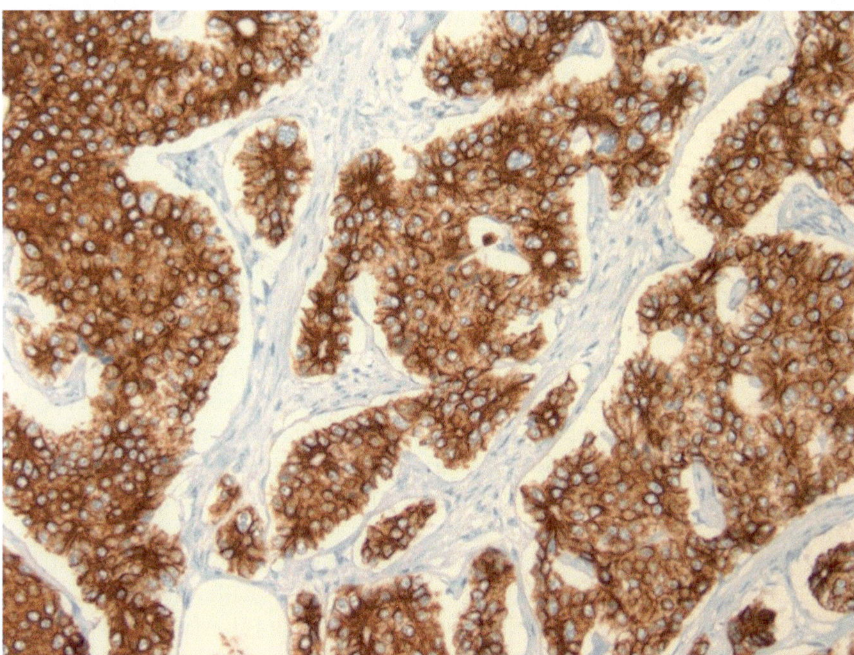

Fig. 5 Well-differentiated NET showing CAM5.2-positive tumor cells [CAM5.2 IHC. Original magnification 200×]

L Cell NETs

These form a minority of primary appendiceal NETs, produce glucagon-like peptides (GLP1, GLP2) and PP/PPY, measure 2–3 mm in size and exhibit tubular or trabecular histologic pattern [1], and resemble similar NETs in the rectum.

Tubular Carcinoid

These affect younger patients and consist of an infiltrative pattern of small tubules with luminal mucin and uniform tumor cells, without any typical nested pattern or mitoses. Tumor cells are often positive for CgA, glucagon, and serotonin but negative for S100 [1]. These tumors originate from basal parts of mucosal crypts and spare primary involvement of the appendiceal mucosa.

The immunologic characterization of gastrointestinal NETs demonstrated a different β-catenin level in appendiceal NETs as compared to NETs localized elsewhere [21].

Molecular Pathology

In contrast to other GI-NETs, loss of heterozygosity (LOH) at the MEN1 gene locus is rare in NETs of the appendix [22–24]. Unlike colonic adenocarcinomas, KRAS mutations are uncommon in appendiceal NETs or GCCs, while immunohistochemical expression of p53 protein or TP53 gene mutations were detected in a fraction (25–31 %) of GCCs [18, 25]. Gene expression profiling has shown overexpression of NAP1L1, MAGED2, and MTA1 as novel markers of aggressive behavior in appendiceal NETs with lymph node or liver metastases, and also in GCCs, but not in incidentally detected small NETs [1].

Prognosis and Postoperative Monitoring

Overall prognosis of small appendiceal NETs is excellent in all ages [3, 4]. Long-term follow-up has revealed that no patient treated by appendectomy died of appendiceal NETs with a diameter <2 cm [8, 26]. Although carcinoid tumors of the appendix rarely metastasize [14, 15, 27], many factors may be associated with increased metastatic potential, the size of the appendiceal NET being the best prognostic factor [2, 16, 26].

According to the North American Neuroendocrine Tumor Society (NANETS) guidelines (2009), low-grade, well-differentiated NETs smaller than 1 cm have a low recurrence rate and do not require further monitoring [4], while in tumors with a diameter of 1–2 cm and presence of aggravating factors (localization at the base, infiltration of the mesoappendix >3 mm, vessel infiltration, grade 2 NET), in which a simple appendectomy was performed, a regular monitoring is recommended [4]. For tumors larger than 2 cm, the National Comprehensive Cancer Network (NCCN) 2013 guidelines propose monitoring by history, physical examination, and imaging every 3 months in the first year and every 6–12 months in the next 10 years and measuring 5-HIAA and CgA [4].

Other prognostic factors include Ki67 index, reduced E-cadherin level, or angioinvasion, but need further investigation [6]. Also, patients with carcinoids of the appendix have up to 33 % risk of developing a synchronous or metachronous colorectal neoplasm [2, 14, 28, 29] and warrant colonoscopic screening as part of their postoperative follow-up [30].

Treatment

Treatment of choice for appendiceal NETs is surgical, and the type of operative procedure is determined by histology and metastatic risk [6]. The majority of patients with an incidental carcinoid are cured by appendectomy [30]. Tumors <1 cm hardly ever metastasize and are treated by appendectomy; tumors >2 cm require right hemicolectomy because of a significant risk of metastatic spread [3, 4]. Treatment for lesions 1–2 cm is controversial and needs further tumor characterization, i.e., mesoappendiceal invasion, vascular invasion, mitotic activity, proliferation markers, and careful patient risk evaluation [3]. Cases with tumor at the base of the appendix with involvement of the surgical margin or cecum are prognostically unfavorable and require at least partial cecal resection to avoid residual tumor or subsequent recurrence [1]. Similarly, transmural infiltration or infiltration of mesoappendix, tumor >2 cm, any high-grade malignant carcinoid (including those with a high mitotic index), and GCC histology require right hemicolectomy or ileocecal resection [2, 26, 31]. Absolute indication for reoperation is the existence of local lymph nodes and the presence of tumor rupture [4].

Appendiceal Carcinoids in Children

Although carcinoids are rare in children, these are the most frequent tumors of the gastrointestinal tract in childhood and adolescence [32].

Demographics

In children the tumor is usually smaller than 2 cm in diameter [33] with a reported incidence of 0.2–0.5 % in surgically removed appendices in children [34]. The tumor is more common in white females with a mean age of 12–13 years [33, 35].

Clinical Features

Generally, carcinoid tumors measuring <10 mm, located at the tip of the appendix, present as acute appendicitis, while tumors measuring more than 20 mm and located at the base of the appendix may present with clinical signs of peritonitis [33]. Metastasis of an appendiceal carcinoid is very rare in children probably because most reported tumors in this age group are small and less aggressive [7].

Prognosis

The appendiceal carcinoids are usually benign, and localized disease has an excellent prognosis. The uncommon occurrence of metastasis is related to the primary tumor size and depth [27]. Clinical awareness and early diagnosis of CT of the appendix may significantly decrease morbidity and mortality [7].

Treatment

The treatment of the carcinoid tumors in the appendix depends on the size and the site of the tumor [7]. Tumors smaller than 2 cm can be adequately treated by appendectomy, while right hemicolectomy is recommended for pediatric patients with appendiceal carcinoid tumors larger than 2 cm, especially when the mesoappendix is involved or if residual tumor is present at the surgical resection margin [36].

Mixed Adenoneuroendocrine Carcinomas (MANECs)

As the name implies, these consist of a mixture of exocrine (signet ring type or poorly differentiated) and endocrine carcinoma components, with one component exceeding 30 % [1]. These are primary carcinomas of the appendix that arise by progression of a pre-existing GCC [37], as explained in a later section. These may involve any part of the appendix; appear as whitish, mucoid induration, 1–5 cm; and exhibit a diffuse infiltrative growth pattern [19, 38]. They generally affect older patients with an average age of 52 years [1]. These are characterized by submucosal concentric growth, mucin positivity, and immunoreactivity of tumor cells for serotonin, somatostatin, and CEA [1]. Histologically, these malignancies are signet ring type or poorly differentiated adenocarcinoma type [37, 39]. The latter tumor type is positive for p53 and MUC1, but negative for MUC2 [37]. These carcinomas usually form in the apparent absence of neoplastic changes in the mucosal epithelium [38]. In a comprehensive GCC and carcinoma study by Tang et al. [37], GCCs were classified as typical GCC (group A) and adenocarcinoma ex-GCC on the basis of the histologic features at the

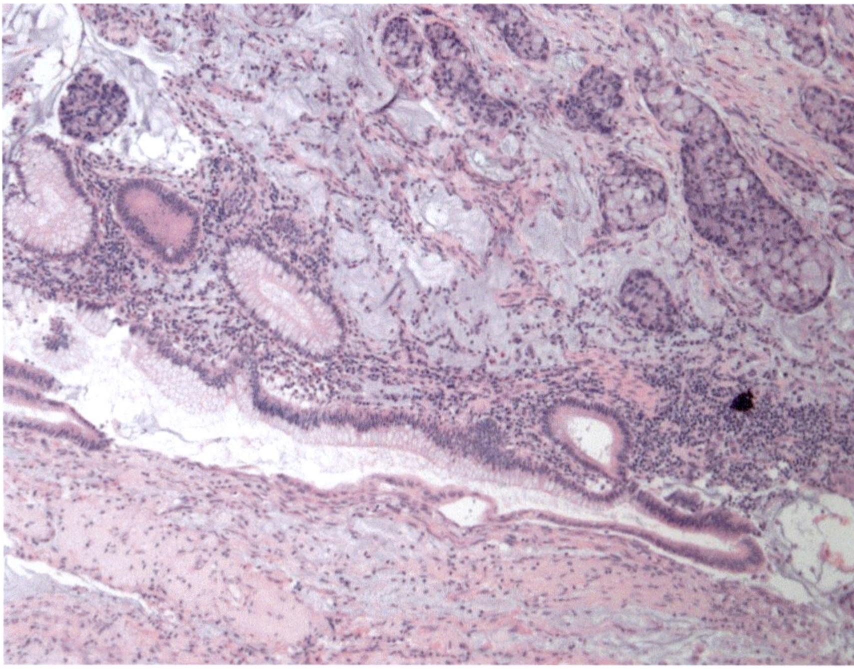

Fig. 6 Adenocarcinoma ex goblet cell carcinoid infiltrating the wall of the appendix [H&E Original magnification 100×]

primary site to help assess prognosis. The adenocarcinoma ex-GCC group was further divided into signet ring cell type (group B) and poorly differentiated adenocarcinoma type (group C). The typical GCC (group A) comprises well-defined goblet cells arranged in clusters with cohesive linear pattern, minimal cytologic atypia, or architectural distortion of appendiceal wall but no desmoplasia. Group B has goblet cells or signet ring cells arranged in irregular large clusters (Figs. 6 and 7), but lacks confluent sheets of cells, discohesive single file, or single cell infiltrating pattern, significant cytologic atypia, stromal desmoplasia, and associated destruction of the appendiceal wall. Group C has at least focal evidence of goblet cell morphology, a component (>1 low-power field or 1 mm^2) not otherwise distinguishable from poorly differentiated adenocarcinoma, which may appear as either (a) gland forming or (b) confluent sheets or signet ring cells or (c) undifferentiated carcinoma.

Primary Neuroendocrine Carcinomas (NECs)

NECs of the appendix, pure or mixed, have been reported [40], but are exceedingly rare [41, 42]. The case described by Rossi et al. [42] was a 35-year-old female with a biphasic malignancy composed of a non-mucinous adenocarcinoma closely juxtaposed with a poorly differentiated (small cell) endocrine carcinoma, who was

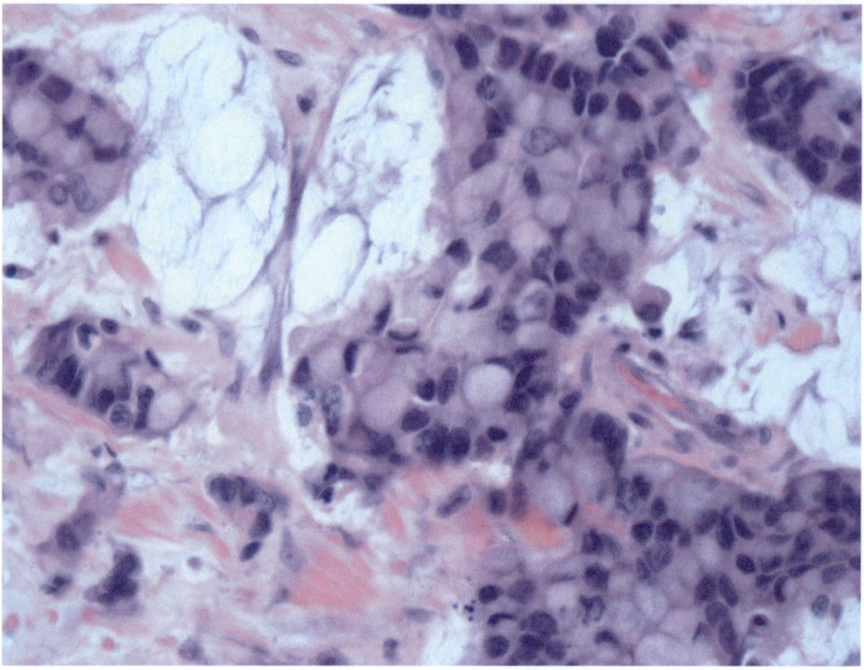

Fig. 7 Adenocarcinoma ex goblet cell carcinoid of the appendix, featuring clusters of signet ring carcinoma cells with highly atypical nuclei in a background of dissecting mucin pools and a few scattered goblet-like cells with smaller, less atypical nuclei [H&E Original magnification 400×]

treated by right hemicolectomy and chemotherapy and was reported to be alive at 65 months of follow-up. Immunohistochemically, the adenocarcinoma component strongly stained for CK20 and CEA, while the endocrine component displayed a dot-like positivity for pan-cytokeratins and Cg. Both components were negative for CDX2 and p53. Genotypic analysis by microsatellite instability showed many microsatellite alterations as well as a normal p53 gene setup. The authors thought of this lesion as a clonal tumor in which the endocrine component was derived from a progressive differentiation of the adenocarcinoma following a glandular-to-endocrine sequence. In general, immunohistopathologic features of primary appendiceal NECs are similar to NECs elsewhere in the GI tract [1]. While these malignancies have aggressive histology, since only a few cases have been reported so far, it is difficult to predict their outcome.

Goblet Cell Carcinoids

The term goblet cell carcinoid was coined by SG Subbuswamy in 1974 for a series of 12 cases of a new entity, in which the principal cell type morphologically resembled goblet cells of the gastrointestinal tract and had a significant population of argentaffin cells [43]. Subsequently, Cooper and Warkel reported a large series of 39 cases using the term "adenocarcinoid" [44] and documented distinct prognostic value for this new entity to be intermediate between carcinoids and the classical adenocarcinoma [45].

Demographics

GCC of the appendix comprises 5 % of all primary appendiceal neoplasms and is more common in Caucasians [11]. The age of presentation ranges from 18 to 89 years with peak incidence in fifth or sixth decades [11, 23, 46]. The reported male to female ratio is 1.4:1–1:2.2 [37, 47]. In a clinicopathologic study of 55 Chinese patients, GCC was more frequent in males and older age and had significantly larger tumor size and greater frequency of mesoappendix infiltration than typical carcinoids (TCs) [48].

Clinical Presentation

Most commonly, GCCs present as acute appendicitis [16, 49, 50]. They may also present as abdominal pain and a palpable lower abdominal mass [37]. Up to 10–20 % of patients may present with distant metastases [51]. About 50 % of the female patients present with metastases to the ovary [50]. Less frequent presentations may be bowel obstruction, intussusception, gastrointestinal bleeding, chronic intermittent lower abdominal pain, and rarely mesenteric adenitis or iron deficiency anemia due to cecal ulceration [47, 50]. In 3 % of cases, it may be an incidental finding [37]. Rarely GCC coexists with conventional mucinous tumors of the appendix [47, 52–54].

Pathogenesis

GCCs are thought to arise from pluripotent intestinal stem cells that reside in appendiceal crypts and can differentiate into mucus cells and also neuroendocrine cells [47, 55]. Initially, they were considered a subtype of carcinoid tumor, based on their basal-glandular/mural location, its well-differentiated nature, and the absence of dysplasia in the surrounding epithelial lining of the appendix [43]. Some cases of GCCs have been reported in patients with appendiceal mucinous neoplasms [56] and schistosomiasis [57]. The latter can lead to GCC by inducing persistent proliferation of pluripotent stem cells in the crypt epithelium. To date no consensus has been reached if GCC is a variant of neuroendocrine tumor or a subtype of mucin-producing adenocarcinoma with neuroendocrine differentiation [45, 48].

Histopathologic Findings

Gross

GCCs generally appear as ill-defined firm nodular thickening of the appendix. Majority of the tumors are >2 cm in size (average 2.4 cm) [37, 58]. Most common location is the tip of the appendix, followed by the base [45]. Circumferential involvement of the appendix wall with longitudinal extension is the most common growth pattern [45], resulting in the formation of an ill-defined tumor mass [38]. For full histopathologic evaluation of this neoplasm and to rule out the presence of adenocarcinoma within the GCC, the entire appendix should be submitted for histopathologic review [37].

Microscopic

In his original description of GCC, Subbuswamy [43] referred to a neoplasm in which mucin-filled cells with crescentic nuclei were arranged in small clumps or rosettes, with no definite lumen, but with striking resemblance to goblet cells or signet ring cells, with the tumor cell clusters resembling Brunner's glands. The bulk of the tumor is in the lamina propria or submucosa of the appendix, surrounding the basal parts of the mucosal crypts. Occasionally goblet cell nests are found in large pools of mucin in the muscularis propria of the appendix. The tumor consists of small, rounded nests of signet ring-like cells, resembling intestinal goblet cells, with mild to moderate atypia, low mitotic activity, and Ki67 index of <20 % [37]. Goblet-like tumor cells and extracellular pools of mucin stain positive with mucin stains [Bosman]. Vascular and perineural invasion and infiltration of the periappendiceal fat are common. The surrounding epithelium either is well preserved or shows fibrous obliteration of the lumen without evidence of adenomatous change. Associated acute appendicitis has been reported in some cases [44].

An unusual mucoid variant of GCC with well-differentiated microacini and rosettes of neuroendocrine cells infiltrating the base of the mucosal glands or the deeper muscle layers without any stromal reaction have been described. In this study an association was found between GCCs and primary carcinomas, which occurred either before or after the appendicular neoplasms [59].

Special Stains

Most neoplastic cell GCCs are argyrophil positive (Sevier-Munger stain), but rarely argentaffin positive (with Fontana-Masson stain) [45]. The vacuolated (goblet-like) cells tend to be positive for mucicarmine, PAS, PAS with diastase, and alcian blue [56].

Immunohistochemistry

Neuroendocrine Markers

Most GCCs show scattered and variable tumor cell positivity for chromogranin A and synaptophysin [25, 37, 55], in contrast to classic appendix carcinoids, in which staining for chromogranin A and synaptophysin is most often homogeneous [60]. The endocrine cell component may also be positive for CD56, serotonin, enteroglucagon, somatostatin, and/or pancreatic polypeptide (PP) [1]. The goblet-like cells express CEA, CK19/CK20, and MUC2 [18, 37], which is also a marker of colonic adenocarcinoma.

Differentiation Markers

Generally GCCs also show strong immunoreactivity for CEA, CDX-2, CAM 5.2, and cytokeratin [18, 55, 61]. CK20 immunoreactivity is present in 100 % and CK7 in 70.5 % of GCCs, while classical appendix carcinoids are CK7 negative and may be CK20 positive in up to 16 % of cases [18, 19]. Based on similar CK7/CK20 immunoprofiles in GCC and colorectal carcinoma, GCCs have also been called crypt cell or amphicrine carcinomas [19], while other authors have proposed the term mucin-producing neuroendocrine tumor of the appendix [62]. Based on their distinctive histology and immunohistochemical profile, GCCs have also been termed term "low-grade adenocarcinoma with neuroendocrine differentiation" [48].

Ki67 Index

Generally, Ki67 index is higher in GCC (4.7 %) relative to classic carcinoids (0.9 %). Using the proliferation index, based on Ki67 immunoreactivity, Tang et al. categorized GCCs in three groups according to histology (groups A, B, and C) and found that the average Ki67 index increases within the groups and that the survival rate is significantly reduced with increasing Ki67 index [37]. In contrast, a more recent study found that Ki67 had no prognostic significance in GCCs [63].

Other Immunohistochemical Markers

Similar to carcinoids and in contrast to adenocarcinoma (E-cadherin negative), E-cadherin staining shows strong membranous staining in GCC [45, 64]. β-catenin staining in GCC is similar to normal appendiceal mucosa and typical carcinoid, with strong membranous staining but without nuclear or cytoplasmic staining, while in adenocarcinoma, β-catenin stain is usually nuclear [64].

Electron Microscopy

The neoplastic cells of GCCs contain both mucin droplets and electron-dense neurosecretory granules [44, 55, 65].

Molecular Pathology

Generally, molecular studies have shown conflicting results in GCCs, although a similarity has been shown between ileal carcinoids and GCCs [45]. Allelic loss of chromosome 11q, 16q, and 18q has been found in 11 %, 11 %, and 39 % of GCCs [23]. This is similar to ileal carcinoids (27, 37, and 56 %), but distinct from appendix carcinoids [45]. Among other molecular alterations, no KRAS, beta-catenin (CTNNB1), or DPC4/SMAD4 mutations or p53 overexpression or loss of DPC4 staining was identified in GCCs [23, 45]. Most GCCs are p53 negative/p16 negative, suggesting its control by a p53 independent pathway [45]. Dysregulation of the cell cycle pathway is likely to be involved, as suggested by overexpression of cyclin D1 (30–70 %) and p21 (40–60 %) [23, 25, 55]. Rb protein expression is preserved in GCCs [37]. Gene expression profiling analysis showed malignant appendiceal carcinoids (APCs) and GCCs to have elevated expression of NAP1L1, MAGE-D2, and MTA1 compared with APCs identified at surgery for appendicitis [66]. These findings and differences in NALP1 gene expression (decreased in GCCs) provide a series of molecular signatures that differentiate various carcinoids of the appendix. The molecular delineation of malignant appendiceal tumor potential provides a scientific basis to define the appropriate surgical management as opposed to morphologic assessment alone [66]. Despite several recent advances, however, molecular studies have failed to settle the controversy around histogenesis of GCCs [45].

Imaging

Computer tomography (CT) scanning or magnetic resonance imaging (MRI) may have low sensitivity for locally advanced disease, but may be used for lymph node and liver metastases [67]. Indium-labeled octreotide scintigraphy is the most sensitive imaging modality for metastasis [45]. FDG-PET is useful for high-grade GCC [45]. Lifelong screening for synchronous or metachronous malignancies is recommended [60], and there may be an increased risk of secondary neoplasms [67, 68].

Diagnosis

The diagnosis of GCC is histologic, which in majority of patients is made during surgery or histopathologic examination of resected specimen for acute appendicitis [60, 69]. A combination of histologic and immunohistopathologic features is needed to confirm the diagnosis [48]. Because of the potential to metastasize to distant sites, including the lungs, contrast CT of the chest, abdomen, and pelvis is recommended for all patients with a GCC regardless of its histologic grade. In equivocal cases, FDG-PET or even guided biopsy of the suspicious lesion may be considered to confirm the diagnosis [51].

Metastatic Spread

The most common route of metastases from GCCs is trans-celomic/peritoneal invasion, and the most common metastatic sites are the ovaries, peritoneal surfaces of the pelvis, and abdominal cavity [45]. Other metastatic sites include the ribs, vertebrae, lymph nodes [70], and rarely prostate [71] and the lung [55]. GCC cells have also been reported in the pleural fluid [72]. In cases of metastatic GCCs [29], the Ki67 proliferation index was >20 %, which, according to the new GCC classification, will be designated as "adenocarcinomas ex-GCC" of "signet ring cell type" or "poorly differentiated adenocarcinoma type" [51]. These authors [51] have also described a first histologically proven lung metastasis and unfavorable outcome from a "typical" GCC with Ki67 index of <5 %.

Prognosis

The prognosis of GCC is intermediate between carcinoids and appendiceal adenocarcinomas with an overall 5-year survival of 76 % [45]. The corresponding survival rates for localized, regional, and distant metastatic disease were 86 %, 74 %, and 18 %, respectively [58]. Stage is the most important prognostic factor, with 5-year disease-specific survival rates of 100 %, 76 %, 22 %, and 14 % for AJCC stages I, II, III, and IV, respectively [50]. Histologic grade is also an important prognostic factor [45], with reported mean survival rates of 119, 43, and 31 months for GCCs in groups A, B, and C, respectively [37]. Histologic features predictive of aggressive behavior in GCCs are high mitotic count (>2/10 hpf), high Ki67 index (>3 %), serosal or mesoappendiceal extension, angioinvasion, lymph node metastases, increased number of Paneth cells, increased mucin secretion, and production of pancreatic polypeptide [29, 38, 64]. Perineural and lymphatic invasion do not correlate with prognosis [49]. Most common cause of death in GCC patients is peritoneal carcinomatosis [45].

Treatment

Primary treatment for GCC is surgical resection. Complete removal of the tumor is recommended because of the unpredictable biological behavior of this tumor, which includes delayed local recurrences and lung metastases [55]. Localized GCCs can be treated with appendectomy, while right hemicolectomy is recommended for higher stage disease due to its unpredictable clinical course and higher risk of nodal metastases [37, 45, 69]. Prophylactic oophorectomy is an option, especially for postmenopausal females due to high incidence of ovarian metastases [37, 50, 73]. Similarly, appendectomy is recommended in females presenting with Krukenberg tumors with unknown primary [74].

Other treatment options include cytoreductive surgery with intraperitoneal chemotherapy for patients with peritoneal carcinomatosis [56, 75], debulking surgery, and adjuvant chemotherapy as for colorectal adenocarcinoma [2], including 5-flourouracil (5FU), leucovorin [50], FOLFOX/FOLFIRI combination (5FU/leucovorin, irinotecan, and oxaliplatin) [60], or streptozotocin with 5FU, cisplatin with etoposide, and interferon [29]. Recent European Neuroendocrine Tumor Society (ENETS) guidelines advocate 5-FU-based combination regimen as first-line therapy for GCCs [67].

Acknowledgements The authors would like to acknowledge excellent support provided by Darlene Sica, Department of Anatomic Pathology, Moffitt Cancer Center, Tampa, FL.

Abbreviations

CEA	Carcinoembryonic antigen
CgA	Chromogranin A
CT	Computer tomography
EC	Enterochromaffin cell
ENC	Epithelial neuroendocrine cells
ENETS	European Neuroendocrine Tumor Society
FDG-PET	Fluorodeoxyglucose (FDG)-positron emission tomography (PET)
GCC	Goblet cell carcinoid
GI	Gastrointestinal
GLP	Glucagon-like peptide
5-HIAA	5-Hydroxyindoleacetic acid
HIPEC	Hyperthermic intraperitoneal chemotherapy
MANEC	Mixed adenoneuroendocrine carcinoma
MEN1	Multiple endocrine neoplasia syndrome 1
MRI	Magnetic resonance imaging
NANETS	The North American Neuroendocrine Tumor Society
NCCN	The National Comprehensive Cancer Network
NETs	Neuroendocrine tumors

PP	Pancreatic polypeptide
RH	Right hemicolectomy
SDHD	Succinate dehydrogenase complex subunit D, integral membrane protein
SNC	Subepithelial neuroendocrine cells
TC	Typical carcinoid
WHO	World Health Organization

References

1. Komminoth P, Arnold R, Capella C. Neuroendocrine neoplasms of the appendix. In: Bosman F, Carneiro F, editors. WHO classification of tumors of the digestive system. Lyon: IARC; 2010.
2. Goede AC, Caplin ME, Winslet MC. Carcinoid tumour of the appendix. Br J Surg. 2003;90(11):1317–22.
3. Stinner B, Rothmund M. Neuroendocrine tumours (carcinoids) of the appendix. Best Pract Res Clin Gastroenterol. 2005;19(5):729–38.
4. Anastasiadis K, Kepertis C, Lampropoulos V, Tsioulas P, Spyridakis I. Carcinoid tumors of the appendix – last decade experience. J Clin Diagn Res. 2014;8(11):NC01–2.
5. Masson P. Carcinoids (argentaffin-cell tumors) and nerve hyperplasia of the appendicular mucosa. Am J Pathol. 1928;4(3):181–212.19.
6. Ploenes T, Borner N, Kirkpatrick CJ, Heintz A. Neuroendocrine tumour, mucinous adenocarcinoma and signet-ring cell carcinoma of the appendix: three cases and review of literature. Indian J Surg. 2013;75 Suppl 1:299–302.
7. Christianakis E, Paschalidis N, Chorti M, Filippou G, Rizos S, Filippou D. Carcinoid tumour of the appendix in children: a case report. Cases J. 2008;1(1):136.
8. Parkes SE, Muir KR, al Sheyyab M, Cameron AH, Pincott JR, Raafat F, et al. Carcinoid tumours of the appendix in children 1957-1986: incidence, treatment and outcome. Br J Surg. 1993;80(4):502–4.
9. Hemminki K, Li X. Incidence trends and risk factors of carcinoid tumors: a nationwide epidemiologic study from Sweden. Cancer. 2001;92(8):2204–10.
10. Sandor A, Modlin IM. A retrospective analysis of 1570 appendiceal carcinoids. Am J Gastroenterol. 1998;93(3):422–8.
11. McCusker ME, Cote TR, Clegg LX, Sobin LH. Primary malignant neoplasms of the appendix: a population-based study from the surveillance, epidemiology and end-results program, 1973-1998. Cancer. 2002;94(12):3307–12.
12. Modlin IM, Lye KD, Kidd M. A 5-decade analysis of 13,715 carcinoid tumors. Cancer. 2003;97(4):934–59.
13. Moyana TN. Carcinoid tumors arising from Meckel's diverticulum. A clinical, morphologic, and immunohistochemical study. Am J Clin Pathol. 1989;91(1):52–6.
14. Moertel CG, Dockerty MB, Judd ES. Carcinoid tumors of the vermiform appendix. Cancer. 1968;21(2):270–8.
15. Tchana-Sato V, Detry O, Polus M, Thiry A, Detroz B, Maweja S, et al. Carcinoid tumor of the appendix: a consecutive series from 1237 appendectomies. World J Gastroenterol. 2006;12(41):6699–701.
16. O'Donnell ME, Carson J, Garstin WI. Surgical treatment of malignant carcinoid tumours of the appendix. Int J Clin Pract. 2007;61(3):431–7.
17. Pickhardt PJ, Levy AD, Rohrmann Jr CA, Kende AI. Primary neoplasms of the appendix: radiologic spectrum of disease with pathologic correlation. Radiographics. 2003;23(3): 645–62.

18. van Eeden S, Offerhaus GJ, Hart AA, Boerrigter L, Nederlof PM, Porter E, et al. Goblet cell carcinoid of the appendix: a specific type of carcinoma. Histopathology. 2007;51(6):763–73.
19. Alsaad KO, Serra S, Schmitt A, Perren A, Chetty R. Cytokeratins 7 and 20 immunoexpression profile in goblet cell and classical carcinoids of appendix. Endocr Pathol. 2007;18(1):16–22.
20. Srivastava A, Hornick JL. Immunohistochemical staining for CDX-2, PDX-1, NESP-55, and TTF-1 can help distinguish gastrointestinal carcinoid tumors from pancreatic endocrine and pulmonary carcinoid tumors. Am J Surg Pathol. 2009;33(4):626–32.
21. Barshack I, Goldberg I, Chowers Y, Horowitz A, Kopolovic J. Different beta-catenin immunoexpression in carcinoid tumors of the appendix in comparison to other gastrointestinal carcinoid tumors. Pathol Res Pract. 2002;198(8):531–6.
22. Perren A, Anlauf M, Komminoth P. Molecular profiles of gastroenteropancreatic endocrine tumors. Virchows Arch. 2007;451 Suppl 1:S39–46.
23. Stancu M, Wu TT, Wallace C, Houlihan PS, Hamilton SR, Rashid A. Genetic alterations in goblet cell carcinoids of the vermiform appendix and comparison with gastrointestinal carcinoid tumors. Mod Pathol Off J U S Can Acad Pathol Inc. 2003;16(12):1189–98.
24. Toliat MR, Berger W, Ropers HH, Neuhaus P, Wiedenmann B. Mutations in the MEN I gene in sporadic neuroendocrine tumours of gastroenteropancreatic system. Lancet. 1997; 350(9086):1223.
25. Ramnani DM, Wistuba II, Behrens C, Gazdar AF, Sobin LH, Albores-Saavedra J. K-ras and p53 mutations in the pathogenesis of classical and goblet cell carcinoids of the appendix. Cancer. 1999;86(1):14–21.
26. Stinner B, Kisker O, Zielke A, Rothmund M. Surgical management for carcinoid tumors of small bowel, appendix, colon, and rectum. World J Surg. 1996;20(2):183–8.
27. Moertel CG, Weiland LH, Nagorney DM, Dockerty MB. Carcinoid tumor of the appendix: treatment and prognosis. N Engl J Med. 1987;317(27):1699–701.
28. Connor SJ, Hanna GB, Frizelle FA. Appendiceal tumors: retrospective clinicopathologic analysis of appendiceal tumors from 7,970 appendectomies. Dis Colon Rectum. 1998;41(1):75–80.
29. Toumpanakis C, Standish RA, Baishnab E, Winslet MC, Caplin ME. Goblet cell carcinoid tumors (adenocarcinoid) of the appendix. Dis Colon Rectum. 2007;50(3):315–22.
30. In't Hof KH, van der Wal HC, Kazemier G, Lange JF. Carcinoid tumour of the appendix: an analysis of 1,485 consecutive emergency appendectomies. J Gastrointest Surg. 2008;12(8):1436–8.
31. Rothmund M, Kisker O. Surgical treatment of carcinoid tumors of the small bowel, appendix, colon and rectum. Digestion. 1994;55 Suppl 3:86–91.
32. Moertel CL, Weiland LH, Telander RL. Carcinoid tumor of the appendix in the first two decades of life. J Pediatr Surg. 1990;25(10):1073–5.
33. Pelizzo G, La Riccia A, Bouvier R, Chappuis JP, Franchella A. Carcinoid tumors of the appendix in children. Pediatr Surg Int. 2001;17(5–6):399–402.
34. Willox SW. Carcinoid tumors of the appendix in childhood. Br J Surg. 1964;51:110–3.
35. Prommegger R, Obrist P, Ensinger C, Profanter C, Mittermair R, Hager J. Retrospective evaluation of carcinoid tumors of the appendix in children. World J Surg. 2002;26(12):1489–92.
36. D'Aleo C, Lazzareschi I, Ruggiero A, Riccardi R. Carcinoid tumors of the appendix in children: two case reports and review of the literature. Pediatr Hematol Oncol. 2001;18(5):347–51.
37. Tang LH, Shia J, Soslow RA, Dhall D, Wong WD, O'Reilly E, et al. Pathologic classification and clinical behavior of the spectrum of goblet cell carcinoid tumors of the appendix. Am J Surg Pathol. 2008;32(10):1429–43.
38. Burke AP, Sobin LH, Federspiel BH, Shekitka KM, Helwig EB. Goblet cell carcinoids and related tumors of the vermiform appendix. Am J Clin Pathol. 1990;94(1):27–35.
39. Wang HL, Dhall D. Goblet or signet ring cells: that is the question. Adv Anat Pathol. 2009;16(4):247–54.

40. Kloppel G, Rindi G, Anlauf M, Perren A, Komminoth P. Site-specific biology and pathology of gastroenteropancreatic neuroendocrine tumors. Virchows Arch. 2007;451 Suppl 1:S9–27.
41. O'Kane AM, O'Donnell ME, Shah R, Carey DP, Lee J. Small cell carcinoma of the appendix. World J Surg Oncol. 2008;6:4.
42. Rossi G, Bertolini F, Sartori G, Bigiani N, Cavazza A, Foroni M, et al. Primary mixed adenocarcinoma and small cell carcinoma of the appendix: a clinicopathologic, immunohistochemical, and molecular study of a hitherto unreported tumor. Am J Surg Pathol. 2004;28(9):1233–9.
43. Subbuswamy SG, Gibbs NM, Ross CF, Morson BC. Goblet cell carcinoid of the appendix. Cancer. 1974;34(2):338–44.
44. Cooper PH, Warkel RL. Ultrastructure of the goblet cell type of adenocarcinoid of the appendix. Cancer. 1978;42(6):2687–95.
45. Roy P, Chetty R. Goblet cell carcinoid tumors of the appendix: an overview. World J Gastrointest Oncol. 2010;2(6):251–8.
46. Anderson NH, Somerville JE, Johnston CF, Hayes DM, Buchanan KD, Sloan JM. Appendiceal goblet cell carcinoids: a clinicopathological and immunohistochemical study. Histopathology. 1991;18(1):61–5.
47. Alsaad KO, Serra S, Chetty R. Combined goblet cell carcinoid and mucinous cystadenoma of the vermiform appendix. World J Gastroenterol. 2009;15(27):3431–3.
48. Jiang Y, Long H, Wang W, Liu H, Tang Y, Zhang X. Clinicopathological features and immunoexpression profiles of goblet cell carcinoid and typical carcinoid of the appendix. Pathol Oncol Res. 2011;17(1):127–32.
49. Warkel RL, Cooper PH, Helwig EB. Adenocarcinoid, a mucin-producing carcinoid tumor of the appendix: a study of 39 cases. Cancer. 1978;42(6):2781–93.
50. Pham TH, Wolff B, Abraham SC, Drelichman E. Surgical and chemotherapy treatment outcomes of goblet cell carcinoid: a tertiary cancer center experience. Ann Surg Oncol. 2006;13(3):370–6.
51. Pericleous M, Lumgair H, Baneke A, Morgan-Rowe L, E Caplin M, Luong TV, et al. Appendiceal goblet cell carcinoid tumour: a case of unexpected lung metastasis. Case Rep Oncol. 2012;5(2):332–8.
52. al-Talib RK, Mason CH, Theaker JM. Combined goblet cell carcinoid and mucinous cystadenoma of the appendix. J Clin Pathol. 1995;48(9):869–70.
53. Carr NJ, Remotti H, Sobin LH. Dual carcinoid/epithelial neoplasia of the appendix. Histopathology. 1995;27(6):557–62.
54. Carr NJ, Sobin LH. Epithelial noncarcinoid tumors and tumor-like lesions of the appendix. Cancer. 1995;76(11):2383–4.
55. Kanthan R, Saxena A, Kanthan SC. Goblet cell carcinoids of the appendix: immunophenotype and ultrastructural study. Arch Pathol Lab Med. 2001;125(3):386–90.
56. Pahlavan PS, Kanthan R. Goblet cell carcinoid of the appendix. World J Surg Oncol. 2005;3:36.
57. Jiang Y, Long H, Li T, Wang W, Liu H, Zhang X. Schistosomiasis may contribute to goblet cell carcinoid of the appendix. J Parasitol. 2012;98(3):565–8.
58. McGory ML, Maggard MA, Kang H, O'Connell JB, Ko CY. Malignancies of the appendix: beyond case series reports. Dis Colon Rectum. 2005;48(12):2264–71.
59. Haqqani MT, Williams G. Mucin producing carcinoid tumours of the vermiform appendix. J Clin Pathol. 1977;30(5):473–80.
60. Holt N, Gronbaek H. Goblet cell carcinoids of the appendix. ScientificWorldJournal. 2013;2013:543696.
61. Lin BT, Gown AM. Mixed carcinoid and adenocarcinoma of the appendix: report of 4 cases with immunohistochemical studies and a review of the literature. Appl Immunohistochem Mol Morphol. 2004;12(3):271–6.
62. Chetty R. Goblet cell carcinoid tumours of the appendix: a unique neuroendocrine tumour. Histopathology. 2008;52(6):770–1.

63. Liu E, Telem DA, Warner RR, Dikman A, Divino CM. The role of Ki-67 in predicting biological behavior of goblet cell carcinoid tumor in appendix. Am J Surg. 2011;202(4):400–3.
64. Li CC, Hirowaka M, Qian ZR, Xu B, Sano T. Expression of E-cadherin, b-catenin, and Ki-67 in goblet cell carcinoids of the appendix: an immunohistochemical study with clinical correlation. Endocr Pathol. 2002;13(1):47–58.
65. Edmonds P, Merino MJ, LiVolsi VA, Duray PH. Adenocarcinoid (mucinous carcinoid) of the appendix. Gastroenterology. 1984;86(2):302–9.
66. Modlin IM, Kidd M, Latich I, Zikusoka MN, Eick GN, Mane SM, et al. Genetic differentiation of appendiceal tumor malignancy: a guide for the perplexed. Ann Surg. 2006;244(1):52–60.
67. Pape UF, Perren A, Niederle B, Gross D, Gress T, Costa F, et al. ENETS Consensus Guidelines for the management of patients with neuroendocrine neoplasms from the jejuno-ileum and the appendix including goblet cell carcinomas. Neuroendocrinology. 2012;95(2):135–56.
68. Bucher P, Gervaz P, Ris F, Oulhaci W, Egger JF, Morel P. Surgical treatment of appendiceal adenocarcinoid (goblet cell carcinoid). World J Surg. 2005;29(11):1436–9.
69. Park K, Blessing K, Kerr K, Chetty U, Gilmour H. Goblet cell carcinoid of the appendix. Gut. 1990;31(3):322–4.
70. Varisco B, McAlvin B, Dias J, Franga D. Adenocarcinoid of the appendix: is right hemicolectomy necessary? A meta-analysis of retrospective chart reviews. Am Surg. 2004; 70(7):593–9.
71. McGregor DH, Cherian R, Weston AP, Lawson L, McAnaw MP. Adenocarcinoid of ileum and appendix, incidentally discovered during exploratory laparotomy for gastric MALT lymphoma, with subsequent diffuse prostatic metastases: report of a case with light, immunohistochemical, and electron microscopic studies. Dig Dis Sci. 1999;44(1):87–95.
72. Zafar S, Chen H, Sun W, Das K. Cytology of metastatic appendiceal goblet cell carcinoid in pleural effusion fluid: a case report. Diagn Cytopathol. 2008;36(12):894–8.
73. Byrn JC, Wang JL, Divino CM, Nguyen SQ, Warner RR. Management of goblet cell carcinoid. J Surg Oncol. 2006;94(5):396–402.
74. Hirschfield LS, Kahn LB, Winkler B, Bochner RZ, Gibstein AA. Adenocarcinoid of the appendix presenting as bilateral Krukenberg's tumor of the ovaries. Immunohistochemical and ultrastructural studies and literature review. Arch Pathol Lab Med. 1985;109(10):930–3.
75. Mahteme H, Sugarbaker PH. Treatment of peritoneal carcinomatosis from adenocarcinoid of appendiceal origin. Br J Surg. 2004;91(9):1168–73.

Neuroendocrine Neoplasms of the Colon and Rectum

Masoumeh Ghayouri, Shabnam Seydafkan, Aejaz Nasir, and Domenico Coppola

Introduction

Neuroendocrine cells within the gastrointestinal (GI) epithelium represent the largest population of hormone-producing cells in the body, and they comprise 1 % of the cells lining the intestinal lumen. These cells are located in crypts, and rarely they are scattered within the lamina propria. The cells that give rise to gastroenteropancreatic-neuroendocrine neoplasms (GEP-NEN) are derived from gastrointestinal stem cells that are able to differentiate into neuroendocrine cells. It is likely that the well- and the poorly differentiated NENs come from different types of tumor stem cells [1].

In poorly differentiated NENs, the cell of origin is most likely close to the intestinal stem cell. If this cell is tackled by mutational hits, multiple profound genetic alterations are initiated, such as p53 mutations, that lead to the development of high-grade malignant, poorly differentiated NENs [1].

M. Ghayouri, MD
Department of Anatomic Pathology, Moffitt Cancer Center, Tampa, FL, USA

Moffitt Cancer Center and Research Institute, University of South Florida, School of Medicine, Tampa, FL, USA
e-mail: Masoumeh.ghayouri@moffitt.org

S. Seydafkan
Department of Anatomic Pathology, Moffitt Cancer Center, Tampa, FL, USA

A. Nasir (✉)
Diagnostic and Experimental Pathology (Tailored Therapeutics), Lilly Research Laboratories, Eli Lilly & Co., Indianapolis, IN, USA
e-mail: nasirae@lilly.com

D. Coppola, MD (✉)
Department of Anatomic Pathology, Moffitt Cancer Center, Tampa, FL, USA
e-mail: domenico.coppola@moffitt.org

A. Nasir, D. Coppola (eds.), *Neuroendocrine Tumors: Review of Pathology, Molecular and Therapeutic Advances*, DOI 10.1007/978-1-4939-3426-3_16

Neuroendocrine neoplasms (NENs) in the colon and rectum are classified by the WHO 2010 as well differentiated neuroendocrine tumors (NETs) and the poorly differentiated NECs (neuroendocrine carcinomas).

The NETs are separated by their proliferative activity into either grade 1(G1) (equivalent to carcinoids) or G2 NETs. The NECs, that are G3 tumors, are subtyped into small cell and large cell type. Mixed adenoneuroendocrine carcinomas (MANEC) are required by WHO 2010 to contain at least 30 % of each component, and components should be recognizable histomorphologically.

NETs are more frequent in the rectum than the colon, whereas NECs are more common in the colon [2]. The rectal NETs that are endoscopically detected are mostly small (1 cm), movable submucosal tumors. They produce glucagon-like peptides and pancreatic polypeptide, but cause no hormonal syndrome. The few colonic NETs are also small; occur in the cecal region, except if they are associated with ulcerative colitis, Crohn's disease [3], and polypous colonic adenomas [4]; and produce serotonin [5].

Neuroendocrine tumors of the colon are rare and account for less than 1 % of all colonic tumors and less than 10 % of gastrointestinal endocrine tumors. Most of these tumors (cecum and transverse colon) are considered to be derived from mid-gut and associated with carcinoid syndrome in about 5 % of cases.

NETs in the left colon and rectosigmoid derived from the hindgut and colorectal NETs are most commonly seen in the rectum (54 % of cases), followed by the cecum (20 %) and sigmoid (7.5 %) [6]. Neuroendocrine carcinomas of the colon are rare and comprise about 0.6 % of colonic carcinomas; however, the colon is the most common site of NEC in GI. The NECs of the colon are usually large and have a high Ki67 index. Synchronous or metachronous colorectal carcinomas are frequently seen in association with NETs or NECs [7].

Rectal and colonic NETs are often incidental findings at endoscopy. Tumor size significantly predicts malignant behavior in NETs of the rectum, but also of the colon. Regional lymph node involvement is very likely, if they are larger than 2 cm and have invaded the muscular wall. In contrast, rectal NETs below 1 cm in size have a very low risk of lymph node metastasis, while those between 1 and 2 cm in size have a risk of 5 %. If the tumors are poorly differentiated, there is a high rate of metastasis at the time of diagnosis [8, 9].

Etiology and Associated Conditions

NET and NEC of the colon are reported in association with ulcerative colitis and Crohn's disease [3]; however, there is no evidence to show direct association between IBD and neuroendocrine carcinogenesis. Multiple rectal NET is reported in diffuse ganglioneurosis [10]. Rarely nests of neuroendocrine cells (microcarcinoids) are found in adenomas of the colon [4], but there is no evidence that the majority of colorectal NETs are etiologically related to adenoma or adenocarcinomas. Neuroendocrine carcinomas can arise in the right colon or left colon and can be large cell type or small cell type or mixed. In the anal canal, they usually are small cell type.

Histopathology

Colon is derived from the embryonic midgut and hindgut. This is reflected in colon NETs. Those which are derived from the midgut (cecum and right colon) that are composed of enterochromaffin cells (EC cells) are serotonin-producing NETs and show histological, cytological, cytochemical, and ultrastructural features that are identical to those of the ileojejunal EC cell NETs. Those derived from hindgut (sigmoid and rectum) are composed of L cells (glucagon-like peptide-producing and PP/PYY-producing NETs). These NETs are histologically composed of trabecular patterns admixed with broad irregular trabeculae with rosettes and occasionally solid nests, while solid nests are most common histological pattern of EC cells NETs (Fig. 1).

Neuroendocrine Carcinomas (NECs)

NECs are usually found in the right colon and are frequently associated with an overlying adenoma (Fig. 2) or adenocarcinoma (Fig. 3) but not associated with NETs. In the colon and rectum, 75 % of NECs are large cell type, whereas in the anus, most of them are small cell type. Primary NECs in the colon without an

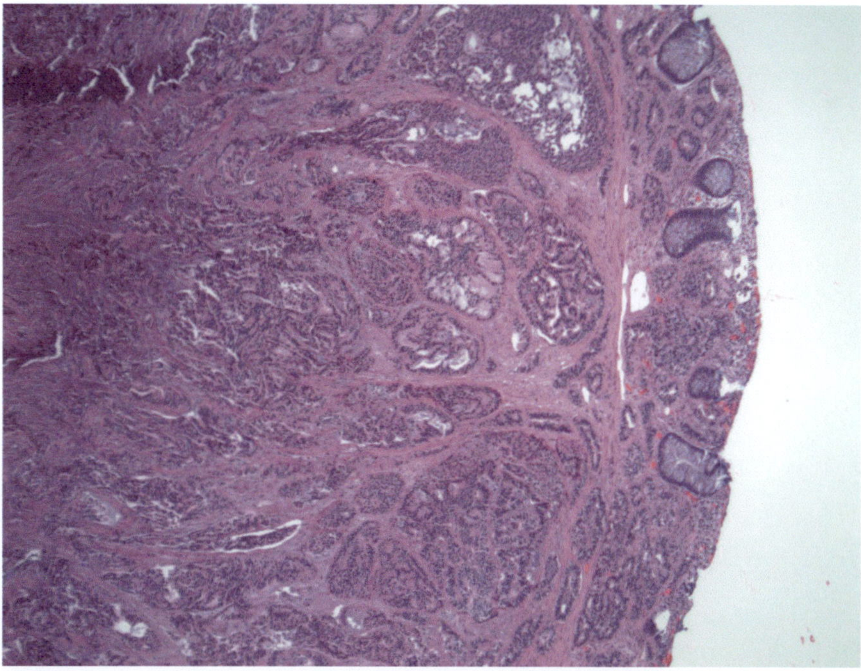

Fig. 1 Neuroendocrine tumor of the rectum with nested, cribriform pattern (×4)

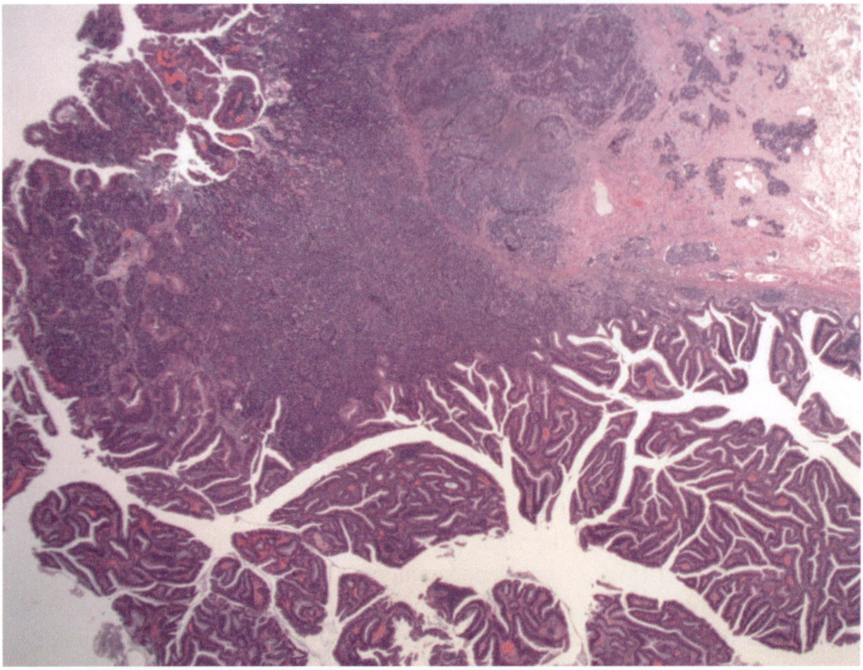

Fig. 2 Neuroendocrine carcinoma arising in a tubulovillous adenoma (×1.25)

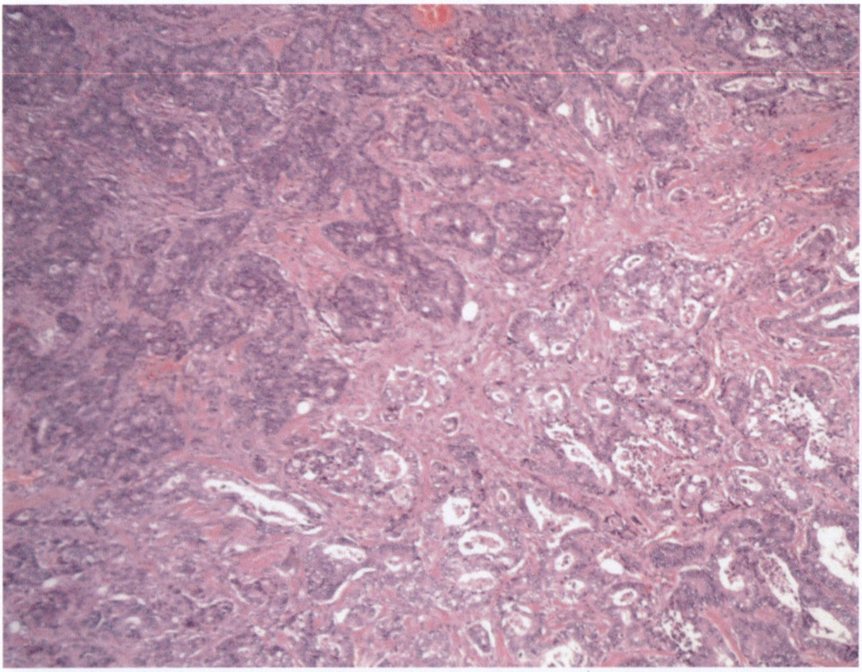

Fig. 3 Mixed adenocarcinoma and neuroendocrine carcinoma (×1.25). Malignant glands separate component of neuroendocrine carcinoma

associated adenoma component must be distinguished from metastasis of pulmonary NECs or cutaneous Merkel cell carcinomas.

Small-Cell NEC

Small cell carcinomas have a diffuse or nesting growth pattern and are composed of small- to medium-sized cells with minimal cytoplasm and fusiform nuclei with granular chromatin and inconspicuous nucleoli. Larger cells (less than 25 % of neoplastic population) are acceptable findings. Necrosis is common. Some cases show component of adenocarcinoma (less than 30 %) or squamous cell carcinoma (in anal cavity). Frequent mitosis is seen, and Ki67 index of more than 50 % and close to 100 % is common.

Large-Cell NEC

These neoplasms show organoid, nesting, trabecular, rosette-like, and palisading pattern that suggest neuroendocrine differentiation (Fig. 4). These cells have abundant cytoplasm, vesicular nuclei, and prominent nucleoli. A component of

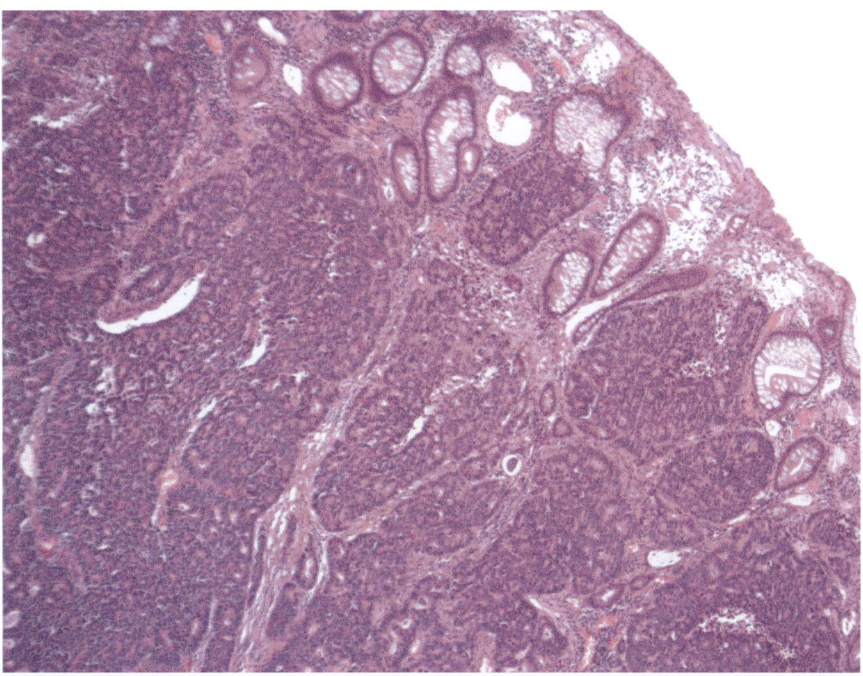

Fig. 4 Neuroendocrine carcinoma, large cell type (4×). Organoid, nested and rosette like pattern of NEC

adenocarcinoma is common (in 61 % of cases), and in some cases, it exceeds 30 % and qualifies for the diagnosis of MANEC.

MANEC

A neoplasm with morphologically recognizable adenocarcinoma and neuroendocrine phenotype (at least 30 % of each component) qualifies as mixed adenoneuroendocrine carcinoma (Fig. 5). Immunohistochemically detectable neuroendocrine cells are commonly seen (in 41 % of colonic adenocarcinomas), most of which have no morphological suggestion of a discrete neuroendocrine component and should not be considered as MANEC. Mixed carcinomas of the anal canal usually contain neuroendocrine carcinoma and squamous cell carcinomas.

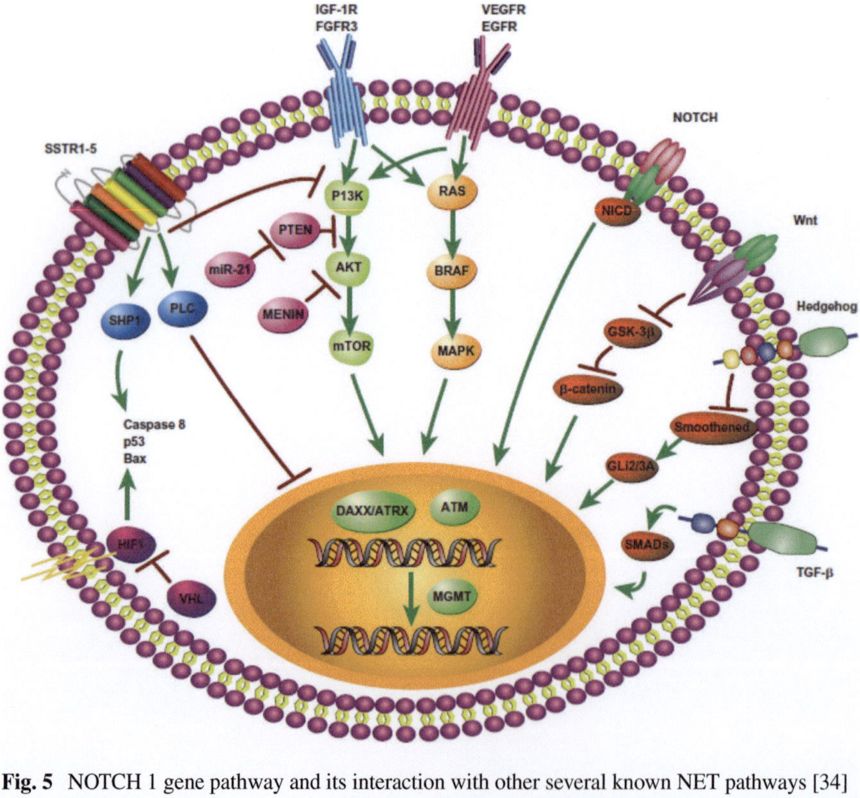

Fig. 5 NOTCH 1 gene pathway and its interaction with other several known NET pathways [34]

Molecular Pathways

The general pathogenesis of neuroendocrine tumor involves the mTOR pathway (the mammalian target of rapamycin, an intracellular serine-threonine kinase), vascular endothelial growth factor (VEGF), insulin-like growth factor receptor (IGFR), phosphoinositol-3-kinase (PI3K)-Akt, somatostatin receptors, and angiogenesis pathways, which are also suggested to be involved in the pathogenesis of colorectal NET [11]. Targeted therapies against aforementioned pathways (e.g., everolimus, octreotide) have been beneficial and have improved outcomes for patients with advanced colorectal NETs further confirming involvement of the same pathway mechanisms in developing colorectal NETS [12].

In addition, TGF-α and the epidermal growth factor (EGF) receptor expression have been reported in neuroendocrine colorectal lesions [13] as well as some suggestions on the existence of a reverse relationship between IL-1 and NE differentia-

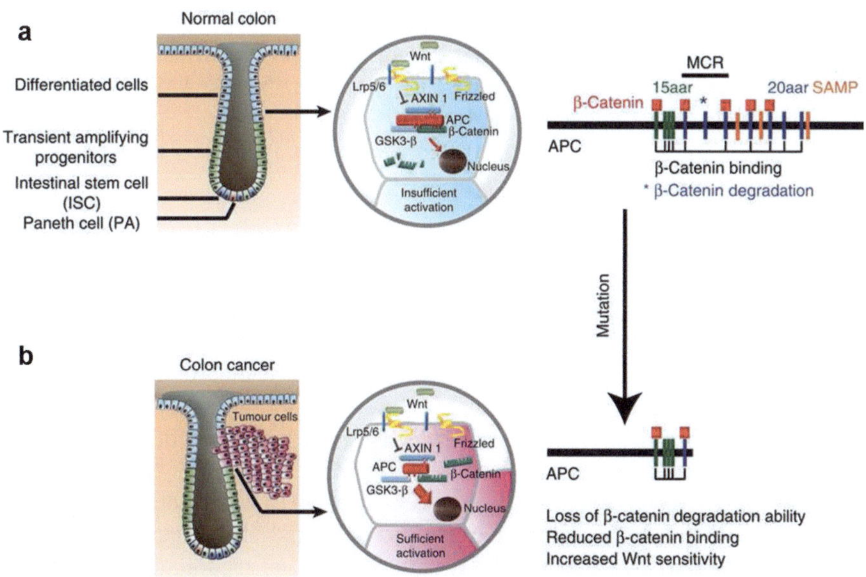

Fig. 6 Schematic model on the role of Wnt secretion in APC mutant cells. (**a**) In normal colon cells, Wnt signaling gradients originating at the bottom of colonic crypts determine cell identity. Low amounts of Wnt signaling lead to differentiation of epithelial cells of the colon. Under these conditions, wild-type APC serves as a scaffold, binding β-catenin and catalytic components of the destruction complex, thus sequestering it in the cytoplasm and causing its degradation. (**b**) In colon cancer cells, APC is truncated but retains some ability to bind β-catenin and act as a scaffold for the destruction complex. However, the efficiency of β-catenin retention is reduced in a manner related to the length of the truncated APC protein. Thus, APC truncations sensitize to canonical Wnts, allowing cancer cells to be more sensitive to activation by Wnt ligands, while retaining regulatory activity. Throughout the signaling cascade. Further, colon cancer cells acquire the ability to secrete Wnts in an autocrine manner, rendering the tumor increasingly independent of the original Wnt sources of the colonic crypts [35]

tion in colorectal carcinomas, in contrast to coexistence of Bcl-2 and chromogranin when differentiating toward neuroendocrine direction within a colorectal cancer [14].

However, colorectal neuroendocrine tumors are argentaffin negative, and their developmental pathways differ from neuroendocrine tumors elsewhere in the GI tract to some extent.

Colorectal cancers (CRCs) are divided to sporadic and hereditary (less than 5 %) subtypes. Germline mutations are responsible for hereditary CRC syndromes, whereas epigenetic alterations result in sporadic CRC [15]. CRC with extensive expression of neuroendocrine markers is defined as a neuroendocrine tumor, and the cancer containing between 2 and 25 % NE component is defined as a carcinoma with neuroendocrine differentiation [14].

The neuroendocrine colorectal carcinoma exhibits poorer prognosis than the adenocarcinoma in sporadic cases [14]. Colorectal poorly differentiated neuroendocrine carcinomas (NECs) and mixed adenoneuroendocrine carcinomas (MANECs) are associated with biological aggressiveness and poor patient survival [16].

To date three molecular pathways are known to be involved in the development of colorectal carcinoma: chromosomal instability (CIN), microsatellite instability (MSI), and CpG island methylator phenotype (CIMP) pathways. A single tumor can exhibit features of more than one pathway [17].

Chromosomal Instability (CIN)

The profile of genetic alterations in colorectal NECs is that of well-differentiated NECs in general, and it is different from the profile seen in CRCs [18]. Chromosomal instability has been shown to be highly involved in malignant progression of endocrine tumors of the GI tract including colorectal tumors. Poorly differentiated endocrine carcinomas of the GI tract demonstrate a high level of chromosomal instability including inactivation of both the p53 and p16/Rb pathways [18]. However, in the colorectum, CIN has been detected also in well-differentiated NETs. Two chromosomal regions, namely, 3p21-p14 and 11p15, appear to be more frequently involved. APC, Wnt pathway and p53 loss, and aneuploidy have roles in CIN during the tumorigenesis process. Whether p53 actively functions to trigger CIN or through promoting a preexisting tendency toward CIN is not yet completely understood [19, 20].

MSI

MSI is common only in sporadic CRC and is not common in neuroendocrine tumors from different anatomical sites [21]. Sporadic (gastroenteropancreatic) GEP-NET is not highly unstable (MSI-H), and only a small number are low-grade unstable

(MSI-L). The majority of tumors show no to minimum mutations of any of the five microsatellite markers and are microsatellite stable (MSS) [22]. Although MSI status and neuroendocrine differentiation had no obvious link, lost expression of mismatch repair gene in sporadic neuroendocrine colorectal tumors has been reported in rare cases suggesting that they might develop secondary to chromosomal instability or that this phenotype may be independent of the developmental pathway in colorectal region (i.e., chromosomal instability vs. MSI) cases [14, 17]. Hereditary cases of colorectal neuroendocrine tumors from HNPCC possess different genetic features of tumor development than sporadic counterpart, but neuroendocrine tumors reported in HNPCC are rare in general [14].

Of the NET from the colon and rectum, only less than 5 % has been reported to be MSI-H, around 20 % can be MSI-L, and the majority are MSS. MSI status is not different in the fore/midgut NETs versus hindgut [21]. However, MSI status has been reported to be correlated with neuroendocrine-CRC prognosis in some studies [16], and colorectal NEC with microsatellite instability has been shown to have a better prognosis than what is generally expected for an NEC [23].

CpG Island Methylator Phenotype (CIMP)

CpG island methylator phenotype (CIMP) is more frequent in poorly differentiated NET, especially in microsatellite stable cases of the colon and rectum than in its well-differentiated fore-/midgut equivalent. Although CIMP phenotype is seen in sporadic CRC as well as in poorly differentiated NET, but it differs between sporadic CRC and poorly differentiated NET of the colon and rectum in its mechanisms in tumor pathogenesis. Sporadic CRC shows higher CIMP in MSI-H subgroup, whereas in colorectal NETs, CIMP is prominent only in MSS or MSI-L groups [21].

Other Genetic Mechanisms

In general, development of NET abnormalities involves different genes, genetic and epigenetic alteration pathways including DNA methylation, point mutations, gene deletions, chromosomal losses, and chromosomal gains.

Mutations

Mutation in SWI/SNF-related, matrix-associated, actin-dependent regulator of chromatin subfamily, a member 4 (SMARCA4), somatic mutations in adenomatous polyposis coli (APC), Kirsten rat sarcoma viral oncogene homolog (KRAS), B-cell CLL/lymphoma 9 (BCL9), and forkhead box P1 (FOXP1) genes have been reported in neuroendocrine differentiation of CRC [24].

Molecular analysis of composite carcinoma of the colon has revealed a G13D KRAS mutation with no BRAF mutation and no microsatellite instability [25]. KRAS and BRAF mutations are more concordant with CRC without neuroendocrine differentiation [26].

Loss of heterozygosity of chromosome 18 as well as at APC, DCC, and p53 genes has been observed in some lesions [14, 27].

Methylation

High levels of methylation have been observed in colorectal neuroendocrine carcinomas [28].

Aberrant methylation of the APC promoter is strongly involved in the molecular tumorigenesis of neuroendocrine GEP tumors [22]. p14 (cyclin-dependent kinase inhibitor 2D), cyclin-dependent kinase inhibitor-2A (p16), MGMT, THBS1, and RAR-β are more frequently methylated in alimentary tract NETs when compared with pancreatic neuroendocrine tumors. ER and cyclooxygenase 2 (COX2) are equally methylated in all types of NETs and normal tissue [29].

Methylation involving p16 patterns involves hindgut tumors in greater extent than other sites within the gut and pancreas. COX2 and O6-methylguanine-DNA-methyl transferase (MGMT) pathways are also involved in hindgut-NET pathogenesis but in lesser amount [21, 30].

Thrombosporin 1 (THBS1), retinoic acid receptor-β 2 (RAR-β), O6-methylguanine-DNA-methyl transferase (MGMT), and p14 are more frequent in the rectum [29].

Other commonly reported genes with significant methylation involving colorectal NETs include MEN1, hMLH1, and TIMP3 [21].

Wnt Pathway/PROX1 Protein

Wnt/β-catenin pathway regulates stem cell pluripotency and cell fate decisions during development in integration with signals from other pathways, including retinoic acid, FGF, TGF-β, and BMP, within different cell types and tissues. PROX1 protein is detected in about half of the rectal NETs, suggesting a role for Wnt pathway in colorectal NET development. Higher immunohistochemical detection of PROX1 correlates with a more malignant variant and metastatic potential in rectal NETs [31].

Notch1

This gene is a member of the Notch family, a 1 transmembrane protein family, and part of an intercellular signaling pathway. They all share structural characteristics including an extracellular domain, multiple epidermal growth factor-like (EGF) repeats, and an intracellular domain. Notch family members have role in cell developmental processes. Specific expression of NOTCH1 has been shown for rectal neuroendocrine tumors (100 %). Besides that, global gene expression of ISL, LIM homeobox 1, cathepsin B, glucagon, and tryptophan hydroxylase 1 genes is different in small intestinal versus rectal neuroendocrine tumors [32].

Insulin-Like Peptide 5 (INSL5)

Insulin-like peptide 5 (INSL5) is a member of the insulin superfamily and a potent agonist for RXFP4. INSL5-RXFP4 signaling might play a role in the colorectal neuroendocrine differentiation, and INSL5 expression has been shown in enteroendocrine cells (EECs) along the colorectum, with a propensity to increased expression toward rectum. Since these EECs with INSL5 expression are not reactive to chromogranin A (CgA), they can be as a unique marker of colorectal EECs [33].

Abbreviations

CIMP	CpG island methylator phenotype
CIN	Chromosomal instability
CRC	Colorectal cancer
EC cells	Enterochromaffin cells
EGF	Epidermal growth factor (EGF)
GEP-NEN	Gastroenteropancreatic-neuroendocrine neoplasms
GI	Gastrointestinal
IGFR	Insulin-like growth factor receptor
MANEC	Mixed adenoneuroendocrine carcinoma
MSI	Microsatellite instability
MSS	Microsatellite stable
mTOR	Mammalian target of rapamycin (an intracellular serine-threonine kinase)
NEC	Neuroendocrine carcinoma
NEN	Neuroendocrine neoplasms
NET	Neuroendocrine tumors
PI3K	Phosphoinositol-3-kinase (PI3K)
PP	Pancreatic polypeptide
PYY	Peptide YY
VEGF	Vascular endothelial growth factor

References

1. Kloppel G. Classification and pathology of gastroenteropancreatic neuroendocrine neoplasms. Endocr Relat Cancer. 2011;18 Suppl 1:S1–16.
2. Anthony LB, Strosberg JR, Klimstra DS, Maples WJ, O'Dorisio TM, Warner RR, Wiseman GA, Benson 3rd AB, Pommier RF. The NANETS consensus guidelines for the diagnosis and

management of gastrointestinal neuroendocrine tumors (nets): well-differentiated nets of the distal colon and rectum. Pancreas. 2010;39:767–74.
3. West NE, Wise PE, Herline AJ, Muldoon RL, Chopp WV, Schwartz DA. Carcinoid tumors are 15 times more common in patients with Crohn's disease. Inflamm Bowel Dis. 2007;13:1129–34.
4. Pulitzer M, Xu R, Suriawinata AA, Waye JD, Harpaz N. Microcarcinoids in large intestinal adenomas. Am J Surg Pathol. 2006;30:1531–6.
5. Berardi RS. Carcinoid tumors of the colon (exclusive of the rectum): review of the literature. Dis Colon Rectum. 1972;15:383–91.
6. Modlin IM, Sandor A. An analysis of 8305 cases of carcinoid tumors. Cancer. 1997;79:813–29.
7. Soga J. Carcinoids of the rectum: an evaluation of 1271 reported cases. Surg Today. 1997;27:112–9.
8. Brenner B, Tang LH, Klimstra DS, Kelsen DP. Small-cell carcinomas of the gastrointestinal tract: a review. J Clin Oncol. 2004;22:2730–9.
9. Brenner B, Tang LH, Shia J, Klimstra DS, Kelsen DP. Small cell carcinomas of the gastrointestinal tract: clinicopathological features and treatment approach. Semin Oncol. 2007;34:43–50.
10. Haraguchi M, Kinoshita H, Koori M, Tsuneoka N, Kosaka T, Ito Y, Furui J, Kanematsu T. Multiple rectal carcinoids with diffuse ganglioneuromatosis. World J Surg Oncol. 2007;5:19.
11. Boussaha T, Rougier P, Taieb J, Lepere C. Digestive neuroendocrine tumors (DNET): the era of targeted therapies. Clin Res Hepatol Gastroenterol. 2013;37:134–41.
12. Castellano D, Bajetta E, Panneerselvam A, Saletan S, Kocha W, O'Dorisio T, Anthony LB, Hobday T, Group R-S. Everolimus plus octreotide long-acting repeatable in patients with colorectal neuroendocrine tumors: a subgroup analysis of the phase III RADIANT-2 study. Oncologist. 2013;18:46–53.
13. Shimizu T, Tanaka S, Haruma K, Kitadai Y, Yoshihara M, Sumii K, Kajiyama G, Shimamoto F. Growth characteristics of rectal carcinoid tumors. Oncology. 2000;59:229–37.
14. Sun MH. Neuroendocrine differentiation in sporadic CRC and hereditary nonpolyosis colorectal cancer. Dis Markers. 2004;20:283–8.
15. Al-Sohaily S, Biankin A, Leong R, Kohonen-Corish M, Warusavitarne J. Molecular pathways in colorectal cancer. J Gastroenterol Hepatol. 2012;27:1423–31.
16. La Rosa S, Marando A, Furlan D, Sahnane N, Capella C. Colorectal poorly differentiated neuroendocrine carcinomas and mixed adenoneuroendocrine carcinomas: insights into the diagnostic immunophenotype, assessment of methylation profile, and search for prognostic markers. Am J Surg Pathol. 2012;36:601–11.
17. Stelow EB, Moskaluk CA, Mills SE. The mismatch repair protein status of colorectal small cell neuroendocrine carcinomas. Am J Surg Pathol. 2006;30:1401–4.
18. Pizzi S, Azzoni C, Bassi D, Bottarelli L, Milione M, Bordi C. Genetic alterations in poorly differentiated endocrine carcinomas of the gastrointestinal tract. Cancer. 2003;98:1273–82.
19. Furlan D, Cerutti R, Uccella S, La Rosa S, Rigoli E, Genasetti A, Capella C. Different molecular profiles characterize well-differentiated endocrine tumors and poorly differentiated endocrine carcinomas of the gastroenteropancreatic tract. Clin Cancer Res Off J Am Assoc Cancer Res. 2004;10:947–57.
20. Pizzi S, Azzoni C, Tamburini E, Bottarelli L, Campanini N, D'Adda T, Fellegara G, Luong TV, Pasquali C, Rossi G, Delle Fave G, Camisa R, Bordi C, Rindi G. Adenomatous polyposis coli alteration in digestive endocrine tumours: correlation with nuclear translocation of beta-catenin and chromosomal instability. Endocr Relat Cancer. 2008;15:1013–24.
21. Arnold CN, Nagasaka T, Goel A, Scharf I, Grabowski P, Sosnowski A, Schmitt-Graff A, Boland CR, Arnold R, Blum HE. Molecular characteristics and predictors of survival in patients with malignant neuroendocrine tumors. Int J Cancer J Int Cancer. 2008;123:1556–64.
22. Arnold CN, Sosnowski A, Blum HE. Analysis of molecular pathways in neuroendocrine cancers of the gastroenteropancreatic system. Ann N Y Acad Sci. 2004;1014:218–9.

23. Sahnane N, Furlan D, Monti M, Romualdi C, Vanoli A, Vicari E, Solcia E, Capella C, Sessa F, La Rosa S. Microsatellite unstable gastrointestinal neuroendocrine carcinomas: a new clinicopathologic entity. Endocr Relat Cancer. 2015;22:35–45.
24. Vanacker L, Smeets D, Hoorens A, Teugels E, Algaba R, Dehou MF, De Becker A, Lambrechts D, De Greve J. Mixed adenoneuroendocrine carcinoma of the colon: molecular pathogenesis and treatment. Anticancer Res. 2014;34:5517–21.
25. Wentz SC, Vnencak-Jones C, Chopp WV. Neuroendocrine and squamous colonic composite carcinoma: case report with molecular analysis. World J Gastroenterol WJG. 2011;17:4729–33.
26. Kleist B, Kempa M, Novy M, Oberkanins C, Xu L, Li G, Loland C, Poetsch M. Comparison of neuroendocrine differentiation and KRAS/NRAS/BRAF/PIK3CA/TP53 mutation status in primary and metastatic colorectal cancer. Int J Clin Exp Pathol. 2014;7:5927–39.
27. Lollgen RM, Hessman O, Szabo E, Westin G, Akerstrom G. Chromosome 18 deletions are common events in classical midgut carcinoid tumors. Int J Cancer J Int Cancer. 2001;92:812–5.
28. Furlan D, Sahnane N, Mazzoni M, Pastorino R, Carnevali I, Stefanoli M, Ferretti A, Chiaravalli AM, La Rosa S, Capella C. Diagnostic utility of MS-MLPA in DNA methylation profiling of adenocarcinomas and neuroendocrine carcinomas of the colon-rectum. Virchows Arch Int J Pathol. 2013;462:47–56.
29. Leotlela PD, Jauch A, Holtgreve-Grez H, Thakker RV. Genetics of neuroendocrine and carcinoid tumours. Endocr Relat Cancer. 2003;10:437–50.
30. Chan AO, Kim SG, Bedeir A, Issa JP, Hamilton SR, Rashid A. Cpg island methylation in carcinoid and pancreatic endocrine tumors. Oncogene. 2003;22:924–34.
31. Jernman J, Kallio P, Hagstrom J, Valimaki MJ, Haapasalo H, Alitalo K, Arola J, Haglund C. Prox1 is involved in progression of rectal neuroendocrine tumors, nets. Virchows Arch Int J Pathol. 2015;467(3):279–84.
32. Wang H, Chen Y, Fernandez-Del Castillo C, Yilmaz O, Deshpande V. Heterogeneity in signaling pathways of gastroenteropancreatic neuroendocrine tumors: a critical look at notch signaling pathway. Mod Pathol Off J U S Can Acad Pathol Inc. 2013;26:139–47.
33. Mashima H, Ohno H, Yamada Y, Sakai T, Ohnishi H. INSL5 may be a unique marker of colorectal endocrine cells and neuroendocrine tumors. Biochem Biophys Res Commun. 2013;432:586–92.
34. Capdevila J, Tabernero J. A shining light in the darkness for the treatment of pancreatic neuroendocrine tumors. Cancer Discov. 2011;1:213–21.
35. Voloshanenko O, Erdmann G, Dubash TD, Augustin I, Metzig M, Moffa G, Hundsrucker C, Kerr G, Sandmann T, Anchang B, Demir K, Boehm C, Leible S, Ball CR, Glimm H, Spang R, Boutros M. Wnt secretion is required to maintain high levels of Wnt activity in colon cancer cells. Nat Commun. 2013;4:2610.

Adrenal Neuroendocrine Tumors: Pheochromocytoma and Neuroblastic Tumors

Carmen M. Perrino and Debra L. Zynger

Pheochromocytoma

Introduction

Chromaffin cells are cells derived from the neural crest which produce catecholamines. These cells are found throughout the body in sympathetic and parasympathetic ganglia and the adrenal medulla. Tumors arising from these cells are termed paraganglioma if extra-adrenal and pheochromocytoma if located within the adrenal gland. Approximately 30 % of pheochromocytomas have a hereditary basis [1, 2]. Seven percent of primary adrenal tumors are pheochromocytomas, and one-quarter of adrenal resections are performed to remove this tumor [3, 4].

Epidemiological and Clinical Features

The estimated annual incidence of pheochromocytoma is 0.8 per 100,000 person years [5]. Sporadic tumors most commonly occur in the fourth and fifth decade, with an equal prevalence in men and women [6, 7]. Patients with familial pheochromocytoma are more likely to have bilateral tumors, and the tumors appear earlier, which may be due to surveillance. Tumors have a mean size of 7.7 cm [8]. The classic triad of symptoms includes episodic headaches, sweating, and tachycardia. About half of patients have sudden intensification of hypertension (paroxysmal

C.M. Perrino, MD (✉)
Department of Pathology and Immunology Campus,Washington University,
St. Louis, MO, USA
e-mail: cmperrino@gmail.com

D.L. Zynger, MD
Department of Pathology, The Ohio State University Wexner Medical Center,
Columbus, OH, USA
e-mail: debra.zynger@osumc.edu

A. Nasir, D. Coppola (eds.), *Neuroendocrine Tumors: Review of Pathology, Molecular and Therapeutic Advances*, DOI 10.1007/978-1-4939-3426-3_17

hypertensive episodes). Some patients have continuously high blood pressure with exacerbations, while 5–15 % are normotensive [9–12]. Other symptoms include palpitations and postural hypotension. Pheochromocytomas discovered incidentally via imaging are more likely to be asymptomatic and/or hereditary [9–12].

Patients clinically suspected to have pheochromocytoma undergo laboratory testing for confirmation. Secretory products can include noradrenaline, adrenaline, and/or dopamine with these catecholamines or their metabolites detected in the serum or urine via high-performance liquid chromatography or tandem mass spectrometry [13, 14]. However, most patients with a workup ultimately prove not to have a pheochromocytoma [15]. Numerous other lesions can produce pheochromocytoma-like symptoms as well as catecholamine elevation ("pseudopheochromocytomas") [16–24].

Imaging can localize the tumor to the adrenal gland and confirm the diagnosis, as pheochromocytoma has a high intensity and hypervascular appearance on T2-weighted MRI. Computed tomography (CT) can also be used and is less expensive although there is radiation exposure. Microscopic evaluation is rarely utilized for diagnosis [25, 26]. Arteriography or needle biopsy is usually not performed as manipulation of the tumor can precipitate a hypertensive crisis due to excessive catecholamine secretion. Biopsy of the tumor is almost never needed but if done requires adrenergic blockade. While rarely encountered, biopsy specimens of unsuspected pheochromocytomas have been reported in several publications [27–35].

Light Microscopic Findings

Pheochromocytomas have a nested ("zellballen") or trabecular appearance at low power light microscopic examination (Fig. 1). The nests are composed of large polygonal cells with abundant cytoplasm and are surrounded by supporting sustentacular cells. The cytoplasm is deeply basophilic to eosinophilic and is finely granular (Fig. 2). Cells sometimes contain hyaline granules. Nuclei are large with occasional pseudoinclusions. Nucleoli are prominent. Rarely, ganglion cells or neural stroma is present forming tumors referred to as *composite pheochromocytomas* (Fig. 3). These tumors have areas that resemble neural tumors including ganglioneuroma, ganglioneuroblastoma, or neuroblastoma.

Predicting the behavior of a pheochromocytoma based on light microscopic findings is difficult. Features worrisome for malignancy include involvement of the periadrenal adipose tissue, capsular invasion, vascular invasion, mitotic figures, atypical mitoses, necrosis, cellular spindling, diffuse growth, high cellularity, cellular monotony, and marked nuclear pleomorphism (Fig. 4; Table 1) [36]. Within extra-adrenal paragangliomas, sustentacular cells detectable with S-100 protein have been associated with a favorable prognosis [37].

Upon biopsy, mistaking pheochromocytoma for normal adrenal medulla has been reported as a diagnostic pitfall [27, 38]. A sample containing uniform basophilic cells reminiscent of the adrenal medulla should raise the differential diagnosis of a pheochromocytoma. In a resection specimen, the diagnosis of a pheochromocy-

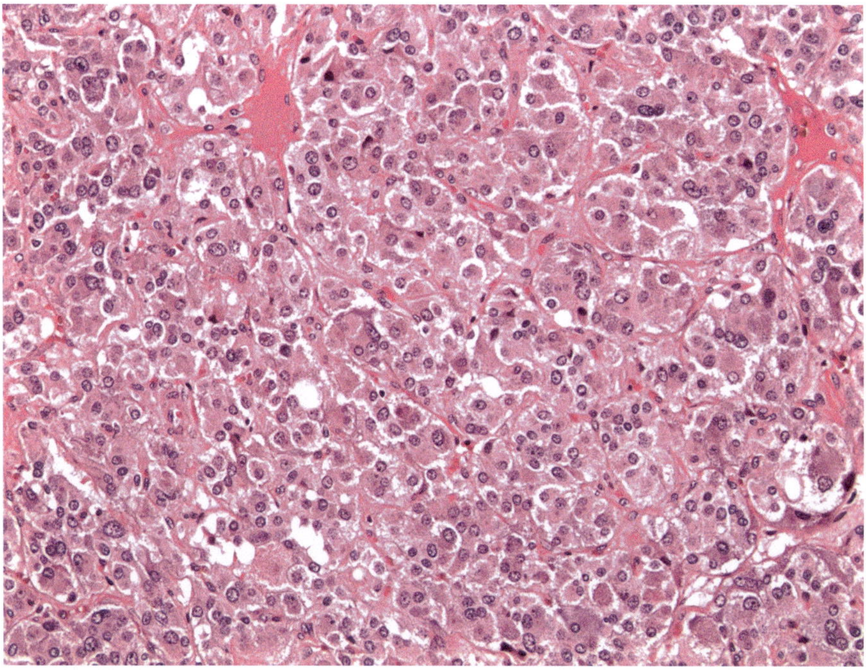

Fig. 1 Pheochromocytoma is composed of nests of tumor separated by thin sustentacular cells

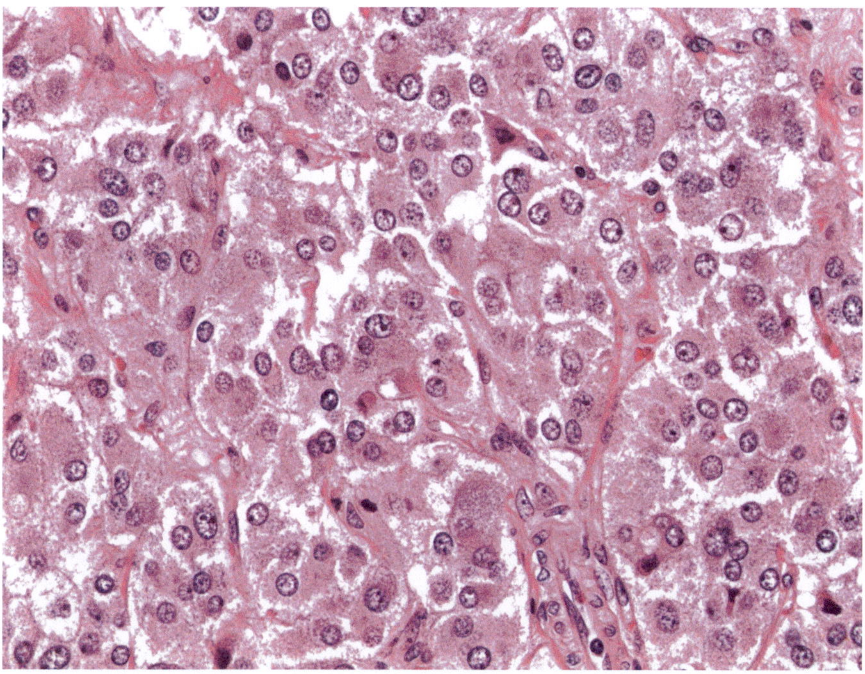

Fig. 2 The cells of pheochromocytoma are polygonal, with abundant deeply colored granular cytoplasm

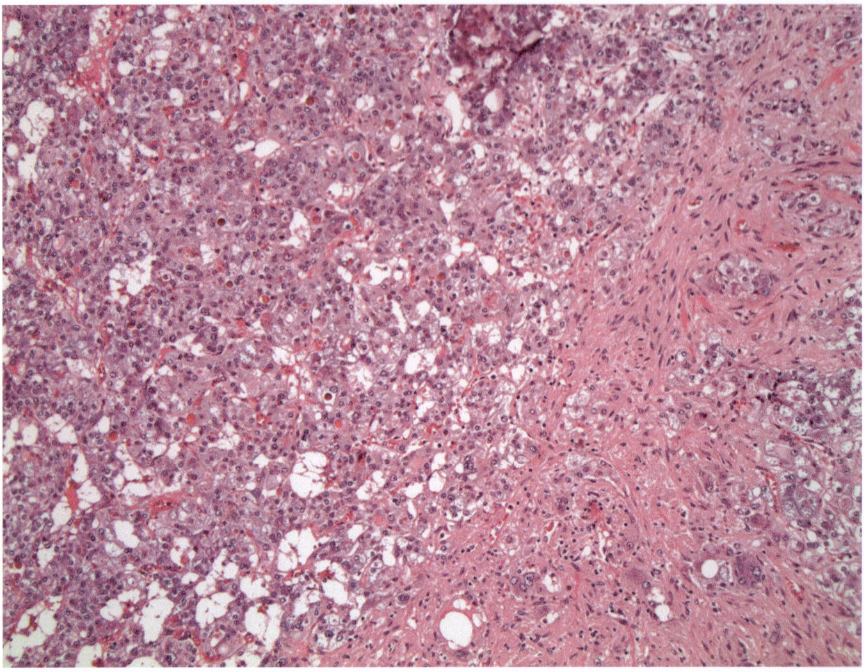

Fig. 3 This composite pheochromocytoma contains ganglion cells in the lower right corner

toma is usually rendered without difficulty. However, tumors with marked pleomorphism and spindling may raise the consideration of adrenal cortical carcinoma (Fig. 5). Adrenal cortical carcinoma typically is more eosinophilic with more readily identifiable mitotic figures and less uniform appearing cells. Immunohistochemical stains can be employed for difficult cases, as described below.

Immunohistochemistry

Synaptophysin and chromogranin A are neuroendocrine proteins that are highly expressed in pheochromocytoma (Fig. 6) [39–43]. Synaptophysin is a glycoprotein found in neuronal presynaptic vesicle membranes and is localized to the cytoplasm. Most pheochromocytomas (91–100 %) have reactivity to synaptophysin [39–41]. The protein chromogranin binds acidic glycoproteins and is located within the secretory vesicles of neurons and endocrine cells. Chromogranin A has similar reliable reactivity (91–100 %) in pheochromocytoma [40–43].

S-100 is highly expressed in the sustentacular cells of pheochromocytoma and also can show expression in the pheochromocytes (Fig. 7) [44, 45]. S-100 is a calcium-binding protein which is found in the nucleus and cytoplasm and is com-

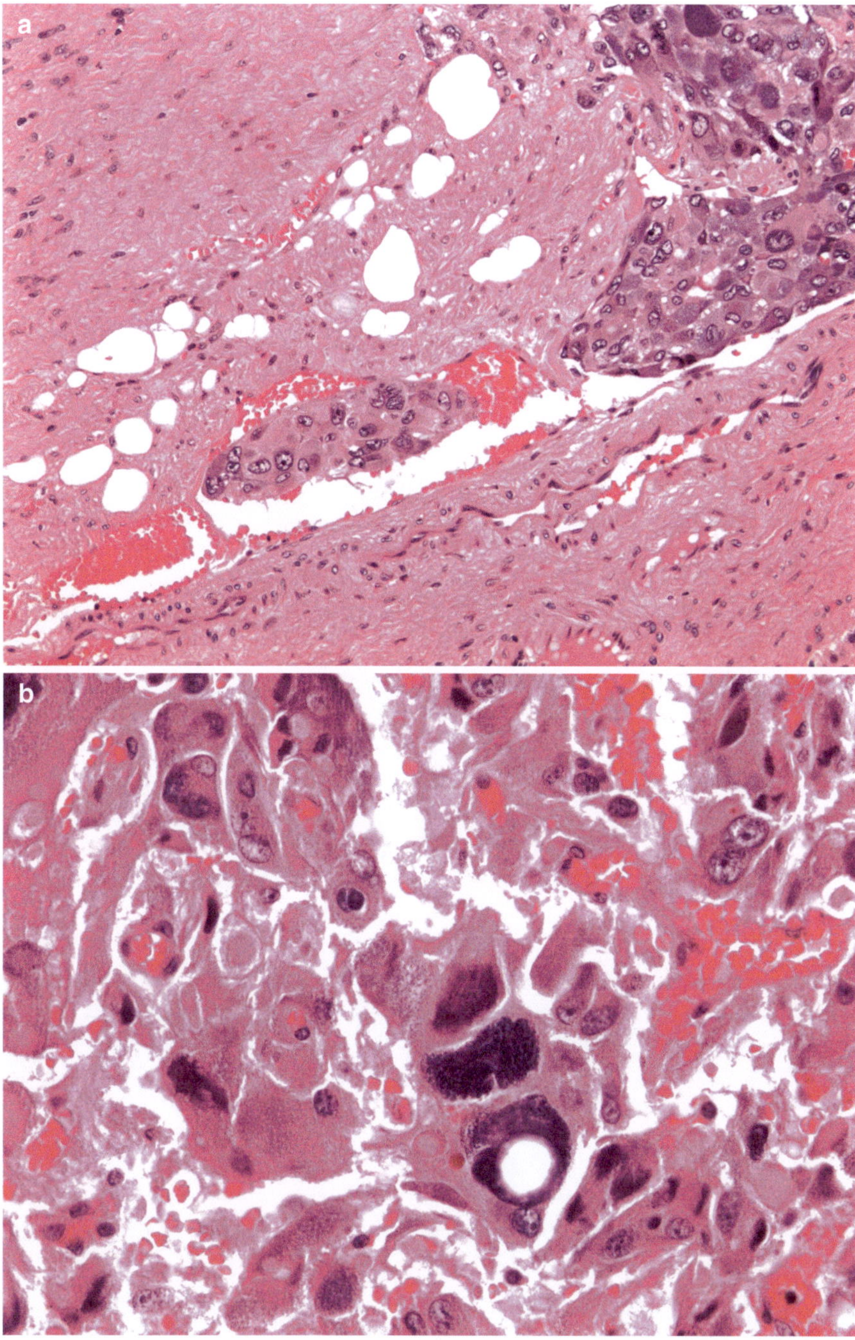

Fig. 4 Features concerning for aggressive behavior in pheochromocytoma. (**a**) Vascular invasion. (**b**) Marked atypia. (**c**) Invasion beyond the capsule. (**d**) Mitotic figure (cell in metaphase in the center of the photo). (**e**) Cellular spindling

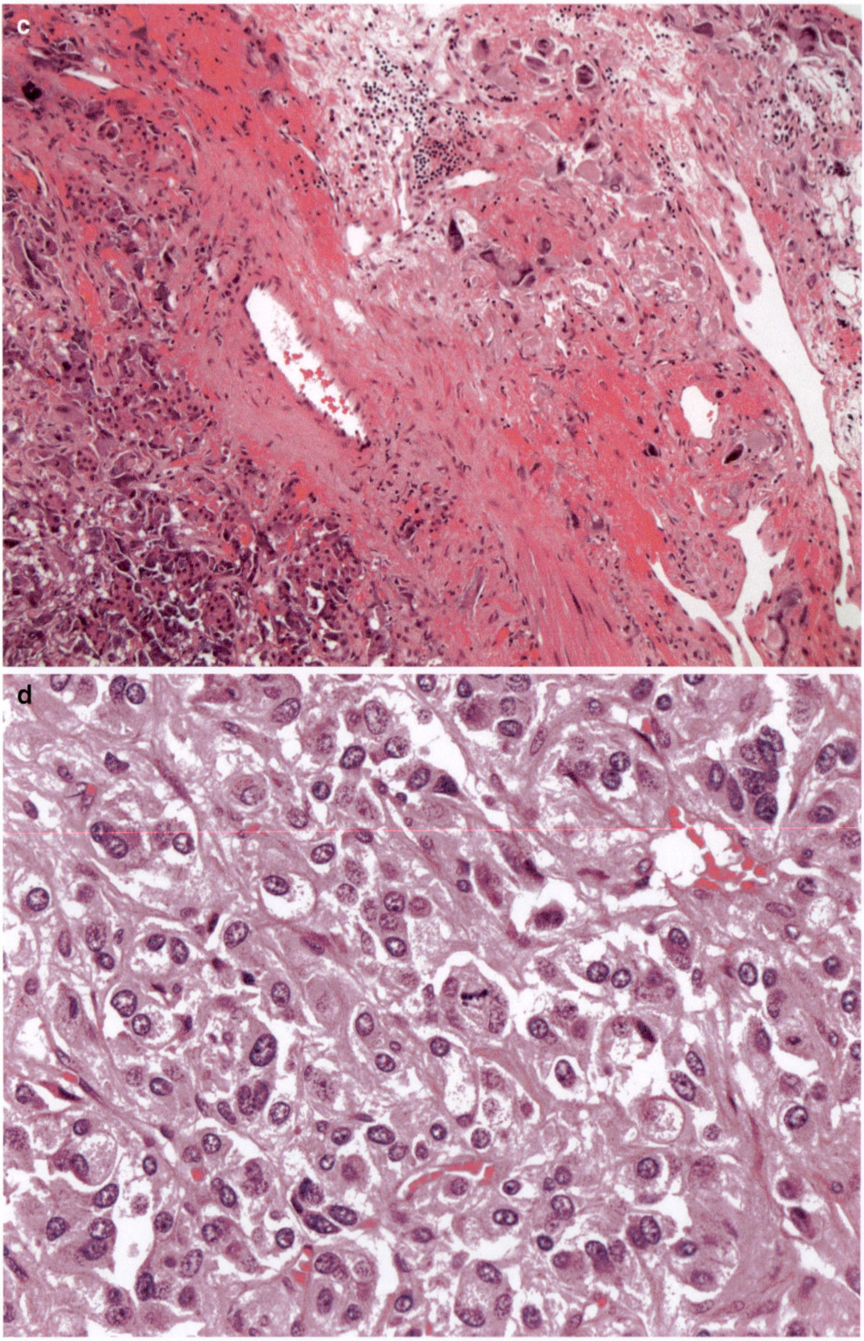

Fig. 4 (continued)

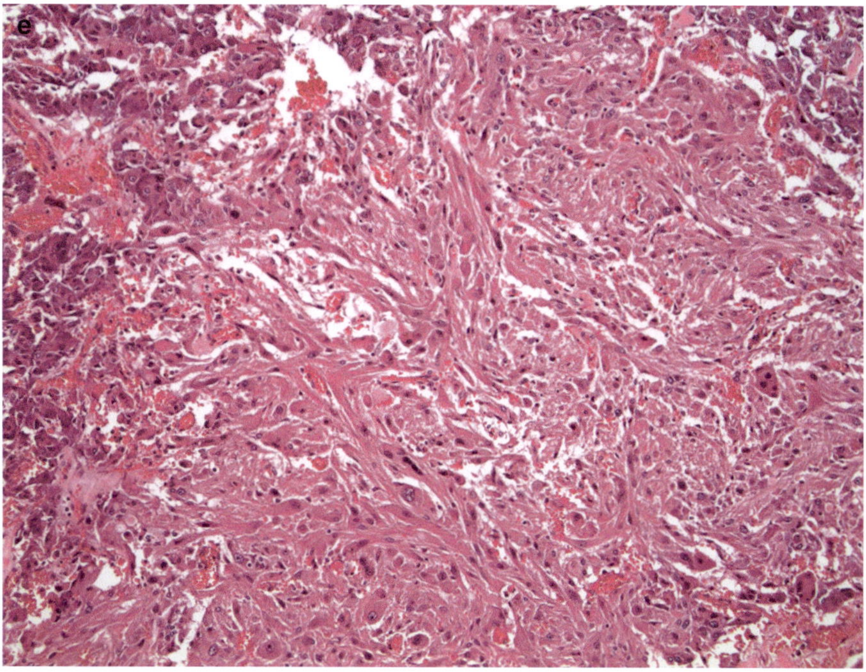

Fig. 4 (continued)

Table 1 Pathologic features of pheochromocytoma worrisome for malignancy

1. Tumor size >5 cm
2. Histologic features
Involvement of the periadrenal adipose tissue
Capsular invasion
Vascular invasion
Mitotic figures (>3/10 high-power fields)
Atypical mitoses
Necrosis
Cellular spindling
Diffuse growth
High cellularity
Cellular monotony
Marked nuclear pleomorphism
Hyperchromasia
Decreased or absent sustentacular cells
3. Ki67 immunoreactivity

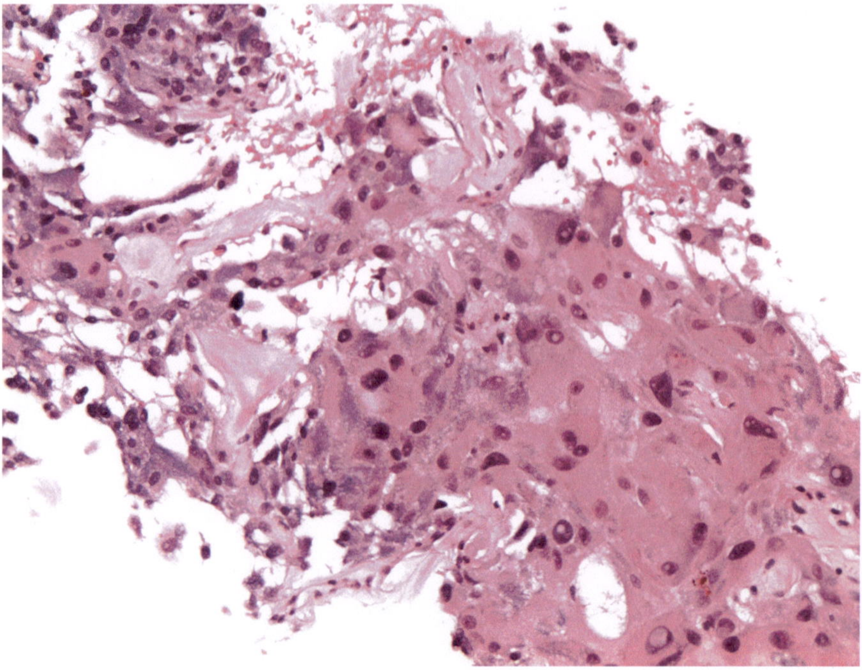

Fig. 5 Biopsy containing pheochromocytoma. This was mistakenly diagnosed as carcinoma

posed of an alpha and beta subunit. Most S-100 protein antibodies used in clinical practice recognize both subunits [46].

If there is a diagnostic dilemma, performing a panel of immunostains to include chromogranin A and S-100 (positive in pheochromocytoma, negative in adrenal cortical tumors) and melan-A, inhibin, and calretinin (negative in pheochromocytoma, positive in adrenal cortical tumors) will allow for discrimination. Synaptophysin is also helpful but often has some weak, patchy expression in adrenal cortical tumors. It is of particular importance to order a sufficiently thorough immunopanel if pheochromocytoma is a diagnostic consideration in a biopsy specimen as a misdiagnosis could have critical consequences during surgical resection if the patient does not receive appropriate adrenergic blockade.

Ultrastructure

Upon ultrastructural examination with transmission electron microscopy, pheochromocytomas have numerous dense secretory granules within the cytoplasm. These granules measure 200–300 nm and store catecholamines [47–49]. Noradrenaline granules have dense cores that are eccentrically placed with a surrounding empty-appearing halo. Adrenaline granules have dense cores that are centrally placed and

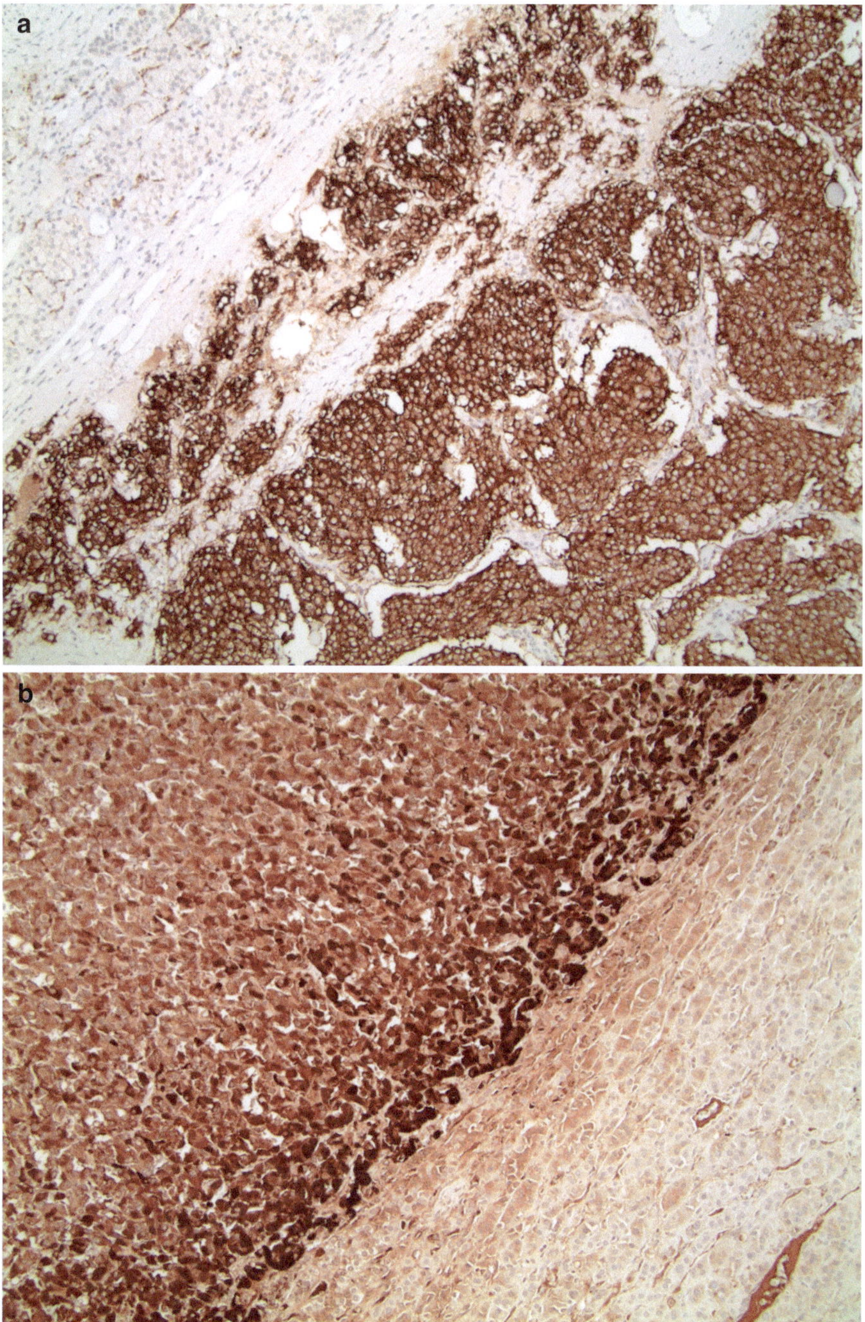

Fig. 6 Pheochromocytoma has strong neuroendocrine expression. (**a**) Synaptophysin is positive (adrenal cortex in *upper left* is negative). (**b**) Chromogranin A is positive (adrenal cortex in *lower right* is weak to negative)

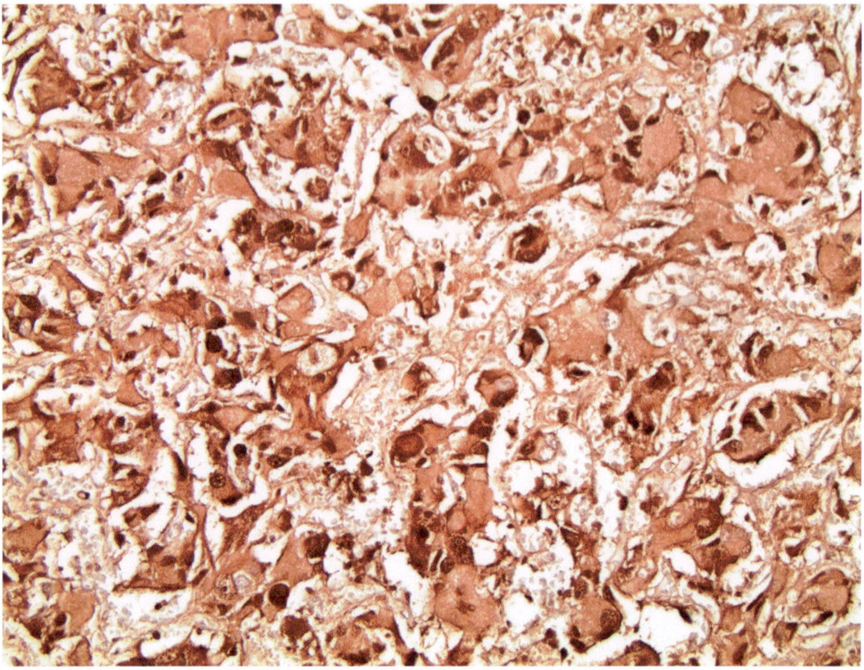

Fig. 7 S-100 is positive in pheochromocytoma

lack a peripheral halo. Most tumors have both types of granules (Fig. 8) [49]. The appearance of the granules which store dopamine is unknown [49]. The number and percentage of each type of granule does not correlate with the type or amount of clinically detected catecholamines [49].

Molecular Pathogenesis and Testing

Hereditary pheochromocytoma accounts for approximately 30 % of cases [50, 51]. These disorders are all autosomal dominant in inheritance and include von Hippel-Lindau syndrome, multiple endocrine neoplasia type 2 (MEN2), neurofibromatosis type 1 (NF1), and familial paraganglioma along with other recently described susceptibility genes (Table 2). Additionally, somatic mutations in genes that lead to these hereditary syndromes are frequent events in nonhereditary pheochromocytoma [52].

von Hippel-Lindau syndrome is caused by a mutation in the *VHL* tumor suppressor gene. The *VHL* gene is located on chromosome 3p25-26. The protein has ubiquitin ligase activity and functions in the regulation of cellular hypoxia via hypoxia-inducible factor alpha (HIF alpha). Loss of function of the VHL protein results in the stabilization of HIF alpha. 10–30 % of von Hippel-Lindau syndrome

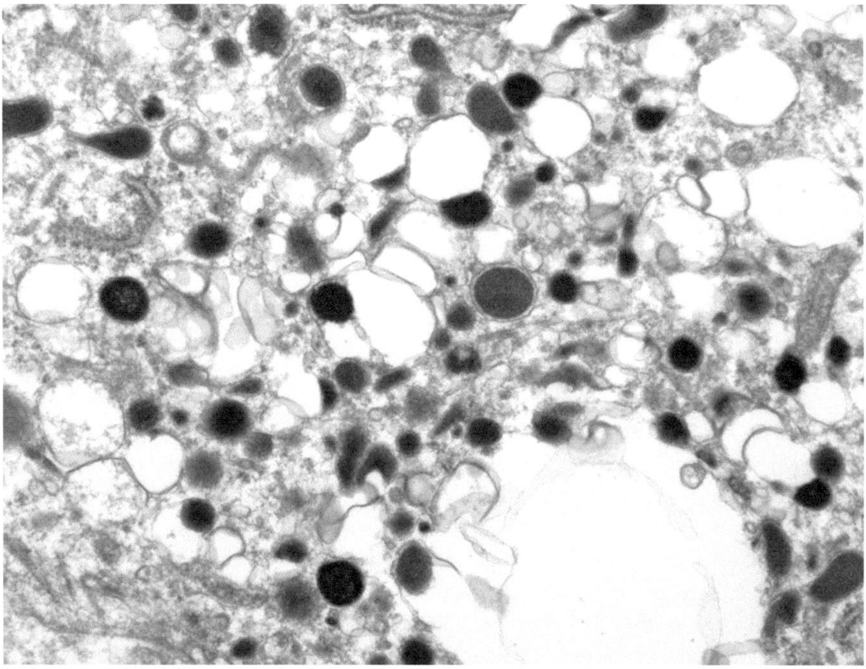

Fig. 8 Ultrastructure of a pheochromocytoma reveals both noradrenaline granules with eccentric dense cores surrounded by an empty-appearing halo and adrenaline granules with centrally placed dense cores that lack a peripheral halo

Table 2 Pheochromocytoma in hereditary genetic disorders

Syndrome/ hereditary mutation	Gene	Location of gene	Percent that develop pheochromocytoma	Age of presentation	Risk for malignancy
von Hippel-Lindau	*VHL*	3p25-26	10–20 %	30's	
Multiple endocrine neoplasia type 2	*RET*	10q11.2	50 %	30's	Low (3–5 %)
Neurofibromatosis 1	*NF1*	17q11.2	1–4 %	40's	
Familial paraganglioma	*SDHB*			30's	High
	SDHD	11q23			
TMEM127	*TMEM127*	2q11		40's	
MAX	*MAX*	14q23		30's	High

patients develop pheochromocytoma. In addition, numerous other tumors can occur including most notably clear cell renal cell carcinoma as well as paraganglioma, hemangioblastoma of the central nervous system, retinal angioma, pancreatic neuroendocrine tumors, middle ear endolymphatic sac tumors, pancreatic serous cystadenoma, and papillary cystadenoma of the epididymis and broad ligament. Several hundred *VHL* germline loss of function mutations have been implicated in von Hippel-Lindau syndrome. Missense mutations are associated with greater risk of pheochromocytoma (type 2 kindreds).

MEN2 is subdivided into MEN2A, MEN2B, and familial medullary thyroid carcinoma. MEN2 is caused by activating mutations in the *RET* proto-oncogene on 10q11.2. The gene encodes for a transmembrane tyrosine kinase receptor that functions in the PI3K signaling pathway and thus regulates cell proliferation and apoptosis [53]. Both types 2A and 2B are characterized by medullary thyroid carcinoma and a 50 % chance of having pheochromocytoma. Pheochromocytoma that develops in MEN2 typically hypersecretes adrenaline. MEN2B accounts for only 5 % of cases and features a marfanoid habitus and skeletal abnormalities [54]. Mutation in one of the cysteine residues of the cysteine-rich extracellular domain coded in exons 10 and 11 accounts for the majority of MEN2A. The mutation disrupts the disulfide bond, increasing the activity of homodimers. In contrast, MEN2B is caused by mutation to the intracellular domain encoded in exon 16, of which most are a missense mutation resulting in a methionine to threonine change. A few percent instead reveal an exon 15 missense mutation yielding an alanine to phenylalanine switch.

NF1 is caused by inactivating mutations in the tumor suppressor gene *NF1* located at 17q11.2. The NF1 protein is a GTPase which regulates the MAPK pathway via interaction with Ras [55]. Patients have a constellation of symptoms including neurofibromas, café au lait spots, axillary and inguinal freckling, and Lisch nodules in the iris. Diagnosis is usually made based on these clinical findings. Genetic testing is difficult due to the size of the gene and lack of mutational hotspots. Approximately 1–4 % of patients develop pheochromocytoma [54, 55]. These tumors typically secrete adrenaline [54].

Familial paraganglioma is a disorder caused by mutations in the succinate dehydrogenase subunit genes (*SDHB, SDHC, SDHD, SDHAF2,* and *SDHA*) [54]. These genes encode proteins which form the mitochondrial complex II that is involved in electron transport chain and tricarboxylic acid cycle [54, 55]. The proteins function as tumor suppressors and regulate HIF alpha. Inactivating mutations lead to the accumulation of succinate and oxygen free radicals [56]. Mutated *SDHB* and *SDHD* lead to an increased risk of pheochromocytoma as well as SDH-deficient renal cell carcinoma. *SDHB* is located on chromosome 1p3, and mutations confer a higher risk of malignant pheochromocytoma, and other tumors may occur including gastrointestinal stromal tumors, breast carcinoma, and papillary thyroid carcinoma with paternal transmission [57, 58].

Other genes have been more recently described to be associated with pheochromocytoma. *TMEM127*, mapped to chromosome 2q11, encodes the TMEM-127 transmembrane tumor suppressor protein [54, 55]. It is hypothesized to be a negative regulator of mammalian target of rapamycin complex 1 (mTOR pathway) in which mutation leads to loss of function and may have a role in protein trafficking [59].

The *MYC-associated factor X* (*MAX*) is a gene whose protein is a transcription factor that functions as a tumor suppressor. It encodes the MAX protein, which forms a part of the MYC/MAX/MXD1 complex that suppresses transcription and thus regulates cell proliferation and apoptosis. Heterodimerization with Myc is speculated to lead to repression of Myc, while *MAX* mutations are thought to cause increased proliferation [60, 61]. A paternal transmission is suggested. MAX-associated pheochromocytomas appear to have a higher risk for malignancy [60]. Additionally, *H-RAS* mutations have been described in a few male patients with pheochromocytoma, and *HIF-2alpha* mutations with gain of function have been identified in rare cases of pheochromocytoma [54].

Genetic testing reveals germline mutations in 25–40 % of pheochromocytomas overall and 2–28 % of sporadic cases with no known family history or evidence of a hereditable disease [51, 53, 62]. Screening patients for known germline mutations is worthwhile because of the relatively high yield of mutations detected, risk of other tumors found in each syndrome, differing risk for aggressive behavior of the pheochromocytoma, and risk to family members [53]. However, due to the large number of genes and genetic heterogeneity encountered, it is cost prohibitive to screen every patient for each mutation. Many of the genes are quite rarely mutated, and therefore, screening every patient would not be helpful [61]. Patients with a known family history of a particular mutation should be initially tested for that mutation. If the patient has symptoms of a particular syndrome, testing should initially focus on the gene implicated in that syndrome. There are no rigid guidelines regarding which patients to test, but a reasonable approach is that in addition to patients with a family history or symptoms of a syndrome, providers may also screen patients with a pheochromocytoma if the patient has bilateral tumors, a pheochromocytoma which presents at <45 years of age, or a concurrent paraganglioma and pheochromocytoma (Table 3). Family members at risk but currently without disease should only be screened if the affected relative has a known mutation identified, and then the screening should be appropriately targeted toward that mutation.

Germline screening is largely accomplished via sequence analysis. Immunohistochemistry can serve as an ancillary technique to evaluate for SDHB-deficient tumors with a loss of expression due to the mutation [54]. Genetic testing for somatic mutations is not clinically performed due to the numerous known mutations and insufficient information regarding the significance of many of the mutations detected. Multiplex sequencing has been used in pheochromocytoma for more efficient evaluation of the genes known to be susceptible [52, 63–65]. In the future, with further advances in sequencing, more in-depth germline testing and possibly also somatic testing may play a role in clinical management.

Table 3 Criteria to determine which patients to screen for pheochromocytoma mutations

1. Screen patient if the patient has a pheochromocytoma and one or more of the following:
Bilateral tumors
Family history
Tumor presents at <45 years of age
Findings suggestive of known syndrome, paraganglioma
2. Screen at-risk family members currently without disease only if affected relative has known mutation identified

Prognostic Factors, Staging, and Management

The mainstay of treatment for organ-confined pheochromocytoma is surgical resection. An adrenalectomy is typically performed. Patients with bilateral disease can undergo subtotal adrenalectomy or a cortical-sparing procedure [66]. The rate of recurrence after adrenalectomy is 6–17 %, and the median time to recurrence is 35 months. Large tumor size (>5 cm) is a predictor of recurrence [67]. One-fourth of recurrences do not have elevated serum or urine metanephrines [67].

For pheochromocytoma, malignancy is defined by metastases. Approximately 10 % of tumors are malignant. Metastases may occur decades after initial diagnosis. The 5-year survival of malignant pheochromocytoma is estimated to be 50 % [68]. Patients with brain, liver, or lung metastases are reported to have worse outcomes compared to those with bone involvement [69].

Initial treatment for metastatic tumor is surgical resection with or without radiopharmaceuticals such as 131-iodine-labeled metaiodobenzylguanidine (^{131}I-MIBG). MIBG is structurally similar to adrenaline. ^{131}I-MIBG is taken up by approximately half of the tumors yielding a response rate of 30 %. Metastatic, unresectable tumor can be treated with a combined chemotherapy regimen such as cyclophosphamide, vincristine, and dacarbazine with progression-free survival of 5 months according to one study [70]. Debulking can be considered to control local and systemic symptoms, although there is little documented long-term benefit [71]. Additionally, external beam radiation therapy, ablative treatments, or ^{131}I-MIBG can be used for local control. External beam radiation therapy reduces the uptake of ^{131}I-MIBG, preventing future efficacy of this therapeutic approach. Small case series have reported the use of the tyrosine kinase inhibitor, sunitinib, in the metastatic setting with a 4-month progression-free survival. Phase II trials are in progress. Other agents are also being tested as survival is poor using current treatments [72].

Predicting malignant behavior is difficult. Large tumor size, in addition to predicting recurrence, is associated with metastatic disease and worse overall survival and is currently the most reliable predictor of behavior [67, 69, 73, 74]. A cutoff of 5 cm is used for concern for future aggressive disease, but this threshold has a high false-negative rate [74]. Histologic features concerning for malignancy were described above and are summarized in Table 1. The Pheochromocytoma of the Adrenal Gland Scaled Score (PASS) is a proposed system in which points are assigned to certain histologic features with an overall score that correlates with malignant behavior according to some reports [36, 75]. The points are assigned as follows: 1 point for vascular invasion, capsular invasion, periadrenal adipose tissue invasion, marked nuclear pleomorphism, and hyperchromasia and 2 points for large nests or diffuse growth, necrosis, high cellularity, tumor spindling, monotony, mitotic figures >3/10 high-power fields, and atypical mitotic figures. Malignant tumors are more likely to have a score of ≥4. Additional scoring systems have been proposed [76, 77]. Proliferation assessed via immunohistochemistry (MIB-1/Ki67) has been reported to correlate with malignancy [75, 78, 79]. Gene expression profiling studies have been performed but have yet to provide one or more useful markers to utilize [74].

Neuroblastic Tumors

Introduction

Neuroblastoma is a primitive neoplasm of neuroectodermal origin. It lies on a spectrum which ranges from neuroblastoma (most primitive) to ganglioneuroblastoma (intermediate) to ganglioneuroma (most mature) tumors. Neuroblastomas arise in the distribution of the sympathoadrenal neuroendocrine system [80].

Epidemiological and Clinical Features

Epidemiological data collected from 1975 to 1995 in the United States showed that the age-adjusted incidence of total neuroblastoma cases in children under 15 years of age was 1492 per million [81]. These tumors are slightly more common in males than females, with this difference most pronounced during infancy (1st year of life) [81]. In infants, tumors were slightly more common in Caucasians, but incidence rates were approximately equal in older children [81]. Regardless of age, most neuroblastomas occurred in the adrenal gland (~40 %), followed by connective/subcutaneous/soft tissue (~20 %), retroperitoneum (~15 %), and mediastinum (~10 %) [81]. Neuroblastoma is the most common malignancy of infancy (<1 year), and the incidence sharply decreases thereafter.

Elevations may be detectable of urinary catecholamine metabolites including homovanillic acid and vanillylmandelic acid and urine or serum dopamine [82]. Clinical symptoms depend on the location of the tumor and are generally due to the effect of compression on surrounding structures [83]. Adrenal neuroblastoma occurs in the abdomen and thus can cause pain, constipation, distension, urinary retention, hypertension, and symptoms of cord compression (urinary retention, paraplegia/paraparesis, clonus) [83]. Paraneoplastic syndromes may occur and include opsoclonus-myoclonus syndrome and vasoactive intestinal peptide-secreting tumors [83].

Light Microscopic Findings

Neuroblastic tumors are categorized on a spectrum of maturation from immature to mature; this spectrum includes neuroblastoma, ganglioneuroblastoma, and ganglioneuroma [84]. These tumors consist of a mixture of neuroblasts, ganglion cells, and Schwannian stroma.

Each of the three main tumor types has several subtypes. Multiple classification schemes have been proposed. The most commonly used system is the Shimada classification initially proposed in 1984, which was later revised by the International

Neuroblastoma Pathology Committee (INPC) and renamed the modified Shimada classification or the INPC classification [84–88].

Features of differentiation of neuroblasts include progressive vesicular nuclear changes, presence of nucleoli, enlarging amphophilic or eosinophilic cytoplasm with/without cytoplasmic processes, and synchronous maturation of the nucleus and cytoplasm. The presence of neuropil signifies that the lesion is at least poorly differentiated. When determining the proportion of neuroblasts in a lesion, only those that are in the intermediate or late stages of maturation are taken into account [84].

The diagnostically relevant terminology often used in neuroblastic tumors is as follows:

Neuroblastomas are composed of neuroblasts and sometimes neuropil (depending on subtype). According to the modified Shimada Classification, three main subtypes exist. *Undifferentiated neuroblastoma* is composed solely of immature neuroblasts of varying sizes, with no evidence of maturation or neuropil. Rarely, undifferentiated or poorly differentiated neuroblastoma *may have a component* composed of large, irregularly shaped neuroblasts with prominent nucleoli and moderate to abundant cytoplasm; cells may be spindled, anaplastic/pleomorphic, bizarre, or even rhabdoid (Fig. 9). In *poorly differentiated neuroblastoma*, <5 % of neuroblasts may show features of differentiation towards ganglion cells (Figs. 10, 11, 12, and 13). In *differentiating neuroblastoma*, ≥5 % of neuroblasts show features of differentiation towards ganglion cells [84].

Ganglioneuroblastoma consists of a mixture of neuroblasts and mature ganglion cells. The ganglioneuromatous component usually comprises >50 % of the lesion. The modified Shimada classification proposed two main subtypes of ganglioneuroblastoma, *nodular* and *intermixed* [84, 87–89]. The classical nodular ganglioneuroblastoma subtype grossly has a neuroblastomatous nodule surrounded by ganglioneuroblastoma, intermixed or ganglioneuroma, and maturing or mature areas (Figs. 14 and 15). Microscopically there is typically an abrupt transition between the nodule and surrounding areas, and the neuroblastoma component is undifferentiated or poorly differentiated [84, 89]. According to the most recent classification system, other subtypes of nodular ganglioneuroblastoma include multiple nodules (≥2 nodules), large (no macroscopically visible nodules, mature component only visible microscopically), and no nodule (primary tumor with features of ganglioneuroblastoma, intermixed, or ganglioneuroma, but metastases show neuroblastoma features) [89]. Lastly, intermixed ganglioneuroblastoma is predominantly composed of ganglioneuroblastoma with well-demarcated microscopic foci of neuroblastoma (Fig. 16) [84].

Ganglioneuroma is composed of mature ganglion cells, and two subtypes are described. *Maturing* ganglioneuroma consists predominantly of mature ganglion cells with a few scattered foci of differentiating neuroblasts, naked neuropil, and maturing ganglion cells. *Mature* ganglioneuroma is composed exclusively of mature ganglion cells (Figs. 17 and 18) [84].

The diagnosis is usually rendered without difficulty in tumors that have evident differentiation. However, in small biopsies with crush artifact or poorly differenti-

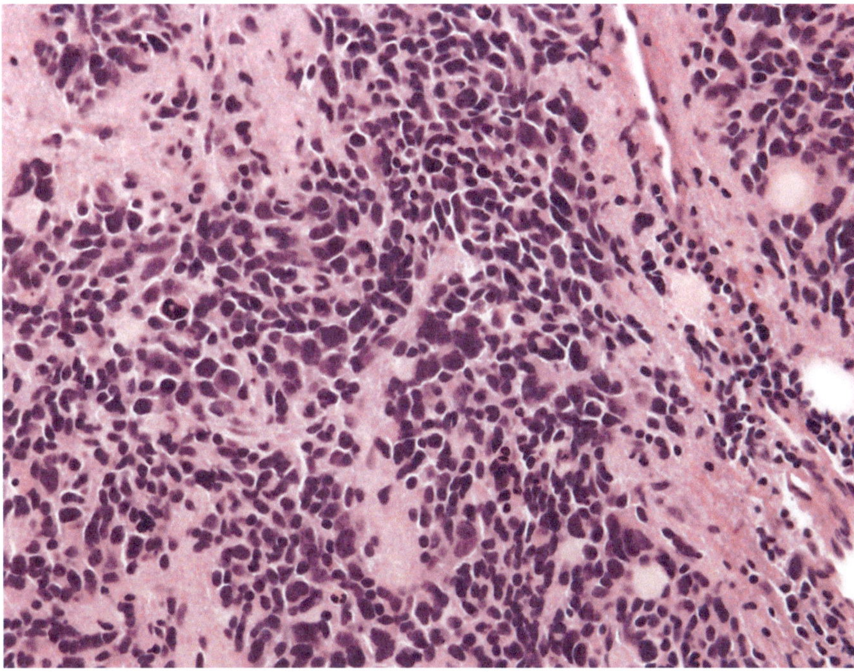

Fig. 9 Neuroblastoma, undifferentiated subtype, with anaplasia

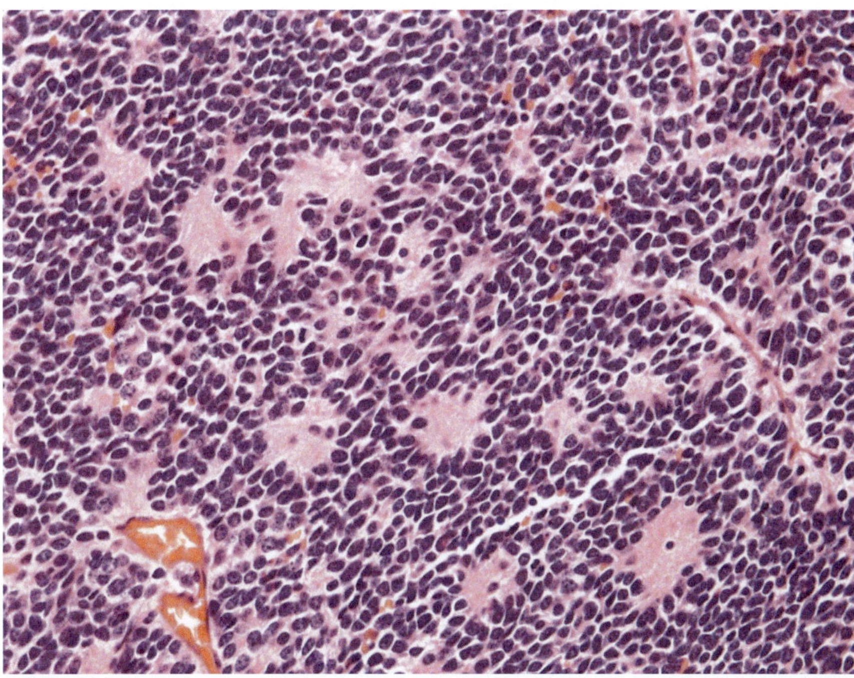

Fig. 10 Neuroblastoma, poorly differentiated subtype with neuroblasts forming Homer-Wright pseudorosettes

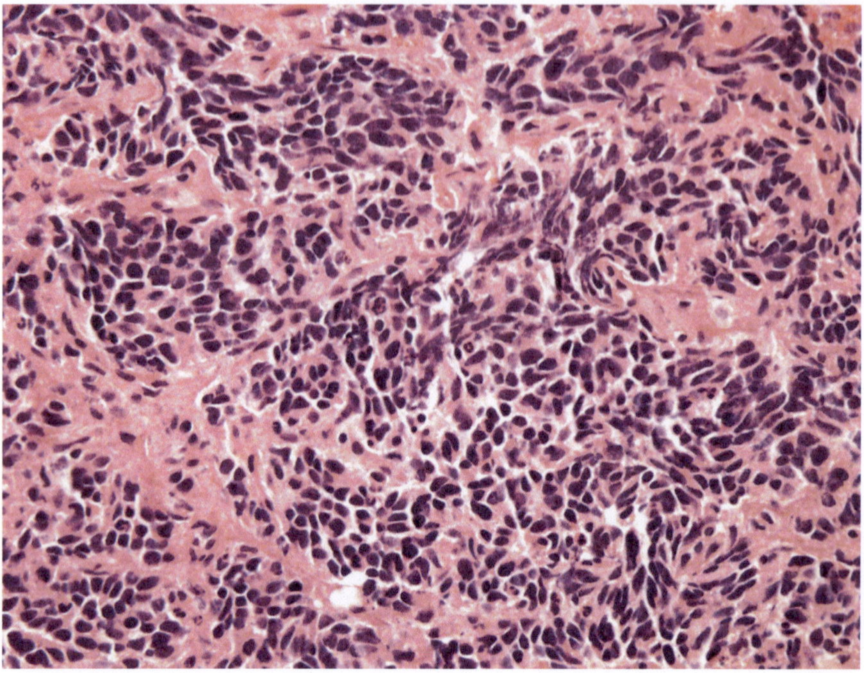

Fig. 11 Neuroblastoma, poorly differentiated subtype, with neuroblasts showing a high mitosis-karyorrhexis index (MKI)

ated tumors, the diagnosis may be challenging. For poorly differentiated neuroblastoma, the differential diagnosis includes other small round blue cell tumors, especially those that occur at a young age and/or nearby the adrenal gland. These tumors include Wilms tumor, lymphoma, leukemia, rhabdomyosarcoma, primitive neuroectodermal tumor/Ewing's sarcoma, malignant rhabdoid tumor, and desmoplastic small round cell tumor. Immunohistochemical stains can be utilized for difficult cases, as described below.

Immunohistochemistry

Neuroblasts stain positive for neuron-specific enolase, CD57/Leu7, CD56, protein gene product 9.5, synaptophysin, chromogranin, neurofilament protein, ALK1 (>90 %), PHOX2B, NB84, and cyclin D1 [90–93]. Neuroblasts are negative for epithelial markers (EMA, cytokeratin), myogenic markers (myogenin, MyoD1, desmin), CD99, vimentin, HMB45, WT1, CD45, glypican-3, and PAX2 [92–95]. Schwannian stroma expresses S-100 [92]. Ganglion cells stain positive for WT1 (cytoplasmic), S-100, synaptophysin, neurofilament protein, glial fibrillary acidic protein, protein gene product 9.5, and type IV collagen [92, 93].

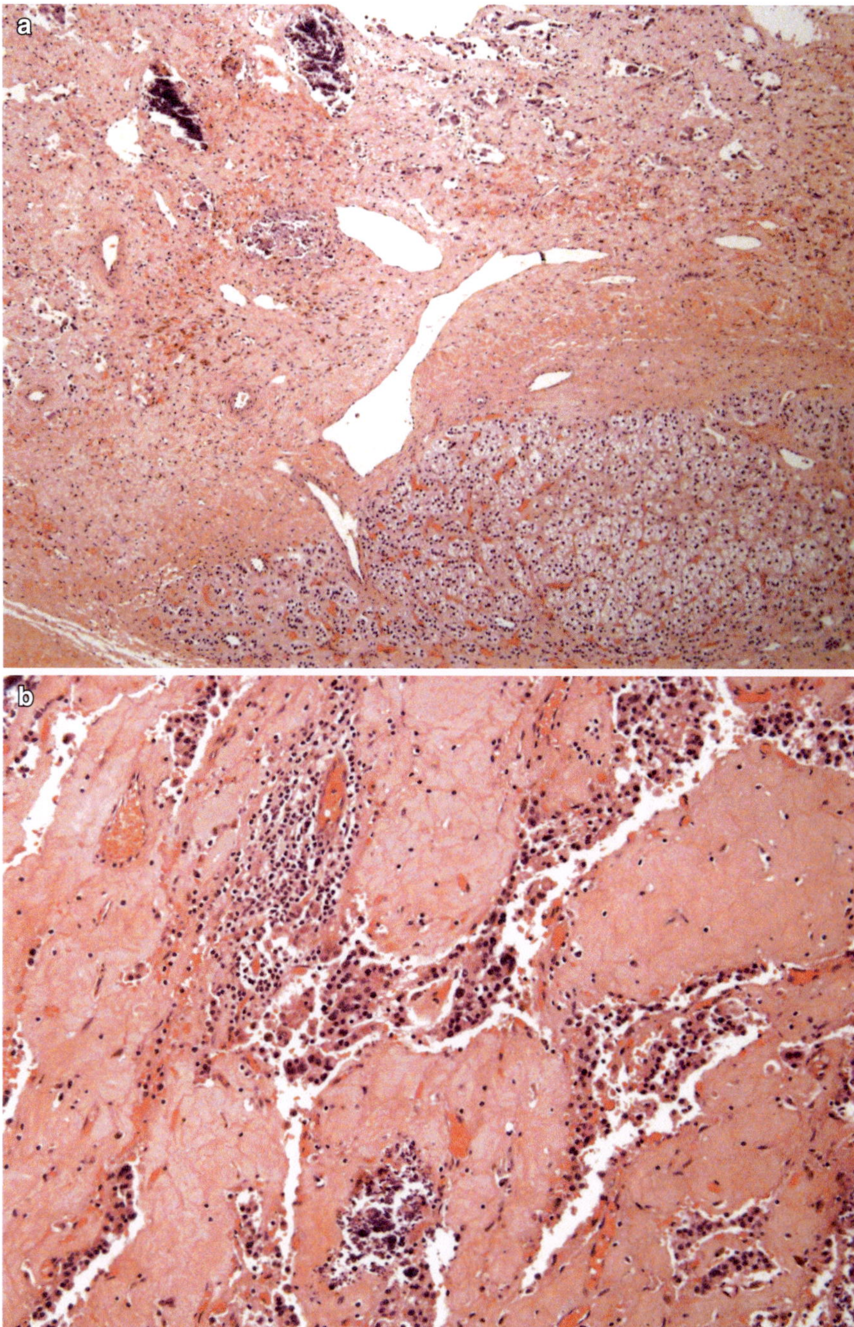

Fig. 12 Neuroblastoma status-post treatment with fibrosis, dystrophic calcification, necrosis, and maturation. (**a**) Low-power view showing adjacent uninvolved adrenal gland (lower right). (**b**) High power

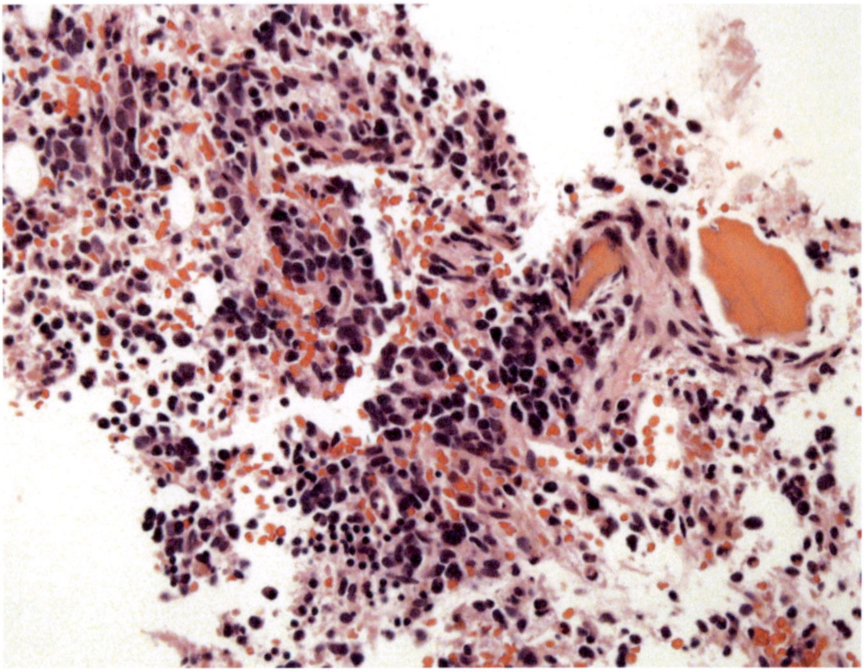

Fig. 13 Neuroblastoma, metastatic to bone marrow

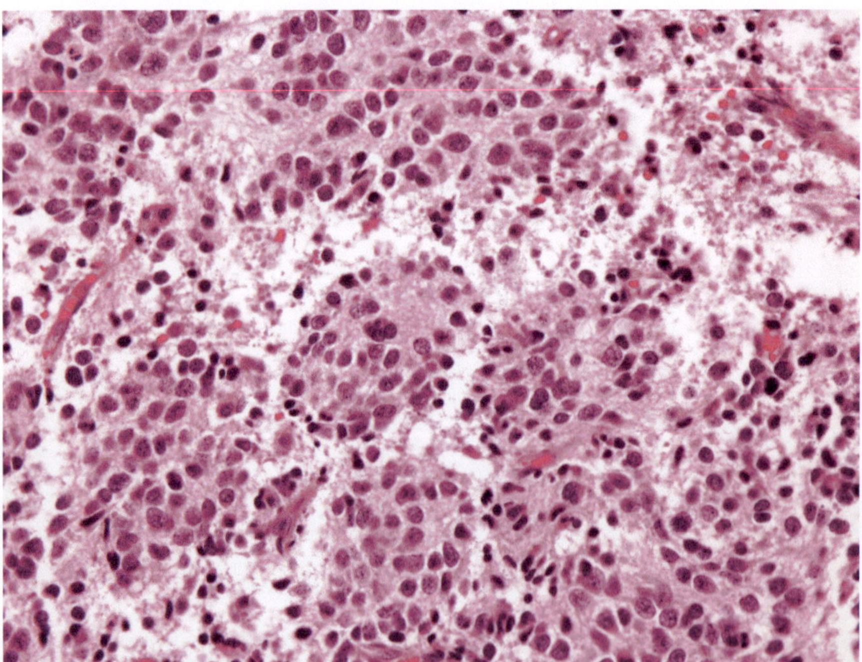

Fig. 14 Ganglioneuroblastoma, nodular variant with an area of immature neuroblasts forming Homer-Wright pseudorosettes with small, round, blue cells surrounding areas of delicate, pink neuropil

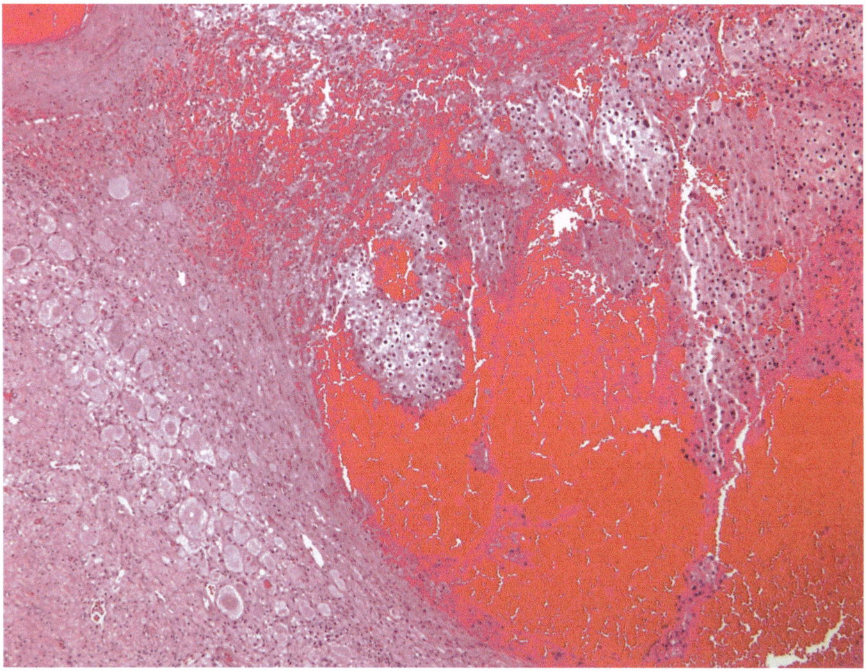

Fig. 15 Ganglioneuroblastoma, nodular variant showing a sharp demarcation between a hemorrhagic nodule containing immature neuroblasts (*right*) and more mature intervening stroma (*left*)

Most other small round blue cell tumors in the differential diagnosis with a poorly differentiated neuroblastoma, such as Wilms tumor, rhabdomyosarcoma, and primitive neuroectodermal tumor/Ewing's sarcoma, do not express neuroendocrine markers (synaptophysin, CD56), and thus, this can be helpful in the distinction of these entities. WT1 is positive in Wilms tumor, unlike neuroblastoma. NB84 is reported to have occasional expression in primitive neuroectodermal tumor, but primitive neuroectodermal tumor will be positive for CD99 while neuroblastoma will be negative. While myogenic markers are negative in neuroblastoma, these are expressed in rhabdomyosarcoma. Hematopoietic markers can discriminate neuroblastoma from lymphoma and leukemia.

Ultrastructure

The most characteristic feature of neuroblastoma on examination with electron microscopy are arrays of neuritic processes containing microtubules, diffuse intermediate filaments, and sparse dense-core neurosecretory granules (average diameter 100 nm) [96]. In differentiated tumors, neuritic processes and rare synapses can be more commonly identified [96]. In undifferentiated neuroblastoma, tumor cells are round to ovoid with large nuclei and an increased nuclear-to-cytoplasmic ratio and scarce cytoplasmic organelles [47]. In more well-differentiated tumors, cells are

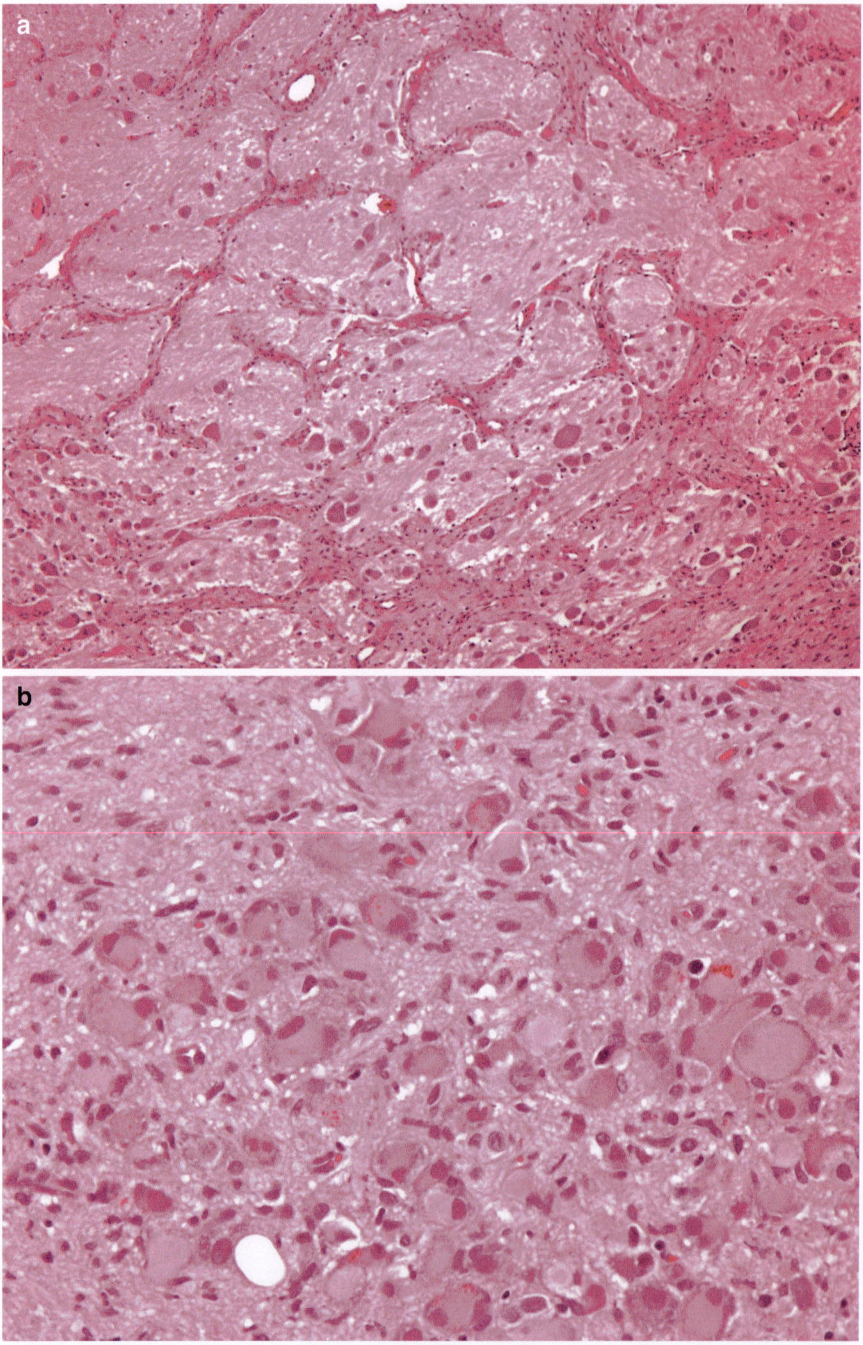

Fig. 16 Ganglioneuroblastoma, intermixed variant with maturing ganglion cells, at both low (**a**) and high (**b**) power

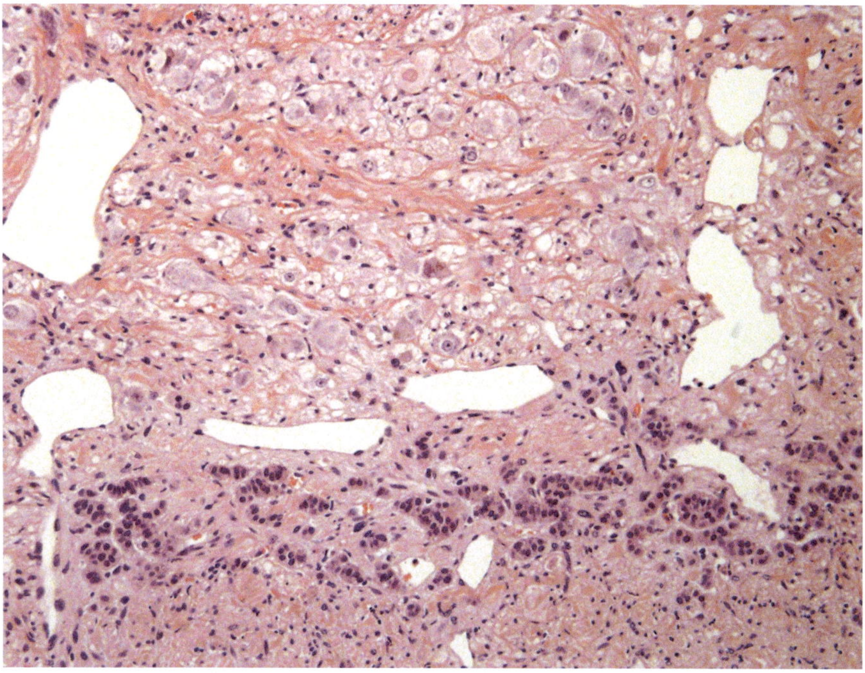

Fig. 17 Ganglioneuroma, mature subtype, with numerous mature ganglion cells (*top*) and residual normal adrenal cortical cells (*bottom*)

larger with increased cytoplasm containing more organelles and a lower nuclear-to-cytoplasmic ratio [47]. Between neuroblastoma cells and at the center of rosettes are varying amounts of cell processes, with more processes found in more well-differentiated tumors [47]. Cell processes contain fine filaments, neurotubules, and synapse-like areas [47]. Smaller catecholamine-like and larger more heterogeneous granules have been noted in the cytoplasm of neuroblastoma [47, 96]. In ganglioneuroblastoma, ganglion cells have a large nucleus with prominent nucleolus and complex cytoplasm with many organelles and granules of varying sizes [47].

Molecular Pathogenesis and Testing

Little is known about the etiology of *neuroblastoma*. During development, primitive clusters of cells within the sympathoadrenal system can remain and may later be the source of neuroblastic tumors. Definitive risk factors have not been established, but exposures before conception or during gestation have been implicated given the early age of occurrence [81].

Amplification of the proto-oncogene *MYCN* of 5 to 100-fold is seen in approximately 20 % of tumors and is associated with a worse prognosis [97]. Amplification of

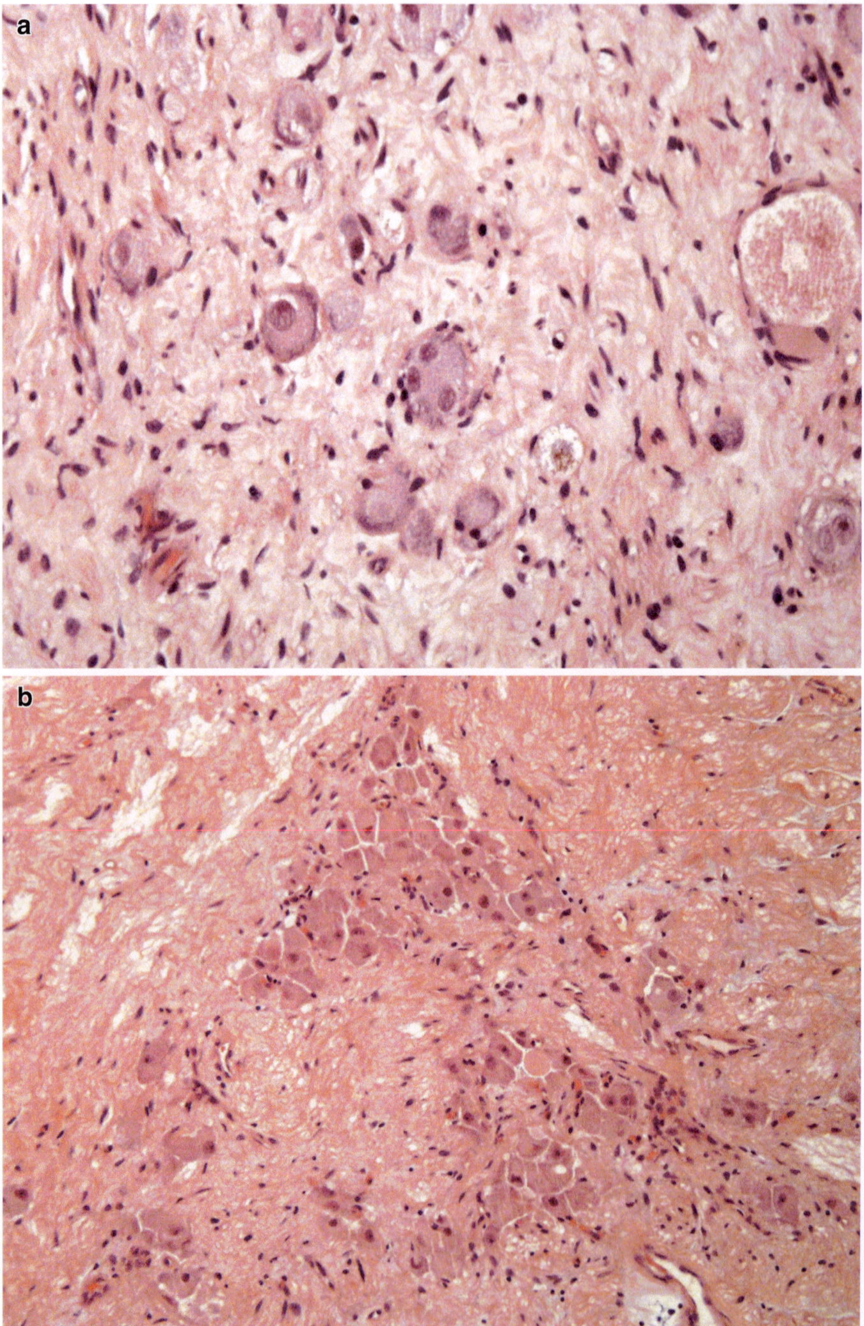

Fig. 18 Ganglioneuroma, mature subtype, with a variety of histologic findings. (**a**) Mature ganglion cells with intervening stroma. (**b**) Cluster of mature ganglion cells. (**c**) Prominent myxoid background

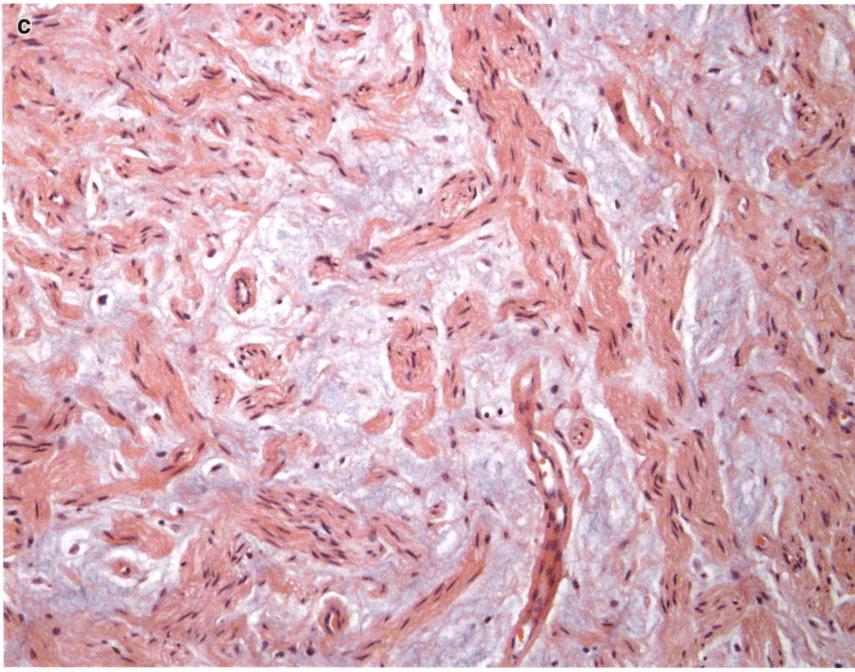

Fig. 18 (continued)

adjacent or more distant genes such as *DDX1*, *NAG*, and *ALK* occurs frequently, but is rare in the absence of *MYCN* amplification [97]. The most common somatic mutation is in *ALK* and is present in about 10 % of neuroblastomas. Familial cases do exist, and the majority are due to germline mutations of *ALK* and *PHOX2B*, the latter of which is associated with Hirschsprung disease or congenital hypoventilation syndrome [98].

Essential testing in all neuroblastoma cases includes *MYCN* amplification, chromosome 11q aberrations, and ploidy status [97, 99]. *MYCN* amplification and 11q23 aberrations can be performed by interphase fluorescence in situ hybridization, polymerase chain reaction (PCR), comparative genomic hybridization array, or multiplex ligation-dependent probe amplification [97]. Ploidy status can be determined by flow or static cytometry [97].

Many genetic markers have been proposed to correlate with prognosis, and future studies are needed to assess how robust these associations are. These genetic markers should be analyzed prospectively and include chromosomes 1p, 2p, 3p, 4p, 7q, 9p, 12p, 14q, and 17q and the *DDX1*, *NAG*, and *ALK* genes [97].

Ganglioneuroblastomas are considered to be molecularly heterogeneous [89, 100, 101]. Ganglioneuroblastoma, nodular subtype, is presumed to consist of different clones; the stroma is comprised of a nonaggressive clone, and the nodular component may have a favorable or unfavorable prognosis [89, 101]. *ALK* mutations were detected by polymerase chain reaction sequencing in 18 % (2/11) of ganglioneuroblastomas in one study, and both cases with mutations were associated with a worse prognosis [91].

Ganglioneuromas do not have a characteristic associated genetic aberration [102]. A review of the literature shows conflicting reports regarding a possible causative role of a *RET* mutation in the pathogenesis of ganglioneuromas [102]. A low level of *RET* expression was detected in only 1 of 3 sporadic ganglioneuromas in one investigation using Northern blot analysis [103]. Another study used direct exon sequencing of the *RET* gene in one adrenal ganglioneuroma and three adrenal composite pheochromocytomas (pheochromocytoma+ganglioneuroma) as well as sequencing of *VHL*, *SDHD*, *SDHB*, and *SDHC* genes in two composite pheochromocytomas (pheochromocytoma+ganglioneuroma) and did not find any mutations [104]. In addition, two pediatric patients with MEN2 syndrome, which results from gain-of-function point mutation of the *RET* proto-oncogene, were reported to each have an isolated adrenal ganglioneuroma [105]. Studies have failed to detect any genetic aberrations involving chromosome 1p36, the *ALK* gene (both associated with neuroblastoma), or chromosome 17p13 (associated with adrenal tumors) in adrenal ganglioneuromas [91, 106].

Prognostic Factors, Staging, and Management

Neuroblastic tumors are most commonly staged according to the International Neuroblastoma Staging System (INSS), a system with four main stages (1 – 4) based on the extent of surgical resection (Table 4) [82]. A second main staging system was proposed more recently, the International Neuroblastoma Risk Group (INRG) criteria; it uses clinical information and imaging features and functions as a presurgical/pretreatment risk assessment tool (Table 5) [99, 107, 108]. The INRG staging system lists numerous “image-defined risk factors” (IDRF) which take the place of information gleaned from surgical resection of the tumor and lymph nodes required for classification with the INSS, thus eliminating dependence on the skill of the surgeon performing the operation and the pathologist sampling the specimen from the staging system [107].

The INSS and INRG staging systems are both incorporated into different risk stratification systems [83]. The Children’s Oncology Group (COG) uses INSS stage, age, *MYCN* status, DNA ploidy, and INPC histology to assign one of three prognostic groups (low, intermediate, or high risk) [83, 98]. The INRG criteria incorporate the INRG staging system along with age, histologic category, grade of differentiation, *MYCN* status, 11q status, and ploidy to assign one of four risk stratification groups (very low, low, intermediate, or high) [99].

A laundry list of additional factors related to tumor histology, urine/serum tumor markers, and genetic features have been correlated with the prognosis of neuroblastic tumors [82]. The most robust of these prognostic markers are histologic subtype, grade of tumor differentiation, stage, age at diagnosis, and *MYCN* status [83, 99]. Worse prognosis is associated with undifferentiated/poorly differentiated tumors, higher stage, older age at diagnosis, *MYCN* amplification, and deletion of chromosome 11q [99, 109, 110]. Favorable prognosis is associated with near-triploid karyotypes with whole chromosome gains [97, 99, 111].

Table 4 International Neuroblastoma Staging System (INSS)

Stage	Description
1	Localized tumor with complete gross excision, with/without microscopic residual disease Ipsilateral lymph nodes negative for tumor microscopically Lymph nodes attached to and removed with primary tumor may be positive
2A	Localized tumor with incomplete gross excision Ipsilateral lymph nodes negative for tumor microscopically
2B	Localized tumor with/without complete gross excision Ipsilateral, nonadherent lymph nodes positive for tumor Enlarged contralateral lymph nodes must be negative for tumor microscopically
3	Unresectable unilateral tumor infiltrating across the midline (midline is defined as the vertebral column) With/without regional lymph node involvement OR Localized unilateral tumor With contralateral regional lymph node involvement OR Midline tumor With bilateral extension by infiltration (unresectable) or by lymph node involvement
4	Disseminated tumor to distant lymph nodes, bone, bone marrow, liver, skin, and/or other organs (except as defined for stage 4S)
4S	Localized primary tumor (as defined for stage 1, 2A, or 2B) with dissemination limited to skin, liver, and/or bone marrow (<10 % of nucleated cells) Only in infants <1 year in age

Table 5 International Neuroblastoma Risk Group (INRG) Staging System

Stage	Description
L1	Localized tumor not involving vital structures as defined by list of image-defined risk factors (IDRF) Confined to one body compartment
L2	Locoregional tumor One/more IDRF
M	Distant metastases (except stage MS)
MS	Children <18 months of age Metastases confined to the skin, liver, and/or bone marrow

The histologic subtypes initially defined by the Shimada classification were correlated with survival status. In the stroma-rich group, ganglioneuroma had the best prognosis (100 % survival) followed by ganglioneuroblastoma, intermixed subtype (92 %), and ganglioneuroblastoma, focal nodular subtype (18 %). In the stroma-poor group, neuroblastoma, differentiating had a better prognosis (72 % survival) than neuroblastoma, undifferentiated subtype (36 %) [85]. Individual histologic features correlating with a better prognosis according to the Shimada classification include differentiating histology, low mitosis-karyorrhexis index (MKI) score, and younger age at diagnosis [85]. The MKI is defined as the total number of both mitoses and karyorrhexis in 5000 cells in random fields and scored as follows: <100 low,

100–200 intermediate, and >200 high [85]. Of note, a recent study explored using immunostaining with MIB-1 (Ki67), tabulating the MIB-1 index manually and with automated software, and converting this score to the MKI with a complex mathematical formula [112]. They found a high correlation between the MKI and both the automated and manual MIB-1 index; however, the authors acknowledged that more studies are needed before this technique should replace routine practice with the manually determined MKI [112]. Likewise, the histologic groups as defined by the more recent INPC system were also shown to have prognostic significance.

Some additional serum/urine prognostic indicators include increased serum ferritin, LDH, neuron-specific enolase, disialoganglioside, chromogranin A, and urine/serum vanillylmandelic acid to homovanillic acid ratio, all of which are associated with a worse outcome [82]. A growing number of genetic factors are being described, including chromosome 1p and 11q deletion by loss of heterozygosity and unbalanced gain of chromosome 17q, which are associated with poor outcome [99, 110, 111].

An appropriate treatment plan is assigned after staging and stratification into risk groups. According to the Children's Oncology Group (COG) risk categories, patients in the low-risk group have >95 %, intermediate group have 80–95 %, and low risk group have 40–50 % event-free survival [83]. Low-risk, localized neuroblastoma is treated with either complete surgical resection or observation; chemotherapy is only given for symptomatic management [83]. The intermediate-risk group consists of localized, unresectable tumor or any tumor plus metastases (without *MYCN* amplification); surgery plus chemotherapy (2–8 cycles) is offered [83]. High-risk disease occurs in patients who are over 18 months in age with metastases or in patients with unfavorable histology and unresectable tumor; these patients are offered multi-agent induction chemotherapy, surgery, external beam radiotherapy, myeloablative consolidation with autologous stem cell rescue, and immunotherapy [83, 98]. Future directions in treatment include reducing cytotoxic therapy in low-risk patients with the same outcomes and development of effective, targeted therapies (*ALK*, anti-disialoganglioside) [98].

Abbreviations

^{131}I-MIBG	131-iodine-labeled metaiodobenzylguanidine
HIF alpha	Hypoxia-inducible factor alpha
IDRF	Image-defined risk factors
INPC	International Neuroblastoma Pathology Committee
INRG	International Neuroblastoma Risk Group
INSS	International Neuroblastoma Staging System
MAX	MYC-associated factor X
MEN2	Multiple endocrine neoplasia type 2
MKI	Mitosis-karyorrhexis
NF1	Neurofibromatosis type 1
PASS	Pheochromocytoma of the Adrenal Gland Scaled Score

References

1. Amar L, Bertherat J, Baudin E, Ajzenberg C, Bressac-de Paillerets B, Chabre O, Chamontin B, Delemer B, Giraud S, Murat A, Niccoli-Sire P, Richard S, Rohmer V, Sadoul JL, Strompf L, Schlumberger M, Bertagna X, Plouin PF, Jeunemaitre X, Gimenez-Roqueplo AP. Genetic testing in pheochromocytoma or functional paraganglioma. J Clin Oncol. 2005;23(34):8812–8.
2. Jiang S, Dahia PL. Minireview: the busy road to pheochromocytomas and paragangliomas has a new member, TMEM127. Endocrinology. 2011;152(6):2133–40.
3. Patócs A, Karádi E, Tóth M, Varga I, Szücs N, Balogh K, Majnik J, Gláz E, Rácz K. Clinical and biochemical features of sporadic and hereditary phaeochromocytomas: an analysis of 41 cases investigated in a single endocrine centre. Eur J Cancer Prev. 2004;13(5):403–9.
4. Kulis T, Knezevic N, Pekez M, Kastelan D, Grkovic M, Kastelan Z. Laparoscopic adrenalectomy: lessons learned from 306 cases. J Laparoendosc Adv Surg Tech A. 2012;22(1):22–6.
5. Beard CM, Sheps SG, Kurland LT, et al. Occurrence of pheochromocytoma in Rochester, Minnesota, 1950 through 1979. Mayo Clin Proc. 1983;58:802.
6. Guerrero MA, Schreinemakers JM, Vriens MR, et al. Clinical spectrum of pheochromocytoma. J Am Coll Surg. 2009;209:727.
7. Lloyd RV. Adrenal cortical tumors, pheochromocytomas and paragangliomas. Mod Pathol. 2011;24 Suppl 2:S58–65.
8. Goffredo P, Sosa JA, Roman SA. Malignant pheochromocytoma and paraganglioma: a population level analysis of long-term survival over two decades. J Surg Oncol. 2013;107(6):659–64.
9. Bravo EL. Pheochromocytoma: new concepts and future trends. Kidney Int. 1991;40:544.
10. Baguet JP, Hammer L, Mazzuco TL, et al. Circumstances of discovery of phaeochromocytoma: a retrospective study of 41 consecutive patients. Eur J Endocrinol. 2004;150:681.
11. Young Jr WF, Maddox DE. Spells: in search of a cause. Mayo Clin Proc. 1995;70:757.
12. Manger WM, Gifford RW. Pheochromocytoma. J Clin Hypertens (Greenwich). 2002;4:62.
13. van Berkel A, Lenders JW, Timmers HJ. Diagnosis of endocrine disease: biochemical diagnosis of phaeochromocytoma and paraganglioma. Eur J Endocrinol. 2014;170(3):R109–19.
14. Taylor RL, Singh RJ. Validation of liquid chromatography-tandem mass spectrometry method for analysis of urinary conjugated metanephrine and normetanephrine for screening of pheochromocytoma. Clin Chem. 2002;48:533.
15. Fogarty J, Engel C, Russo J, et al. Hypertension and pheochromocytoma testing: the association with anxiety disorders. Arch Fam Med. 1994;3:55.
16. Alsabeh R, Mazoujian G, Goates J, Mederios LJ, Weiss LM. Adrenal cortical tumors clinically mimicking pheochromocytoma. Am J Clin Pathol. 1995;104(4):382–90.
17. Ivsic T, Komorowski RA, Sudakoff GS, Wilson SD, Datta MW. Adrenal cortical adenoma with adrenalin-type neurosecretory granules clinically mimicking a pheochromocytoma. Arch Pathol Lab Med. 2002;126(12):1530–3.
18. Kiriakopoulos A, Papaioannou D, Linos D. Adrenal cortical oncocytoma mimicking pheochromocytoma. Hormones (Athens). 2011;10(1):76–9.
19. Lee JA, Zarnegar R, Shen WT, Kebebew E, Clark OH, Duh QY. Adrenal incidentaloma, borderline elevations of urine or plasma metanephrine levels, and the "subclinical" pheochromocytoma. Arch Surg. 2007;142(9):870–3. p6.
20. Simon S, Tötsch M, Schmidlin F, Iselin CE, Meier CA. Adrenal cortical phaeochromocytoma: a case report of a rare entity. Exp Clin Endocrinol Diabetes. 2003;111(2):111–4.
21. Walters G, Wyatt GB, Kelleher J. Carcinoma of the adrenal cortex presenting as a pheochromocytoma: report of a case. J Clin Endocrinol Metab. 1962;22:575–80.
22. Perrino CM, Prall DN, Calomeni EP, Nadasdy T, Zynger DL. Ultrastructural findings in adrenal cortical adenomas clinically mimicking pheochromocytoma: a comparison with other adrenal tumors and tissue preparation techniques. Ultrastruct Pathol. 2012;36(5):287–93.

23. Morse MO, Schwartz FL, Zynger DL. First report of adrenal cortical endothelial (vascular) cyst mimicking phaeochromocytoma (pseudophaeochromocytoma). Pathology. 2014;46(4):364–5.
24. Horchani A, Nouira Y, Nouira K, et al. Hydatid cyst of the adrenal gland: a clinical study of six cases. Scientific World Journal. 2006;6:2420–5.
25. Sharma KV, Venkatesan AM, Swerdlow D, DaSilva D, Beck A, Jain N, Wood BJ. Image-guided adrenal and renal biopsy. Tech Vasc Interv Radiol. 2010;13(2):100–9.
26. Musella M, Conzo G, Milone M, Corcione F, Belli G, De Palma M, Tricarico A, Santini L, Palazzo A, Bianco P, Biondi B, Pivonello R, Colao A. Preoperative workup in the assessment of adrenal incidentalomas: outcome from 282 consecutive laparoscopic adrenalectomies. BMC Surg. 2013;13:57.
27. Villelli NW, Jayanti MK, Zynger DL. Use and usefulness of adrenal core biopsies without FNA or on-site evaluation of adequacy: a study of 204 cases for a 12-year period. Am J Clin Pathol. 2012;137(1):124–31.
28. Quayle FJ, Spitler JA, Pierce RA, Lairmore TC, Moley JF, Brunt LM. Needle biopsy of incidentally discovered adrenal masses is rarely informative and potentially hazardous. Surgery. 2007;142(4):497–502.
29. Paulsen SD, Nghiem HV, Korobkin M, et al. Changing role of imaging-guided percutaneous biopsy of adrenal masses: evaluation of 50 adrenal biopsies. Am J Roentgenol. 2004;182:1033–7.
30. Mazzaglia PJ, Monchik JM. Limited value of adrenal biopsy in the evaluation of adrenal neoplasm: a decade of experience. Arch Surg. 2009;144:465–70.
31. Harisinghani MG, Maher MM, Hahn PF, et al. Predictive value of benign percutaneous adrenal biopsies in oncology patients. Clin Radiol. 2002;57:898–901.
32. Lumachi F, Borsato S, Tregnaghi A, et al. CT-scan, MRI and image-guided FNA cytology of incidental adrenal masses. Eur J Surg Oncol. 2003;29:689–92.
33. Bernardino ME, Walther MM, Phillips VM, Graham Jr SD, Sewell CW, Gedgaudas-McClees K, Baumgartner BR, Torres WE, Erwin BC. CT-guided adrenal biopsy: accuracy, safety, and indications. AJR Am J Roentgenol. 1985;144(1):67–9.
34. DeWitt J, Alsatie M, LeBlanc J, McHenry L, Sherman S. Endoscopic ultrasound-guided fine-needle aspiration of left adrenal gland masses. Endoscopy. 2007;39(1):65–71.
35. de Agustín P, López-Ríos F, Alberti N, Pérez-Barrios A. Fine-needle aspiration biopsy of the adrenal glands: a ten-year experience. Diagn Cytopathol. 1999;21(2):92–7.
36. Thompson LD. Pheochromocytoma of the Adrenal gland Scaled Score (PASS) to separate benign from malignant neoplasms: a clinicopathologic and immunophenotypic study of 100 cases. Am J Surg Pathol. 2002;26(5):551–66.
37. Montresor E, Iacono C, Nifosi F, Zanza A, Modena S, Zamboni G, Bernardello F, Serio G. Retroperitoneal paragangliomas: role of immunohistochemistry in the diagnosis of malignancy and in assessment of prognosis. Eur J Surg. 1994;160(10):547–52.
38. Fassina AS, Borsato S, Fedeli U. Fine needle aspiration cytology (FNAC) of adrenal masses. Cytopathology. 2000;11:302–11.
39. Sangoi AR, McKenney JK. A tissue microarray-based comparative analysis of novel and traditional immunohistochemical markers in the distinction between adrenal cortical lesions and pheochromocytoma. Am J Surg Pathol. 2010;34(3):423–32.
40. Fraga M, García-Caballero T, Antúnez J, Couce M, Beiras A, Forteza J. A comparative immunohistochemical study of phaeochromocytomas and paragangliomas. Histol Histopathol. 1993;8(3):429–36.
41. Lam KY, Chan AC, Wong WM, Lam KS. A review of clinicopathologic features of pheochromocytomas in Hong Kong Chinese. Eur J Surg Oncol. 1993;19(5):421–7.
42. Kimura N, Sasano N, Yamada R, Satoh J. Immunohistochemical study of chromogranin in 100 cases of pheochromocytoma, carotid body tumour, medullary thyroid carcinoma and carcinoid tumour. Virchows Arch A Pathol Anat Histopathol. 1988;413(1):33–8.
43. Weiler R, Fischer-Colbrie R, Schmid KW, Feichtinger H, Bussolati G, Grimelius L, Krisch K, Kerl H, O'Connor D, Winkler H. Immunological studies on the occurrence and properties of chromogranin A and B and secretogranin II in endocrine tumors. Am J Surg Pathol. 1988;12(11):877–84.

44. Busam KJ, Iversen K, Coplan KA, Old LJ, Stockert E, Chen YT, McGregor D, Jungbluth A. Immunoreactivity for A103, an antibody to melan-A (Mart-1), in adrenocortical and other steroid tumors. Am J Surg Pathol. 1998;22(1):57–63.
45. Schröder S, Padberg BC, Achilles E, Holl K, Dralle H, Klöppel G. Immunocytochemistry in adrenocortical tumours: a clinicomorphological study of 72 neoplasms. Virchows Arch A Pathol Anat Histopathol. 1992;420(1):65–70.
46. Loeffel SC, Gillespie GY, Mirmiran SA, Miller EW, Golden P, Askin FB, Siegal GP. Cellular immunolocalization of S100 protein within fixed tissue sections by monoclonal antibodies. Arch Pathol Lab Med. 1985;109(2):117–22.
47. Tannenbaum M. Ultrastructural pathology of adrenal medullary tumors. Pathol Annu. 1970;5:145–71.
48. Gómez RR, Osborne BM, Ordoñez NG, Mackay B. Pheochromocytoma. Ultrastruct Pathol. 1991;15(4–5):557–62.
49. Mihai R, Wong NA, Luckett M, Sheffield E, Farndon JR. No correlation between phaeochromocytoma catecholamine secretion and granule ultrastructure. Br J Surg. 1998;85(12):1681–5.
50. Fishbein L, Nathanson KL. Pheochromocytoma and paraganglioma: understanding the complexities of the genetic background. Cancer Genet. 2012;205(1–2):1–11.
51. Gimenez-Roqueplo AP, Burnichon N, Amar L, Favier J, Jeunemaitre X, Plouin PF. Recent advances in the genetics of phaeochromocytoma and functional paraganglioma. Clin Exp Pharmacol Physiol. 2008;35(4):376–9.
52. Crona J, Nordling M, Maharjan R, Granberg D, Stålberg P, Hellman P, Björklund P. Integrative genetic characterization and phenotype correlations in pheochromocytoma and paraganglioma tumours. PLoS One. 2014;9(1):e86756.
53. Fishbein L, Merrill S, Fraker DL, Cohen DL, Nathanson KL. Inherited mutations in pheochromocytoma and paraganglioma: why all patients should be offered genetic testing. Ann Surg Oncol. 2013;20(5):1444–50.
54. King KS, Pacak K. Familial pheochromocytomas and paragangliomas. Mol Cell Endocrinol. 2014;386(1–2):92–100.
55. Shuch B, Ricketts CJ, Metwalli AR, Pacak K, Linehan WM. The genetic basis of pheochromocytoma and paraganglioma: implications for management. Urology. 2014;83(6):1225–32.
56. Astuti D, Latif F, Dallol A, Dahia PL, Douglas F, George E, Sköldberg F, Husebye ES, Eng C, Maher ER. Gene mutations in the succinate dehydrogenase subunit SDHB cause susceptibility to familial pheochromocytoma and to familial paraganglioma. Am J Hum Genet. 2001;69(1):49–54.
57. Ricketts CJ, Forman JR, Rattenberry E, Bradshaw N, Lalloo F, Izatt L, Cole TR, Armstrong R, Kumar VK, Morrison PJ, Atkinson AB, Douglas F, Ball SG, Cook J, Srirangalingam U, Killick P, Kirby G, Aylwin S, Woodward ER, Evans DG, Hodgson SV, Murday V, Chew SL, Connell JM, Blundell TL, Macdonald F, Maher ER. Tumor risks and genotype-phenotype-proteotype analysis in 358 patients with germline mutations in SDHB and SDHD. Hum Mutat. 2010;31(1):41–51.
58. Hensen EF, Jordanova ES, van Minderhout IJ, Hogendoorn PC, Taschner PE, van der Mey AG, Devilee P, Cornelisse CJ. Somatic loss of maternal chromosome 11 causes parent-of-origin-dependent inheritance in SDHD-linked paraganglioma and phaeochromocytoma families. Oncogene. 2004;23(23):4076–83.
59. Qin Y, Yao L, King EE, Buddavarapu K, Lenci RE, Chocron ES, Lechleiter JD, Sass M, Aronin N, Schiavi F, Boaretto F, Opocher G, Toledo RA, Toledo SP, Stiles C, Aguiar RC, Dahia PL. Germline mutations in TMEM127 confer susceptibility to pheochromocytoma. Nat Genet. 2010;42(3):229–33.
60. Comino-Méndez I, Gracia-Aznárez FJ, Schiavi F, Landa I, Leandro-García LJ, Letón R, Honrado E, Ramos-Medina R, Caronia D, Pita G, Gómez-Graña A, de Cubas AA, Inglada-Pérez L, Maliszewska A, Taschin E, Bobisse S, Pica G, Loli P, Hernández-Lavado R, Díaz JA, Gómez-Morales M, González-Neira A, Roncador G, Rodríguez-Antona C, Benítez J, Mannelli M, Opocher G, Robledo M, Cascón A. Exome sequencing identifies MAX mutations as a cause of hereditary pheochromocytoma. Nat Genet. 2011;43(7):663–7.

61. Crona J, Maharjan R, Delgado Verdugo A, Stålberg P, Granberg D, Hellman P, Björklund P. MAX mutations status in Swedish patients with pheochromocytoma and paraganglioma tumours. Fam Cancer. 2014;13(1):121–5.
62. Rana HQ, Rainville IR, Vaidya A. Genetic testing in the clinical care of patients with pheochromocytoma and paraganglioma. Curr Opin Endocrinol Diabetes Obes. 2014;21(3):166–76.
63. McInerney-Leo AM, Marshall MS, Gardiner B, Benn DE, McFarlane J, Robinson BG, Brown MA, Leo PJ, Clifton-Bligh RJ, Duncan EL. Whole exome sequencing is an efficient and sensitive method for detection of germline mutations in patients with phaeochromcytomas and paragangliomas. Clin Endocrinol (Oxf). 2014;80(1):25–33.
64. Welander J, Andreasson A, Juhlin CC, Wiseman RW, Bäckdahl M, Höög A, Larsson C, Gimm O, Söderkvist P. Rare germline mutations identified by targeted next-generation sequencing of susceptibility genes in pheochromocytoma and paraganglioma. J Clin Endocrinol Metab. 2014;99(7):E1352–60.
65. Rattenberry E, Vialard L, Yeung A, Bair H, McKay K, Jafri M, Canham N, Cole TR, Denes J, Hodgson SV, Irving R, Izatt L, Korbonits M, Kumar AV, Lalloo F, Morrison PJ, Woodward ER, Macdonald F, Wallis Y, Maher ER. A comprehensive next generation sequencing-based genetic testing strategy to improve diagnosis of inherited pheochromocytoma and paraganglioma. J Clin Endocrinol Metab. 2013;98(7):E1248–56.
66. Grubbs EG, Rich TA, Ng C, Bhosale PR, Jimenez C, Evans DB, Lee JE, Perrier ND. Long-term outcomes of surgical treatment for hereditary pheochromocytoma. J Am Coll Surg. 2013;216(2):280–9.
67. Press D, Akyuz M, Dural C, Aliyev S, Monteiro R, Mino J, Mitchell J, Hamrahian A, Siperstein A, Berber E. Predictors of recurrence in pheochromocytoma. Surgery. 2014; 156(6):1523–7.
68. Pommier RF, Vetto JT, Billingsly K, Woltering EA, Brennan MF. Comparison of adrenal and extraadrenal pheochromocytomas. Surgery. 1993;114(6):1160–5.
69. Ayala-Ramirez M, Feng L, Johnson MM, Ejaz S, Habra MA, Rich T, Busaidy N, Cote GJ, Perrier N, Phan A, Patel S, Waguespack S, Jimenez C. Clinical risk factors for malignancy and overall survival in patients with pheochromocytomas and sympathetic paragangliomas: primary tumor size and primary tumor location as prognostic indicators. J Clin Endocrinol Metab. 2011;96(3):717–25.
70. Deutschbein T, Fassnacht M, Weismann D, Reincke M, Mann K, Petersenn S. Treatment of malignant phaeochromocytoma with a combination of cyclophosphamide, vincristine and dacarbazine: own experience and overview of the contemporary literature. Clin Endocrinol (Oxf). 2015;82(1):84–90.
71. Ellis RJ, Patel D, Prodanov T, Sadowski S, Nilubol N, Adams K, Steinberg SM, Pacak K, Kebebew E. Response after surgical resection of metastatic pheochromocytoma and paraganglioma: can postoperative biochemical remission be predicted? J Am Coll Surg. 2013;217(3):489–96.
72. Hadoux J, Favier J, Scoazec JY, Leboulleux S, Al Ghuzlan A, Caramella C, Déandreis D, Borget I, Loriot C, Chougnet C, Letouzé E, Young J, Amar L, Bertherat J, Libé R, Dumont F, Deschamps F, Schlumberger M, Gimenez-Roqueplo AP, Baudin E. SDHB mutations are associated with response to temozolomide in patients with metastatic pheochromocytoma or paraganglioma. Int J Cancer. 2014;135(11):2711–20.
73. Schovanek J, Martucci V, Wesley R, Fojo T, Del Rivero J, Huynh T, Adams K, Kebebew E, Frysak Z, Stratakis CA, Pacak K. The size of the primary tumor and age at initial diagnosis are independent predictors of the metastatic behavior and survival of patients with SDHB-related pheochromocytoma and paraganglioma: a retrospective cohort study. BMC Cancer. 2014;14:523.
74. Korevaar TI, Grossman AB. Pheochromocytomas and paragangliomas: assessment of malignant potential. Endocrine. 2011;40(3):354–65.

75. Strong VE, Kennedy T, Al-Ahmadie H, Tang L, Coleman J, Fong Y, Brennan M, Ghossein RA. Prognostic indicators of malignancy in adrenal pheochromocytomas: clinical, histopathologic, and cell cycle/apoptosis gene expression analysis. Surgery. 2008;143(6):759–68.
76. Kimura N, Watanabe T, Noshiro T, Shizawa S, Miura Y. Histological grading of adrenal and extra-adrenal pheochromocytomas and relationship to prognosis: a clinicopathological analysis of 116 adrenal pheochromocytomas and 30 extra-adrenal sympathetic paragangliomas including 38 malignant tumors. Endocr Pathol. 2005;16(1):23–32.
77. Kimura N, Takayanagi R, Takizawa N, Itagaki E, Katabami T, Kakoi N, Rakugi H, Ikeda Y, Tanabe A, Nigawara T, Ito S, Kimura I, Naruse M, Phaeochromocytoma Study Group in Japan. Pathological grading for predicting metastasis in phaeochromocytoma and paraganglioma. Endocr Relat Cancer. 2014;21(3):405–14.
78. Kumaki N, Kajiwara H, Kameyama K, DeLellis RA, Asa SL, Osamura RY, Takami H. Prediction of malignant behavior of pheochromocytomas and paragangliomas using immunohistochemical techniques. Endocr Pathol. 2002;13(2):149–56.
79. Elder EE, Xu D, Höög A, Enberg U, Hou M, Pisa P, Gruber A, Larsson C, Bäckdahl M. KI-67 AND hTERT expression can aid in the distinction between malignant and benign pheochromocytoma and paraganglioma. Mod Pathol. 2003;16(3):246–55.
80. Lack EE. Tumors of the adrenal glands and extraadrenal paraganglia. 4th ed. Silver Spring: ARP Press; 2007, Print.
81. Ries LAG, Smith MA, Gurney JG, Linet M, Tamra T, Young JL, Bunin GR, editors. Cancer incidence and survival among children and adolescents: United States SEER program 1975–1995. Bethesda: National Cancer Institute, SEER Program; 1999. NIH Pub. No. 99-4649.
82. Brodeur GM, Pritchard J, Berthold F, Carlsen NL, Castel V, Castelberry RP, De Bernardi B, Evans AE, Favrot M, Hedborg F, et al. Revisions of the international criteria for neuroblastoma diagnosis, staging, and response to treatment. J Clin Oncol. 1993;11(8):1466–77.
83. Irwin MS, Park JR. Neuroblastoma: paradigm for precision medicine. Pediatr Clin North Am. 2015;62(1):225–56.
84. Joshi VV. Peripheral neuroblastic tumors: pathologic classification based on recommendations of international neuroblastoma pathology committee (Modification of shimada classification). Pediatr Dev Pathol. 2000;3(2):184–99.
85. Shimada H, Chatten J, Newton Jr WA, Sachs N, Hamoudi AB, Chiba T, Marsden HB, Misugi K. Histopathologic prognostic factors in neuroblastic tumors: definition of subtypes of ganglioneuroblastoma and an age-linked classification of neuroblastomas. J Natl Cancer Inst. 1984;73(2):405–16.
86. Castleberry RP. Neuroblastoma. Eur J Cancer. 1997;33(9):1430–7; discussion 1437–8.
87. Shimada H, Ambros IM, Dehner LP, Hata J, Joshi VV, Roald B. Terminology and morphologic criteria of neuroblastic tumors: recommendations by the International Neuroblastoma Pathology Committee. Cancer. 1999;86(2):349–63.
88. Shimada H, Ambros IM, Dehner LP, Hata J, Joshi VV, Roald B, Stram DO, Gerbing RB, Lukens JN, Matthay KK, Castleberry RP. The International Neuroblastoma Pathology Classification (the Shimada system). Cancer. 1999;86(2):364–72.
89. Peuchmaur M, d'Amore ES, Joshi VV, Hata J, Roald B, Dehner LP, Gerbing RB, Stram DO, Lukens JN, Matthay KK, Shimada H. Revision of the International Neuroblastoma Pathology Classification: confirmation of favorable and unfavorable prognostic subsets in ganglioneuroblastoma, nodular. Cancer. 2003;98(10):2274–81.
90. Bielle F, Fréneaux P, Jeanne-Pasquier C, Maran-Gonzalez A, Rousseau A, Lamant L, Paris R, Pierron G, Nicolas AV, Sastre-Garau X, Delattre O, Bourdeaut F, Peuchmaur M. PHOX2B immunolabeling: a novel tool for the diagnosis of undifferentiated neuroblastomas among childhood small round blue-cell tumors. Am J Surg Pathol. 2012;36(8):1141–9.
91. Duijkers FA, Gaal J, Meijerink JP, Admiraal P, Pieters R, de Krijger RR, van Noesel MM. High anaplastic lymphoma kinase immunohistochemical staining in neuroblastoma and ganglioneuroblastoma is an independent predictor of poor outcome. Am J Pathol. 2012;180(3):1223–31.

92. Dabbs DJ, Thompson L. Diagnostic immunohistochemistry: theranostic and genomic applications. 4th ed. Philadelphia: Elsevier Saunders; 2013 Print.
93. Magro G, Longo FR, Angelico G, Spadola S, Amore FF, Salvatorelli L. Immunohistochemistry as potential diagnostic pitfall in the most common solid tumors of children and adolescents. Acta Histochem. 2015;117(4–5):397–414.
94. Davis JL, Matsumura L, Weeks DA, Troxell ML. PAX2 expression in Wilms tumors and other childhood neoplasms. Am J Surg Pathol. 2011;35(8):1186–94.
95. Chan ES, Pawel BR, Corao DA, Venneti S, Russo P, Santi M, Sullivan LM. Immunohistochemical expression of glypican-3 in pediatric tumors: an analysis of 414 cases. Pediatr Dev Pathol. 2013;16(4):272–7.
96. Erlandson RA, Nesland JM. Tumors of the endocrine/neuroendocrine system: an overview. Ultrastruct Pathol. 1994;18(1–2):149–70.
97. Ambros PF, Ambros IM, Brodeur GM, Haber M, Khan J, Nakagawara A, Schleiermacher G, Speleman F, Spitz R, London WB, Cohn SL, Pearson AD, Maris JM. International consensus for neuroblastoma molecular diagnostics: report from the International Neuroblastoma Risk Group (INRG) Biology Committee. Br J Cancer. 2009;100(9):1471–82.
98. Park JR, Bagatell R, London WB, Maris JM, Cohn SL, Mattay KK, Hogarty M, COG Neuroblastoma Committee. Children's Oncology Group's 2013 blueprint for research: neuroblastoma. Pediatr Blood Cancer. 2013;60(6):985–93.
99. Cohn SL, Pearson AD, London WB, Monclair T, Ambros PF, Brodeur GM, Faldum A, Hero B, Iehara T, Machin D, Mosseri V, Simon T, Garaventa A, Castel V, Matthay KK, INRG Task Force. The International Neuroblastoma Risk Group (INRG) classification system: an INRG Task Force report. J Clin Oncol. 2009;27(2):289–97.
100. Schmidt ML, Salwen HR, Chagnovich D, Bauer KD, Crawford SE, Cohn SL. Evidence for molecular heterogeneity in human ganglioneuroblastoma. Pediatr Pathol. 1993;13(6):787–96.
101. Umehara S, Nakagawa A, Matthay KK, Lukens JN, Seeger RC, Stram DO, Gerbing RB, Shimada H. Histopathology defines prognostic subsets of ganglioneuroblastoma, nodular. Cancer. 2000;89(5):1150–61.
102. Shawa H, Elsayes KM, Javadi S, Morani A, Williams MD, Lee JE, Waguespack SG, Busaidy NL, Vassilopoulou-Sellin R, Jimenez C, Habra MA. Adrenal ganglioneuroma: features and outcomes of 27 cases at a referral cancer centre. Clin Endocrinol (Oxf). 2014;80(3):342–7.
103. Takaya K, Yoshimasa T, Arai H, Tamura N, Miyamoto Y, Itoh H, Nakao K. Expression of the RET proto-oncogene in normal human tissues, pheochromocytomas, and other tumors of neural crest origin. J Mol Med (Berl). 1996;74(10):617–21.
104. Rondeau G, Nolet S, Latour M, Braschi S, Gaboury L, Lacroix A, Panzini B, Arjane P, Cohade C, Bourdeau I. Clinical and biochemical features of seven adult adrenal ganglioneuromas. J Clin Endocrinol Metab. 2010;95(7):3118–25.
105. Lora MS, Waguespack SG, Moley JF, Walvoord EC. Adrenal ganglioneuromas in children with multiple endocrine neoplasia type 2: a report of two cases. J Clin Endocrinol Metab. 2005;90(7):4383–7.
106. Koch CA, Brouwers FM, Rosenblatt K, Burman KD, Davis MM, Vortmeyer AO, Pacak K. Adrenal ganglioneuroma in a patient presenting with severe hypertension and diarrhea. Endocr Relat Cancer. 2003;10(1):99–107.
107. Monclair T, Brodeur GM, Ambros PF, Brisse HJ, Cecchetto G, Holmes K, Kaneko M, London WB, Matthay KK, Nuchtern JG, von Schweinitz D, Simon T, Cohn SL, Pearson AD, INRG Task Force. The International Neuroblastoma Risk Group (INRG) staging system: an INRG Task Force report. J Clin Oncol. 2009;27(2):298–303.
108. Murphy JM, La Quaglia MP. Advances in the surgical treatment of neuroblastoma: a review. Eur J Pediatr Surg. 2014;24(6):450–6.
109. Brodeur GM, Seeger RC, Schwab M, Varmus HE, Bishop JM. Amplification of N-myc in untreated human neuroblastomas correlates with advanced disease stage. Science. 1984;224(4653):1121–4.

110. Fischer M, Spitz R, Oberthür A, Westermann F, Berthold F. Risk estimation of neuroblastoma patients using molecular markers. Klin Padiatr. 2008;220(3):137–46.
111. Brodeur GM. Neuroblastoma: biological insights into a clinical enigma. Nat Rev Cancer. 2003;3(3):203–16.
112. Atikankul T, Atikankul Y, Santisukwongchote S, Marrano P, Shuangshoti S, Thorner PS. MIB-1 Index as a Surrogate for Mitosis-Karyorrhexis Index in Neuroblastoma. Am J Surg Pathol. 2015;39(8):1054–60.

Neuroendocrine Tumors of the Urinary Bladder and Molecular Features

Jasreman Dhillon

There are more than 500,000 people in the United States who are bladder cancer survivors. Bladder cancer is the fourth most common cancer diagnosed in men after prostate, lung, and colorectal cancers. Men are about 3–4 times more likely to get bladder cancer during their lifetime than women [1]. More than 90 % of bladder cancers are urothelial carcinomas. Primary bladder adenocarcinomas and squamous cell carcinomas are relatively less common. Neuroendocrine tumors are even rarer with neuroendocrine carcinomas accounting for less than 1 % of primary bladder malignancies. WHO has histologically classified the neuroendocrine tumors of the urinary tract as carcinoid, small cell carcinoma, and paraganglioma [2]. Large cell neuroendocrine carcinoma (LCNEC) of the bladder is not yet classified as a variant of neuroendocrine tumors of the urinary tract by WHO. LCNEC of the bladder is rarely encountered with only few case reports being documented in the literature. We herein discuss the histopathological spectrum of different neuroendocrine tumors that are encountered in the bladder.

Carcinoid Tumors

Primary carcinoid tumors of the urinary bladder are very rare. This tumor is recognized as a distinct entity of neuroendocrine neoplasms that is potentially malignant. These tumors usually occur in middle-aged adults with a slight male predominance [3]. The most common presenting symptom is hematuria with occasional cases found as incidental findings on cystoscopy [4]. These tumors predominantly involve the trigone and bladder neck regions and are usually very small and rarely invade past the lamina propria. The size of this tumor ranges from 2 mm up to 10 mm in

J. Dhillon, MD
Department of Anatomic Pathology, Moffitt Cancer Center, Tampa, FL, USA
e-mail: Jasreman.dhillon@moffitt.org

A. Nasir, D. Coppola (eds.), *Neuroendocrine Tumors: Review of Pathology, Molecular and Therapeutic Advances*, DOI 10.1007/978-1-4939-3426-3_18

the reported literature. On cystoscopic examination, the tumors appear as polyps and small submucosal nodules and may be sometimes associated with changes suggestive of an inflammatory process [3].

On microscopic examination, the tumor exhibits pseudoglandular architecture with tumor cells present in cribriform and acinar patterns. The tumor cells are monomorphic with finely stippled salt and pepper chromatin and inconspicuous nucleoli. The tumor cells generally have abundant cytoplasm containing eosinophilic granules. Mitotic figures are infrequent. Necrosis is absent. These tumors are positive for neuroendocrine markers such as synaptophysin and chromogranin and for cytokeratins AE1–AE3.

Mixed carcinoid tumors are also known to occur where the carcinoid tumor may coexist with small cell carcinoma, primary bladder adenocarcinoma, or urothelial carcinoma [5, 6].

Pure carcinoid tumors are generally associated with a very favorable outcome. Some of the tumors are so small that they are probably completely removed by biopsies and hence are cured. However, more than 25 % of patients are reported to have regional lymph node or distant metastasis [2].

Small Cell Carcinoma

Small cell carcinoma (SCC) of the urinary bladder is an extremely rare malignancy. Its reported incidence is between 0.5 and 1 % of all bladder malignancies [7–9]. This tumor is associated with tobacco smoking and predominantly occurs in men in their sixth to seventh decade of life [10]. Hematuria with or without dysuria is the most common presenting symptom. Occasionally, patients have paraneoplastic syndromes with hypercalcemia, hypophosphatemia, or ectopic secretion of adrenocorticotropic hormone (ACTH) [11].

The tumor most commonly presents as a large solid, polypoid mass. Histologically, the tumor is similar to its lung counterpart. The tumor cells are intermediate to small in size and are present in diffuse sheets (Fig. 1). The tumor cells have scant cytoplasm and exhibit nuclear molding, inconspicuous nucleoli, and salt and pepper chromatin (Fig. 2). There is brisk mitotic activity. Foci of necrosis are admixed. Tumor cells may also have crush artifact. Lymphovascular invasion is almost always present. A great majority of the tumors extensively involve the detrusor muscle. In approximately 7090 % of cases, small cell carcinoma coexists with urothelial carcinoma, adenocarcinoma, or squamous cell carcinoma [7, 8]. Pure small cell carcinoma is present in approximately 10–30 % of cases. These tumors usually express the neuroendocrine markers synaptophysin, chromogranin, CD56, and neuron-specific enolase (NSE) and have a dot like reactivity for CAM5.2. Up to 40 % of bladder small cell carcinomas can be positive for immunohistochemical stain TTF1 [12]. The diagnosis of small cell carcinoma can be made on the typical morphologic features alone even if neuroendocrine differentiation cannot be demonstrated [2, 13].

The majority of patients present with metastatic disease at the time of diagnosis to regional lymph nodes, bones, liver, and lungs [7]. Overall prognosis correlates with the stage of the disease at presentation. The presence of coexisting non-small

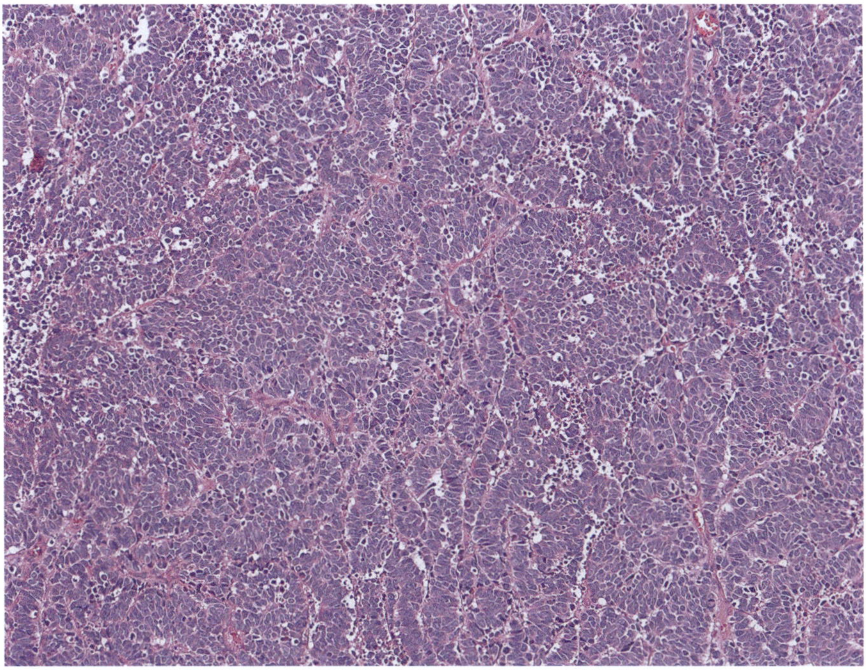

Fig. 1 Small cell carcinoma of the bladder showing organoid and nested pattern

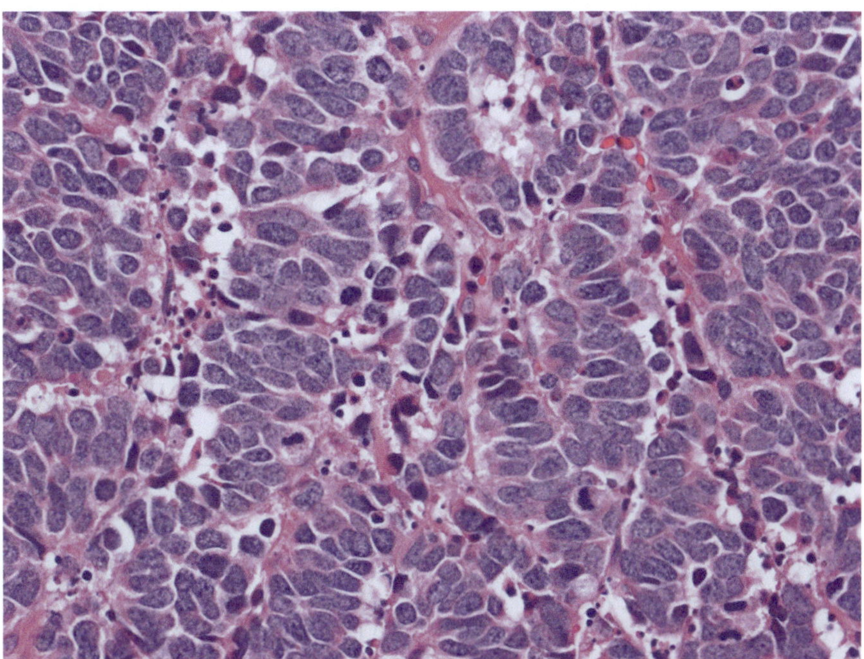

Fig. 2 Small cell carcinoma of the bladder exhibiting nuclear molding and salt and pepper chromatin with many apoptotic bodies in the background

cell carcinoma component is not associated significantly with survival [7, 14]. The 5-year survival rate for all stages is variable and ranges between 8 % and 40 %.

Large Cell Neuroendocrine Carcinoma (LCNEC)

Primary LCNEC is rare and relatively new histologic subtype which is not yet included in the 2004 WHO classification of the neuroendocrine tumors of the urinary tract. Patients usually present at a late stage and have a very poor prognosis. Median survival for these patients is 20–23 months [15]. The most common presenting symptom is hematuria [16].

LCNEC shows typical features of a neuroendocrine tumor such as organoid nesting, palisading, rosettes, and trabecular patterns. The tumor is admixed with foci of necrosis, has a high mitotic rate, and immunohistochemically stains for neuroendocrine markers (Figs. 3 and 4). This tumor is different from small cell carcinoma cytologically. The tumor cells are large in size with a low nuclear to cytoplasm ratio, coarse chromatin, and frequent nucleoli (Fig. 5). LCNEC can occur as a pure tumor but is usually admixed with other components such as primary adenocarcinoma of the bladder, squamous cell carcinoma, carcinosarcoma, or urothelial carcinoma [16].

LCNEC is considered to be as aggressive as small cell carcinoma and tends to develop distant metastases despite treatment soon after diagnosis [17].

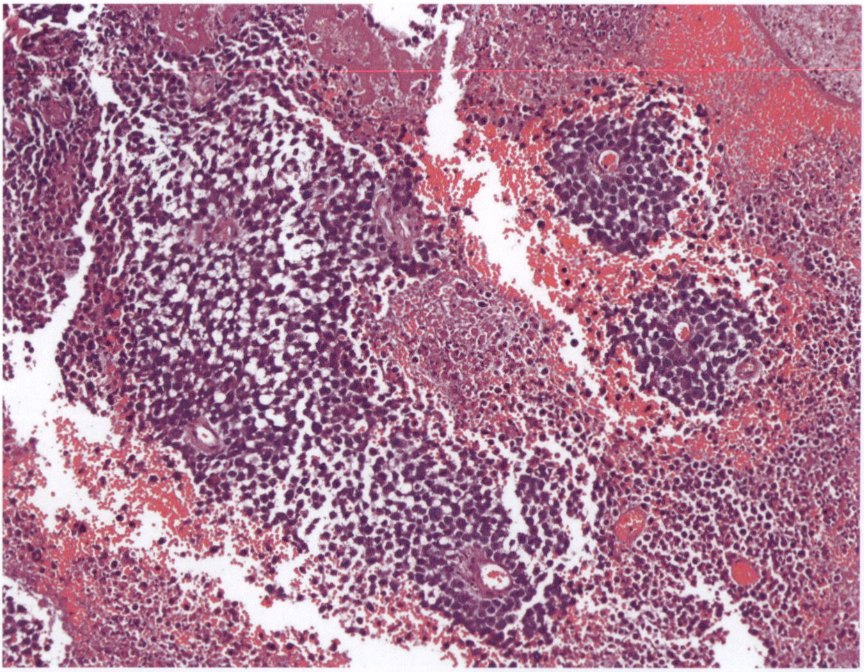

Fig. 3 Large cell neuroendocrine tumor of the bladder admixed with foci of hemorrhage and necrosis

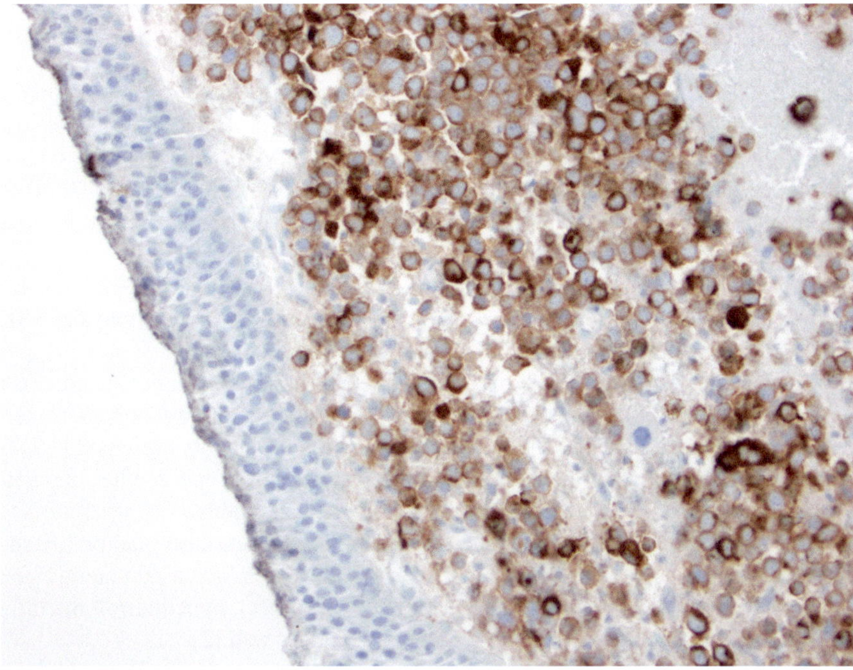

Fig. 4 Large cell neuroendocrine tumor of the bladder staining positive for synaptophysin

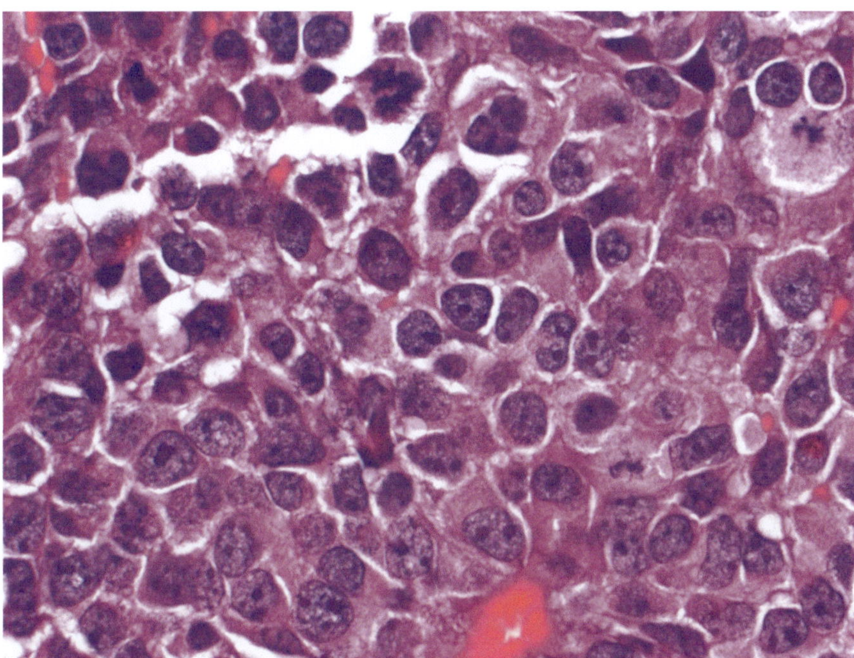

Fig. 5 Large cell neuroendocrine tumor of the bladder showing large nuclei with prominent nucleoli and many mitotic figures

Paragangliomas

Paragangliomas of the urinary bladder are rare. These tumors arise from the paraganglionic cells that are located in the wall of the bladder [18]. On cystoscopy, these tumors look like polyps which can be removed by simple excision [19]. These tumors are sometimes accidental findings in radical cystectomy specimens for other lesions. Paragangliomas may present with hematuria or with attacks of hypertension during micturition [20, 21].

Paragangliomas are characterized by the "zellballen" pattern with cells that are positive for neuroendocrine markers like chromogranin and synaptophysin NSE and contain sustentacular cells which are positive for S100 protein (Figs. 6, 7, and 8). The tumor is multifocal in 20 % of cases. Of the 16 cases of bladder paragangliomas analyzed by Cheng et al., one patient presented in T1 stage, nine patients presented at T2 stage, two patients presented at T3 stage, and four patients presented at T4b stage [22]. One patient in their series had distant metastases and another one had lymph node metastases. One of the patients died after 18 months.

The criteria for diagnosing malignant paraganglia are metastases and/or "extensive local disease" [23]. Features that appear to indicate an increased potential for malignant behavior are younger age (second decade of life), hypertension micturition attacks, and invasive dispersion through the bladder wall [2].

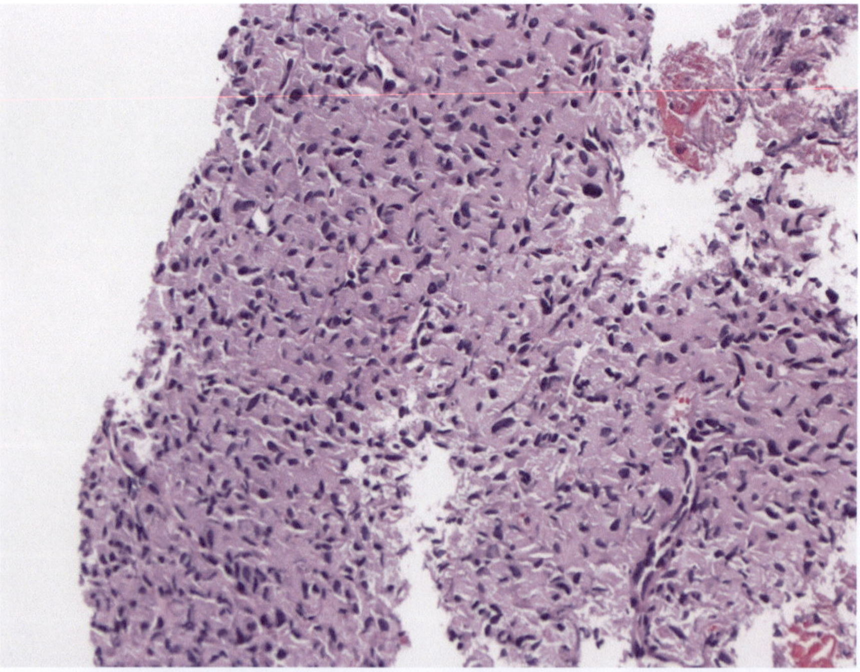

Fig. 6 Paraganglioma of the bladder exhibiting round to oval nuclei with moderate amount of eosinophilic granular cytoplasm

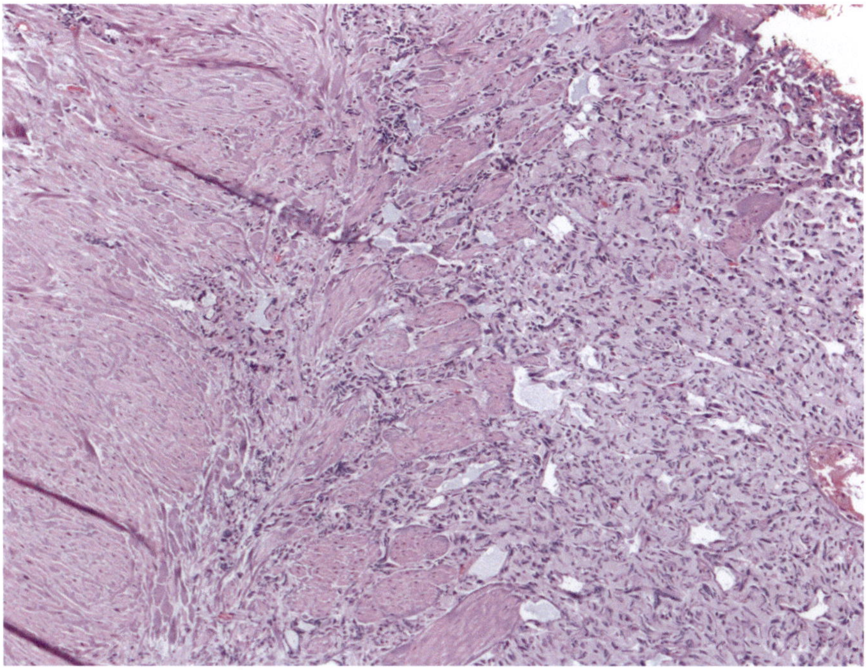

Fig. 7 Paraganglioma infiltrating into muscularis propria

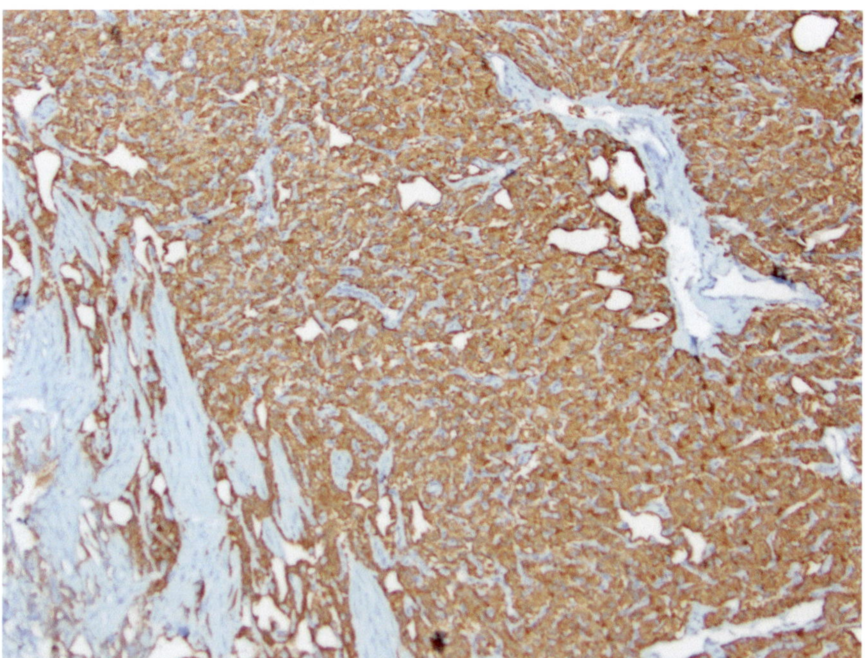

Fig. 8 Paraganglioma of the bladder showing diffuse reactivity for synaptophysin

Therapy for these tumors is surgical excision. Neither radiation nor chemotherapy is effective against these tumors as they are terminally differentiated [19].

Besides the entities described, very often, there are carcinomas which are histologically not pure neuroendocrine carcinoma subtypes as described above but have a neuroendocrine differentiation. These carcinomas are usually admixed with urothelial carcinoma of the bladder. Such cases are currently diagnosed as urothelial carcinomas with neuroendocrine differentiation.

Molecular Features

Telomerase reverse transcriptase (TERT) promoter mutations have recently been discovered in tumors like melanoma and urothelial carcinoma by next generation sequencing. Zheng et al. [24] have demonstrated high frequency of TERT promoter mutation in small cell carcinoma (SCC) of the urinary bladder but not in SCC of other origin, such as the prostate. These findings illustrate molecular differences between SCC of the urinary bladder and SCC of other origins, despite their shared morphologic and immunophenotypic similarities. The TERT promoter mutation may be used for differentiating SCC of the urinary bladder from SCC of non-bladder origin.

Prominent pathways altered in cases of bladder cancer include PI3K/AKT/mTOR pathway, MAPK pathway, and chromatin regulatory genes [25]. These, however, are not specific for bladder cancer with neuroendocrine differentiation.

References

1. http://www.cancer.org. Cancer facts and figures. American Cancer Society. 2013.
2. Eble JN, Sauter G, Epstein JI, editors. Pathology and genetics of tumours of the urinary system and male genital organs. Lyon: IARC Press; 2004. World Health Organization classification of tumors.
3. Chen Y, Epstein JI. Primary carcinoid tumors of the urinary bladder and prostatic urethra: a clinicopathologic study of 6 cases. Am J Surg Pathol. 2011;35:442–6.
4. Sugihara A, Kajio K, Yoshimoto T, et al. Primary carcinoid tumor of the urinary bladder. Int Urol Nephrol. 2002;33:53–7.
5. Mills SE, Wolfe III JT, Weiss MA, et al. Small cell undifferentiated carcinoma of the urinary bladder: a light-microscopic, immunocytochemical, and ultrastructural study of 12 cases. Am J Surg Pathol. 1987;11:606–17.
6. Ordonez NG, Khorsand J, Ayala AG, et al. Oat cell carcinoma of the urinary tract: an immunohistochemical and electron microscopic study. Cancer. 1986;58:2519–30.
7. Cheng L, Pan CX, Yang XJ, et al. Small cell carcinoma of the urinary bladder: a clinicopathologic analysis of 64 patients. Cancer. 2004;101:957–62.
8. Abrahams NA, Moran C, Reyes AO, et al. Small cell carcinoma of the bladder: a contemporary clinicopathological study of 51 vases. Histopathology. 2005;46:57–63.
9. Blomjous CE, Vos W, De Voogt HJ, et al. Small cell carcinoma of the urinary bladder. A clinicopathologic, morphometric, immunohistochemical, and ultrastructural study of 18 cases. Cancer. 1989;64:1347–57.

10. Holmang S, Borghede G, Johansson SL. Primary small cell carcinoma of the bladder: a report of 25 cases. J Urol. 1995;153:1820–2.
11. Reyes CV, Soneru I. Small cell carcinoma of the urinary bladder with hypercalcemia. Cancer. 1985;56:2530–3.
12. Jones TD, Kernek KM, Yang XJ, et al. Thyroid transcription factor 1 expression in small cell carcinoma of the urinary bladder: an immunohistochemical profile of 44 cases. Hum Pathol. 2005;36:718–23.
13. Wang X, MacLennan GT, Lopez-Beltran A, et al. Small cell carcinoma of the urinary bladder – Histogenesis, genetics, diagnosis, biomarkers, treatment, and prognosis. Appl Immunohistochem Mol Morphol. 2007;15:8–18.
14. Choong NW, Wuevedo JF, Kaur JS. Small cell carcinoma of the urinary bladder. The Mayo Clinic experience. Cancer. 2005;103:1172–8.
15. Sehgal SS, Wein AJ, Bing Z, et al. Neuroendocrine tumor of the bladder. Rev Urol. 2010;12:197–201.
16. Akamatsu S, Kanamaru S, Ishihara M, et al. Primary large cell neuroendocrine carcinoma of the bladder. Int J Urol. 2008;15:1080–3.
17. Mazzucchelli R, Morichetti D, Lopez-Beltran A, et al. Neuroendocrine tumours of the urinary system and male genital organs: clinical significance. BJU Int. 2009;103:1464–70.
18. Hervonen A, Vaalasti A, Partanen M. Paraganglia of the bladder. J Urol. 1978;119:335–7.
19. Helpap H, Kloppel G. Neuroendocrine carcinomas of the prostate and urinary bladder: a diagnostic and therapeutic challenge. Virchows Arch. 2002;440:241–8.
20. Davaris P, Petraki K, Arvanitis D, et al. Urinary bladder paraganglioma. Pathol Res Pract. 1986;181:101–6.
21. Sweetser PM, Ohl DA, Thompson NW. Phaeochromocytoma of the urinary bladder. Surgery. 1991;109:677–81.
22. Cheng L, Leibovich BC, Cheville JC, et al. Paraganglioma of the urinary bladder: can biologic potential be predicted? Cancer. 2000;88:844–52.
23. Linnoila RI, Keiser HR, Steinberg SM, et al. Histopathology of benign versus malignant sympathoadrenal paragangliomas: clinicopathologic study of 1200 cases including unusual histologic features. Hum Pathol. 1990;21:1168–80.
24. Zheng X, Zhuge J, Bezerra SM, et al. High frequency of TERT promoter mutation in small cell carcinoma of bladder, but not in small cell carcinoma of other origins. J Hematol Oncol. 2014;7:47.
25. Carneiro BA, Meeks JJ, Kuzel TM, et al. Emerging therapeutic targets in bladder cancer. Cancer Treat Rev. 2015;2:170–8.

Neuroendocrine Tumors of the Prostate and Molecular Features

Jasreman Dhillon

Introduction

Prostate cancer is the third most common carcinoma among men. According to the American Cancer Society's estimate, 1 in 7 men will be diagnosed with prostate cancer during their lifetime. Prostate cancer is the second leading cause of cancer death in American men, behind only lung cancer. About 1 man in 38 will die of prostate cancer [1]. The World Health Organization (WHO) currently divides neuroendocrine (NE) tumors into conventional prostatic adenocarcinoma, carcinoid tumor (WHO's well-differentiated neuroendocrine tumor), small cell carcinoma, large cell neuroendocrine carcinoma, and paraganglioma. Recently, the working committee for the Prostate Cancer Foundation has proposed a classification of NE differentiation in prostate cancer [2]. According to this committee, the NE differentiation in prostate carcinoma can be divided into usual prostate adenocarcinoma with NE differentiation, adenocarcinoma with Paneth cell NE differentiation, carcinoid tumor, small cell carcinoma, large-cell neuroendocrine carcinoma (LCNEC), and mixed (small or large) NE carcinoma–acinar adenocarcinoma.

Endocrine Differentiation Within Adenocarcinoma

Normal prostate glands contain NE cells randomly scattered within the epithelial cells. On microscopic examination, these are small cells resting on the basal cell layer and in between the secretory cells. These cells may have a bright granular eosinophilic cytoplasm on hematoxylin and eosin staining (Fig. 1). A variety of peptide hormones like serotonin, histamine, chromogranin A, calcitonin, vasoactive

J. Dhillon, MD
Department of Anatomic Pathology, Moffitt Cancer Center, Tampa, FL 33612, USA
e-mail: Jasreman.dhillon@moffitt.org

A. Nasir, D. Coppola (eds.), *Neuroendocrine Tumors: Review of Pathology, Molecular and Therapeutic Advances*, DOI 10.1007/978-1-4939-3426-3_19

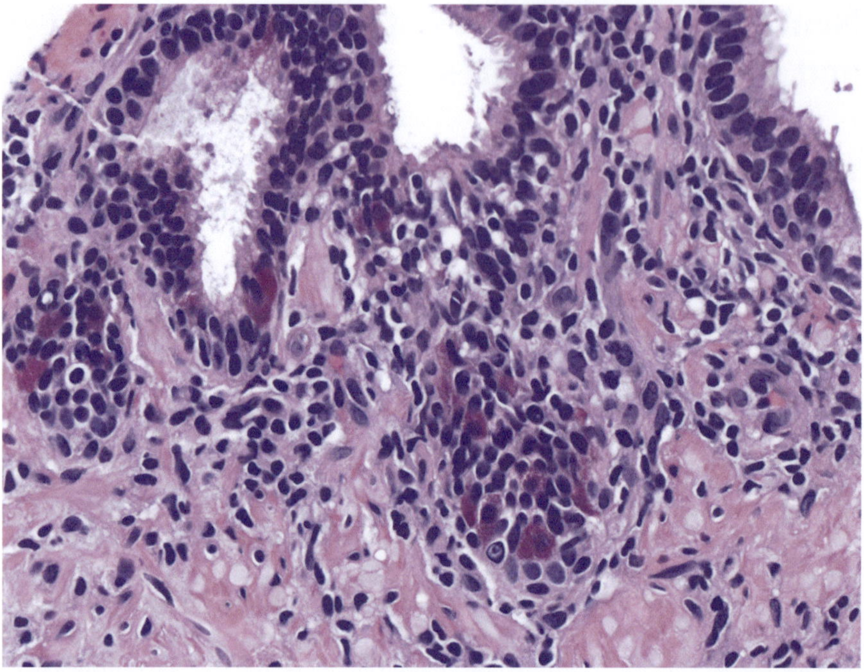

Fig. 1 Benign prostatic glands with scattered neuroendocrine cells having bright, granular eosinophilic cytoplasm

intestinal peptide, and bombesin/gastrin-releasing peptide besides others are secreted by these cells [3–5]. Prostate is the organ in the genitourinary system with the highest number of NE cells.

Usual prostate adenocarcinoma with NE differentiation is defined as the usual acinar or ductal adenocarcinoma of the prostate in which NE differentiation is demonstrated by immunohistochemical (IHC) stains (synaptophysin, chromogranin, and CD56) alone [2]. All prostate cancers can show focal NE differentiation [6, 7]. Majority show only rare or sparse single NE cells demonstrated by NE markers immunohistochemically (Fig. 2). Most of the studies have not shown any prognostic relationship in tumors exhibiting focal NE differentiation [8–10]. Hence, it is not recommended to routinely use IHC stains to detect NE differentiation in a typical prostatic adenocarcinoma.

Carcinoid Tumor

Carcinoid tumor is defined as a well-differentiated NE tumor occurring in the prostate gland that meets the diagnostic criteria for carcinoid tumor elsewhere (Fig. 3). It should not be closely associated with usual prostatic adenocarcinoma and should

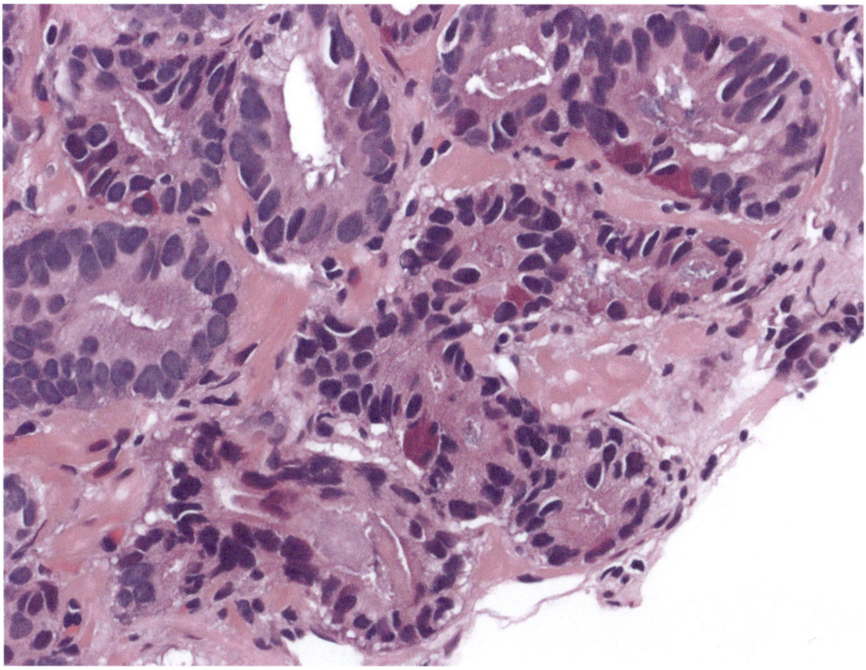

Fig. 2 Prostatic adenocarcinoma, Gleason score 6 (3 + 3) with scattered neuroendocrine cells having bright, granular eosinophilic cytoplasm

not arise from the urethra or extend from the bladder [2]. It is an extremely rare tumor of the prostate gland. These tumors are diffusely positive for NE markers synaptophysin, chromogranin, and CD56 and are negative for PSA (Figs. 4 and 5). Proliferation marker Ki67 is reported to be low (<5–20 %). Carcinoid tumors have to be differentiated from "carcinoid-like tumors" that most commonly include the usual acinar prostatic adenocarcinoma with an organoid appearance and focal neuroendocrine immunoreactivity. The "carcinoid-like tumor" is usually strongly positive for prostate-specific antigen (PSA), whereas carcinoid tumor is negative for PSA. Carcinoid tumors occur in younger patients including children as compared to the prostatic adenocarcinoma patients and may be associated with multiple endocrine neoplasia IIB syndrome [11, 12].

Small Cell Carcinoma

Small cell carcinoma is a high-grade neuroendocrine tumor that is histologically identical to small cell carcinoma of the lung [13]. On microscopic examination, the tumor cells exhibit lack of prominent nucleoli, nuclear molding, crush artifact, high nuclear-to-cytoplasmic ratio, and indistinct cell borders (Fig. 6). There is brisk

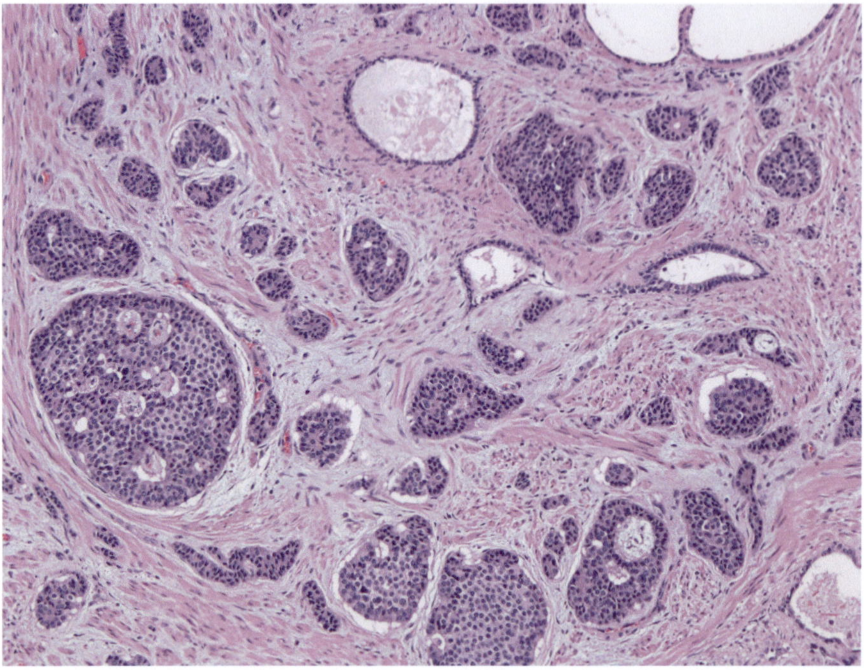

Fig. 3 Carcinoid tumor of the prostate showing tumor cells exhibiting little cytologic variability

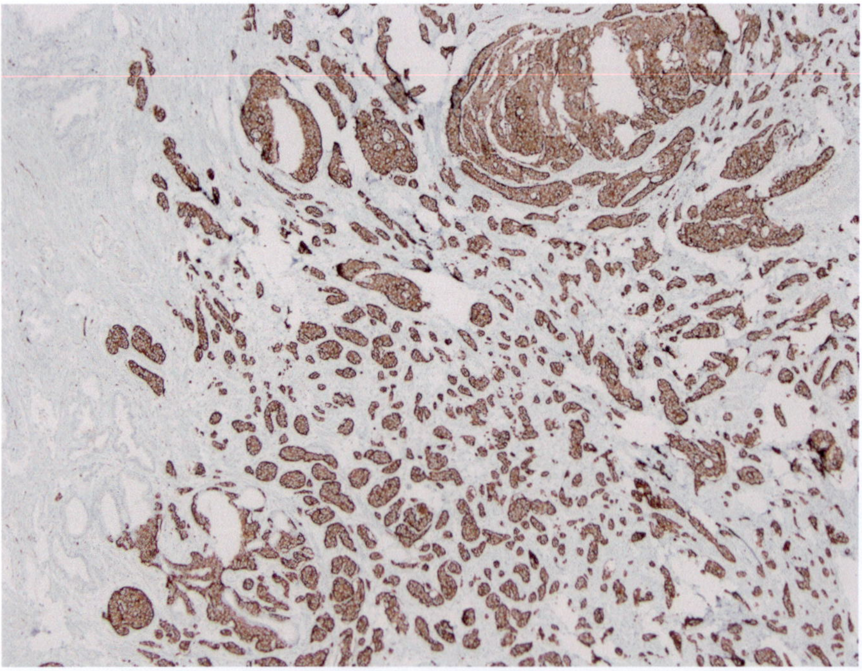

Fig. 4 Synaptophysin with strong positivity in the carcinoid tumor to the right and negative staining in the benign prostate glands to the left

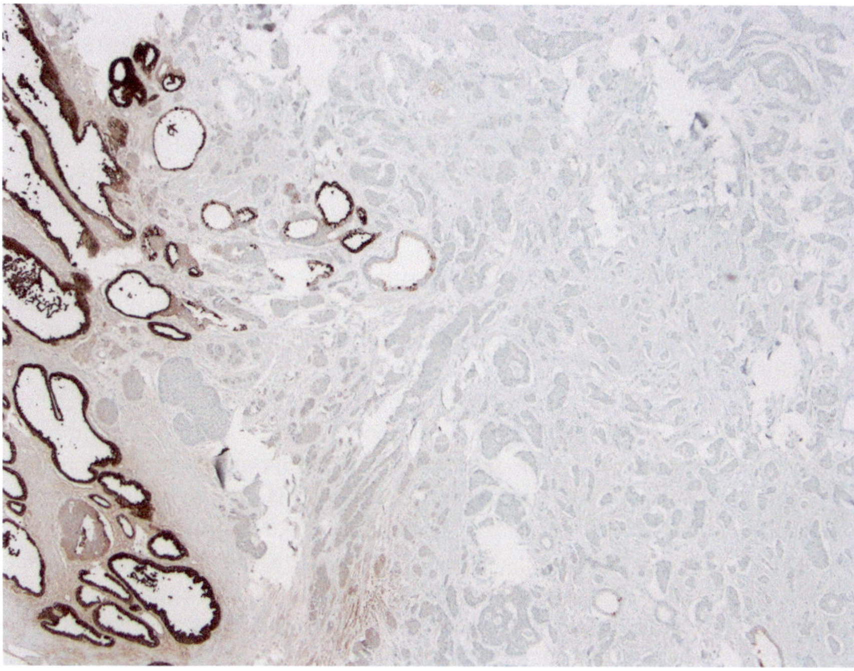

Fig. 5 PSA with no staining in the carcinoid tumor to the right and strong staining in the normal prostatic glands to the left

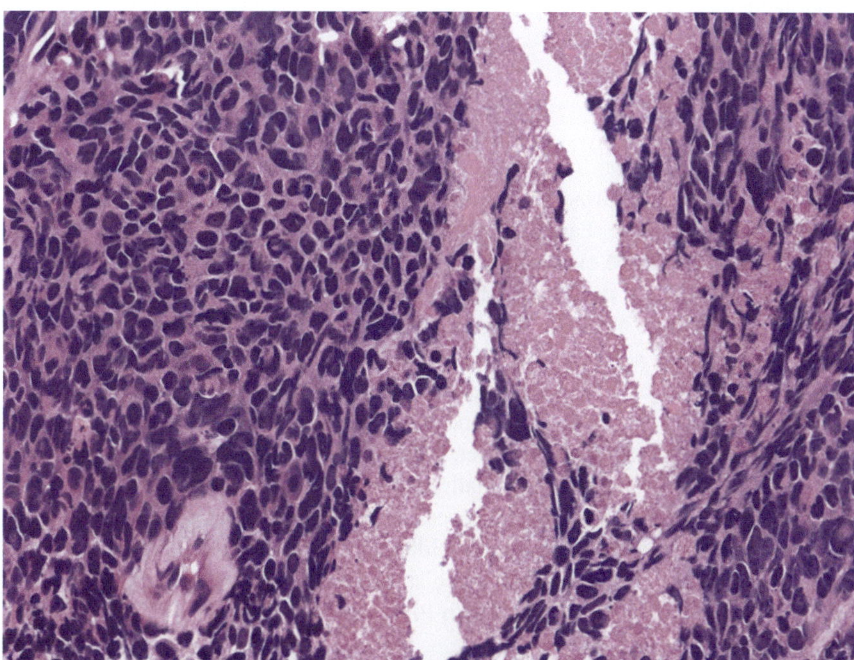

Fig. 6 Small cell carcinoma of the prostate admixed with necrosis

mitotic activity with numerous apoptotic bodies. Proliferation marker Ki67 is usually positive in >80 % of the tumor cell nuclei. Geographic foci of necrosis are frequently present in prostatectomy specimens. Morphologic variations include intermediate cell type with open chromatin and small visible nucleoli, tumor giant cells, and Indian filing [14]. Almost 90 % of the tumors express NE markers synaptophysin, chromogranin, and CD56 [14, 15]. Prostate-specific markers PSA and prostein are positive in about 17–25 % of cases [14, 15]. Immunohistochemical stain TTF1 is reported to be positive in >50 % of cases, making it difficult to distinguish prostate from a lung primary [14–16]. Fluorescence in situ hybridization (FISH) testing for TMPRSS2 and ERG (ETS-related gene) gene fusion is relatively specific for prostatic origin and is present in approximately 50 % of the small cell carcinomas of the prostate [17, 18].

Approximately half of small cell carcinomas have previous history of a hormonally treated acinar prostatic adenocarcinoma. As the small cell component predominates, serum PSA levels fall. Small cell carcinomas account for majority of prostatic tumors with clinical evidence of ACTH or antidiuretic hormone production. Patients with emergence of small cell carcinoma during progression of prostatic adenocarcinoma usually present with visceral metastasis. The median cancer-specific survival of patients with small cell carcinoma of the prostate according to the SEER database from 1973 to 2004 was reported to be 19 months. Two- and 5-year survival rates were reported to be 27.5 % and 14.3 %, respectively [19].

Small cell carcinoma of the prostate is treated aggressively with chemotherapy and radiation. Metastatic small cell carcinoma is treated with platinum-based combination chemotherapy [20, 21].

Paraganglioma

Paragangliomas of the prostate are extremely rare tumors with only seven cases reported in the literature. Paragangliomas are slow-growing usually benign tumors thought to arise from the extra-adrenal chromaffin cells. The tumor is composed of small nests (zellballen) or clusters of round cells surrounded by fibrous trabeculae. The tumor cells have abundant, granular, eosinophilic cytoplasm and are uniform and mostly round. The nuclei have a salt-and-pepper appearance, with occasional nuclear pleomorphism. Histopathological features associated with malignant behavior of the tumor are confluent tumoral necrosis, vascular invasion, capsular invasion, and increased mitotic activity. However, presence of metastases is the only currently widely accepted criterion to define malignant paraganglioma. On needle core biopsies, paragangliomas may be misdiagnosed as prostatic adenocarcinoma due to rarity of these tumors. However, this can be avoided if attention is paid to the morphologic features and utilizing pertinent immunohistochemical stains. Paragangliomas may stain like prostatic adenocarcinoma with PIN4 immunostaining which is a cocktail of AMACR, p63, and high molecular weight cytokeratin (HMWCK) exhibiting no staining with basal cell markers p63 and HMWCK. However, these tumors are negative for prostate-specific markers like PSA and prostate-specific acid phosphatase and are strongly positive for chromogranin and synaptophysin [22]. Immunostain S100 highlights the sustentacular cells that surround the nests of tumor cells.

Clinical presentation is variable and depends if the tumor is functional or nonfunctional. Functional tumors may present with symptoms of catecholamine overproduction such as hypertension, headaches, sweating, tachycardia, or anxiety. These symptoms may be precipitated by micturition. Nonfunctioning tumors may present with hematuria, obstructive symptoms, or a palpable nodule [23, 24]. Nonfunctioning tumors may not be clinically detected until at advanced stage. Of the reported five cases of nonfunctioning prostatic paraganglioma, two were surgically unresectable. Paragangliomas are treated either surgically or by radiation. Radiation is used as a palliative treatment in bone metastasis.

Adenocarcinoma with Paneth Cell-Like NE Differentiation

The working committee of the Prostate Cancer Foundation has proposed adenocarcinoma with Paneth cell-like NE differentiation as one of the subtypes of prostate cancer with NE differentiation. This tumor subtype is composed of typical adenocarcinoma of the prostate containing varying proportions of cells with prominent eosinophilic cytoplasmic granules on microscopic examination. These Paneth cell-like foci stain positive for NE markers [2]. Paneth cell-like NE differentiation is usually associated with lower-grade conventional adenocarcinoma. The current recommendation of the working committee is not to assign a Gleason score to these tumors and to add a comment to the generally favorable prognosis of this morphologic variant based on the limited data available [25].

Large-Cell Neuroendocrine Carcinoma (LCNEC)

LCNEC is a recently described entity which is included in the recent 4th edition of the WHO classification of the neuroendocrine tumors of the prostate. This is an aggressive, high-grade NE tumor that is composed of large nests with peripheral palisading and large foci of necrosis. The tumor cells have prominent nucleoli, abundant cytoplasm, and a high mitotic rate. Ki67 stains usually >50 % of the tumor cell nuclei. These tumors are diffusely positive for NE markers and usually negative for PSA.

LCNEC of the prostate is rare and usually represents progression from prior typical prostate adenocarcinoma after long-standing androgen deprivation therapy [26]. In a study by Evans et al., patients had a mean survival of 7 months and rapid metastases. It can also be present in association with small cell carcinoma and prostate adenocarcinoma.

Mixed NE Carcinoma: Acinar Adenocarcinoma

This subgroup is defined by the working committee as a biphasic carcinoma that is composed of a mixture of NE carcinoma (small cell or large cell) and usual conventional acinar adenocarcinoma [2]. Both the components should be distinct and recognizable. Most of the cases encountered are mixed small cell carcinoma–acinar adenocarcinoma where the patients usually have metastatic castration-resistant disease. It is a high-grade and aggressive tumor. The working committee recommends that the percentage and grade of the acinar component be provided when reporting these tumors.

Molecular Features

Approximately half of the usual prostatic adenocarcinomas and small cell carcinomas of the prostate have fusion of the androgen-responsive gene transmembrane serine 2 (TMPRSS2) with ETS-related genes in particular estrogen-regulated gene (ERG), both of which are located on chromosome 21 [17, 18, 27]. This fusion can be detected by fluorescence in situ hybridization (FISH) or reverse transcription polymerase chain reaction. The overexpression of ERG in these cases can also be detected immunohistochemically. However, small cell carcinomas with TMPRSS2-ERG rearrangements are not reliably positive for ERG protein by IHC [17], requiring the use of FISH for confirmation. This fusion when present helps to distinguish small cell carcinoma of the prostate from other small cell carcinomas.

Prognostic value of TMPRSS2-ERG gene fusion is hotly debated with most studies indicating an unfavorable outcome. In prostate cancer, overexpression of ERG and loss of PTEN (phosphatase and tensin) homolog deleted on chromosome 10 are two common events involved in the molecular pathogenesis of this disease [27, 28]. PTEN is a tumor suppressor gene, whose disruption leads to activation of downstream components of the phosphatidylinositol-3-kinase pathway. Besides upregulation of ERG and loss of PTEN, other molecular alterations identified in small cell prostate cancer include loss of androgen receptor (AR) and androgen-regulated protein expression and loss of tumor suppressor genes p53 and RB1. Loss of RB1 may be a useful potential therapeutic target [29]. p53 mutation leads to Aurora kinase A (AURKA) overexpression which is critically important for rapid proliferation and aggressive behavior of small cell prostate cancer and is considered to be a viable therapeutic target [30]. Molecular alterations such as PLK1 upregulation and c-MYC PCDH-PC, EZH2, IL-6, MIF, FAK, Siah2, and c-Kit overexpression in small cell prostate cancer are other potential therapeutic targets.

Abbreviations

AR	Androgen receptor
AURKA	Aurora kinase A
ERG	Estrogen regulated gene
HMWCK	High molecular weight cytokeratin
IHC	Immunohistochemical
LCNEC	Large-cell neuroendocrine carcinoma
NE	Neuroendocrine
PSA	Prostate-specific antigen
PTEN	Phosphatase and tensin
TMPRSS2	Transmembrane serine 2
WHO	World Health Organization

References

1. http://www.cancer.org. Cancer Statistics. American Cancer Society. 2015.
2. Epstein JI, Amin MB, Beltran H, Lotan TL, Mosquera JM, Reuter VE, Robinson BD, Troncoso P, Rubin MA. Proposed morphologic classification of prostate cancer with neuroendocrine differentiation. Am J Surg Pathol. 2014;38(6):756–67.
3. Abrahamsson PA. Neuroendocrine cells in tumour growth of the prostate. Endocr Relat Cancer. 1999;6:503–19.
4. Abrahamsson PA, Wadstrom LB, Alumets J, et al. Peptide hormone- and serotonin-immunoreactive tumour cells in carcinoma of the prostate. Pathol Res Pract. 1987;182:298–307.
5. Sun B, Halmos G, Schally AV, Wang X, Martinez M. Presence of receptors for bombesin/gastrin-releasing peptide and mRNA for three receptor subtypes in human prostate cancers. Prostate. 2000;42:295–303.
6. Komiya A, Suzuki H, Imamoto T, et al. Neuroendocrine differentiation in the progression of prostate cancer. Int J Urol. 2009;16:37–44.
7. Vashchenko N, Abrahamsson PA. Neuroendocrine differentiation in prostate cancer: implications for new treatment modalities. Eur Urol. 2005;47:147–55.
8. Shariff AH, Ather MH. Neuroendocrine differentiation in prostate cancer. Urology. 2006;68:2–8.
9. Cohen MK, Arber DA, Coffield KS, et al. Neuroendocrine differentiation in prostatic adenocarcinoma and its relationship to tumor progression. Cancer. 1994;74:1899–903.
10. Jeetle SS, Fisher G, Yang ZH, et al. Neuroendocrine differentiation does not have independent prognostic value in conservatively treated prostate cancer. Virchows Arch. 2012;461:103–7.
11. Goulet-Salmon B, Berthe E, Franc S, et al. Prostatic neuroendocrine tumor in multiple endocrine neoplasia type 2B. J Endocrinol Invest. 2004;27:570–3.
12. Whelan T, Gatfield CT, Robertson S, et al. Primary carcinoid of the prostate in conjunction with multiple endocrine neoplasia IIb in a child. J Urol. 1995;153:1080–2.
13. Tetu B, Ro JY, Ayala AG, et al. Small cell carcinoma of the prostate. Part I. A clinicopathologic study of 20 cases. Cancer. 1987;59:1803–9.
14. Wang W, Epstein JI. Small cell carcinoma of the prostate. A morphologic and immunohistochemical study of 95 cases. Am J Surg Pathol. 2008;32:65–71.
15. Yao JL, Madeb R, Bourne P, et al. Small cell carcinoma of the prostate: an immunohistochemical study. Am J Surg Pathol. 2006;30:705–12.

16. Agoff SN, Lamps SW, Philip AT, et al. Thyroid transcription factor-1 is expressed in extrapulmonary small cell carcinomas but not in other extrapulmonary neuroendocrine tumors. Mod Pathol. 2000;13:238–42.
17. Lotan TL, Gupta NS, Wang W, et al. ERG gene rearrangements are common in prostatic small cell carcinomas. Mod Pathol. 2011;24:820–8.
18. Guo CC, Dancer JY, Wang Y, et al. TMPRSS2-ERG gene fusion in small cell carcinoma of the prostate. Hum Pathol. 2011;42:11–7.
19. Deorah S, Rao MB, Raman R, et al. Survival of patients with small cell carcinoma of the prostate during 1973–2003: a population based study. BJU Int. 2012;109:824–30.
20. Aparicio AM, Harzstark AL, Corn PG, et al. Platinum-based chemotherapy for variant castrate-resistant prostate cancer. Clin Cancer Res. 2013;19:3621–30.
21. Papandreou CN, Daliani DD, Thall PF, et al. Results of a phase II study with doxorubicin, etoposide, and cisplatin in patients with fully characterized small-cell carcinoma of the prostate. J Clin Oncol. 2002;20:3072–80.
22. Parwani AV, Cao D, Epstein JI. Pathologic quiz case: a 35-year-old man with hematuria. Paraganglioma involving the prostate. Arch Pathol Lab Med. 2004;128:e104–6.
23. Mehta M, Nodel NS, Lanni Y, et al. Malignant paraganglioma of the prostate and retroperitoneum. J Urol. 1979;121:376–8.
24. Campodonico F, Bandelloni R, Maffezzinni M. Paraganglioma of the prostate in a young adult. Urology. 2005;66:657.
25. Tamas EF, Epstein JI. Prognostic significance of paneth cell-like neuroendocrine differentiation in adenocarcinoma of the prostate. Am J Surg Pathol. 2006;30:980–5.
26. Evans AJ, Humphrey PA, Belani J, et al. Large cell neuroendocrine carcinoma of prostate: a clinicopathologic summary of 7 cases of a rare manifestation of advanced prostate cancer. Am J Surg Pathol. 2006;30:684–93.
27. Tomlins SA, Rhodes DR, Perner S, et al. Recurrent fusion of TMPRSS2 and ETS transcription factor genes in prostate cancer. Science. 2005;310:644–8.
28. Di Cristofano A, Pandolfi PP. The multiple roles of PTEN in tumor suppression. Cell. 2000;100:387–90.
29. Tan HL, Sood A, Rahimi HA, et al. Rb loss is characteristic of prostatic small cell neuroendocrine carcinoma. Clin Cancer Res. 2014;20:890–903.
30. Li Z, Sun Y, Chen X, et al. p53 mutation directs AURKA overexpression via miR-25 and FBXW7 in prostatic small cell neuroendocrine carcinoma. Mol Cancer Res. 2015;13(3):584–91.

Neuroendocrine Tumors of the Female Genital Tract

Ozlen Saglam and Ardeshir Hakam

Neuroendocrine tumors (NET) and tumors with focal neuroendocrine differentiation can arise throughout the female genital tract. NET can be pure or associated with various epithelial tumors such as ovarian mucinous, endometrioid, brenner and serous neoplasms, endometrial endometrioid adenocarcinoma, and endocervical adenocarcinomas [1–5]. Altogether these are rare entities, and pure NET does not comprise more than 2 % of female genital tract neoplasms [6]. The origin of neuroendocrine tumors was related to neural crest-derived amine precursor update and decarboxylation (APUD) cells until recent past. This concept was discarded mainly by LeDouarin' s work on chick-quail chimeras [7]. Current evidence is conclusive for endodermal origin of the gut and pancreatic neuroendocrine neoplasms [8]. Neuroendocrine cells have been identified within normal epithelium of the female genital tract [9]. These cells, as a part of diffuse neuroendocrine system, are likely to be the origin of neuroendocrine neoplasms other than tumors arising within teratomas.

Some NETs such as primary carcinoid tumors of the female genital tract share similar morphology to that of carcinoid tumors arising in other organ systems. It may be difficult to differentiate a primary disease from metastatic lesions in certain cases. There is no separate histologic grading system for NET arising in female genital tract. They are graded in a similar way to primary NET of the lung. NET can be functioning and produce hormones. Patients with these lesions may present with clinical syndromes as a result of ectopic hormone production. Here we discussed pathologic features and some of the clinical presentations of the female genital tract NET in specific anatomic sites.

O. Saglam, MD (✉) • A. Hakam, MD, MBA
Department of Pathology, Moffitt Cancer Center, Tampa, FL, USA
e-mail: ozlen.saglam@moffitt.org

A. Nasir, D. Coppola (eds.), *Neuroendocrine Tumors: Review of Pathology, Molecular and Therapeutic Advances*, DOI 10.1007/978-1-4939-3426-3_20

Ovaries

NETs arising in the ovaries are carcinoid tumors; small cell carcinoma hypercalcemic type; and small cell carcinoma pulmonary type. Primary ovarian large-cell neuroendocrine carcinoma has also been described in case reports [10]. Carcinoid tumors (well-differentiated neuroendocrine carcinoma) can be primary or metastatic from other anatomic sites. The morphologic subtypes include insular, trabecular, strumal, and mucinous carcinoids. They can also present with mixed morphologic features. Strumal and mucinous carcinoids contain epithelial elements which are thyroid tissue and mucinous epithelium, respectively. Primary ovarian insular and trabecular carcinoids are similar to intestinal counterparts. They can be observed in teratomas, mucinous tumors, and Sertoli-Leydig cell tumors [11]. Pure carcinoid tumors (strumal carcinoid) can be considered as monodermal teratomas. Most patients with carcinoid tumors are either postmenopausal or perimenopausal [12]. One-third of insular carcinoids are associated with carcinoid syndrome [13]. The rate of developing carcinoid syndrome was calculated around 8 % for the trabecular carcinoids in a study which used multiple tumor registries as a database [11].

Insular carcinoids are composed of solid nests of cells and small acini which may have eosinophilic secretions. Neoplastic cells have ample cytoplasm and centrally located round nuclei with finely stippled chromatin. The mitotic activity is low. Trabecular carcinoids are composed of one- to two-cell layered wavy ribbons and cords that are surrounded by fibromatous stroma (Fig. 1). Trabecular and mixed trabecular-insular carcinoids should be sampled thoroughly to rule out a strumal component. They are found in close proximity of thyroid tissue. Ultrastructurally, neurosecretory granules show variation in size and shape in the insular carcinoid

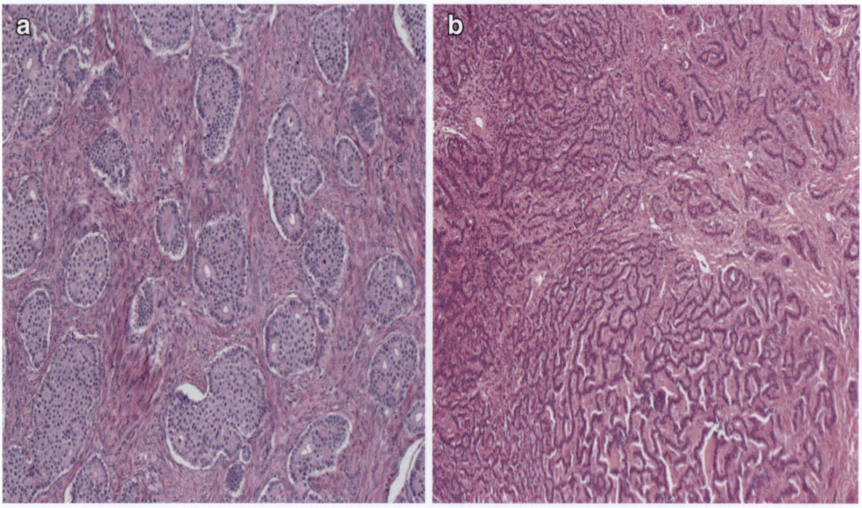

Fig. 1 Ovarian carcinoid tumors. (**a**) Insular pattern. (**b**) Trabecular pattern (10×)

tumors. On the other hand, relatively uniform and round secretory granules are observed in the trabecular type [14].

Mucinous carcinoids (goblet cell carcinoid) are rarely diagnosed in the ovary. A metastatic lesion should be ruled out before establishing the diagnosis of a primary ovarian neoplasm. Some morphologic features including presence of teratomatous elements or a surface epithelial tumor in combination, unilateral involvement of the ovaries, and absence of lymphovascular invasion are in favor of a primary neoplasm [15]. Mucinous carcinoid tumors are composed of numerous small glands and acini with small lumens. Neoplastic cells appear distended with intracytoplasmic mucin. There may be extracellular mucinous pools. Immunostains for chromogranin, CK20, and CK7 can be positive in mucinous carcinoids in varying percentages [16, 17].

Insular carcinoids are considered as potentially malignant tumors. In a series containing only insular, trabecular, and strumal subtypes, surgical treatment gave excellent results when the tumor was confined to the ovaries [12]. Mucinous carcinoids behave more aggressively than both insular and trabecular carcinoid tumors [18]. The degree of differentiation and presence of associated carcinoma are also related to overall prognosis [15]. Limited number of reported strumal carcinoid cases followed benign clinical course [19]. When a carcinoid tumor was part of cystic teratoma (Fig. 2), a significant difference was observed in multiple prognostic indicators compared to pure NET. The first group had smaller tumor size, lower rates of distant metastases, and hepatic involvement [11].

Metastatic carcinoid tumors almost always affect bilateral ovaries. They form well-circumscribed tumor nodules (Fig. 3), in contrast to single diffuse mass lesion of primary neoplasms. There is no definite morphologic feature or immunohistochemical panel that can differentiate primary versus metastatic carcinoid tumors of the ovary. Immunostain for CDX2 was proposed to use for discriminating primary disease from gastrointestinal metastasis [20]. There was weak staining in about 20 % of cases with CDX2 in this study. In another, diffuse CDX2 expression was reported in four out of six insular, one out of six strumal, and one out of one primary ovarian mucinous carcinoid tumors [21].

Small cell carcinoma of hypercalcemic type (SSC-H) is considered as undifferentiated carcinoma by some authors. These lesions are classified under miscellaneous category in the current World Health Organization's (WHO) book on classification of tumors of female reproductive organs [22]. They are highly aggressive tumors and commonly occur in young patients under 40 years of age. About two-thirds of cases are associated with elevated levels of calcium. They are usually unilateral fleshy white and solid lesions on gross examination. Diffuse small epithelial cells are separated by follicle-like spaces containing eosinophilic secretions. Brisk mitotic activity is observed throughout the lesion. Necrosis is also common. There are variants with large plasmacytoid/rhabdoid-appearing cells. They have glassy eosinophilic cytoplasm and nuclei with prominent nucleoli. Immunostains for WT-1, CD10, cytokeratins, and calretinin are useful in diagnosing SSC-H [23]. The staining pattern can be diffuse or focal with these markers. Recent whole-genome sequencing studies performed on SSC-H cases showed frequent inactivating germline and/or somatic

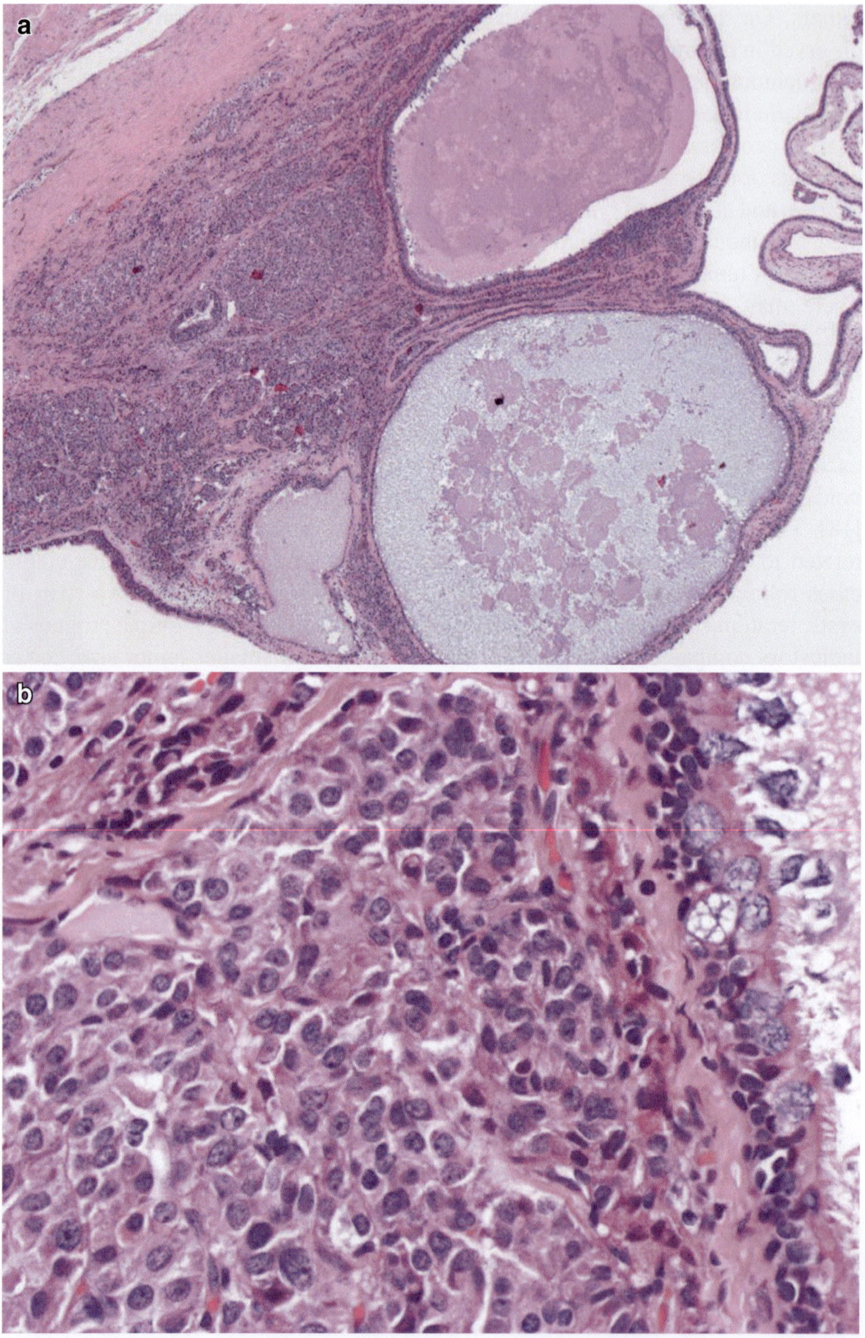

Fig. 2 (**a**) Incidental neuroendocrine tumor within a cystic teratoma (5×). (**b**) Neuroendocrine neoplasm and mucinous-type epithelium (20×)

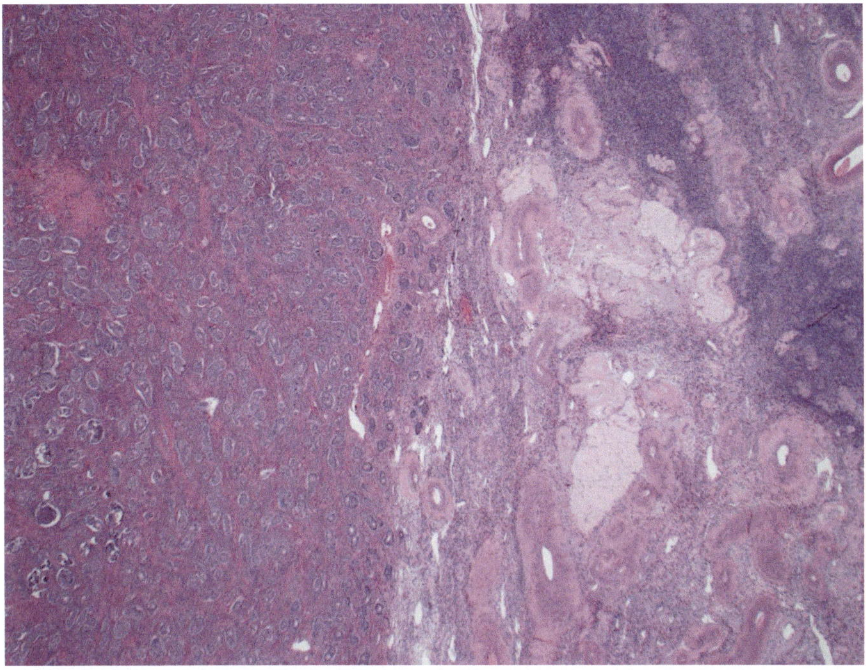

Fig. 3 Metastatic carcinoid tumor to the ovaries. Well-demarcated border between benign ovarian tissue and carcinoid tumor is characteristic for metastatic lesions (5×)

mutations in *SMARCA4* gene [24]. This mutation is also shared with malignant rhabdoid tumor arising in other anatomic sites. In addition to shared mutation, presence of some morphologic similarities brought the possibility of common cell origin for both neoplasms [25].

Small cell carcinoma of the ovary-pulmonary type (SSC-P) shows identical morphologic features to that of small cell carcinoma of the lung and can express TTF1 [4]. Clinical correlation is required before diagnosing a primary ovarian disease. They can be associated with other epithelial tumors such as endometrioid carcinoma, brenner tumor, and teratoma [26, 27]. Paraneoplastic syndromes are less common compared to primary lung disease. Cushing's syndrome and inappropriate secretion of antidiuretic hormone were described in the SSC-P type [28].

Fallopian Tube

Primary NET in the fallopian tubes is extremely rare. It was described in a postmenopausal woman with adnexal torsion [29].

Uterine Cervix

Cervical NETs were divided into low-grade and high-grade tumors in the current WHO's book on classifications of tumors of female reproductive organs [30]. Low-grade tumors are carcinoid and atypical carcinoid tumors. High-grade NETs of the uterine cervix are small-cell neuroendocrine carcinoma (SmCC) and large-cell neuroendocrine carcinoma. Low-grade NETs are extremely rare in the uterine cervix. Morphologic features of atypical carcinoid tumors include mild to moderate nuclear atypia, a mitotic count of 5–10 per high-power field (HPF), and focal necrosis [31]. High-risk human papillomavirus infection was detected in both low- and high-grade NETs of the cervix [32]. HPV 18 is more commonly identified compared to other subtypes. NET of the cervix can be diagnosed as mixed carcinoma with other epithelial tumors.

The mean age at diagnosis is 49 for endocrine tumors and 52 years for squamous cell carcinoma of the cervix [33]. Between 1977 and 2003, the mean annual incidence for SmCC of the uterine cervix was reported as 0.06 per 100,000 women. In comparison, the incidence of squamous cell carcinoma and adenocarcinoma was 6.6 and 1.2 per 100,000, respectively [34]. SmCC occurs most frequently in the cervix but can also involve the endometrium, ovary, fallopian tube, vagina, and vulva [35]. Majority of patients presents with vaginal bleeding [36]. There is a tendency for early hematogenous and lymphatic spread. Evaluation of the chest, abdomen, and pelvis by imaging studies is required as an initial diagnostic workup [37]. The morphology of SmCC is similar in all anatomic sites including the female genital tract. Tumor cells are composed of monotonous population of small cells with ovoid hyperchromatic nuclei and scant cytoplasm. Nuclear molding is frequently observed. There are abundant mitotic figures and apoptotic bodies. Prominent necrosis is also commonly seen. NET of the cervix can be associated with in situ and invasive endocervical adenocarcinoma and squamous cell carcinomas [38] (Fig. 4). One of the neuroendocrine markers such as synaptophysin, chromogranin, and CD56 is usually positive in NET of the cervix. However, negative results do not exclude the diagnosis of SmCC. By microsatellite analysis, loss of heterozygosity at several loci including 3p14, 5q31, 13q14, 17p13, 17q22, and 18q21 was detected in five out of ten SmCC components of mixed cervical cancers [39].

SmCC of the cervix is highly malignant tumor, and combination therapies are used in the treatment [40]. Patients with early-stage disease (I–II) showed significantly better survival rates compared with late-stage cancer (III–IV) in a small series [41]. A population-based study of Surveillance, Epidemiology, and End Results (SEER) reported worse prognosis in any kind of neuroendocrine tumors at all stages compared to squamous cell carcinoma of the cervix [33]. Patients with endocrine tumors presented at higher FIGO stage. The median survival for women with endocrine tumors was 22 months and for women with squamous cell carcinoma was 10 years.

High-grade neuroendocrine carcinomas of large cell type can have diffuse, organoid, trabecular, or cord-like patterns. Neoplastic cells have abundant cytoplasm, large nuclei, and prominent nuclei. The mitotic count is very high. Large-cell

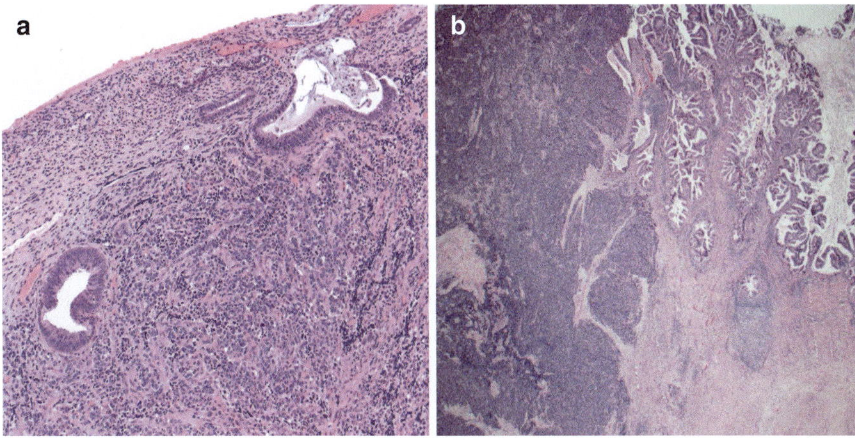

Fig. 4 Cervical NET. (**a**) Cervical adenocarcinoma in situ and NET (10×). (**b**) Invasive adenocarcinoma and NET (5×)

NET may also have glandular differentiation [42]. They are reactive with synaptophysin and chromogranin [43]. Microsatellite instability (MSI) was found in nine out of nine cases in a series. There were MSI and MMR defects. MSI-H was observed in around 89 % of cases. The latter was related to resistance to chemotherapy and radiation therapy [44]. By comparative genomic hybridization (CGH), amplification of 3q was the most remarkable chromosomal aberration detected in a case report [45].

Endometrium

NETs of the endometrium are usually observed in premenopausal and postmenopausal women [46]. They can present in combination with other common epithelial neoplasms. Small-cell NET, carcinoid, and large-cell NET were reported with papillary serous carcinoma of the endometrium [47–49]. The latter report describes epithelial pagetoid extension of neuroendocrine cells within benign and malignant endometrial glands. We observed similar phenomenon in the cervical and endometrial NET. Malignant tumor cells extended to benign endocervical and endometrial glands (Fig. 5). One can also assume that neoplastic cells are dropping down from the epithelium into the stroma rather than extending into it since their benign counterpart is present within the normal epithelium [9].

Large-cell neuroendocrine carcinoma was also observed in combination with grade 1 and 3 endometrioid adenocarcinoma [50]. A common tumor cell origin for epithelial and NET versus collision tumors is a proposed theory in the literature. Mhawech-Fauceglia et al. studied four mixed adenocarcinoma and high-grade neuroendocrine carcinomas arising from uterine corpus and the ovary by array CGH. Both components of all four cases showed almost similar genetic

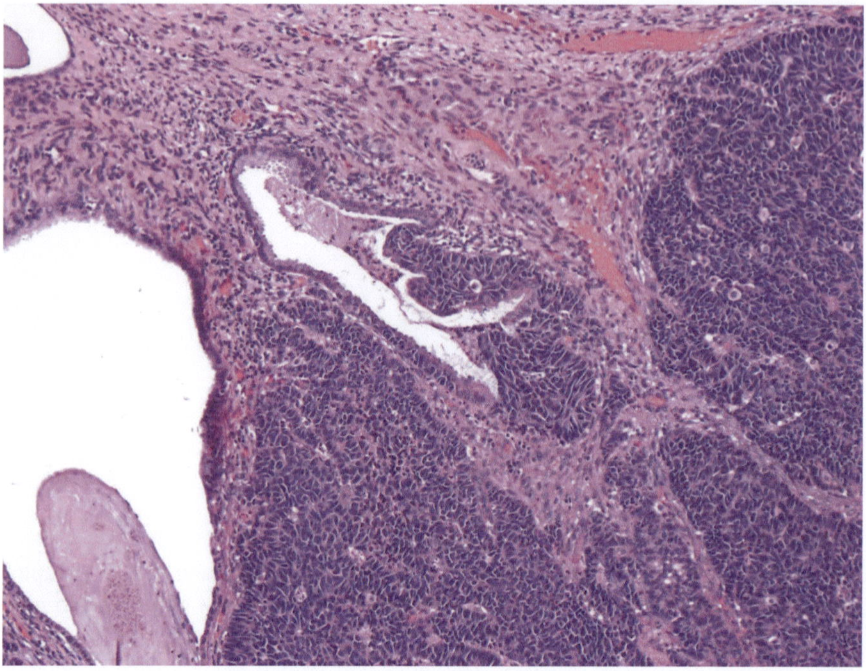

Fig. 5 Extension of NET to benign-appearing endometrial glands (10×)

abnormalities. In addition, NEC component demonstrated numerous additional genetic alterations including gain on 6p25.3-p21.2 and 19q12 and losses on 6q24.2-q27, 19q13.11-13.2, and 19q13.31-13.41 [51]. Their data indicate that high-grade neuroendocrine carcinoma and adenocarcinoma are genetically similar. However, neuroendocrine carcinoma component may be more dedifferentiated by acquiring more genetic abnormalities.

Taraif et al. reported neuroendocrine differentiation in 40 % of undifferentiated carcinoma of the endometrium. Most of these tumors had focal expression of neuroendocrine markers [52]. There was no survival difference in the group with neuroendocrine differentiation compared to the group without neuroendocrine features. This may be related to overall poor prognosis of undifferentiated carcinoma. Pure large-cell neuroendocrine and small-cell neuroendocrine carcinomas of the endometrium have a guarded prognosis [35, 53] (Fig. 6).

Vagina and Vulva

Primary small cell carcinoma and Merkel cell carcinoma (MCC) of the vagina are extremely rare [54, 55]. One of the small cell carcinoma cases occurred in a pregnant patient [56], and another was found in association with atypical vaginal

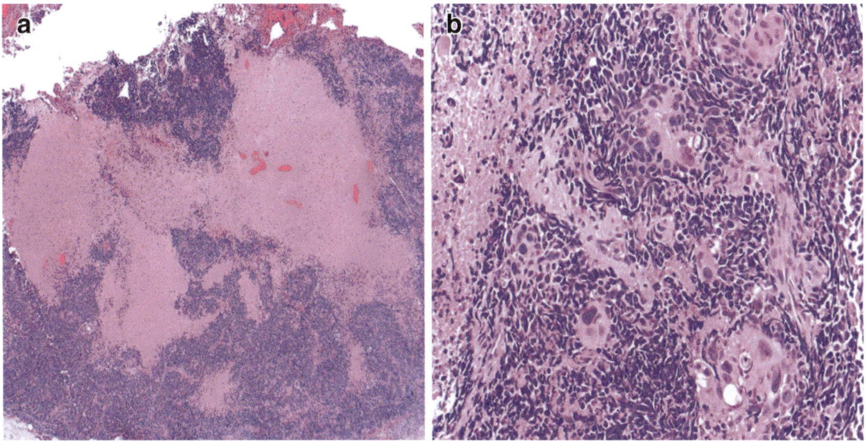

Fig. 6 Endometrial NET. (**a**) Areas of necrosis (5×). (**b**) Large cell features (10×)

adenosis [57]. Vaginal lesions should not be in continuity with the cervical tissue in order to rule out local extension of a cervical primary disease. There is no standard therapy for these aggressive tumors, and patients are treated in different combination of surgery, radiation, and chemotherapy [37].

Majority of neuroendocrine tumors of the vulva are MCC [37]. They have the same morphology and immunostaining profile with tumors arising in other anatomical sites. There is diffuse infiltration of dermis with uniform, small round cells with scant cytoplasm. Nuclei are pale and finely granular. Apoptotic bodies and mitotic figures are easily found. Characteristically cytokeratins highlight paranuclear cytoplasm in a dot-like pattern. Two out of 3778 MCCs occurred in the vulva in a population-based study [58]. Given the rarity of the lesion, it is difficult to estimate their behavior in this anatomic site. Primary clear cell carcinoid tumor of the vulva was also described [59]. These should be differentiated from other neoplasms with clear cell features such as malignant melanoma, metastatic renal cell carcinoma, and perivascular epithelioid cell tumor.

Conclusion

NET of the female genital tract is comprised of a spectrum of tumors with different clinical, prognostic, and pathologic features. It is important to differentiate primary and metastatic lesions since there is an overlap in the morphology of neuroendocrine tumors arising in different anatomical sites. Clinical and imaging correlation and appropriate amount of tissue sampling especially in mixed lesions are important for accurate diagnosis and clinical management of the disease.

Abbreviations

NET	Neuroendocrine tumors
SSC-H	Small cell carcinoma of hypercalcemic type
WHO	World Health Organization
SSC-P	Small cell carcinoma of the ovary-pulmonary type
SmCC	Small-cell neuroendocrine carcinoma
SEER	Surveillance, Epidemiology, and End Results
FIGO	International Federation of Gynecology and Obstetrics
MSI	Microsatellite instability
CGH	Comparative genomic hybridization
MCC	Merkel cell carcinoma

References

1. Roth LM, Goheen MP, Broshears JR. Malignant Brenner tumor of the ovary with transformation to trabecular carcinoid: an immunocytochemical and electron microscopic study. Int J Gynecol Pathol. 2012;31(1):91–7. PubMed Epub 2011/11/30. eng.
2. Ramalingam P, Malpica A, Deavers MT. Mixed endocervical adenocarcinoma and high-grade neuroendocrine carcinoma of the cervix with ovarian metastasis of the former component: a report of 2 cases. Int J Gynecol Pathol. 2012;31(5):490–6. PubMed Epub 2012/07/27. eng.
3. Chenevert J, Bessette P, Plante M, Tetu B, Dube V. Mixed ovarian large cell neuroendocrine carcinoma, mucinous adenocarcinoma, and teratoma: a report of two cases and review of the literature. Pathol Res Pract. 2009;205(9):657–61. PubMed Epub 2009/07/07. eng.
4. Grandjean M, Legrand L, Waterkeyn M, Baurain JF, Jadoul P, Donnez J, et al. Small cell carcinoma of pulmonary type inside a microinvasive mucinous cystadenocarcinoma of the ovary: a case report. Int J Gynecol Pathol. 2007;26(4):426–31. PubMed Epub 2007/09/22. eng.
5. Veras E, Deavers MT, Silva EG, Malpica A. Ovarian nonsmall cell neuroendocrine carcinoma: a clinicopathologic and immunohistochemical study of 11 cases. Am J Surg Pathol. 2007;31(5):774–82. PubMed Epub 2007/04/27. eng.
6. Rouzbahman M, Clarke B. Neuroendocrine tumors of the gynecologic tract: select topics. Semin Diagn Pathol. 2013;30(3):224–33. PubMed Epub 2013/10/23. eng.
7. Rosai J. The origin of neuroendocrine tumors and the neural crest saga. Modern Pathol. 2011;24 Suppl 2:S53–7. PubMed Epub 2011/04/06. eng.
8. Andrew A, Kramer B, Rawdon BB. The origin of gut and pancreatic neuroendocrine (APUD) cells – the last word? J Pathol. 1998;186(2):117–8. PubMed Epub 1999/01/30. eng.
9. Scully RE, Aguirre P, DeLellis RA. Argyrophilia, serotonin, and peptide hormones in the female genital tract and its tumors. Int J Gynecol Pathol. 1984;3(1):51–70. PubMed Epub 1984/01/01. eng.
10. Voutsadakis IA. Large cell neuroendocrine carcinoma of the ovary: a pathologic entity in search of clinical identity. World J Clin Oncol. 2014;5(2):36–8. PubMed Pubmed Central PMCID: PMC4014794, Epub 2014/05/16. eng.
11. Soga J, Osaka M, Yakuwa Y. Carcinoids of the ovary: an analysis of 329 reported cases. J Exp Clin Cancer Res. 2000;19(3):271–80. PubMed Epub 2001/01/06. eng.
12. Davis KP, Hartmann LK, Keeney GL, Shapiro H. Primary ovarian carcinoid tumors. Gynecol Oncol. 1996;61(2):259–65. PubMed Epub 1996/05/01. eng.
13. Robboy SJ, Scully RE, Norris HJ. Carcinoid metastatic to the ovary. A clinicopathologic analysis of 35 cases. Cancer. 1974;33(3):798–811. PubMed Epub 1974/03/01. eng.

14. Serratoni FT, Robboy SJ. Ultrastructure of primary and metastatic ovarian carcinoids: analysis of 11 cases. Cancer. 1975;36(1):157–60. PubMed Epub 1975/07/01. eng.
15. Baker PM, Oliva E, Young RH, Talerman A, Scully RE. Ovarian mucinous carcinoids including some with a carcinomatous component: a report of 17 cases. Am J Surg Pathol. 2001;25(5):557–68. PubMed Epub 2001/05/09. eng.
16. Vang R, Gown AM, Zhao C, Barry TS, Isacson C, Richardson MS, et al. Ovarian mucinous tumors associated with mature cystic teratomas: morphologic and immunohistochemical analysis identifies a subset of potential teratomatous origin that shares features of lower gastrointestinal tract mucinous tumors more commonly encountered as secondary tumors in the ovary. Am J Surg Pathol. 2007;31(6):854–69. PubMed Epub 2007/05/29. eng.
17. Jiang Y, Long H, Wang W, Liu H, Tang Y, Zhang X. Clinicopathological features and immunoexpression profiles of goblet cell carcinoid and typical carcinoid of the appendix. Pathol Oncol Res. 2011;17(1):127–32. PubMed Epub 2010/07/20. eng.
18. Talerman A. Carcinoid tumors of the ovary. J Cancer Res Clin Oncol. 1984;107(2):125–35. PubMed Epub 1984/01/01. eng.
19. Snyder RR, Tavassoli FA. Ovarian strumal carcinoid: immunohistochemical, ultrastructural, and clinicopathologic observations. Int J Gynecol Pathol. 1986;5(3):187–201. PubMed Epub 1986/01/01. eng.
20. Desouki MM, Lioyd J, Xu H, Cao D, Barner R, Zhao C. CDX2 may be a useful marker to distinguish primary ovarian carcinoid from gastrointestinal metastatic carcinoids to the ovary. Hum Pathol. 2013;44(11):2536–41. PubMed Epub 2013/09/14. eng.
21. Rabban JT, Lerwill MF, McCluggage WG, Grenert JP, Zaloudek CJ. Primary ovarian carcinoid tumors may express CDX-2: a potential pitfall in distinction from metastatic intestinal carcinoid tumors involving the ovary. Int J Gynecol Pathol. 2009;28(1):41–8. PubMed Epub 2008/12/03. eng.
22. Robert J, Kurman MLC, Simon Herrington C, Young RH. WHO classification of tumours of female reproductive organs. Lyon, France: WHO; 2014. p. 69–73.
23. McCluggage WG, Oliva E, Connolly LE, McBride HA, Young RH. An immunohistochemical analysis of ovarian small cell carcinoma of hypercalcemic type. Int J Gynecol Pathol. 2004;23(4):330–6. PubMed Epub 2004/09/24. eng.
24. Ramos P, Karnezis AN, Craig DW, Sekulic A, Russell ML, Hendricks WP, et al. Small cell carcinoma of the ovary, hypercalcemic type, displays frequent inactivating germline and somatic mutations in SMARCA4. Nat Genet. 2014;46(5):427–9. PubMed Epub 2014/03/25. eng.
25. Foulkes WD, Clarke BA, Hasselblatt M, Majewski J, Albrecht S, McCluggage WG. No small surprise – small cell carcinoma of the ovary, hypercalcaemic type, is a malignant rhabdoid tumour. J Pathol. 2014;233(3):209–14. PubMed Epub 2014/04/23. eng.
26. Eichhorn JH, Young RH, Scully RE. Primary ovarian small cell carcinoma of pulmonary type. A clinicopathologic, immunohistologic, and flow cytometric analysis of 11 cases. Am J Surg Pathol. 1992;16(10):926–38. PubMed Epub 1992/10/01. eng.
27. Fukunaga M, Endo Y, Miyazawa Y, Ushigome S. Small cell neuroendocrine carcinoma of the ovary. Virchows Arch. 1997;430(4):343–8. PubMed Epub 1997/04/01. eng.
28. Brown H, Lane M. Cushing's and malignant carcinoid syndromes from ovarian neoplasm. Arch Intern Med. 1965;115:490–4. PubMed Epub 1965/04/01. eng.
29. Crochet P, Luneau F, Rojat-Habib MC, Agostini A. Primary neuroendocrine carcinoma of the fallopian tube: a case report. Gynecol Oncol Case Rep. 2012;4:38–40. PubMed Pubmed Central PMCID: PMC3862233, Epub 2012/01/01. eng.
30. Robert J, Kurma MLC, Simon Herrington C, Young RH. WHO classification of tumours of female reproductive organs. WHO; 2014. p. 196–8.
31. Yasuoka T, Hashimoto H, Hamada K, Fujioka T, Nawa A. Atypical carcinoid of the uterine cervix with aggressive clinical behavior: a case report. Gynecol Oncol Case Rep. 2014;7:4–6. PubMed Pubmed Central PMCID: PMC3895285, Epub 2014/03/14. eng.
32. Mannion C, Park WS, Man YG, Zhuang Z, Albores-Saavedra J, Tavassoli FA. Endocrine tumors of the cervix: morphologic assessment, expression of human papillomavirus, and

evaluation for loss of heterozygosity on 1p,3p, 11q, and 17p. Cancer. 1998;83(7):1391–400. PubMed Epub 1998/10/08. eng.
33. McCusker ME, Cote TR, Clegg LX, Tavassoli FJ. Endocrine tumors of the uterine cervix: incidence, demographics, and survival with comparison to squamous cell carcinoma. Gynecol Oncol. 2003;88(3):333–9. PubMed Epub 2003/03/22. eng.
34. Chen J, Macdonald OK, Gaffney DK. Incidence, mortality, and prognostic factors of small cell carcinoma of the cervix. Obstet Gynecol. 2008;111(6):1394–402. PubMed Epub 2008/06/03. eng.
35. Atienza-Amores M, Guerini-Rocco E, Soslow RA, Park KJ, Weigelt B. Small cell carcinoma of the gynecologic tract: a multifaceted spectrum of lesions. Gynecol Oncol. 2014;134(2): 410–8. PubMed Epub 2014/05/31. Eng.
36. Tsunoda S, Jobo T, Arai M, Imai M, Kanai T, Tamura T, et al. Small-cell carcinoma of the uterine cervix: a clinicopathologic study of 11 cases. Int J Gynecol Cancer. 2005;15(2): 295–300. PubMed Epub 2005/04/13. eng.
37. Crowder S, Tuller E. Small cell carcinoma of the female genital tract. Semin Oncol. 2007;34(1):57–63. PubMed Epub 2007/02/03. eng.
38. Abeler VM, Holm R, Nesland JM, Kjorstad KE. Small cell carcinoma of the cervix. A clinicopathologic study of 26 patients. Cancer. 1994;73(3):672–7. PubMed Epub 1994/02/01. eng.
39. Ishida GM, Kato N, Hayasaka T, Saito M, Kobayashi H, Katayama Y, et al. Small cell neuroendocrine carcinomas of the uterine cervix: a histological, immunohistochemical, and molecular genetic study. Int J Gynecol Pathol. 2004;23(4):366–72. PubMed Epub 2004/09/24. eng.
40. Dongol S, Tai Y, Shao Y, Jiang J, Kong B. A retrospective clinicopathological analysis of small-cell carcinoma of the uterine cervix. Mol Clin Oncol. 2014;2(1):71–5. PubMed Pubmed Central PMCID: PMC3915860, Epub 2014/03/22. Eng.
41. Wang Y, Mei K, Xiang MF, Li JM, Xie RM. Clinicopathological characteristics and outcome of patients with small cell neuroendocrine carcinoma of the uterine cervix: case series and literature review. Eur J Gynaecol Oncol. 2013;34(4):307–10. PubMed Epub 2013/09/12. eng.
42. Rhemtula H, Grayson W, van Iddekinge B, Tiltman A. Large-cell neuroendocrine carcinoma of the uterine cervix – a clinicopathological study of five cases. South African Med J. 2001;91(6):525–8. PubMed Epub 2001/07/18. eng.
43. Sato Y, Shimamoto T, Amada S, Asada Y, Hayashi T. Large cell neuroendocrine carcinoma of the uterine cervix: a clinicopathological study of six cases. Int J Gynecol Pathol. 2003; 22(3):226–30. PubMed Epub 2003/06/24. eng.
44. Mhawech-Fauceglia P, Chan A, Keitz B, Lele S, Cheney RT, Starostik P. Microsatellite instability in large cell neuroendocrine carcinoma of the female genital tract. Histopathology. 2009;55(5):621–5. PubMed Epub 2009/11/17. eng.
45. Kawauchi S, Okuda S, Morioka H, Iwasaki F, Fukuma F, Chochi Y, et al. Large cell neuroendocrine carcinoma of the uterine cervix with cytogenetic analysis by comparative genomic hybridization: a case study. Hum Pathol. 2005;36(10):1096–100. PubMed Epub 2005/10/18. eng.
46. Katahira A, Akahira J, Niikura H, Ito K, Moriya T, Matsuzawa S, et al. Small cell carcinoma of the endometrium: report of three cases and literature review. Int J Gynecol Cancer. 2004;14(5):1018–23. PubMed Epub 2004/09/14. eng.
47. Shaco-Levy R, Manor E, Piura B, Ariel I. An unusual composite endometrial tumor combining papillary serous carcinoma and small cell carcinoma. Am J Surg Pathol. 2004;28(8):1103–6. PubMed Epub 2004/07/15. eng.
48. Van Eeden S, Nederlof PM, Taal BG, Offerhaus GJ, Van Velthuysen ML. A tumour with a neuroendocrine and papillary serous component: two or a pair? J Clin Pathol. 2002;55(9): 710–4. PubMed Pubmed Central PMCID: PMC1769742, Epub 2002/08/27. eng.
49. Posligua L, Malpica A, Liu J, Brown J, Deavers MT. Combined large cell neuroendocrine carcinoma and papillary serous carcinoma of the endometrium with pagetoid spread. Arch Pathol Lab Med. 2008;132(11):1821–4. PubMed Epub 2008/11/04. eng.
50. Mulvany NJ, Allen DG. Combined large cell neuroendocrine and endometrioid carcinoma of the endometrium. Int J Gynecol Pathol. 2008;27(1):49–57. PubMed Epub 2007/12/25.eng.

51. Mhawech-Fauceglia P, Odunsi K, Dim D, Nowak N, Lele S, Cheney RT, et al. Array-comparative genomic hybridization analysis of primary endometrial and ovarian high-grade neuroendocrine carcinoma associated with adenocarcinoma: mystery resolved? Int J Gynecol Pathol. 2008;27(4):539–46. PubMed Epub 2008/08/30.eng.
52. Tafe LJ, Garg K, Chew I, Tornos C, Soslow RA. Endometrial and ovarian carcinomas with undifferentiated components: clinically aggressive and frequently underrecognized neoplasms. Modern Pathol. 2010;23(6):781–9. PubMed Epub 2010/03/23. eng.
53. Nguyen ML, Han L, Minors AM, Bentley-Hibbert S, Pradhan TS, Pua TL, et al. Rare large cell neuroendocrine tumor of the endometrium: a case report and review of the literature. Int J Surg Case Rep. 2013;4(8):651–5. PubMed Pubmed Central PMCID: PMC3710906, Epub 2013/06/25. eng.
54. Tamura R, Yokoyama Y, Kobayashi A, Osawa Y, Shigeto T, Futagami M, et al. A case of small cell carcinoma of the vagina. Rare Tumors. 2013;5(4):e58. PubMed Pubmed Central PMCID: PMC3882930, Epub 2014/01/15. eng.
55. Coleman NM, Smith-Zagone MJ, Tanyi J, Anderson ML, Coleman RL, Dyson SW, et al. Primary neuroendocrine carcinoma of the vagina with Merkel cell carcinoma phenotype. Am J Surg Pathol. 2006;30(3):405–10. PubMed Epub 2006/03/16. eng.
56. ElNaggar AC, Patil AS, Singh K, Reed ME. Neuroendocrine carcinoma of the vagina in pregnancy. Obstet Gynecol. 2012;119(2 Pt 2):445–7. PubMed Epub 2012/01/25. eng.
57. Khurana A, Gupta G, Gupta M, Kaur M. Primary neuroendocrine carcinoma of the vagina with coexistent atypical vaginal adenosis: a rare entity. J Cancer Res Ther. 2013;9(2):328–30. PubMed Epub 2013/06/19. eng.
58. Albores-Saavedra J, Batich K, Chable-Montero F, Sagy N, Schwartz AM, Henson DE. Merkel cell carcinoma demographics, morphology, and survival based on 3870 cases: a population based study. J Cutan Pathol. 2010;37(1):20–7. PubMed Epub 2009/07/30. eng.
59. Srivastava SA, Wang Y, Vallone J, Felix JC. Primary clear cell carcinoid tumors of the vulva. Am J Surg Pathol. 2012;36(9):1371–5. PubMed Epub 2012/08/17. eng.

Pathology of Merkel Cell Carcinoma (Primary Neuroendocrine Carcinoma of the Skin)

Carlos N. Prieto-Granada and Jane L. Messina

Introduction

Merkel cell carcinoma (MCC), also known as primary cutaneous neuroendocrine carcinoma and historically as trabecular carcinoma and as "APUDoma," is a rare skin tumor with an aggressive clinical behavior and a predilection for the elderly and the immunosuppressed. Dr. Cyril Toker first described this entity in 1972 under the rubric of trabecular carcinoma [1]. Dr. Toker characterized this tumor as a primary cutaneous carcinoma composed of small round blue cells that could be potentially confused for metastatic carcinoma. In subsequent papers, he attributed sudoriferous and neurosecretory features to the tumor cells, speculating that the tumor may have originated from normal Merkel cells, sweat glands, or a pluripotential precursor [2]. The term Merkel cell carcinoma, the most widely accepted name for the entity, was coined by De Wolff-Peeters in 1980 [3]. The question of the "cell of origin" from which MCC arises has been a matter of much controversy. Since MCC tumor cells share many immunophenotypic and ultrastructural features with normal Merkel cells, it was long believed that these cells act as a precursor for MCC. This notion has been further reinforced by the fact that a fraction of MCC cases can exhibit a prominent intraepidermal component as well as by the existence of an in situ MCC variant.

C.N. Prieto-Granada, MD (✉)
Dermatopathology, Department of Cutaneous Surgery and Oncology, Moffitt Cancer Center/
USF Morsani College of Medicine, 12902 USF Magnolia Dr., Tampa, FL 33612, USA
e-mail: carlos.prietogranada@moffitt.org

J.L. Messina, MD
Departments of Anatomic Pathology and Cutaneous Oncology, Moffitt Cancer Center,
12902 USF Magnolia Dr., Tampa, FL 33612, USA

Pathology and Cell Biology, Oncologic Sciences, and Dermatology, USF Morsani
College of Medicine, Tampa, FL, USA
e-mail: jane.messina@moffitt.org

A. Nasir, D. Coppola (eds.), *Neuroendocrine Tumors: Review of Pathology, Molecular and Therapeutic Advances*, DOI 10.1007/978-1-4939-3426-3_21

Normal Merkel cells, first characterized by Friedrich Sigmund Merkel in 1875, are intraepidermal neural crest-derived cells that are thought to serve as slow-acting mechanoreceptors responsible for touch and hair movement sensitivity. They occur singly or in clusters in touch domes (*haarscheibe*) in close relationship with sensory axons and along the basilar layer of the epidermis, in hair disks, and in the bulge region of the follicle [4]. As far as anatomical distribution of Merkel cells is concerned, they are widely and numerously present in sensitive areas of the skin as well as of the oral and anal mucosal surfaces. Merkel cells can also be found in high numbers populating tongue taste buds, whisker pads, palatine mucosa rugae, and the vermillion border of the lips and in hairy and glabrous sensitive skin and even in sweat glands [5]. Interestingly enough, normal Merkel cells tend to be more abundant in sun-exposed areas [5].

Recently, the concept that MCC most likely originates from a pluripotential stem cell precursor with acquired immunophenotypic and ultrastructural characteristics akin to normal Merkel cells has gained more traction [6]. This concept is further supported by the presence of divergent differentiation in some MCC cases, a phenomenon to be discussed below. Some authors have recently proposed that a possible precursor of MCC could be represented by pre-/pro-B lymphoid stem cells [7], particularly after the observation that MCC cells can express primitive B-cell markers such as PAX5 and TdT [8, 9]. It is important to point out that the discovery of the Merkel cell polyomavirus (MCPyV) [10] has truly revolutionized our understating of MCC. MCPyV is a polyomavirus, first characterized in 2008, that is found in about 80 % of MCC cases. This finding prompted a classification of MCC into two groups: the MCPyV-positive MCCs and the MCPyV-negative MCCs. This dichotomous view of MCC will be expanded below.

Epidemiological and Clinical Features

Due to the combination of an aging population, increased disease awareness, and improved diagnostic tools and criteria, the yearly incidence rate of MCC in the United States has been steadily increasing from less than 0.1 cases per 100,000 in the 1980s to 0.24 cases per 10,000 toward the end of the twentieth century [11] to up to 0.6 cases per 10,000 in 2006 [12]. A similar trend has been observed in other industrialized nations [13]. Caucasian men are the most frequently affected, with MCC only rarely affecting blacks and other ethnic groups. MCC is a tumor of the elderly with average age at presentation being 76 years old for women and 72 years old for men [12]. This entity thrives in an immunosuppressed milieu [14], and patients with HIV/AIDS [15], hematologic conditions [16], and in the post-transplant status [17–19] are at increased risk of developing MCC. The frequent link between MCC and immunosuppression triggered a suspicion for an infective agent being an etiologic factor, ultimately leading to the discovery of the MCPyV [10]. Individuals afflicted by MCC are also at increased risk of developing additional malignancies [13, 20, 21], a finding likely related to the above-mentioned fact that

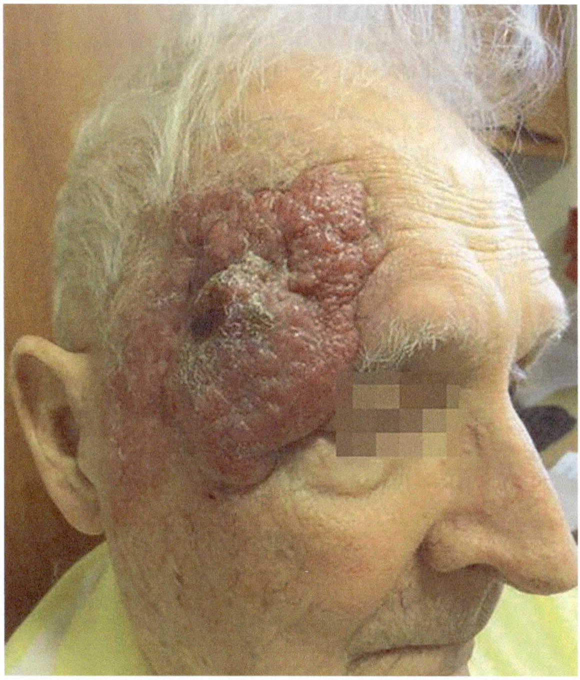

Fig. 1 Clinical presentation of MCC. Image representing the most commonly seen clinical features of MCC: a non-ulcerated erythematous head and neck mass arising in an elderly individual

these patients are frequently immunosuppressed. With regard to anatomic location, MCC frequently arises on chronically sun-damaged skin of the head and neck and extremities with rare cases arising from the trunk [12, 22–25]. However, MCC can arise in a variety of non-sun-exposed sites such as mucosal surfaces of the mouth [26–29], tongue [30], nasopharynx [31], and skin from the external genitalia [32, 33]. Lymph nodes are also mentioned as primary sites for MCC [34–37], probably representing nodal metastases from completely regressed cutaneous tumors. Rare cases of MCC-like tumors have been documented arising from the parotid gland [37–39], stomach [40], and vagina [41, 42]. Clinically, MCC often presents as a rapidly-growing painless and often firm nodule or mass with erythematous, pink, violaceous, or even bruise-like-colored overlying skin that is often non-ulcerated [14, 43] (Fig. 1). Some tumors can even exhibit a pigmented appearance [44, 45]. Due to this relatively nonspecific clinical presentation, MCC is more often included as part of a clinical differential diagnosis that includes basal cell carcinoma (BCC), squamous cell carcinoma (SCC), amelanotic melanoma, cyst, adnexal tumor, or lymphoma cutis [46]. Multicentric presentations [47] and in-transit metastatic spread [48, 49] have been reported. MCC is characterized by frequent regional nodal metastasis, and a positive lymph node status, particularly if clinically detected, is negatively correlated with outcome [50, 51]. Distant metastatic spread can affect a wide variety of organs and anatomical sites including the iris [52], brain [53–55], meninges [56, 57], gingiva [58],oropharynx [59], heart [60–63], gastrointestinal tract [64–66] (Fig. 2), pancreas [67, 68], genitourinary system [69–73], and soft

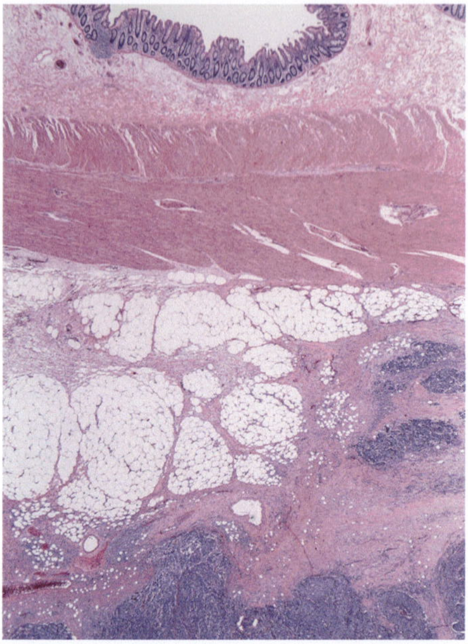

Fig. 2 MCC can metastasize to a variety of anatomical sites, including the gastrointestinal tract as in this case where tumor nodules can be appreciated involving the pericolic adipose tissue (H&E, 1.5×)

tissue [74]. Cases of MCC exhibiting massive involvement of bone marrow [75] and leukemic dissemination [76] have been described, and although they are extremely rare events, such occurrences carry an obvious dismal prognosis. Spontaneous regression of MCC is an unusual but well-documented phenomenon [77–86] that may account for a good proportion of cases described as "primary" lymph node MCCs [34–36, 87–90] as well as for cases with unknown primary [91–94]. As is the case with other small cell carcinomas with neuroendocrine features, MCC can very rarely exhibit paraneoplastic manifestations such as thrombocytopenia [95], hyponatremia from ectopic ACTH production [96], and Lambert-Eaton syndrome [97].

Light Microscopic Findings

MCC is most often a dermal tumor, centered in the mid-dermis and exhibiting a Grenz zone. A fraction of the cases (up to 10 %) will display a prominent intraepidermal component, sometimes even more prominent than the dermal component [18, 98–102]. Pure in situ intraepidermal variants can be rarely encountered [103, 104]. On H&E-stained tissue sections, the presence of dark-blue dermal nodules "grossly" distinguishable on the glass slide section even before placing it under the microscope is a characteristic of this tumor. The tumor's deeply basophilic hue reflects the fact that it represents a "small round blue cell" (SRBC) proliferation, thus composed of monomorphic small- to medium-sized cells bearing hyperchromatic nuclei and scant cytoplasm. These cells can be arranged in a variety of

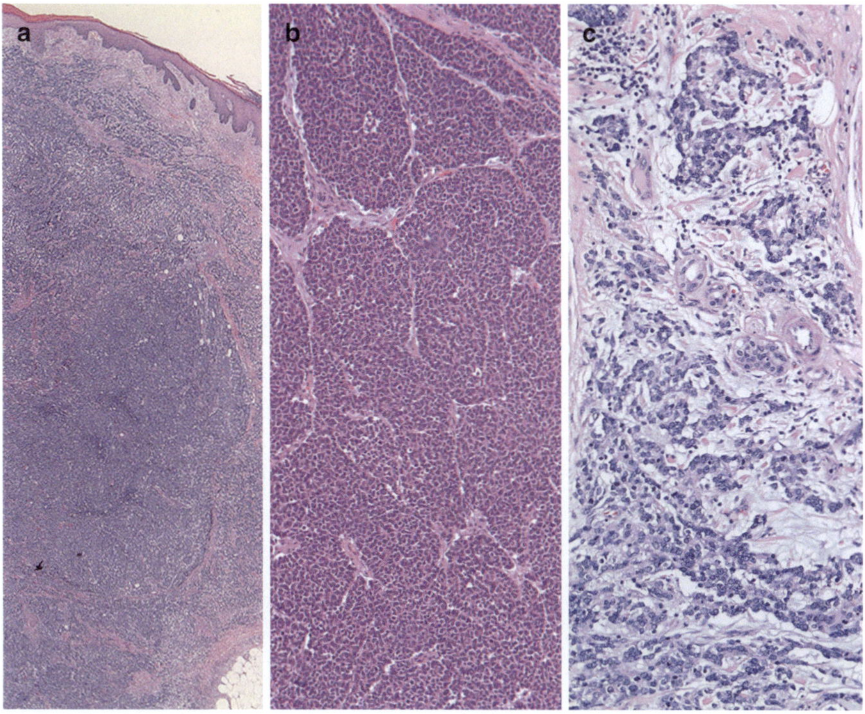

Fig. 3 Panel exhibiting some of the growth patterns seen with MCC including sheets (**a**), nests (**c**), and trabecular (**c**). Note the Grenz zone on image **a** (H&E, **a**: 1.5×, **b**: 100×, **c**: 200×)

patterns: large sheets, nests, and cords or the characteristic trabeculae that prompted the tumor's first moniker (Fig. 3). As is characteristic of small cell carcinomas and SRBC tumors, the lesional cells are often closely packed but lack intercellular cohesion, a consequence of dysfunctional E-cadherin/beta-catenin machinery, which mediates intercellular adhesion [105, 106]. This growth pattern can make evaluation for lymphovascular invasion (LVI) and margin status a quite difficult task. Nevertheless, *Bona fide* LVI is a frequent finding in MCC, particularly in thick tumors (Fig. 4). The tumor borders can be pushing or infiltrative, a distinction that might carry prognostic significance, as will be discussed below. Other features akin to SRBC and high-grade neuroendocrine tumors can be often seen in MCC, such as nuclear molding as well as signs of high cell turnover with numerous readily identifiable mitotic figures and apoptotic bodies. Classically, three morphologic patterns have been recognized: trabecular, intermediate, and small cell (Fig. 5). However, these morphologic variants have no correlation with clinical outcome [107] and are commonly found in combination in a single tumor. Furthermore, MCCs can exhibit a myriad of additional growth patterns, including organoid [108] and spindle cell patterns (Fig. 6), as well as tumors forming Homer-Wright rosettes [18, 98, 109] and some exhibiting a pseudo-follicular type of arrangement (Fig. 7). Cytologically distinctive tumor cell features include pleomorphic and plasmacytoid forms and

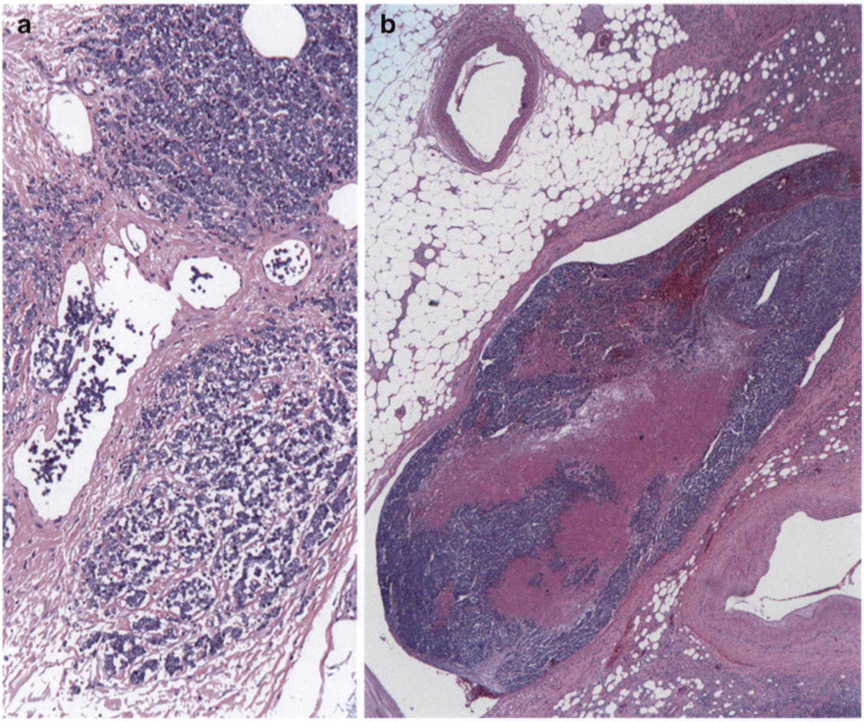

Fig. 4 Lymphovascular invasion (LVI) is a frequent finding in MCC and is an adverse prognostic factor. One can either find intravascular small nests and tumor cells at the edge of the tumor (**a**) or even extreme cases of large tumor emboli (**b**) (H&E, **a**: 100×, **b**: 1.5×)

cells with "washed-out" nuclear chromatin (Fig. 5) [110]. The so-called Azzopardi phenomenon, a feature frequently seen in SRBC and high-grade neuroendocrine tumors that relates to the increased cell fragility due to a practically absent cytoplasm, can be identified in MCCs [111, 112]. The stroma surrounding the tumor cells often shows a mucinous/myxoid appearance (Fig. 5), but it can also be sclerotic or show deposition of amyloid-like material [110]. Varying amounts of newly formed vessels, a product of reactive angiogenesis, can be identified surrounding MCCs [112]. In addition, it is not unusual to find prominent peri-tumoral lymphocytic infiltrates [110], sometimes adopting a follicular pattern [113]. Since MCC likely originates from a pluripotential stem cell precursor [6], this entity has the potential to exhibit quite varied types of divergent differentiation. Some of the described associated divergent phenotypes associated with MCC include squamous, glandular (Fig. 8), basal cell carcinoma, melanocytic, rhabdomyosarcomatous, leiomyosarcomatous, fibrosarcomatous, neuroblastic, and even atypical fibroxanthoma-like [114–128]. The most common associated neoplasm identified closely associated with MCC is squamous cell carcinoma (either in situ or invasive), which is recognized in approximately one-third of cases. Rare variants of MCC mimicking other

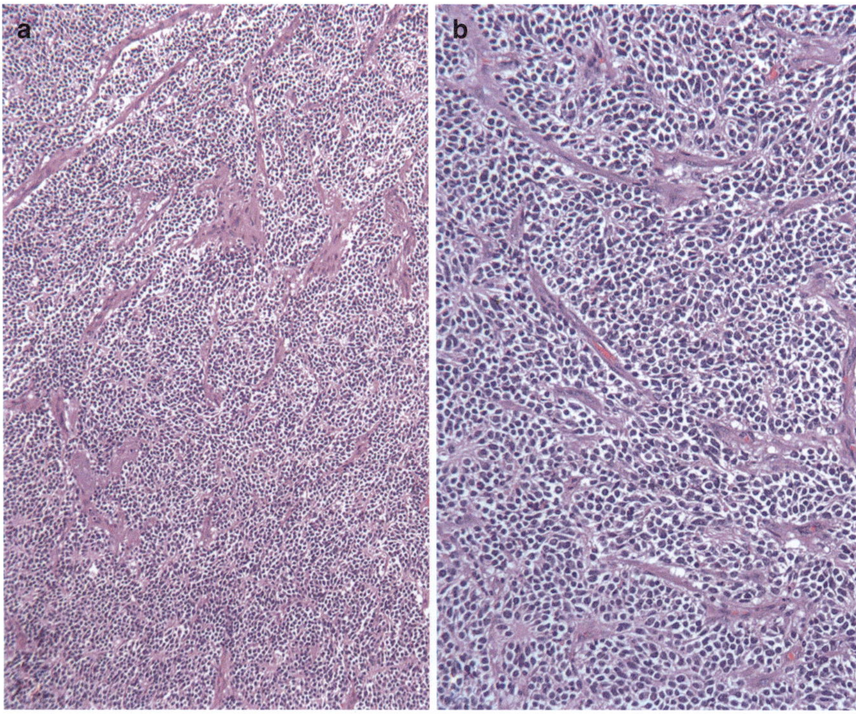

Fig. 5 MCC with small cell pattern, indistinguishable from other small cell carcinomas. Some authors claim it corresponds to the MCPyV-positive tumors. Note the nuclear molding (H&E, **a**: 40×, **b**: 200×).

skin neoplasms have been described, such as lymphoepithelioma-like [129, 130] and microcystic adnexal carcinoma-like [131] patterns.

As previously mentioned, MCC tends to arise in chronically sun-damaged skin. Thus, concomitant actinic keratosis, both invasive and in situ SCC (Fig. 9) and BCC, is often recognized [18, 103, 115, 128, 132–141]. In fact, similar UV-signature *TP53* mutations can be found in both squamous cell carcinoma and MCC [142] suggesting a similar tumorigenesis pathway, and these MCC examples are often MCPyV negative [133, 141, 143]. Recent studies claim that there are somewhat specific morphologic features that will distinguish MCPyV-positive from MCPyV-negative MCCs, with a decent correlation when compared against immunohistochemical and molecular tests for the virus. The features associated with MCPyV-negative MCC include an association with SCC, cells with abundant cytoplasm, and larger pleomorphic and irregular nuclei, roughly corresponding to the "intermediate cell" type. On the other hand, MCPyV-positive MCC will have smaller cells with higher nuclear to cytoplasmic ratio and round nuclei, corresponding to the previously described "small cell variant" [144, 145]. Aside from the above-mentioned association between MCC and SCC, several other cutaneous lesions have been described to arise in conjunction with MCC including sebaceous

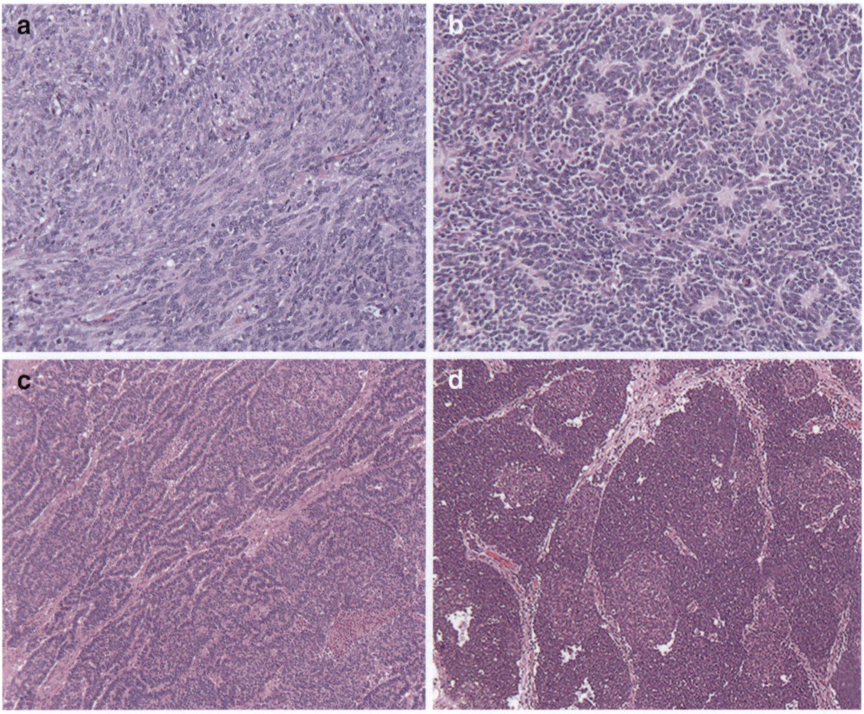

Fig. 6 Composite image demonstrating less frequent growth patterns in MCC, a spindle cell (**a**), an example with well-formed Homer-Wright rosettes (**b**), an example with a striking organoid arrangement (**c**), and a tumor exhibiting a "pseudo-follicular" pattern, in the manner of medulloblastoma (**d**) (H&E, **a** and **b** 200×, **c** and **d**: 100×)

carcinoma [146], atypical fibroxanthoma [147], and trichilemmal [148, 149] and infundibular follicular [150] cysts. Another well-documented and worth mentioning association is that with chronic lymphocytic leukemia/small lymphocytic lymphoma (CLL/SLL) (Fig. 10) [13, 16, 151–154]. As commented above this phenomenon is likely related to both the immunosuppressed milieu and the older population of patients in which MCC arises. Interestingly, although recent findings have suggested shared molecular events between CLL/SLL and MCC [16], it is likely that these two entities do not share the same pathogenesis [155].

The main morphologic differential diagnosis of MCC includes metastases from small cell carcinomas of other origins, particularly pulmonary, from which it can be practically indistinguishable by morphology. The possibility of a lymphoid neoplasm should also be ruled out. Other less frequently encountered differential diagnostic possibilities include other primary SRBC tumors that can rarely arise in the skin such as the superficial variant of Ewing sarcoma [156–159] and the rare small cell melanoma. In the unique and unusual occurrence of a purely in situ MCC, one should consider the differential of pagetoid entities such as superficial spreading melanoma and cutaneous T-cell lymphoma [98, 99, 103]. Fortunately, in the majority of the

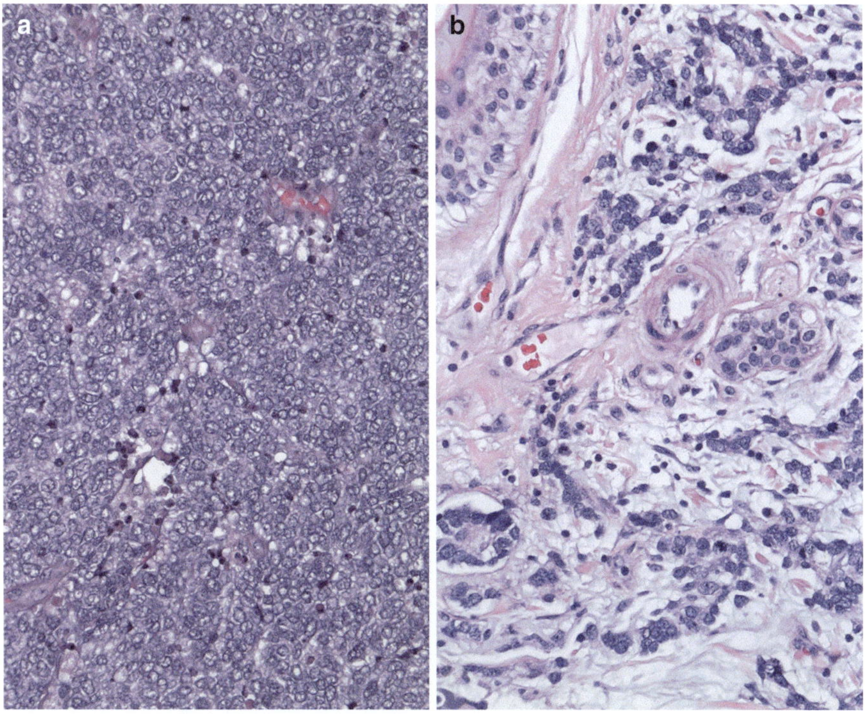

Fig. 7 "Cleared out" chromatin in MCC tumor cells (**a**) and the frequently encountered myxoid stromal reaction adjacent to MCC (H&E, **a** and **b**: 400×)

cases, immunohistochemical staining patterns differ between these entities, allowing for correct classification. Please refer to the immunohistochemistry section for a complete discussion.

Immunohistochemical Aspects of MCC

Just like their normal "counterparts," MCC cells usually and characteristically express cytokeratins and neuroendocrine markers with the prototypical immunoprofile of CK7 negative, CK20 positive, synaptophysin, and chromogranin positive [160]. Albeit quite nonspecific and thus rarely used, another neuroendocrine/neural marker that is frequently described as positive in MCC is neuron-specific enolase (NSE). Regarding the cytokeratins, it is important to emphasize the quite distinctive staining pattern with CK20 found in MCC cells: a strong, paranuclear dot-like signal that either can be found in its "pure" form or accompanied by a diffuse perinuclear or membranous staining. In the latter case, the pattern is best characterized as paranuclear dot-like "accentuation" [107, 161, 162] (Fig. 11) (Importantly, *peri* is a Greek prefix for "around" or "about," while the *para* prefix means "alongside" or

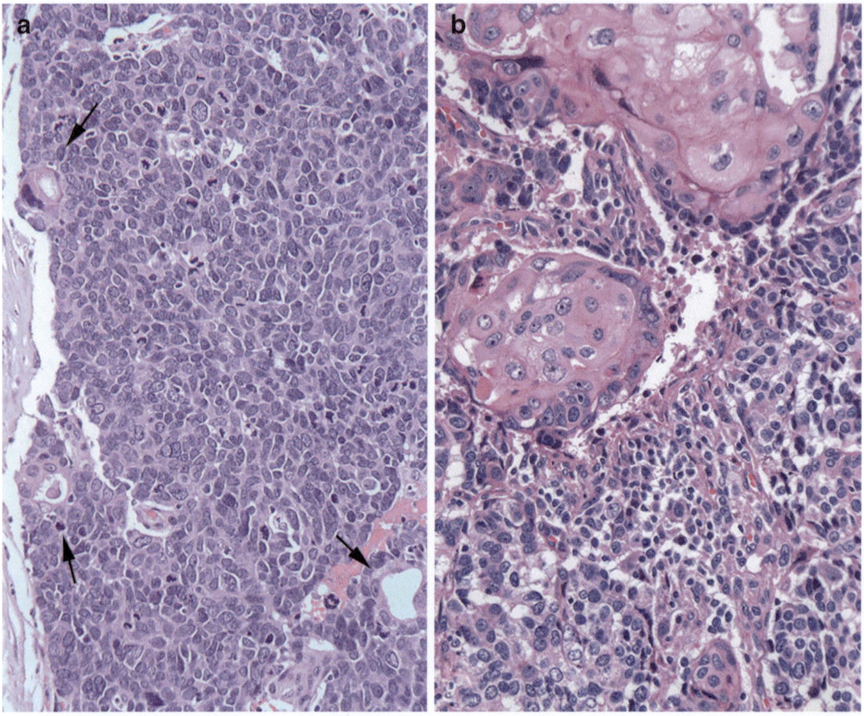

Fig. 8 Glandular (**a**, *arrows*) and squamous (**b**) differentiations in MCC tumors are rarely encountered features (H&E, **a** and **b**: 400×)

"beside"). CK20 and keratin cocktails (CAM 5.2 and AE1:AE3) are particularly useful when evaluating lymph nodes for metastatic disease [163], a procedure that can be quite challenging if one were to use only morphology, particularly in small metastatic deposits (Fig. 12). The distinctive staining pattern with CK20 is replicated in staining for neurofilament [164, 165] and/or CAM 5.2 and AE1:AE3 keratin cocktails and translates to paranuclear accumulation of intermediate filaments, a constant ultrastructural feature of MCC tumor cells. Nevertheless, it is worth emphasizing that both of these immunohistochemical and ultrastructural features can also be observed in a wide variety of other SRBC tumors and small cell (high-grade neuroendocrine) carcinomas from other organs [166–170]. Another important caveat to take in account is that up to 38 % of MCCs can exhibit CK7 positivity [171] with some cases having a CK7+/CK20− immunophenotype [172, 173]. Interestingly enough, normal Merkel cells exhibit a strong, diffuse, and homogeneous cytoplasmic pattern when stained with CK20 and keratin cocktails, and they can also exhibit CK7 positivity [174]. Other epithelial markers expressed in MCC include BerEP4 [100] and p63. Expression of p63 in early-stage MCC has been correlated with progression of disease and worse prognosis [175–177]; however, subsequent studies yielded only a small fraction of MCC expressing p63 without correlation with survival, raising questions about the prognostic utility of this

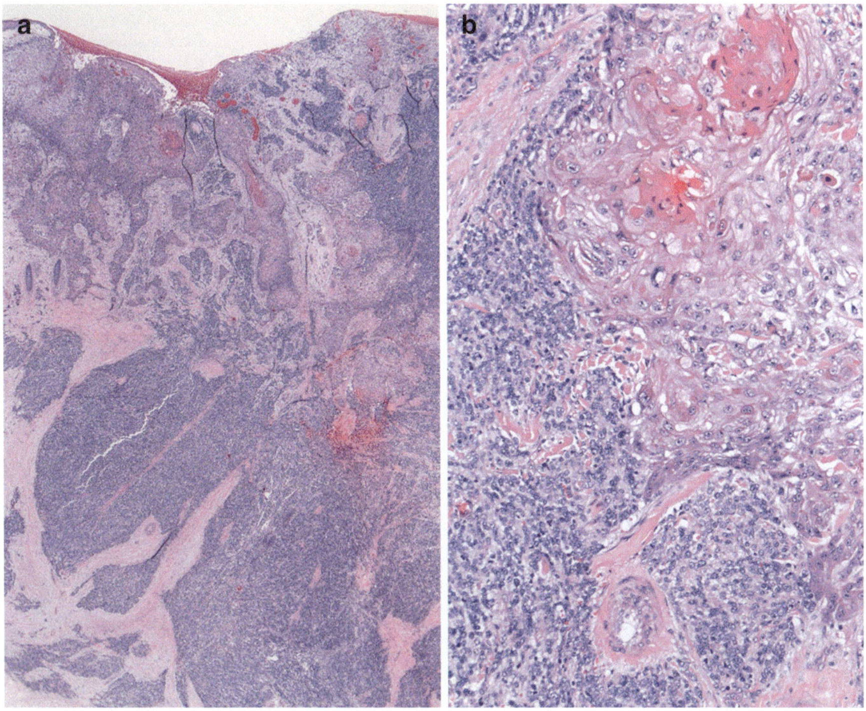

Fig. 9 MCC arising in association with a squamous cell carcinoma (SCC). These tumors tend to be MCPyV negative (H&E, **a**:1.5×, **b**: 200×)

marker [176, 178]. Following the discovery of the MCPyV [10], an antibody clone directed to the large T antigen (LT-Ag) of the virus (CM2B4) was developed [179]. This antibody shows a diffuse nuclear signal by immunohistochemistry (Fig. 13) and performs fairly well and has been shown to have a sensitivity ranging from 77 to 95 % and specificity of 83 %, when compared to MCPyV detection via molecular techniques [133, 145, 179]. The Ab3 clone, a recently developed antibody directed to a different epitope of LT-Ag, has allegedly outperformed CM2B4, with a sensitivity of 97 % [180]. Importantly, these antibodies can certainly be used as diagnostic tools since it is usually not expressed in tumors within the differential diagnosis [133, 180]. Along the lines of the proposed dichotomous model of two tumor pathways (UV-damage *TP53* mutated and MCPyV driven), expression of p53 has been more frequently found in the context of MCPyV-negative MCC tumors, with the p53-positive cases accounting for around 20 % [181] which corresponds to both the proportion of MCPyV-negative tumors and the *TP53*-mutated tumors [142, 182, 183]. Likewise, loss of expression of Rb protein by immunohistochemistry has been related to the MCPyV-negative group of tumors; however, recent data suggest that an underlying dysfunction of the *RB* gene is present in both MCC groups (MCPyV positive and negative) via two different mechanisms [184]. This interplay will be further discussed in the pathogenesis and prognosis sections. Several studies have

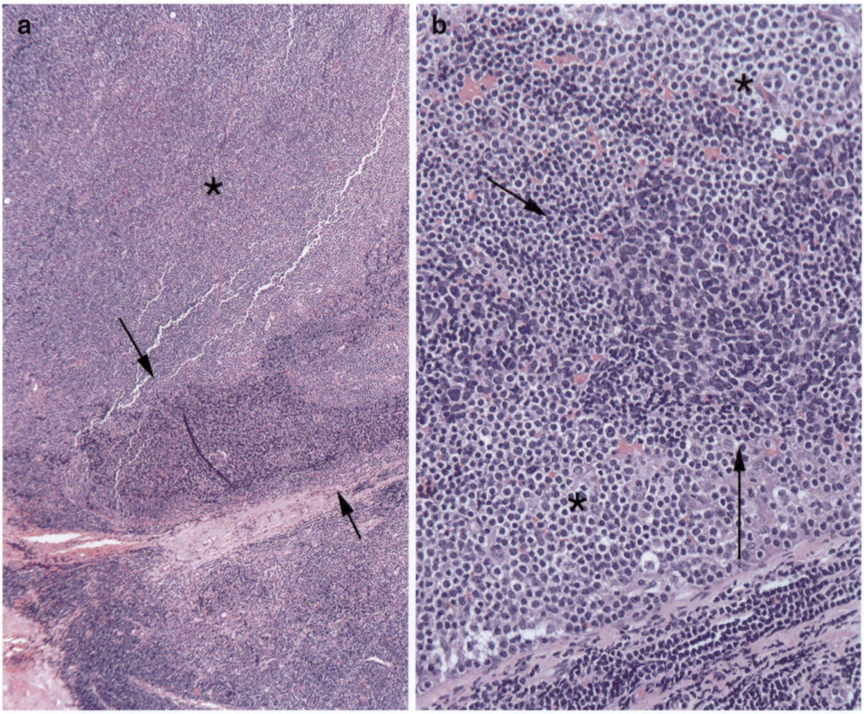

Fig. 10 MCC metastatic deposits (*arrows*) in a lymph node affected by CLL/SLL (*asterisks*). This association is not surprising due to MCC relationship with immunosuppressed and older individuals (H&E, **a**: 40×, **b**: 200×)

demonstrated that MCC is positive for c-kit (CD117) immunohistochemical staining in approximately 50 % of patients [185–188], without a clear correlation with clinical outcome. Unfortunately, this feature is not related to activating *KIT* mutations; MCC is virtually unresponsive to small molecule tyrosine kinase inhibitor therapeutic agents such as imatinib [181, 189–191].

As previously mentioned, the morphologic differential diagnosis of MCC includes several completely unrelated entities requiring immunohistochemical evaluation to be solved. In the following section, we will describe these entities and their different staining patterns. Please see Table 1 for a concise review of the main immunohistochemical differential diagnosis of MCC. First and foremost, a crucial distinction to be made is between MCC and metastatic small cell carcinoma, particularly of pulmonary origin. In this setting, immunohistochemistry for thyroid transcription factor 1 (TTF-1) is of paramount importance. The great majority of MCC are negative for TTF-1, while a large proportion of pulmonary small cell carcinomas and other small cell carcinomas will be positive with this marker [167, 171, 192, 193]. There are rare but well-documented examples of TTF-1-positive MCC, with two cases in which the TTF-1 positivity was present in MCC metastases [55, 194–196]. These unusual examples comprise about 1.1 % of the MCC cases that

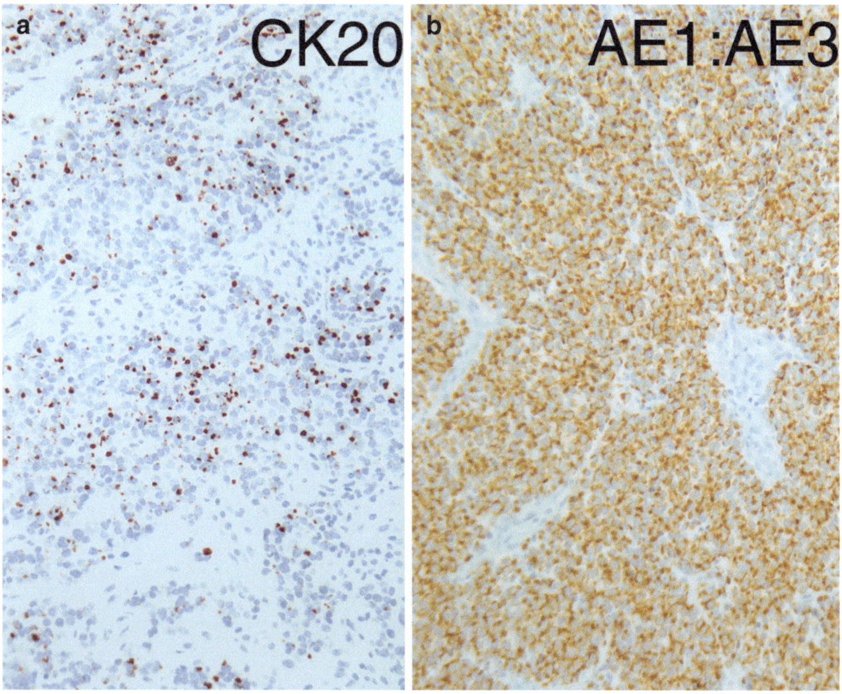

Fig. 11 Cytokeratin immunohistochemistry for MCC, either CK20 or cytokeratin cocktails (AE1:AE3 and Cam 5.2) can potentially exhibit these patterns, the "globular" or "dot-like" paranuclear signal (**a**) or the "dot-like" paranuclear accentuation of the signal (**b**) (**a**: CK20 immunohistochemistry, 400×, **b**: AE1: AE3 immunohistochemistry, 400×)

were tested for TTF-1 according to a recent review [143]. A newly described marker that has been deemed as helpful in the MCC versus small cell lung carcinoma (SCLC) differential is the mammalian/human achaete-scute complex homolog 1 (MASH1/hASH1). This is a transcription factor related to neuroendocrine development that is retained in the majority of SCLCs tested, suggesting that it may be more specific than TTF-1 [195] in this differential diagnosis. Interestingly enough, Notch-1, which is a transcription factor that suppresses MASH1/hASH1, is expressed in MCC and is negative in other neuroendocrine tumors including SCLC [105], yet another available diagnostic tool for this differential diagnosis. Lymphoid neoplasms are also included in the differential diagnosis. Although MCC is consistently negative for CD45 (LCA) [8], it can exhibit considerable overlap with hematologic malignancies in terms of immunohistochemical markers, since MCCs can express a variety of lymphoid-related markers such as CD56 (NCAM) [171, 197], the B-cell-associated transcription factor PAX5 and the primitive lymphoid marker TdT [7–9, 194, 198]. Additionally, the majority of MCC will express the apoptosis-related marker bcl-2 [8, 106, 199], an apparently major player in MCC tumor cell survival [200]. Furthermore, another lymphoid-related marker that can be expressed by MCC cells is anaplastic lymphoma kinase (ALK), specifically with the D5F3

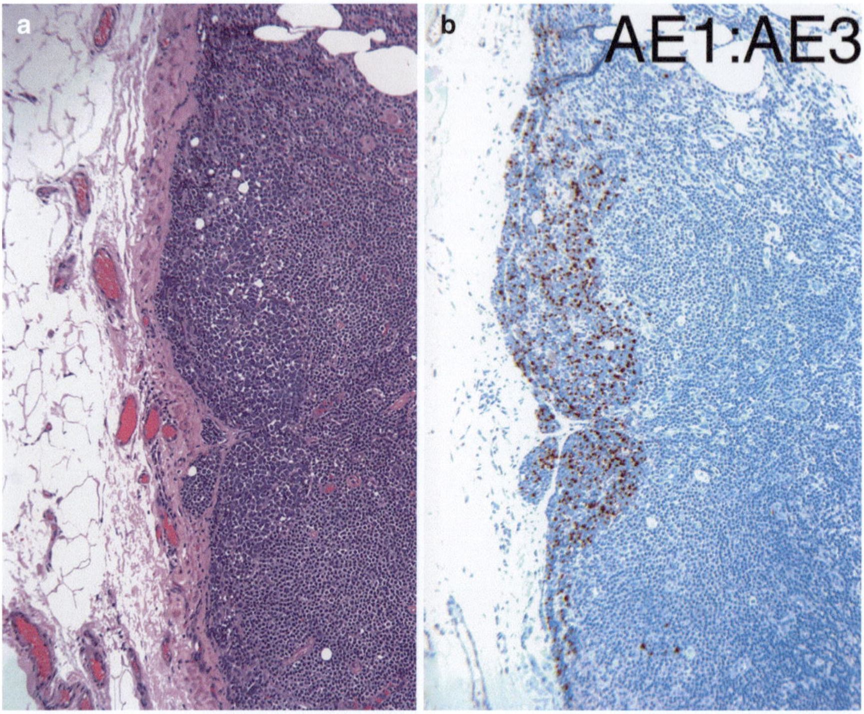

Fig. 12 Cytokeratin immunohistochemistry is an invaluable tool when evaluating for lymph node metastatic disease, particularly if they are small deposits (**a**: H&E and **b**: AE1: AE3, both 100×)

clone but less so with the ALK-1 clone [201]. Finally, consideration must be given to the SRBC group of tumors, particularly the superficial variant of Ewing sarcoma/primitive neuroectodermal tumor (PNET) group, since MCC can frequently express CD99 and Friend leukemia integration 1 (FLI1), while conversely up to 20 % of Ewing sarcoma/PNET can show expression of keratins, particularly with CAM 5.2 and AE1:AE3 cocktails [170]. In potential cases of PNET that are indistinguishable morphologically and immunohistochemically from MCC, one could resort to cytogenetic studies, since MCCs completely lack the cytogenetic aberrations found in those tumors [159].

Ultrastructural Features of MCC

As previously stated, MCC tumor cells exhibit many shared ultrastructural characteristics with normal Merkel cells, the main reason behind the tumor's nomenclature. Under the transmission electron microscope, normal Merkel cells are identified as cells measuring about 15 μm size, oval shaped with their long axis oriented parallel to the basement membrane plane [4, 5]. Close relationship to a sensory axon is

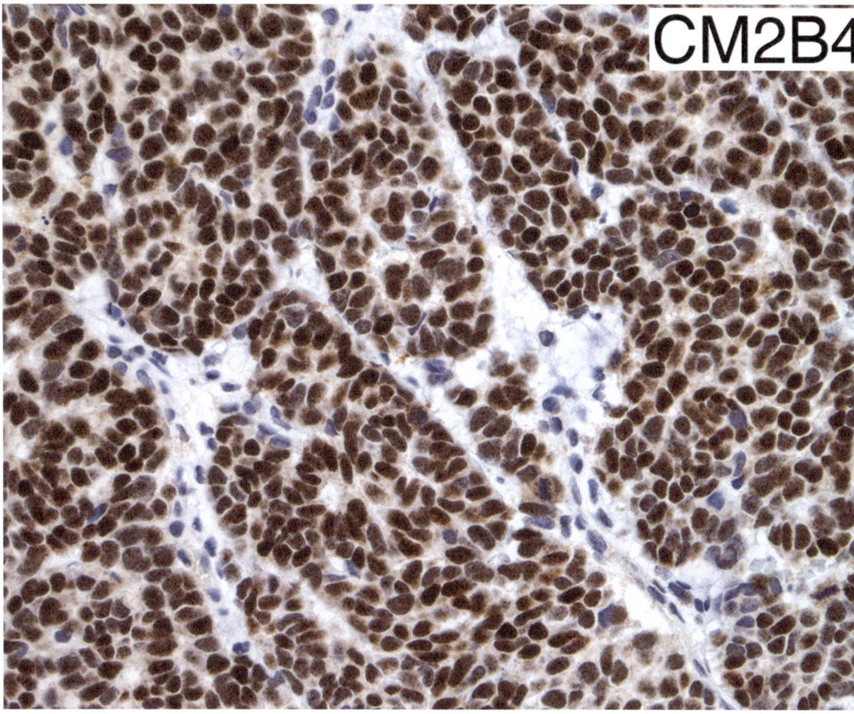

Fig. 13 Immunohistochemistry directed to the LT-Ag of MCPyV in an MCC case. Note the clean and strong nuclear signal denoting integration of the viral genome in the tumor cells (MCPyV immunohistochemistry (CM2B4 clone, 400×) (Image courtesy of Gauri Panse M.D. from Baystate Medical Center-Tufts University, Springfield, MA)

Table 1 Immunohistochemical differential diagnosis between MCC and mimickers

Tumor type	Cam 5.2	CK7	CK20	TTF-1	S100	LCA	CD99	PAX5	MASH1
MCC	100 %	27 %	92 %	1.1 %	20 %	0 %	25 % (C)	91 %	0 %
Small cell carcinoma	60–80 %	40 %	3 %	91 %	0 %	0 %	12 % (C)	78 %	83 %[a]
EWS/PNET	20 %	ND	ND	ND	50 %	0 %	92 % (M)	0 %	ND
Lymphoma	0 %	0 %	0 %	ND	6 %	98 %	7 %	Near 100 %[b]	ND
Small cell melanoma	0 %	0 %	0 %	0 %	97 %	0 %	8 %	0 %	ND

Table constructed with data from the following references: McKee's Pathology of the Skin [45], Kuwamoto [143], Fan [240], Desouki et al. [241]

Abbreviations: *MCC* Merkel cell carcinoma, *EWS/PNET* Ewing sarcoma/primitive neuroectodermal tumor, *C* cytoplasmic, *M* membranous, *ND* no data

[a]Specifically in small cell lung carcinoma origin

[b]Particularly in B-cell processes and classic Hodgkin lymphoma

often evident. Normal Merkel cell bears a large, usually bilobulated nuclei, and their cytoplasm is scant, relatively scarcely populated by organelles but containing many free ribosomes. Numerous neurosecretory granules can be appreciated close to the area where the cell is in relationship with a sensory axon. Other salient ultrastructural features of normal Merkel cells are the abundant spikelike spinous cytoplasmic processes interdigitating with the surrounding keratinocytes to which they are attached by sparse, small, and poorly formed desmosomes [4, 5, 202]. Interestingly, melanosomes have been described to occur in normal Merkel cells.

Neoplastic Merkel cells replicate the majority of the above-cited ultrastructural features of normal Merkel cells, including the very characteristic spinous processes and the neurosecretory granules. However, MCC tumor cells exhibit a prominent perinuclear ball-like collection of intermediate filaments contrasting to the sparse collections of simple keratin-intermediate filaments found in the cytoplasm of normal Merkel cells [4, 5]. This cytoplasmic ball of intermediate filaments is an ultrastructural feature common among neuroendocrine tumors and small cell carcinomas. This accumulation of intermediate filaments translates to the immunohistochemical pattern that is observed in MCC with CK20, keratin cocktails, and neurofilament immunostains.

Molecular Aspects, Pathogenesis, and Association with the Merkel Cell Polyomavirus (MCPyV)

The discovery of the MCPyV has indeed completely changed our understanding of MCC pathogenesis and behavior. MCPyV is a novel polyomavirus that belongs to the same family as the JC, BK, KI, and WU as well as the recently discovered trichodysplasia-associated polyomavirus (TSPyV) [203]. However, so far, only MCPyV has an associated oncogenic potential. Several recent studies have demonstrated that MCPyV is quite prevalent in the healthy adult population, and it is detected in peripheral blood both by molecular DNA amplification techniques and serology. Evidence of the virus has also demonstrated from cutaneous swabs [143, 204–208]. A recent prospective study has correlated high serum MCPyV antibody titers in healthy individuals with an increased risk of subsequent MCC development in older age [209]. Transmission is likely to occur in early childhood, especially between family members [210], and the virus remains dormant in a wide variety of tissues [211] until immunosuppression-triggered reactivation, as is characteristic of this viral group. The importance of MCPyV resides in that it is part of the two proposed models of MCC pathogenesis, the other being a UV-damage-induced pathway, which involves *TP53* mutations and is to MCPyV. The causative oncogenic role of MCPyV in MCC is nowadays widely accepted, since the viral genetic material is integrated and clonally expanded in viral-positive MCC tumor cells [10]. Numerous studies on the subject have shown that MCPyV can be detected in about 70–80 % of MCC tumors [133, 145, 205, 207, 211–218]. However, a recent study claims that if one were to use sensitive enough molecular techniques, all MCC tumors will show integrated MCPyV genome [180]. Along this line of thought, some authors claim that the two pathways could be unified into one that is driven by mutagenic effects of preexisting MCPyV, which has been reactivated itself in an immunosuppressed host that has been accumulating deleterious UV-induced mutations [219]. As we discussed before in this chapter, there is a well-documented and clear link between MCC and various types of immunosuppressive states, including chronic solar damage. The main oncogenic mechanism of MCPyV is exerted via the interaction between LT-Ag and the retinoblastoma (Rb) group of proteins. It is important to understand the fact that the oncogenic gene LT-Ag present in the infected MCC tumor cells has undergone a signature truncating mutation [179, 220]. The product of this mutated LT-Ag, through its LxCxE motif, binds and sequesters hypophosphorylated Rb leading to its accumulation and thus allowing E2F-mediated transcription that leads to the entry of the cell into S-phase [221]. The p53 protein system also becomes affected by LT-Ag, albeit in an indirect fashion [220, 222]. Additionally, the LT-Ag protein also serves to allow detection of MCPyV by immunohistochemistry. Regarding the MCPyV-negative MCC group, Rb function is also impaired but through different mechanisms that include hypermethylation and heterozygous deletions [184]. Characteristically, p53 is more often suppressed and immunohistochemically overexpressed (accumulated) in this particular group. These alterations in Rb are reflected on immunohistochemistry with LT-Ag-positive MCC tumors expressing the accumulated Rb and conversely with 87 % of LT-Ag-negative tumors being predominantly Rb negative due to the deletions and silencing hypermethylation [212, 223]. Likewise, it seems that there is an inverse relationship between p53 overexpression and MCPyV viral abundance [181, 224] with overexpression of p53 being also negatively related to survival. Furthermore, recent studies have correlated both tumor positivity for MCPyV and an effective viral-directed immune response with better survival [15, 181, 223–225]. After reviewing these models, one could draw comparisons with what occurs in other organ systems such as in the lower female genital tract SCC (HPV driven versus p53 driven) and head and neck SCC (p16-positive/HPV-positive tumors having better prognosis than HPV-negative tumors).

Prognostic Factors, Staging, and Management

Several clinical and histopathologic features in MCC are associated with clinical outcome. In terms of clinical features, a large Surveillance, Epidemiology, and End Results (SEER)-based National Cancer Institute (NCI) study [12] demonstrated that women have a 10-year survival advantage compared to men with the rates being 64.8 % and 50.5 %, respectively. Additionally, tumor location yielded survival differences, and if one were to align the anatomical sites from best to worse prognosis, it would show the following pattern: upper limbs, head and neck, lower limbs, and trunk. Furthermore, this study added tumor diameter to the prognostic factors, demonstrating that tumors equal or less than 2 cm have statistically significant better survival (61 %) than tumors larger than 2 cm (39.6 %). In fact, tumor size is the main focus of tumor staging [14, 226]. In the 2010 American Joint Committee on Cancer (AJCC) guidelines, a four-tier staging system is used for MCC: tumors are designated as stage I or stage II if they are localized to the skin at the primary site (stage I/T1 is less or equal than 2 cm in diameter, and stage II/T2 is more than 2 cm in size); stage III denotes spread to regional lymph nodes; and stage IV indicates spread beyond the regional lymph nodes. According to some recent studies, tumor thickness measured utilizing the Breslow technique has emerged as a strong and important independent prognostic factor. Studies indicate that thicker tumors are related to advanced stage [185], predict positive sentinel lymph node (SLN) status [227, 228], and are associated with both higher recurrence rate and worse survival [178, 229, 230]. A suggested cutoff of equal or greater than 10 mm in thickness [178] was proposed to indicate increased risk for the mentioned complications. Tumor growth pattern and tumor borders have also been reported to be associated with prognosis with both infiltrative tumor borders [229] and diffuse growth pattern [230] being negatively associated with survival. It is likely that the development of thick tumors with irregular borders is correlated with higher expression of several types of metalloproteinases by the tumor cells, which has been found to impact prognosis by itself [186, 231]. The presence of LVI, a rather frequent finding in MCC, is also considered a strong adverse prognostic factor [228, 229, 232]. Unsurprisingly, a high proliferative rate, represented by either an elevated Ki-67 proliferation index of equal or more than 35 or 50 % and/or a high mitotic rate, has also been correlated with both disease progression and worse survival [24, 185, 233, 234].

While a comprehensive discussion of management is beyond the scope of this chapter, the mainstay of treatment, particularly in localized disease, is surgical. The data related to the role of the sentinel lymph node biopsy is somewhat less clear in MCC in comparison to melanoma and breast carcinoma. Current National Comprehensive Cancer Network (NCCN) treatment recommendations include surgical excision of the primary tumor with wide margins (1–2 cm) followed by sentinel lymph node biopsy (SLNB) or elective lymphadenectomy (for clinically node-negative cases), as 25–30 % patients have regional nodal disease at presentation [22, 227, 235]. Chemotherapy and radiation therapy are reserved for advanced stage patients. A recent study from a large cohort of patients underscored the beneficial impact of SLNB and completion lymphadenectomy on survival while finding that chemotherapy and radiotherapy had no effect on survival in node-negative patients [235]. Other studies pointed out that clinically detectable metastatic lymph node deposits were more predictive of outcome than lymph nodes with microscopic deposits [232]. More data need to be accumulated in this regard to be able to make stronger evidence-based management recommendations.

MCC tumors can be accompanied by a brisk immune response. However, as is the case with other highly immunogenic tumors such as melanoma, the relationship between this immune host response and survival has had conflicting results in the literature, with some studies attributing a worse prognosis to either the presence [230] or absence [185] of immune response, while in other study the presence of an immune response was associated with good prognosis particularly in lymph node-negative tumors with nodular growth pattern [229]. It appears that

MCPyV might play a role in this issue since it has been recently suggested that the MCPyV status of the tumor is reflected in patient survival with patients with a higher viral load and mounting an appropriate immune response having better clinical outcome [15, 181, 223, 224]. Another interesting new finding is that in MCPyV-positive tumors, there is evidence of tumor-driven immune suppression, as a high proportion of PD-L1-positive tumor-infiltrating lymphocytes (TILs) and macrophages found particularly at the tumor-stroma interface [236]. Furthermore, the same study showed that expression of PD-L1 in MCC tumor cells is correlated with better survival. The innate immune system is apparently also affected by the tumor [237]. In addition, it has been shown that specific T-cell populations directed to MCPyV are detected peripherally in MCC patients and also express the immune exhaustion markers PD-1 and Tim-3 [238]. Other studies demonstrated that presence of specific T-cell [239] TIL subpopulations without impaired function might also predict improved survival. These observations open exciting opportunities for potential immune modulatory therapy with recently developed monoclonal antibodies [219] in this particular group of virus-driven MCC.

Abbreviations

AJCC	American Joint Committee on Cancer
APUD	Amine precursor uptake and decarboxylation
BCC	Basal cell carcinoma
CK	Cytokeratin
CLL	Chronic lymphocytic leukemia
ACTH	Adrenocorticotropic hormone
HIV/AIDS	Human immunodeficiency virus/acquired immunodeficiency syndrome
LT-Ag	Large T antigen
LVI	Lymphovascular invasion
MASH1/hASH1	Mammalian/human achaete-scute complex homolog 1
MCC	Merkel cell carcinoma
MCPyV	Merkel cell polyomavirus
NCCN	National Comprehensive Cancer Network
NSE	Neuron-specific enolase
PNET	Peripheral neuroectodermal tumor
Rb	Retinoblastoma
SCC	Squamous cell carcinoma
SCLC	Small cell lung carcinoma
SEER	Surveillance, Epidemiology, and End Results
SLN	Sentinel lymph node
SRBC	Small round blue cell
TILs	Tumor-infiltrating lymphocytes
TTF-1	Thyroid transcription factor 1

References

1. Toker C. Trabecular carcinoma of the skin. Arch Dermatol. 1972;105(1):107–10.
2. Toker C. Trabecular carcinoma of the skin. A question of title. Am J Dermatopathol. 1982;4(6):497–500.
3. De Wolff-Peeters C, Marien K, Mebis J, Desmet V. A cutaneous APUDoma or Merkel cell tumor? A morphologically recognizable tumor with a biological and histological malignant aspect in contrast with its clinical behavior. Cancer. 1980;46(8):1810–6.
4. Sidhu GS, Chandra P, Cassai ND. Merkel cells, normal and neoplastic: an update. Ultrastruct Pathol. 2005;29(3–4):287–94.
5. Boulais N, Misery L. Merkel cells. J Am Acad Dermatol. 2007;57(1):147–65.
6. Lemasson G, Coquart N, Lebonvallet N, Boulais N, Galibert MD, Marcorelles P, et al. Presence of putative stem cells in Merkel cell carcinomas. J Eur Acad Dermatol Venereol. 2012;26(6):789–95.
7. Zur Hausen A, Rennspiess D, Winnepenninckx V, Speel EJ, Kurz AK. Early B-cell differentiation in Merkel cell carcinomas: clues to cellular ancestry. Cancer Res. 2013;73(16):4982–7.
8. Sur M, AlArdati H, Ross C, Alowami S. TdT expression in Merkel cell carcinoma: potential diagnostic pitfall with blastic hematological malignancies and expanded immunohistochemical analysis. Mod Pathol. 2007;20(11):1113–20.
9. Dong HY, Liu W, Cohen P, Mahle CE, Zhang W. B-cell specific activation protein encoded by the PAX-5 gene is commonly expressed in Merkel cell carcinoma and small cell carcinomas. Am J Surg Pathol. 2005;29(5):687–92.
10. Feng H, Shuda M, Chang Y, Moore PS. Clonal integration of a polyomavirus in human Merkel cell carcinoma. Science. 2008;319(5866):1096–100.
11. Agelli M, Clegg LX. Epidemiology of primary Merkel cell carcinoma in the United States. J Am Acad Dermatol. 2003;49(5):832–41.
12. Albores-Saavedra J, Batich K, Chable-Montero F, Sagy N, Schwartz AM, Henson DE. Merkel cell carcinoma demographics, morphology, and survival based on 3870 cases: a population based study. J Cutan Pathol. 2010;37(1):20–7.
13. Kaae J, Hansen AV, Biggar RJ, Boyd HA, Moore PS, Wohlfahrt J, et al. Merkel cell carcinoma: incidence, mortality, and risk of other cancers. J Natl Cancer Inst. 2010;102(11):793–801.
14. Heath M, Jaimes N, Lemos B, Mostaghimi A, Wang LC, Penas PF, et al. Clinical characteristics of Merkel cell carcinoma at diagnosis in 195 patients: the AEIOU features. J Am Acad Dermatol. 2008;58(3):375–81.
15. Paulson KG, Iyer JG, Blom A, Warton EM, Sokil M, Yelistratova L, et al. Systemic immune suppression predicts diminished Merkel cell carcinoma-specific survival independent of stage. J Invest Dermatol. 2013;133(3):642–6.
16. Tadmor T, Aviv A, Polliack A. Merkel cell carcinoma, chronic lymphocytic leukemia and other lymphoproliferative disorders: an old bond with possible new viral ties. Ann Oncol. 2011;22(2):250–6.
17. Penn I, First MR. Merkel's cell carcinoma in organ recipients: report of 41 cases. Transplantation. 1999;68(11):1717–21.
18. Walsh NM. Primary neuroendocrine (Merkel cell) carcinoma of the skin: morphologic diversity and implications thereof. Hum Pathol. 2001;32(7):680–9.
19. Kanitakis J, Euvrard S, Chouvet B, Butnaru AC, Claudy A. Merkel cell carcinoma in organ-transplant recipients: report of two cases with unusual histological features and literature review. J Cutan Pathol. 2006;33(10):686–94.
20. Brenner B, Sulkes A, Rakowsky E, Feinmesser M, Yukelson A, Bar-Haim E, et al. Second neoplasms in patients with Merkel cell carcinoma. Cancer. 2001;91(7):1358–62.
21. Gass JK, Chan SK, Rytina E, Greenberg DC, Burrows NP. Multiple primary malignancies in patients with Merkel cell carcinoma. J Eur Acad Dermatol Venereol. 2010;24(5):601–3.

22. Hitchcock CL, Bland KI, Laney 3rd RG, Franzini D, Harris B, Copeland 3rd EM. Neuroendocrine (Merkel cell) carcinoma of the skin. Its natural history, diagnosis, and treatment. Ann Surg. 1988;207(2):201–7.
23. Gollard R, Weber R, Kosty MP, Greenway HT, Massullo V, Humberson C. Merkel cell carcinoma: review of 22 cases with surgical, pathologic, and therapeutic considerations. Cancer. 2000;88(8):1842–51.
24. Skelton HG, Smith KJ, Hitchcock CL, McCarthy WF, Lupton GP, Graham JH. Merkel cell carcinoma: analysis of clinical, histologic, and immunohistologic features of 132 cases with relation to survival. J Am Acad Dermatol. 1997;37(5 Pt 1):734–9.
25. Hohaus K, Kostler E, Schonlebe J, Klemm E, Wollina U. Merkel cell carcinoma – a retrospective analysis of 17 cases. J Eur Acad Dermatol Venereol. 2003;17(1):20–4.
26. Inoue T, Shimono M, Takano N, Saito C, Tanaka Y. Merkel cell carcinoma of palatal mucosa in a young adult: immunohistochemical and ultrastructural features. Oral Oncol. 1997;33(3):226–9.
27. Longo F, Califano L, Mangone GM, Errico ME. Neuroendocrine (Merkel cell) carcinoma of the oral mucosa: report of a case with immunohistochemical study and review of the literature. J Oral Pathol Med. 1999;28(2):88–91.
28. Baker P, Alguacil-Garcia A. Moderately differentiated neuroendocrine carcinoma in the floor of the mouth: a case report. J Oral Maxillofac Surg. 1999;57(9):1143–7.
29. Prabhu S, Smitha RS, Punnya VA. Merkel cell carcinoma of the alveolar mucosa in a young adult: a rare case report. Br J Oral Maxillofac Surg. 2010;48(1):48–50.
30. Yom SS, Rosenthal DI, El-Naggar AK, Kies MS, Hessel AC. Merkel cell carcinoma of the tongue and head and neck oral mucosal sites. Oral Surg Oral Med Oral Pathol Oral Radiol Endod. 2006;101(6):761–8.
31. Snow SN, Larson PO, Hardy S, Bentz M, Madjar D, Landeck A, et al. Merkel cell carcinoma of the skin and mucosa: report of 12 cutaneous cases with 2 cases arising from the nasal mucosa. Dermatol Surg. 2001;27(2):165–70.
32. Hierro I, Blanes A, Matilla A, Muñoz S, Vicioso L, Nogales FF. Merkel cell (neuroendocrine) carcinoma of the vulva. Pathol Res Pract. 2000;196(7):503–9.
33. Tomic S, Warner TF, Messing E, Wilding G. Penile Merkel cell carcinoma. Urology. 1995;45(6):1062–5.
34. Eusebi V, Capella C, Cossu A, Rosai J. Neuroendocrine carcinoma within lymph nodes in the absence of a primary tumor, with special reference to Merkel cell carcinoma. Am J Surg Pathol. 1992;16(7):658–66.
35. Fotia G, Barni R, Bellan C, Neri A. Lymph nodal Merkel cell carcinoma: primary or metastatic disease? A clinical case. Tumori. 2002;88(5):424–6.
36. Kim EJ, Kim HS, Kim HO, Jung CK, Ko YH, Kim TH, et al. Merkel cell carcinoma of the inguinal lymph node with an unknown primary site. J Dermatol. 2009;36(3):170–3.
37. de Biase D, Ragazzi M, Asioli S, Eusebi V. Extracutaneous Merkel cell carcinomas harbor polyomavirus DNA. Hum Pathol. 2012;43(7):980–5.
38. Fornelli A, Eusebi V, Pasquinelli G, Quattrone P, Rosai J. Merkel cell carcinoma of the parotid gland associated with Warthin tumour: report of two cases. Histopathology. 2001;39(4):342–6.
39. Chernock RD, Duncavage EJ, Gnepp DR, El-Mofty SK, Lewis Jr JS. Absence of Merkel cell polyomavirus in primary parotid high-grade neuroendocrine carcinomas regardless of cytokeratin 20 immunophenotype. Am J Surg Pathol. 2011;35(12):1806–11.
40. Capella C, Marando A, Longhi E, Bernasconi B, Finzi G, Parravicini C, et al. Primary gastric Merkel cell carcinoma harboring DNA polyomavirus: first description of an unusual high-grade neuroendocrine carcinoma. Hum Pathol. 2014;45(6):1310–4.
41. Bing Z, Levine L, Lucci JA, Hatch SS, Eltorky MA. Primary small cell neuroendocrine carcinoma of the vagina: a clinicopathologic study. Arch Pathol Lab Med. 2004;128(8):857–62.
42. Coleman NM, Smith-Zagone MJ, Tanyi J, Anderson ML, Coleman RL, Dyson SW, et al. Primary neuroendocrine carcinoma of the vagina with Merkel cell carcinoma phenotype. Am J Surg Pathol. 2006;30(3):405–10.

43. Ratner D, Nelson BR, Brown MD, Johnson TM. Merkel cell carcinoma. J Am Acad Dermatol. 1993;29(2 Pt 1):143–56.
44. Perdikis G, TerKonda SP. Pigmented skin lesions of the upper extremity. Hand Clin. 2004;20(3):283–91. vi.
45. McKee PH, Calonje E, Granter SR. Pathology of the skin: with clinical correlations/[edited by] Phillip H. McKee, Eduardo Calonje, Scott R. Granter. 3rd ed. Edinburgh: Philadelphia Elsevier Mosby; 2005. v <1 >p.
46. Smith PD, Patterson JW. Merkel cell carcinoma (neuroendocrine carcinoma of the skin). Am J Clin Pathol. 2001;115(Suppl):S68–78.
47. Satter EK, Derienzo DP. Synchronous onset of multiple cutaneous neuroendocrine (Merkel cell) carcinomas localized to the scalp. J Cutan Pathol. 2008;35(7):685–91.
48. Grandpeix C, Bonvalot S, Petrow P, Fraitag S, Gounod N, Avril MF. Continued complete remission of Merkel cell carcinoma with in-transit metastasis after treatment with isolated limb perfusion regional chemotherapy. Ann Dermatol Venereol. 2006;133(8–9 Pt 1):700–3.
49. Grotz TE, Tarantola TI, Otley CC, Weaver AL, McGree ME, Jakub JW. Natural history of Merkel cell carcinoma following locoregional recurrence. Ann Surg Oncol. 2012;19(8):2556–62.
50. Howle JR, Veness MJ. Outcome of patients with microscopic and macroscopic metastatic nodal Merkel cell carcinoma: an Australian experience. Dermatol Surg. 2014;40(1):46–51.
51. Iyer JG, Storer BE, Paulson KG, Lemos B, Phillips JL, Bichakjian CK, et al. Relationships among primary tumor size, number of involved nodes, and survival for 8044 cases of Merkel cell carcinoma. J Am Acad Dermatol. 2014;70(4):637–43.
52. Kirwan C, Carney D, O'Keefe M. Merkel cell carcinoma metastasis to the iris in a 23 year old female. Ir Med J. 2009;102(2):53–4.
53. Ikawa F, Kiya K, Uozumi T, Yuki K, Takeshita S, Hamasaki O, et al. Brain metastasis of Merkel cell carcinoma. Case report and review of the literature. Neurosurg Rev. 1999;22(1):54–7.
54. Feletti A, Marton E, Rossi S, Canal F, Longatti P, Billeci D. Pituitary metastasis of Merkel cell carcinoma. J Neurooncol. 2010;97(2):295–9.
55. Shalin SC, Cifarelli CP, Suen JY, Gao L. Loss of cytokeratin 20 and acquisition of thyroid transcription factor-1 expression in a Merkel cell carcinoma metastasis to the brain. Am J Dermatopathol. 2014.
56. Chang DT, Mancuso AA, Riggs Jr CE, Mendenhall WM. Merkel cell carcinoma of the skin with leptomeningeal metastases. Am J Otolaryngol. 2005;26(3):210–3.
57. Abul-Kasim K, Soderstrom K, Hallsten L. Extensive central nervous system involvement in Merkel cell carcinoma: a case report and review of the literature. J Med Case Rep. 2011;5:35.
58. Schmidt-Westhausen A, Reichart PA, Gross UM. Gingival metastasis of Merkel cell carcinoma: a case report. J Oral Pathol Med. 1996;25(1):44–7.
59. Reichel OA, Mayr D, Issing WJ. Oropharyngeal metastasis of a Merkel cell carcinoma of the skin. Eur Arch Otorhinolaryngol. 2003;260(5):258–60.
60. Jongbloed MR, Kanen BL, Visser M, Niessen H, Flens MJ, Loffeld RJ. Case 2. Intracardiac metastasis from a Merkel cell carcinoma. J Clin Oncol. 2004;22(6):1153–6.
61. Yamana N, Sueyama H, Hamada M. Cardiac metastasis from Merkel cell skin carcinoma. Int J Clin Oncol. 2004;9(3):210–2.
62. Fong LS, Mathur M, Bhindi R, Figtree GA. Right atrial Merkel cell tumour metastasis characterization using a multimodality approach. Eur Heart J. 2012;33(17):2205.
63. Suttie CF, Hruby G, Horvath L, Thompson J. Cardiac metastasis in Merkel cell carcinoma. J Clin Oncol. 2014;32(13):e52–3.
64. Idowu MO, Contos M, Gill S, Powers C. Merkel cell carcinoma: a report of gastrointestinal metastasis and review of the literature. Arch Pathol Lab Med. 2003;127(3):367–9.
65. Syal NG, Dang S, Rose J, Chen C, Aduli F. Gastric metastasis of Merkel cell cancer – uncommon complication of a rare neoplasm. J Ark Med Soc. 2012;109(7):134–6.
66. Parikh MP, Samo S, Ganipisetti V, Krishnan S, Dhandha M, Yungbluth M, et al. Gastric metastasis of Merkel cell carcinoma, a rare cause of gastrointestinal bleeding: case report and review of the literature. J Gastrointest Oncol. 2014;5(4):E68–72.

67. Ouellette JR, Woodyard L, Toth L, Termuhlen PM. Merkel cell carcinoma metastatic to the head of the pancreas. JOP. 2004;5(2):92–6.
68. Bachmann J, Kleeff J, Bergmann F, Shrikhande SV, Hartschuh W, Buchler MW, et al. Pancreatic metastasis of Merkel cell carcinoma and concomitant insulinoma: case report and literature review. World J Surg Oncol. 2005;3:58.
69. Woo HH, Kencian JD. Metastatic Merkel cell tumour to the bladder. Int Urol Nephrol. 1995;27(3):301–5.
70. Santis WF, Billings EJ, DeWolf WC. Metastatic Merkel cell tumor to bladder presenting as an encroachment tumor with gross hematuria. Urology. 1999;54(1):163.
71. Mack DP, Moussa M, Cook A, Izawa JI. Metastatic Merkel cell tumor to the prostate and bladder. Urology. 2004;64(1):156–8.
72. Gleason JM, Kohler TS, Monga M. Merkel cell carcinoma metastatic to testis. Urology. 2006;67(2):423.e13–e14.
73. Strasser H, Amann K, Schrott KM, Krause FS. Solitary metastasis of a Merkel cell tumor to the urinary bladder. Anticancer Res. 2008;28(2b):1361–4.
74. Wang W, Veness M. Metastatic Merkel cell carcinoma to the soft tissues of the lower back. Australas J Dermatol. 2004;45(1):38–41.
75. Lentz SR, Krewson L, Zutter MM. Recurrent neuroendocrine (Merkel cell) carcinoma of the skin presenting as marrow failure in a man with systemic lupus erythematosus. Med Pediatr Oncol. 1993;21(2):137–41.
76. Nemoto I, Sato-Matsumura KC, Fujita Y, Natsuga K, Ujiie H, Tomita Y, et al. Leukaemic dissemination of Merkel cell carcinoma in a patient with systemic lupus erythematosus. Clin Exp Dermatol. 2008;33(3):270–2.
77. Kayashima K, Ono T, Johno M, Kojo Y, Yamashita N, Matsunaga W. Spontaneous regression in Merkel cell (neuroendocrine) carcinoma of the skin. Arch Dermatol. 1991;127(4):550–3.
78. Duncan WC, Tschen JA. Spontaneous regression of Merkel cell (neuroendocrine) carcinoma of the skin. J Am Acad Dermatol. 1993;29(4):653–4.
79. Yanguas I, Goday JJ, Gonzalez-Guemes M, Oleaga JM, Lozano M, Soloeta R. Spontaneous regression of Merkel cell carcinoma of the skin. Br J Dermatol. 1997;137(2):296–8.
80. Connelly TJ, Cribier B, Brown TJ, Yanguas I. Complete spontaneous regression of Merkel cell carcinoma: a review of the 10 reported cases. Dermatol Surg. 2000;26(9):853–6.
81. Maruo K, Kayashima KI, Ono T. Regressing Merkel cell carcinoma-a case showing replacement of tumour cells by foamy cells. Br J Dermatol. 2000;142(6):1184–9.
82. Sais G, Admella C, Soler T. Spontaneous regression in primary cutaneous neuroendocrine (Merkel cell) carcinoma: a rare immune phenomenon? J Eur Acad Dermatol Venereol. 2002;16(1):82–3.
83. Junquera L, Torre A, Vicente JC, Garcia-Consuegra L, Fresno MF. Complete spontaneous regression of Merkel cell carcinoma. Ann Otol Rhinol Laryngol. 2005;114(5):376–80.
84. Missotten GS, de Wolff-Rouendaal D, de Keizer RJ. Merkel cell carcinoma of the eyelid review of the literature and report of patients with Merkel cell carcinoma showing spontaneous regression. Ophthalmology. 2008;115(1):195–201.
85. Karkos PD, Sastry A, Hampal S, Al-Jafari M. Spontaneous regression of Merkel cell carcinoma of the nose. Head Neck. 2010;32(3):411–4.
86. Wooff JC, Trites JR, Walsh NM, Bullock MJ. Complete spontaneous regression of metastatic Merkel cell carcinoma: a case report and review of the literature. Am J Dermatopathol. 2010;32(6):614–7.
87. Warnick M, Singh S, Boisvert ME, Peck GL. Merkel cell carcinoma presenting as lymphadenopathy without a primary cutaneous lesion: a report of 2 cases. Arch Dermatol. 2008;144(10):1397–8.
88. Cozzolino I, Zeppa R, Zeppa P. Lymph nodal Merkel cell carcinoma: primary tumor or metastasis from unknown primary site? J Cutan Pathol. 2011;38(10):836–7.
89. de Zeeuw S, Schouten van der Velden AP, de Wilt HJ, Wetzels CT, Bonenkamp HJ. A Merkel cell carcinoma presenting as a solitary lymph node metastasis without a primary lesion. Report of a case and review of the literature. Acta Chir Belg. 2012;112(4):317–21.

90. Deneve JL, Messina JL, Marzban SS, Gonzalez RJ, Walls BM, Fisher KJ, et al. Merkel cell carcinoma of unknown primary origin. Ann Surg Oncol. 2012;19(7):2360–6.
91. Boghossian V, Owen ID, Nuli B, Xiao PQ. Neuroendocrine (Merkel cell) carcinoma of the retroperitoneum with no identifiable primary site. World J Surg Oncol. 2007;5:117.
92. Nazarian Y, Shalmon B, Horowitz Z, Bedrin L, Pfeffer MR, Talmi YP. Merkel cell carcinoma of unknown primary site. J Laryngol Otol. 2007;121(4), e1.
93. Tarantola TI, Vallow LA, Halyard MY, Weenig RH, Warschaw KE, Weaver AL, et al. Unknown primary Merkel cell carcinoma: 23 new cases and a review. J Am Acad Dermatol. 2013;68(3):433–40.
94. Rossini D, Caponnetto S, Lapadula V, De Filippis L, Del Bene G, Emiliani A, et al. Merkel cell carcinoma of the retroperitoneum with no identifiable primary site. Case Rep Oncol Med. 2013;2013:131695.
95. Haider K, Hu Q, McFadden AJ, Shoker A, Barton JW, Ahmed S. Thrombocytopenia: an unusual manifestation of advanced composite Merkel cell carcinoma and in situ squamous cell carcinoma. Am J Clin Oncol. 2007;30(4):442–3.
96. Anzai S, Sato T, Takayasu S, Asada Y, Terashi H, Takasaki S. Postoperative hyponatremia in a patient with ACTH-producing Merkel cell carcinoma. J Dermatol. 2000;27(6):397–400.
97. Eggers SD, Salomao DR, Dinapoli RP, Vernino S. Paraneoplastic and metastatic neurologic complications of Merkel cell carcinoma. Mayo Clin Proc. 2001;76(3):327–30.
98. Rocamora A, Badia N, Vives R, Carrillo R, Ulloa J, Ledo A. Epidermotropic primary neuroendocrine (Merkel cell) carcinoma of the skin with Pautrier-like microabscesses. Report of three cases and review of the literature. J Am Acad Dermatol. 1987;16(6):1163–8.
99. LeBoit PE, Crutcher WA, Shapiro PE. Pagetoid intraepidermal spread in Merkel cell (primary neuroendocrine) carcinoma of the skin. Am J Surg Pathol. 1992;16(6):584–92.
100. Smith KJ, Skelton 3rd HG, Holland TT, Morgan AM, Lupton GP. Neuroendocrine (Merkel cell) carcinoma with an intraepidermal component. Am J Dermatopathol. 1993;15(6):528–33.
101. Ball NJ, Tanhuanco-Kho G. Merkel cell carcinoma frequently shows histologic features of basal cell carcinoma: a study of 30 cases. J Cutan Pathol. 2007;34(8):612–9.
102. D'Agostino M, Cinelli C, Willard R, Hofmann J, Jellinek N, Robinson-Bostom L. Epidermotropic Merkel cell carcinoma: a case series with histopathologic examination. J Am Acad Dermatol. 2010;62(3):463–8.
103. Al-Ahmadie HA, Mutasim DF, Mutema GK. A case of intraepidermal Merkel cell carcinoma within squamous cell carcinoma in-situ: Merkel cell carcinoma in-situ? Am J Dermatopathol. 2004;26(3):230–3.
104. Ferringer T, Rogers HC, Metcalf JS. Merkel cell carcinoma in situ. J Cutan Pathol. 2005;32(2):162–5.
105. Panelos J, Batistatou A, Paglierani M, Zioga A, Maio V, Santi R, et al. Expression of Notch-1 and alteration of the E-cadherin/beta-catenin cell adhesion complex are observed in primary cutaneous neuroendocrine carcinoma (Merkel cell carcinoma). Mod Pathol. 2009;22(7):959–68.
106. Knapp CF, Sayegh Z, Schell MJ, Rawal B, Ochoa T, Sondak VK, et al. Expression of CXCR4, E-cadherin, Bcl-2, and survivin in Merkel cell carcinoma: an immunohistochemical study using a tissue microarray. Am J Dermatopathol. 2012;34(6):592–6.
107. Pilotti S, Rilke F, Bartoli C, Grisotti A. Clinicopathologic correlations of cutaneous neuroendocrine Merkel cell carcinoma. J Clin Oncol. 1988;6(12):1863–73.
108. Wick MR, Goellner JR, Scheithauer BW, Thomas 3rd JR, Sanchez NP, Schroeter AL. Primary neuroendocrine carcinomas of the skin (Merkel cell tumors). A clinical, histologic, and ultrastructural study of thirteen cases. Am J Clin Pathol. 1983;79(1):6–13.
109. Silva EG, Mackay B, Goepfert H, Burgess MA, Fields RS. Endocrine carcinoma of the skin (Merkel cell carcinoma). Pathol Annu. 1984;19(Pt 2):1–30.
110. Plaza JA, Suster S. The Toker tumor: spectrum of morphologic features in primary neuroendocrine carcinomas of the skin (Merkel cell carcinoma). Ann Diagn Pathol. 2006;10(6):376–85.
111. Vazmitel M, Michal M, Kazakov DV. Merkel cell carcinoma and Azzopardi phenomenon. Am J Dermatopathol. 2007;29(3):314–5.

112. Vazmitel M, Michal M, Shelekhova KV, Sima R, Mukensnabl P, Kazakov DV. Vascular changes in Merkel cell carcinoma based on a histopathological study of 92 cases. Am J Dermatopathol. 2008;30(2):106–11.
113. Vazmitel M, Michal M, Kempf W, Mukensnabl P, Kazakov DV. Merkel cell carcinoma with a follicular lymphocytic infiltrate: report of 2 cases. Am J Dermatopathol. 2008;30(4):389–91.
114. Gould E, Albores-Saavedra J, Dubner B, Smith W, Payne CM. Eccrine and squamous differentiation in Merkel cell carcinoma. An immunohistochemical study. Am J Surg Pathol. 1988;12(10):768–72.
115. Iacocca MV, Abernethy JL, Stefanato CM, Allan AE, Bhawan J. Mixed Merkel cell carcinoma and squamous cell carcinoma of the skin. J Am Acad Dermatol. 1998;39(5 Pt 2):882–7.
116. Cooper L, Debono R, Alsanjari N, Al-Nafussi A. Merkel cell tumour with leiomyosarcomatous differentiation. Histopathology. 2000;36(6):540–3.
117. Foschini MP, Eusebi V. Divergent differentiation in endocrine and nonendocrine tumors of the skin. Semin Diagn Pathol. 2000;17(2):162–8.
118. Boutilier R, Desormeau L, Cragg F, Roberts P, Walsh N. Merkel cell carcinoma: squamous and atypical fibroxanthoma-like differentiation in successive local tumor recurrences. Am J Dermatopathol. 2001;23(1):46–9.
119. Fernandez-Figueras MT, Puig L, Gilaberte M, Gomez-Plaza Mdel C, Rex J, Ferrandiz C, et al. Merkel cell (primary neuroendocrine) carcinoma of the skin with nodal metastasis showing rhabdomyosarcomatous differentiation. J Cutan Pathol. 2002;29(10):619–22.
120. Hwang JH, Alanen K, Dabbs KD, Danyluk J, Silverman S. Merkel cell carcinoma with squamous and sarcomatous differentiation. J Cutan Pathol. 2008;35(10):955–9.
121. Tan KB, Murali R, Karim RZ, Dutta B, Dutta R, McCarthy SW, et al. Merkel cell carcinoma with fibrosarcomatous differentiation. Pathology. 2008;40(3):314–6.
122. Lau PP, Ting SH, Ip YT, Tsang WY, Chan JK. Merkel cell carcinosarcoma: Merkel cell carcinoma with embryonal rhabdomyosarcoma-like component. Ann Diagn Pathol. 2012;16(5):388–91.
123. Adhikari LA, McCalmont TH, Folpe AL. Merkel cell carcinoma with heterologous rhabdomyoblastic differentiation: the role of immunohistochemistry for Merkel cell polyomavirus large T-antigen in confirmation. J Cutan Pathol. 2012;39(1):47–51.
124. Martin B, Poblet E, Rios JJ, Kazakov D, Kutzner H, Brenn T, et al. Merkel cell carcinoma with divergent differentiation: histopathological and immunohistochemical study of 15 cases with PCR analysis for Merkel cell polyomavirus. Histopathology. 2013;62(5):711–22.
125. Koba S, Misago N, Nagase K, Tsuruta N, Inoue T, Ikeda S, et al. Triphasic differentiations of Merkel cell carcinoma in primary and metastatic lesions. J Cutan Pathol. 2014;41(5):469–74.
126. Roncaroli F, Mauri F, Pasquinelli G. Primary neuroendocrine carcinoma with ganglion cell differentiation in a crural lymph node. Virchows Arch. 2000;437(6):675–9.
127. Vanchinathan V, Marinelli EC, Kartha RV, Uzieblo A, Ranchod M, Sundram UN. A malignant cutaneous neuroendocrine tumor with features of Merkel cell carcinoma and differentiating neuroblastoma. Am J Dermatopathol. 2009;31(2):193–6.
128. Iwasaki T, Kodama H, Matsushita M, Kuroda N, Yamasaki Y, Murakami I, et al. Merkel cell polyomavirus infection in both components of a combined Merkel cell carcinoma and basal cell carcinoma with ductal differentiation; each component had a similar but different novel Merkel cell polyomavirus large T antigen truncating mutation. Hum Pathol. 2013;44(3):442–7.
129. Rosso R, Paulli M, Carnevali L. Neuroendocrine carcinoma of the skin with lymphoepithelioma-like features. Am J Dermatopathol. 1998;20(5):483–6.
130. Ben Abdelkrim S, Dhouibi A, Moussa A, Hadhri R, Njim L, Mighri K, et al. Merkel cell carcinoma with lymphoepithelioma-like pattern: a case report of an exceedingly rare variant of Merkel cell carcinoma with lymph node metastases at presentation. Case Rep Pathol. 2011;2011:840575.
131. Li N, Wolgamot G, Argenyi Z. Primary cutaneous neuroendocrine cell carcinoma (Merkel cell carcinoma) with prominent microcystic features, mimicking eccrine carcinoma. J Cutan Pathol. 2007;34(5):410–4.

132. Aydin A, Kocer NE, Bekerecioglu M, Sari I. Cutaneous undifferentiated small (Merkel) cell carcinoma, that developed synchronously with multiple actinic keratoses, squamous cell carcinomas and basal cell carcinoma. J Dermatol. 2003;30(3):241–4.
133. Busam KJ, Jungbluth AA, Rekthman N, Coit D, Pulitzer M, Bini J, et al. Merkel cell polyomavirus expression in Merkel cell carcinomas and its absence in combined tumors and pulmonary neuroendocrine carcinomas. Am J Surg Pathol. 2009;33(9):1378–85.
134. Cerroni L, Kerl H. Primary cutaneous neuroendocrine (Merkel cell) carcinoma in association with squamous- and basal-cell carcinoma. Am J Dermatopathol. 1997;19(6):610–3.
135. Gomez LG, DiMaio S, Silva EG, Mackay B. Association between neuroendocrine (Merkel cell) carcinoma and squamous carcinoma of the skin. Am J Surg Pathol. 1983;7(2):171–7.
136. Hewitt JB, Sherif A, Kerr KM, Stankler L. Merkel cell and squamous cell carcinomas arising in erythema ab igne. Br J Dermatol. 1993;128(5):591–2.
137. Iwafuchi M, Watanabe H, Ishihara N, Takahashi Y, Yoshimura M. A neuroendocrine (Merkel) cell carcinoma with coexisting intraepidermal squamous cell carcinoma of the skin. Its growth accelerated by an extrinsic factor. Acta Pathol Jpn. 1986;36(7):1099–108.
138. Jones CS, Tyring SK, Lee PC, Fine JD. Development of neuroendocrine (Merkel cell) carcinoma mixed with squamous cell carcinoma in erythema ab igne. Arch Dermatol. 1988;124(1):110–3.
139. Sirikanjanapong S, Melamed J, Patel RR. Intraepidermal and dermal Merkel cell carcinoma with squamous cell carcinoma in situ: a case report with review of literature. J Cutan Pathol. 2010;37(8):881–5.
140. Vieites B, Suarez-Penaranda JM, Delgado V, Vazquez-Veiga H, Varela J, Forteza J. Merkel cell carcinoma associated with in situ and invasive squamous cell carcinoma. Acta Derm Venereol. 2009;89(2):184–6.
141. Tan BH, Busam KJ, Pulitzer MP. Combined intraepidermal neuroendocrine (Merkel cell) and squamous cell carcinoma in situ with CM2B4 negativity and p53 overexpression(*). J Cutan Pathol. 2012;39(6):626–30.
142. Popp S, Waltering S, Herbst C, Moll I, Boukamp P. UV-B-type mutations and chromosomal imbalances indicate common pathways for the development of Merkel and skin squamous cell carcinomas. Int J Cancer. 2002;99(3):352–60.
143. Kuwamoto S. Recent advances in the biology of Merkel cell carcinoma. Hum Pathol. 2011;42(8):1063–77.
144. Iwasaki T, Matsushita M, Kuwamoto S, Kato M, Murakami I, Higaki-Mori H, et al. Usefulness of significant morphologic characteristics in distinguishing between Merkel cell polyomavirus-positive and Merkel cell polyomavirus-negative Merkel cell carcinomas. Hum Pathol. 2013;44(9):1912–7.
145. Kuwamoto S, Higaki H, Kanai K, Iwasaki T, Sano H, Nagata K, et al. Association of Merkel cell polyomavirus infection with morphologic differences in Merkel cell carcinoma. Hum Pathol. 2011;42(5):632–40.
146. Tanahashi J, Kashima K, Daa T, Yada N, Fujiwara S, Yokoyama S. Merkel cell carcinoma co-existent with sebaceous carcinoma of the eyelid. J Cutan Pathol. 2009;36(9):983–6.
147. Youker SR, Billingsley EM. Combined Merkel cell carcinoma and atypical fibroxanthoma. J Cutan Med Surg. 2005;9(1):6–9.
148. Ivan D, Bengana C, Lazar AJ, Diwan AH, Prieto VG. Merkel cell tumor in a trichilemmal cyst: collision or association? Am J Dermatopathol. 2007;29(2):180–3.
149. Su W, Kheir SM, Berberian B, Cockerell CJ. Merkel cell carcinoma in situ arising in a trichilemmal cyst: a case report and literature review. Am J Dermatopathol. 2008;30(5):458–61.
150. Requena L, Jaqueti G, Rutten A, Mentzel T, Kutzner H. Merkel cell carcinoma within follicular cysts: report of two cases. J Cutan Pathol. 2008;35(12):1127–33.
151. Craig PJ, Calonje JE, Harries M, Stefanato CM. Incidental chronic lymphocytic leukaemia in a biopsy of Merkel cell carcinoma. J Cutan Pathol. 2009;36(6):706–10.
152. Koljonen V, Kukko H, Pukkala E, Sankila R, Bohling T, Tukiainen E, et al. Chronic lymphocytic leukaemia patients have a high risk of Merkel-cell polyomavirus DNA-positive Merkel-cell carcinoma. Br J Cancer. 2009;101(8):1444–7.

153. Li Z, Yang JJ, Wu M. Collision tumor of primary Merkel cell carcinoma and chronic lymphocytic leukemia/small lymphocytic lymphoma, diagnosed on ultrasound-guided fine-needle aspiration biopsy: A unique case report and review of literature. Diagn Cytopathol. 2015;43:66–71.
154. Papalas JA, McKinney MS, Kulbacki E, Dave SS, Wang E. Merkel cell carcinoma with partial B-cell blastic immunophenotype: a potential mimic of cutaneous richter transformation in a patient with chronic lymphocytic lymphoma. Am J Dermatopathol. 2014;36(2):148–52.
155. Tolstov YL, Arora R, Scudiere SC, Busam K, Chaudhary PM, Chang Y, et al. Lack of evidence for direct involvement of Merkel cell polyomavirus (MCV) in chronic lymphocytic leukemia (CLL). Blood. 2010;115(23):4973–4.
156. Shingde MV, Buckland M, Busam KJ, McCarthy SW, Wilmott J, Thompson JF, et al. Primary cutaneous Ewing sarcoma/primitive neuroectodermal tumour: a clinicopathological analysis of seven cases highlighting diagnostic pitfalls and the role of FISH testing in diagnosis. J Clin Pathol. 2009;62(10):915–9.
157. Terrier-Lacombe MJ, Guillou L, Chibon F, Gallagher G, Benhattar J, Terrier P, et al. Superficial primitive Ewing's sarcoma: a clinicopathologic and molecular cytogenetic analysis of 14 cases. Mod Pathol. 2009;22(1):87–94.
158. Machado I, Llombart B, Calabuig-Farinas S, Llombart-Bosch A. Superficial Ewing's sarcoma family of tumors: a clinicopathological study with differential diagnoses. J Cutan Pathol. 2011;38(8):636–43.
159. Fernandez-Flores A, Suarez-Penaranda JM, Alonso S. Study of EWS/FLI-1 rearrangement in 18 cases of CK20+/CM2B4+ Merkel cell carcinoma using FISH and correlation to the differential diagnosis of Ewing sarcoma/peripheral neuroectodermal tumor. Appl Immunohistochem Mol Morphol. 2013;21(5):379–85.
160. Lloyd RV, Cano M, Rosa P, Hille A, Huttner WB. Distribution of chromogranin A and secretogranin I (chromogranin B) in neuroendocrine cells and tumors. Am J Pathol. 1988;130(2):296–304.
161. Leong AS, Milios J. Cytokeratin distribution in Merkel cell tumor of the skin. Hum Pathol. 1987;18(3):308–9.
162. Battifora H, Silva EG. The use of antikeratin antibodies in the immunohistochemical distinction between neuroendocrine (Merkel cell) carcinoma of the skin, lymphoma, and oat cell carcinoma. Cancer. 1986;58(5):1040–6.
163. Allen PJ, Busam K, Hill AD, Stojadinovic A, Coit DG. Immunohistochemical analysis of sentinel lymph nodes from patients with Merkel cell carcinoma. Cancer. 2001;92(6):1650–5.
164. Miettinen M. Synaptophysin and neurofilament proteins as markers for neuroendocrine tumors. Arch Pathol Lab Med. 1987;111(9):813–8.
165. Narisawa Y, Hashimoto K, Kohda H. Immunohistochemical demonstration of the expression of neurofilament proteins in Merkel cells. Acta Derm Venereol. 1994;74(6):441–3.
166. Arnold MA, Schoenfield L, Limketkai BN, Arnold CA. Diagnostic pitfalls of differentiating desmoplastic small round cell tumor (DSRCT) from Wilms tumor (WT): overlapping morphologic and immunohistochemical features. Am J Surg Pathol. 2014;38(9):1220–6.
167. Jerome Marson V, Mazieres J, Groussard O, Garcia O, Berjaud J, Dahan M, et al. Expression of TTF-1 and cytokeratins in primary and secondary epithelial lung tumours: correlation with histological type and grade. Histopathology. 2004;45(2):125–34.
168. Rund CR, Fischer EG. Perinuclear dot-like cytokeratin 20 staining in small cell neuroendocrine carcinoma of the ovary (pulmonary-type). Appl Immunohistochem Mol Morphol. 2006;14(2):244–8.
169. Schmidt U, Muller U, Metz KA, Leder LD. Cytokeratin and neurofilament protein staining in Merkel cell carcinoma of the small cell type and small cell carcinoma of the lung. Am J Dermatopathol. 1998;20(4):346–51.
170. Gu M, Antonescu CR, Guiter G, Huvos AG, Ladanyi M, Zakowski MF. Cytokeratin immunoreactivity in Ewing's sarcoma: prevalence in 50 cases confirmed by molecular diagnostic studies. Am J Surg Pathol. 2000;24(3):410–6.

171. Bobos M, Hytiroglou P, Kostopoulos I, Karkavelas G, Papadimitriou CS. Immunohistochemical distinction between Merkel cell carcinoma and small cell carcinoma of the lung. Am J Dermatopathol. 2006;28(2):99–104.
172. Calder KB, Coplowitz S, Schlauder S, Morgan MB. A case series and immunophenotypic analysis of CK20-/CK7+ primary neuroendocrine carcinoma of the skin. J Cutan Pathol. 2007;34(12):918–23.
173. Beer TW. Merkel cell carcinomas with CK20 negative and CK7 positive immunostaining. J Cutan Pathol. 2009;36(3):385–6; author reply 7.
174. Lundquist K, Kohler S, Rouse RV. Intraepidermal cytokeratin 7 expression is not restricted to Paget cells but is also seen in Toker cells and Merkel cells. Am J Surg Pathol. 1999;23(2):212–9.
175. Asioli S, Righi A, de Biase D, Morandi L, Caliendo V, Picciotto F, et al. Expression of p63 is the sole independent marker of aggressiveness in localised (stage I-II) Merkel cell carcinomas. Mod Pathol. 2011;24(11):1451–61.
176. Dabner M, McClure RJ, Harvey NT, Budgeon CA, Beer TW, Amanuel B, et al. Merkel cell polyomavirus and p63 status in Merkel cell carcinoma by immunohistochemistry: Merkel cell polyomavirus positivity is inversely correlated with sun damage, but neither is correlated with outcome. Pathology. 2014;46(3):205–10.
177. Fleming KE, Ly TY, Pasternak S, Godlewski M, Doucette S, Walsh NM. Support for p63 expression as an adverse prognostic marker in Merkel cell carcinoma: report on a Canadian cohort. Hum Pathol. 2014;45(5):952–60.
178. Lim CS, Whalley D, Haydu LE, Murali R, Tippett J, Thompson JF, et al. Increasing tumor thickness is associated with recurrence and poorer survival in patients with Merkel cell carcinoma. Ann Surg Oncol. 2012;19(11):3325–34.
179. Shuda M, Arora R, Kwun HJ, Feng H, Sarid R, Fernandez-Figueras MT, et al. Human Merkel cell polyomavirus infection I. MCV T antigen expression in Merkel cell carcinoma, lymphoid tissues and lymphoid tumors. Int J Cancer. 2009;125(6):1243–9.
180. Rodig SJ, Cheng J, Wardzala J, DoRosario A, Scanlon JJ, Laga AC, et al. Improved detection suggests all Merkel cell carcinomas harbor Merkel polyomavirus. J Clin Invest. 2012;122(12):4645–53.
181. Waltari M, Sihto H, Kukko H, Koljonen V, Sankila R, Bohling T, et al. Association of Merkel cell polyomavirus infection with tumor p53, KIT, stem cell factor, PDGFR-alpha and survival in Merkel cell carcinoma. Int J Cancer. 2011;129(3):619–28.
182. Van Gele M, Kaghad M, Leonard JH, Van Roy N, Naeyaert JM, Geerts ML, et al. Mutation analysis of P73 and TP53 in Merkel cell carcinoma. Br J Cancer. 2000;82(4):823–6.
183. Lassacher A, Heitzer E, Kerl H, Wolf P. p14ARF hypermethylation is common but INK4a-ARF locus or p53 mutations are rare in Merkel cell carcinoma. J Invest Dermatol. 2008;128(7):1788–96.
184. Sahi H, Savola S, Sihto H, Koljonen V, Bohling T, Knuutila S. RB1 gene in Merkel cell carcinoma: hypermethylation in all tumors and concurrent heterozygous deletions in the polyomavirus-negative subgroup. APMIS. 2014;122:1157–66.
185. Llombart B, Monteagudo C, Lopez-Guerrero JA, Carda C, Jorda E, Sanmartin O, et al. Clinicopathological and immunohistochemical analysis of 20 cases of Merkel cell carcinoma in search of prognostic markers. Histopathology. 2005;46(6):622–34.
186. Fernandez-Figueras MT, Puig L, Musulen E, Gilaberte M, Lerma E, Serrano S, et al. Expression profiles associated with aggressive behavior in Merkel cell carcinoma. Mod Pathol. 2007;20(1):90–101.
187. Su LD, Fullen DR, Lowe L, Uherova P, Schnitzer B, Valdez R. CD117 (KIT receptor) expression in Merkel cell carcinoma. Am J Dermatopathol. 2002;24(4):289–93.
188. Feinmesser M, Halpern M, Kaganovsky E, Brenner B, Fenig E, Hodak E, et al. c-kit expression in primary and metastatic Merkel cell carcinoma. Am J Dermatopathol. 2004;26(6):458–62.
189. Andea AA, Patel R, Ponnazhagan S, Kumar S, DeVilliers P, Jhala D, et al. Merkel cell carcinoma: correlation of KIT expression with survival and evaluation of KIT gene mutational status. Hum Pathol. 2010;41(10):1405–12.

190. Swick BL, Ravdel L, Fitzpatrick JE, Robinson WA. Merkel cell carcinoma: evaluation of KIT (CD117) expression and failure to demonstrate activating mutations in the C-KIT proto-oncogene – implications for treatment with imatinib mesylate. J Cutan Pathol. 2007;34(4):324–9.
191. Kartha RV, Sundram UN. Silent mutations in KIT and PDGFRA and coexpression of receptors with SCF and PDGFA in Merkel cell carcinoma: implications for tyrosine kinase-based tumorigenesis. Mod Pathol. 2008;21(2):96–104.
192. Ordonez NG. Value of thyroid transcription factor-1 immunostaining in distinguishing small cell lung carcinomas from other small cell carcinomas. Am J Surg Pathol. 2000;24(9):1217–23.
193. Byrd-Gloster AL, Khoor A, Glass LF, Messina JL, Whitsett JA, Livingston SK, et al. Differential expression of thyroid transcription factor 1 in small cell lung carcinoma and Merkel cell tumor. Hum Pathol. 2000;31(1):58–62.
194. Buresh CJ, Oliai BR, Miller RT. Reactivity with TdT in Merkel cell carcinoma: a potential diagnostic pitfall. Am J Clin Pathol. 2008;129(6):894–8.
195. Ralston J, Chiriboga L, Nonaka D. MASH1: a useful marker in differentiating pulmonary small cell carcinoma from Merkel cell carcinoma. Mod Pathol. 2008;21(11):1357–62.
196. Sierakowski A, Al-Janabi K, Dam H, Sood M. Metastatic Merkel cell carcinoma with positive expression of thyroid transcription factor-1 – a case report. Am J Dermatopathol. 2009;31(4):384–6.
197. McNiff JM, Cowper SE, Lazova R, Subtil A, Glusac EJ. CD56 staining in Merkel cell carcinoma and natural killer-cell lymphoma: magic bullet, diagnostic pitfall, or both? J Cutan Pathol. 2005;32(8):541–5.
198. Kolhe R, Reid MD, Lee JR, Cohen C, Ramalingam P. Immunohistochemical expression of PAX5 and TdT by Merkel cell carcinoma and pulmonary small cell carcinoma: a potential diagnostic pitfall but useful discriminatory marker. Int J Clin Exp Pathol. 2013;6(2):142–7.
199. Feinmesser M, Halpern M, Fenig E, Tsabari C, Hodak E, Sulkes J, et al. Expression of the apoptosis-related oncogenes bcl-2, bax, and p53 in Merkel cell carcinoma: can they predict treatment response and clinical outcome? Hum Pathol. 1999;30(11):1367–72.
200. Verhaegen ME, Mangelberger D, Weick JW, Vozheiko TD, Harms PW, Nash KT, et al. Merkel cell carcinoma dependence on bcl-2 family members for survival. J Invest Dermatol. 2014;134(8):2241–50.
201. Filtenborg-Barnkob BE, Bzorek M. Expression of anaplastic lymphoma kinase in Merkel cell carcinomas. Hum Pathol. 2013;44(8):1656–64.
202. Rickelt S, Moll I, Franke WW. Intercellular adhering junctions with an asymmetric molecular composition: desmosomes connecting Merkel cells and keratinocytes. Cell Tissue Res. 2011;346(1):65–77.
203. Kazem S, van der Meijden E, Wang RC, Rosenberg AS, Pope E, Benoit T, et al. Polyomavirus-Associated Trichodysplasia Spinulosa Involves Hyperproliferation, pRB Phosphorylation and Upregulation of p16 and p21. PLoS One. 2014;9(10):e108947.
204. Tolstov YL, Pastrana DV, Feng H, Becker JC, Jenkins FJ, Moschos S, et al. Human Merkel cell polyomavirus infection II. MCV is a common human infection that can be detected by conformational capsid epitope immunoassays. Int J Cancer. 2009;125(6):1250–6.
205. Touze A, Gaitan J, Maruani A, Le Bidre E, Doussinaud A, Clavel C, et al. Merkel cell polyomavirus strains in patients with Merkel cell carcinoma. Emerg Infect Dis. 2009;15(6):960–2.
206. Touze A, Le Bidre E, Laude H, Fleury MJ, Cazal R, Arnold F, et al. High levels of antibodies against Merkel cell polyomavirus identify a subset of patients with Merkel cell carcinoma with better clinical outcome. J Clin Oncol. 2011;29(12):1612–9.
207. Foulongne V, Kluger N, Dereure O, Mercier G, Moles JP, Guillot B, et al. Merkel cell polyomavirus in cutaneous swabs. Emerg Infect Dis. 2010;16(4):685–7.
208. Pancaldi C, Corazzari V, Maniero S, Mazzoni E, Comar M, Martini F, et al. Merkel cell polyomavirus DNA sequences in the buffy coats of healthy blood donors. Blood. 2011;117(26):7099–101.
209. Faust H, Andersson K, Ekstrom J, Hortlund M, Robsahm TE, Dillner J. Prospective study of Merkel cell polyomavirus and risk of Merkel cell carcinoma. Int J Cancer. 2014;134(4):844–8.

210. Martel-Jantin C, Pedergnana V, Nicol JT, Leblond V, Tregouet DA, Tortevoye P, et al. Merkel cell polyomavirus infection occurs during early childhood and is transmitted between siblings. J Clin Virol. 2013;58(1):288–91.
211. Loyo M, Guerrero-Preston R, Brait M, Hoque MO, Chuang A, Kim MS, et al. Quantitative detection of Merkel cell virus in human tissues and possible mode of transmission. Int J Cancer. 2010;126(12):2991–6.
212. Bhatia K, Goedert JJ, Modali R, Preiss L, Ayers LW. Merkel cell carcinoma subgroups by Merkel cell polyomavirus DNA relative abundance and oncogene expression. Int J Cancer. 2010;126(9):2240–6.
213. Garneski KM, Warcola AH, Feng Q, Kiviat NB, Leonard JH, Nghiem P. Merkel cell polyomavirus is more frequently present in North American than Australian Merkel cell carcinoma tumors. J Invest Dermatol. 2009;129(1):246–8.
214. Kassem A, Schopflin A, Diaz C, Weyers W, Stickeler E, Werner M, et al. Frequent detection of Merkel cell polyomavirus in human Merkel cell carcinomas and identification of a unique deletion in the VP1 gene. Cancer Res. 2008;68(13):5009–13.
215. Becker JC, Houben R, Ugurel S, Trefzer U, Pfohler C, Schrama D. MC polyomavirus is frequently present in Merkel cell carcinoma of European patients. J Invest Dermatol. 2009;129(1):248–50.
216. Andres C, Puchta U, Flaig MJ. Detection of Merkel cell polyomavirus DNA in atypical fibroxanthoma in correlation to clinical features. Am J Dermatopathol. 2010;32(8):799–803.
217. Sastre-Garau X, Peter M, Avril MF, Laude H, Couturier J, Rozenberg F, et al. Merkel cell carcinoma of the skin: pathological and molecular evidence for a causative role of MCV in oncogenesis. J Pathol. 2009;218(1):48–56.
218. Sihto H, Kukko H, Koljonen V, Sankila R, Bohling T, Joensuu H. Clinical factors associated with Merkel cell polyomavirus infection in Merkel cell carcinoma. J Natl Cancer Inst. 2009;101(13):938–45.
219. Bhatia S, Afanasiev O, Nghiem P. Immunobiology of Merkel cell carcinoma: implications for immunotherapy of a polyomavirus-associated cancer. Curr Oncol Rep. 2011;13(6):488–97.
220. Borchert S, Czech-Sioli M, Neumann F, Schmidt C, Wimmer P, Dobner T, et al. High-affinity Rb binding, p53 inhibition, subcellular localization, and transformation by wild-type or tumor-derived shortened Merkel cell polyomavirus large T antigens. J Virol. 2014;88(6):3144–60.
221. Houben R, Adam C, Baeurle A, Hesbacher S, Grimm J, Angermeyer S, et al. An intact retinoblastoma protein-binding site in Merkel cell polyomavirus large T antigen is required for promoting growth of Merkel cell carcinoma cells. Int J Cancer. 2012;130(4):847–56.
222. Houben R, Dreher C, Angermeyer S, Borst A, Utikal J, Haferkamp S, et al. Mechanisms of p53 restriction in Merkel cell carcinoma cells are independent of the Merkel cell polyoma virus T antigens. J Invest Dermatol. 2013;133(10):2453–60.
223. Sihto H, Kukko H, Koljonen V, Sankila R, Bohling T, Joensuu H. Merkel cell polyomavirus infection, large T antigen, retinoblastoma protein and outcome in Merkel cell carcinoma. Clin Cancer Res. 2011;17(14):4806–13.
224. Bhatia K, Goedert JJ, Modali R, Preiss L, Ayers LW. Immunological detection of viral large T antigen identifies a subset of Merkel cell carcinoma tumors with higher viral abundance and better clinical outcome. Int J Cancer. 2010;127(6):1493–6.
225. Paulson KG, Carter JJ, Johnson LG, Cahill KW, Iyer JG, Schrama D, et al. Antibodies to Merkel cell polyomavirus T antigen oncoproteins reflect tumor burden in Merkel cell carcinoma patients. Cancer Res. 2010;70(21):8388–97.
226. Allen PJ, Bowne WB, Jaques DP, Brennan MF, Busam K, Coit DG. Merkel cell carcinoma: prognosis and treatment of patients from a single institution. J Clin Oncol. 2005;23(10):2300–9.
227. Schwartz JL, Griffith KA, Lowe L, Wong SL, McLean SA, Fullen DR, et al. Features predicting sentinel lymph node positivity in Merkel cell carcinoma. J Clin Oncol. 2011;29(8):1036–41.
228. Fields RC, Busam KJ, Chou JF, Panageas KS, Pulitzer MP, Kraus DH, et al. Recurrence and survival in patients undergoing sentinel lymph node biopsy for Merkel cell carcinoma: analysis of 153 patients from a single institution. Ann Surg Oncol. 2011;18(9):2529–37.

229. Andea AA, Coit DG, Amin B, Busam KJ. Merkel cell carcinoma: histologic features and prognosis. Cancer. 2008;113(9):2549–58.
230. Mott RT, Smoller BR, Morgan MB. Merkel cell carcinoma: a clinicopathologic study with prognostic implications. J Cutan Pathol. 2004;31(3):217–23.
231. Suomela S, Koljonen V, Skoog T, Kukko H, Bohling T, Saarialho-Kere U. Expression of MMP-10, MMP-21, MMP-26, and MMP-28 in Merkel cell carcinoma. Virchows Arch. 2009;455(6):495–503.
232. Fields RC, Busam KJ, Chou JF, Panageas KS, Pulitzer MP, Allen PJ, et al. Five hundred patients with Merkel cell carcinoma evaluated at a single institution. Ann Surg. 2011;254(3):465–73; discussion 73–5.
233. Fernandez-Figueras MT, Puig L, Musulen E, Gilaberte M, Ferrandiz C, Lerma E, et al. Prognostic significance of p27Kip1, p45Skp2 and Ki67 expression profiles in Merkel cell carcinoma, extracutaneous small cell carcinoma, and cutaneous squamous cell carcinoma. Histopathology. 2005;46(6):614–21.
234. Koljonen V, Tukiainen E, Haglund C, Bohling T. Proliferative activity detected by Ki67 correlates with poor outcome in Merkel cell carcinoma. Histopathology. 2006;49(5):551–3.
235. Tseng J, Dhungel B, Mills JK, Diggs BS, Weerasinghe R, Fortino J, et al. Merkel cell carcinoma: what makes a difference? Am J Surg. 2015;209:342–6.
236. Lipson EJ, Vincent JG, Loyo M, Kagohara LT, Luber BS, Wang H, et al. PD-L1 expression in the Merkel cell carcinoma microenvironment: association with inflammation, Merkel cell polyomavirus and overall survival. Cancer Immunol Res. 2013;1(1):54–63.
237. Shahzad N, Shuda M, Gheit T, Kwun HJ, Cornet I, Saidj D, et al. The T antigen locus of Merkel cell polyomavirus downregulates human Toll-like receptor 9 expression. J Virol. 2013;87(23):13009–19.
238. Afanasiev OK, Yelistratova L, Miller N, Nagase K, Paulson K, Iyer JG, et al. Merkel polyomavirus-specific T cells fluctuate with Merkel cell carcinoma burden and express therapeutically targetable PD-1 and Tim-3 exhaustion markers. Clin Cancer Res. 2013;19(19):5351–60.
239. Sihto H, Bohling T, Kavola H, Koljonen V, Salmi M, Jalkanen S, et al. Tumor infiltrating immune cells and outcome of Merkel cell carcinoma: a population-based study. Clin Cancer Res. 2012;18(10):2872–81.
240. Fan R. PAX immunoreactivity in poorly differentiated small round cell tumors of childhood. Fetal Pediatr Pathol. 2014;33(4):244–52.
241. Desouki MM, Post GR, Cherry D, Lazarchick J. PAX-5: a valuable immunohistochemical marker in the differential diagnosis of lymphoid neoplasms. Clin Med Res. 2010;8(2):84–8.

Extraskeletal Ewing Sarcoma/Primitive Neuroectodermal Tumor

Rania Shamekh, Vicky Pham, and Marilyn M. Bui

Introduction

Ewing sarcoma (ES)/primitive neuroectodermal tumor (PNET) is the most common bone tumor between the age of 0–4 years [1], the second most common bone malignancy in children and adolescents [2–5], and the third most common bone sarcoma among adults [5]. ES/PNET is a family of tumor that shares hallmark molecular signature and varying degrees of neuroectodermal differentiation, which is now designated as ES by the 2013 *WHO Classification of Tumours of Soft Tissue and Bone* [3]. ES is more common among males compared to females with a male to female ratio of 3.4:1.6 [1]. The incidence of ES is higher among white population and is low among black and Asian populations [1]. Eighty to 90 % of ES affect the bony skeleton, commonly involving the diaphysis and metaphysis of long bones [3]. ES can also be seen in the pelvis, scapula, ribs, and skull. The remaining 10–20 % are extraskeletal. ES have been described in the lung [6], gastrointestinal tract [7], pancreas [8], breast [9], uterus [10], cervix [11], and pineal gland [12, 13].

R. Shamekh, MD
Department of Cell Biology and Pathology, University of South Florida Morsani College of Medicine, Tampa, FL 33612, USA

V. Pham, MS
Research Scholar Concentration Program, University of South Florida Morsani College of Medicine, Tampa, FL 33612, USA

M.M. Bui, MD, PhD (✉)
Department of Cell Biology and Pathology, University of South Florida Morsani College of Medicine, Tampa, FL 33612, USA

Department of Anatomic Pathology, Moffitt Cancer Center, Tampa, FL 33612, USA

Department of Sarcoma, Moffitt Cancer Center, Tampa, FL 33612, USA

Departments of Oncological Sciences, University of South Florida, Tampa, FL 33612, USA
e-mail: Marilyn.Bui@Moffitt.org

A. Nasir, D. Coppola (eds.), *Neuroendocrine Tumors: Review of Pathology, Molecular and Therapeutic Advances*, DOI 10.1007/978-1-4939-3426-3_22

Pathogenesis

ES shows neuroectodermal differentiation with a pathognomonic translocation of the *EWSR1* gene on chromosome 22 with one of the ETS transcription factors. This specific translocation results in fusion oncogenes that is very characteristic for the Ewing/PNET (ES/PNET) pathogenesis [3], which is summarized in Table 1.

Microscopic Appearance

ES is mostly composed of small, blue, round cells with scant cytoplasm and indistinct cytoplasmic membrane. The nuclei are uniform and round with finely granular chromatin [3]. Ewing sarcoma is divided into several subtypes: (1) Classic Ewing sarcoma, which is the most common subtype. It is comprised of nests or sheets of small uniform cells with round nuclei, smooth nuclear contours, fine granular chromatin, and inconspicuous nucleoli. The cytoplasm is scant and eosinophilic. Mitosis and necrosis are infrequent. (2) PNET is composed of Ewing sarcoma with various degrees of neuroectodermal differentiation (confirmed by immunohistochemistry) together with true and pseudorosettes rendering the diagnosis of Ewing/PNET. (3) Atypical Ewing sarcoma is composed of large cells with large pleomorphic nuclei, irregular nuclear contour, coarse chromatin, and prominent nuclei. Mitosis and necrosis are common [4, 14]. Other rare ES subtypes include: (4) Adamantinoma Ewing sarcoma, which consists of nests of pleomorphic, hyperchromatic cells with peripheral palisading within a desmoplastic stroma [14, 15]. (5) Spindle cell Ewing sarcoma, this subtype is characterized by greater degree of spindling admixed with branching vasculature, reminiscent of a spindle

Table 1 Chromosomal rearrangement and fusion genes of ES [3]

Chromosomal rearrangement	Fusion gene
t(11;22)(q24;q12)	*EWSR1-FLI1*
t(21;22)(q22;q12)	*EWSR1-ERG*
t(7;22)(p22;q12)	*EWSR1-ETV1*
t(17;22)(q21;q12)	*EWSR1-ETV4*
t(2;22)(q35;q12)	*EWSR1-FEV*
t(16;21)(p11;q22)	*FUS-ERG*
t(2;16)(q35;p11)	*FUS-FEV*
t(20;22)(q13;q12)	*EWSR1-NFATC2*
t(6;22)(p21;q12)	*EWSR1-POU5F1*
t(4;22)(q31;q12)	*EWSR1-SMARCA5*
Submicroscopic inv (22) in t(1;22)(p36.1;q12)	*EWSR1-PATZ*
t(2;22)(q31;q12)	*EWSR1-SP3*
t(4;19)(q35;q13)	*CIC-DUX4*

cell sarcoma. (6) Sclerosing Ewing sarcoma, the neoplastic cells resembled the cells of typical ES but is distinguished by the presence of abundant, hyalinized, eosinophilic matrix [14].

Immunophenotype

The classic Ewing, which lacks neuroendocrine differentiation, expresses strong membranous staining for CD99 [3–16]. The FLI-1 protein expression, resulting in fusion of the *EWS* gene on chromosome 22 to the *FLI-1* gene on chromosome 11 (*EWSR1-FLI-1*), is another diagnostic marker of the classic Ewing sarcoma [16–18] (representative case shown in Fig. 1). FLI-1 has been expressed in more than 70 % of ES/PNET with greater than 90 % specificity [15]. Therefore, FLI-1 is useful for the diagnosis of ES/PNET. *NKX2*, a member of the NK2 family of

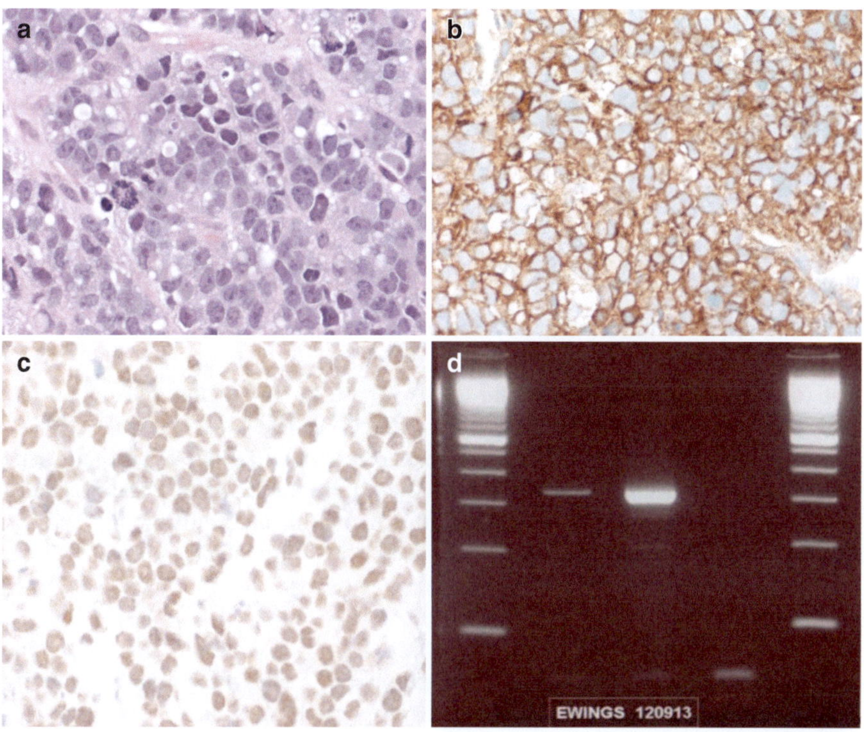

Fig. 1 A Ewing sarcoma in the right posterior shoulder of a 71-year-old man. (**a**) HE stain of the tumor exhibiting blue round cell tumor with epithelioid morphology. 200×. (**b**) CD99 immunostain reveals strong membrane reactivity. (**c**) FLI-1 immunostain is positive in the tumor nuclei. (**d**) The tumor harbors an EWSR1/FLI fusion transcript, type II, by RT-PCR confirming the diagnosis. Lane 1 and 4 DNA, size controls. Lane 3, positive control. Lane 4, patient sample

transcription, has an essential role in neuronal differentiation [19]. The *NKX2.2* gene has been recently identified as another important factor, similar to EWS/FLI in Ewing sarcoma oncogenesis [20]. For ES with *EWS-ERG* rearrangement, ERG protein expression, using the newly discovered anti-ERG antibody, is helpful for the diagnosis [21].

The PNET differentiation can be assessed by the expression of all classes of intermediate filament proteins [22], as well as synaptophysin, chromograin, CD56, CD57, CD99, neuron-specific enolase (NSE) [23].

Classic ES Versus ES/PNET

In 1991, a report by Schmidt and colleagues stated that neuroectodermal differentiation in ES (ES/PNET) has the worst prognosis and a significant decrease in disease-free survival compared to classic ES [24]. However, recent articles found that neuroectodermal differentiation in Ewing sarcoma (ES/PNET) had no prognostic impact when compared to classic ES [25]. These contradicting results may be due to the use of modern, more effective combined multiagent chemotherapy, radiation, and/or surgery which has improved the prognosis and outcome of ES/PNET dramatically [26]. Therefore, histological classification of ES is not neither necessary nor essential for proper management.

Differential Diagnosis

As small, blue, round cell tumors that may express neuroendocrine differentiation, ES overlaps morphologically and histologically with a group of malignant neoplasms that can occur in both children and adults. These tumors include neuroblastoma (NB), rhabdomyosarcoma (RMS), poorly differentiated synovial sarcomas (PDSS), lymphoblastic lymphoma (LBL), esthesioneuroblastoma (ENB), and desmoplastic round cell tumor (DRCT), mesenchymal chondrosarcoma (MCS), and blastemal predominant Wilms' tumor (WT). These tumors are histologically similar and can only be distinguished by their immunohistochemical profile and molecular profile [15, 27]. Useful immunohistochemical and molecular profiles for the above tumors are summarized in Table 2.

ES may present as a diagnostic pitfall mimicking a neuroendocrine carcinoma when neuroendocrine differentiation is expressed in conjunction with cytokeratin aberrant expression. In fact, ES can express the high molecular weight cytokeratin AE1/AE3 in almost 40 % of cases [31]. Therefore, in the proper histological and molecular setting, the expression of cytokeratin does not exclude the diagnosis of ES.

Table 2 Immunohistochemical and molecular characteristics of tumors mimic ES [3, 28–30]

Diagnosis	Translocation/molecular characteristics	Immunohistochemical positivity
Ewing-like sarcomas (undifferentiated round cell sarcomas)	*CIC-DUX4*, t(4:19)(q35;q13) or t(10;19)(q26;q13) CIC-FOXO4, t(X;19)(q13;q13.3)	CD 99 (patchy) Variable stains for CD34 Keratin, EMA, actin, and desmin
Alveolar rhabdomyosarcoma	*PAX3-FOXO1*, t(2;13)(q35;q14) *PAX7-FOXO1*, t(1;13)(p36;q14)	Desmin Myoglobin Myogenin Actin
Desmoplastic small round cell tumor	*WT1-EWSR1*, t(11;22)(p13;q12)	Multilineage markers such as: EMA and cytokeratin Vimentin and desmin NSE Desmin (dot-like) WT-1 carboxy-terminus
Extraskeletal myxoid chondrosarcoma	*NR4A3-EWSR1*, t(9:22)(q22;q12) *NR4A3-TAF15*, t(9;17)(q22;q11)	S100 (20 %) CD117 (CKIT) (30 %) Synaptophysin and NSE Loss of INI (tumors with rhabdoid features)
Clear cell sarcoma	*ATF1-EWSR1*, t(12;22)(q13;q12)	S100 HMB-45 MITF1 Other melanocytic markers

Management and Some Biomarkers

Five-year survival rates of ES were 68 % in males and 65 % in females [2, 32]. Decrease in survival rate can be due to tumor size (>8 cm) and presence of metastatic disease [32]. Management of localized disease includes wide surgical excision +/− chemotherapy to irradiate disease and prevent recurrence. Management of metastatic disease include chemotherapy, radiotherapy, and possible resection of limited metastasis [32].

Studies of additional biomarkers are underway to discover diagnostic, prognostic, and predictive information. Interestingly, the M3 and M5 subtypes of muscarinic acetylcholine receptor as well as the alpha 7 subunit of nicotinic acetylcholine receptor have been expressed in a significant number of ES/PNET family of tumors [33]. However, the clinical significance of these findings is yet to be determined. It was recently suggested that the expression of the gap junction protein connexin 43 in EWS/PNETs is reminiscent of a more aggressive clinical behavior [34].

Genomic technologies have identified genes that are modulated by EWS/FLI in Ewing sarcoma. The study of various chromosomes copy number alterations in Ewing sarcoma using karyotyping, comparative genomic hybridization, and single nucleotide polymorphism (SNP) microarray technologies has been previously reported. The summary of chromosomal aberration in Ewing sarcoma has been reviewed [35].

Tumor cells can be detected in the peripheral blood and/or bone marrow where they circulate. Circulating tumor cell (CTC) detection has been reported in epithelial neoplasms such as breast and colorectal carcinoma [36–39]; however, only few studies have been reported regarding CTC in ES. Analysis of bone marrow (BM) and peripheral blood (PB) of patients with ES using RT-PCR showed positive CTC in metastatic (46 % in BM and 22 % in PB) and nonmetastatic disease (19 % in BM and 20 % in PB) [40]. MicroRNAs (miRNAs) are short noncoding RNA which regulate gene expression, promote proliferation and differentiation, and may predispose to various human malignancies [41]. The role of microRNAs in ES pathogenesis has been investigated in the last few years. Studies have been targeted and aimed at microRNAs mediated by the *EWS-FLI-1* translocations. In vitro studies on human pediatric mesenchymal cell lines (hpMSCs) expressing EWS-FLI-1 showed that repression of miRNA-145 and the *SOX2* gene modulation induced ES pathogenesis [42]. Another in vitro study showed that hsa-miR-145 suppresses EWS-FLI-1 translation and therefore has a major role in ES pathogenesis [43]. In vivo studies on an ES mouse model showed that the *EWS-FLI-1* translocation induces CD99 expression by the inhibition of miRNA-30a-5p expression [44]. These new data may propose the utilization of miRNA as a future therapeutic target in the management of Ewing sarcoma.

Conclusion

ES should be considered as a rare but important differential diagnosis when working up a blue round cell tumor of soft tissue with neuroendocrine differentiation. Hallmark genetic marker can confirm the diagnosis, while some new immunostains are also helpful. New biomarkers are under investigation.

Abbreviations

DRCT	Desmoplastic round cell tumor
ENB	Esthesioneuroblastoma
ES	Ewing sarcoma
LBL	Lymphoblastic lymphoma
MCS	Mesenchymal chondrosarcoma
NB	Neuroblastoma

NSE	Neuron-specific enolase
PDSS	Poorly differentiated synovial sarcomas
PNET	Primitive neuroectodermal tumor
RMS	Rhabdomyosarcoma
WT	Blastemal predominant Wilms' tumor

References

1. Parkin DM, Stiller CA, Nectoux J. International variations in the incidence of childhood bone tumours. Int J Cancer. 1993;53(3):371–6.
2. Linabery AM, Ross JA. Childhood and adolescent cancer survival in the US by race and ethnicity for the diagnostic period 1975-1999. Cancer. 2008;113(9):2575–96.
3. Fletcher CDM, Bridge JA, Hogendoorn PCW, Mertens F, editors. WHO classification of tumours of soft tissue and bone. 4th ed. Lyon Cedex: International Agency for Research on Cancer (IARC) Press; 2013. International Agency for Research on Cancer. Fred T. Bosman ESJ, Sunii R. Lakhani, Hiroko Ohgaki, ed.
4. Choi EY, Gardner JM, Lucas DR, McHugh JB, Patel RM. Ewing sarcoma. Semin Diagn Pathol. 2014;31(1):39–47.
5. Herzog CE. Overview of sarcomas in the adolescent and young adult population. J Pediatr Hematol Oncol. 2005;27(4):215–8.
6. Kahn AG, Avagnina A, Nazar J, Elsner B. Primitive neuroectodermal tumor of the lung. Arch Pathol Lab Med. 2001;125(3):397–9.
7. Stockman DL, Miettinen M, Suster S, et al. Malignant gastrointestinal neuroectodermal tumor: clinicopathologic, immunohistochemical, ultrastructural, and molecular analysis of 16 cases with a reappraisal of clear cell sarcoma-like tumors of the gastrointestinal tract. Am J Surg Pathol. 2012;36(6):857–68.
8. Movahedi-Lankarani S, Hruban RH, Westra WH, Klimstra DS. Primitive neuroectodermal tumors of the pancreas: a report of seven cases of a rare neoplasm. Am J Surg Pathol. 2002;26(8):1040–7.
9. Potier B, Arnaud D, Paillocher N, Darsonval V, Rousseau P. Primitive neuroendocrine cancer of the breast. Post-traumatic discovery of a man. Ann Chir Plast Esthet. 2012;57(6):630–3.
10. Akbayir O, Gungorduk K, Rafioglu G, et al. Primary primitive neuroectodermal tumor of the uterus: a case report. Arch Gynecol Obstet. 2008;277(4):345–8.
11. Tsao AS, Roth LM, Sandler A, Hurteau JA. Cervical primitive neuroectodermal tumor. Gynecol Oncol. 2001;83(1):138–42.
12. Saab R, Rodriguez-Galindo C, Matmati K, et al. p18Ink4c and p53 Act as tumor suppressors in cyclin D1-driven primitive neuroectodermal tumor. Cancer Res. 2009;69(2):440–8.
13. Schwartz AM, Ghatak NR, Laine FJ. Intrasellar primitive neuroectodermal tumor (PNET) in familial retinoblastoma: a variant of "trilateral retinoblastoma". Clin Neuropathol. 1990;9(2):55–9.
14. Pinto A, Dickman P, Parham D. Pathobiologic markers of the ewing sarcoma family of tumors: state of the art and prediction of behaviour. Sarcoma. 2011;2011:856190.
15. Folpe AL, Hill CE, Parham DM, O'Shea PA, Weiss SW. Immunohistochemical detection of FLI-1 protein expression: a study of 132 round cell tumors with emphasis on CD99-positive mimics of Ewing's sarcoma/primitive neuroectodermal tumor. Am J Surg Pathol. 2000;24(12):1657–62.
16. Olsen SH, Thomas DG, Lucas DR. Cluster analysis of immunohistochemical profiles in synovial sarcoma, malignant peripheral nerve sheath tumor, and Ewing sarcoma. Mod Pathol. 2006;19(5):659–68.
17. Rossi S, Orvieto E, Furlanetto A, Laurino L, Ninfo V, Dei Tos AP. Utility of the immunohistochemical detection of FLI-1 expression in round cell and vascular neoplasm using a monoclonal antibody. Mod Pathol. 2004;17(5):547–52.

18. Bui MM, Zhang P. Ewing sarcoma: molecular characterization and potential molecular therapeutic targets. In: Coppola D, editor. Mechanisms of oncogenesis – an update on tumorgenesis, vol. 12. Dordrecht/London: Springer; 2010.
19. Yoshida A, Sekine S, Tsuta K, Fukayama M, Furuta K, Tsuda H. NKX2.2 is a useful immunohistochemical marker for Ewing sarcoma. Am J Surg Pathol. 2012;36(7):993–9.
20. Smith R, Owen LA, Trem DJ, et al. Expression profiling of EWS/FLI identifies NKX2.2 as a critical target gene in Ewing's sarcoma. Cancer Cell. 2006;9(5):405–16.
21. Wang WL, Patel NR, Caragea M, et al. Expression of ERG, an Ets family transcription factor, identifies ERG-rearranged Ewing sarcoma. Mod Pathol. 2012;25(10):1378–83.
22. Gould VE, Jansson DS, Molenaar WM, et al. Primitive neuroectodermal tumors of the central nervous system. Patterns of expression of neuroendocrine markers, and all classes of intermediate filament proteins. Lab Invest. 1990;62(4):498–509.
23. Wick MR. Immunohistology of neuroendocrine and neuroectodermal tumors. Semin Diagn Pathol. 2000;17(3):194–203.
24. Schmidt D, Herrmann C, Jurgens H, Harms D. Malignant peripheral neuroectodermal tumor and its necessary distinction from Ewing's sarcoma. A report from the Kiel Pediatric Tumor Registry. Cancer. 1991;68(10):2251–9.
25. Parham DM, Hijazi Y, Steinberg SM, et al. Neuroectodermal differentiation in Ewing's sarcoma family of tumors does not predict tumor behavior. Hum Pathol. 1999;30(8):911–8.
26. Wexler LH, Meyer WH, Parham DM, Tsokos M. Neural differentiation and prognosis in peripheral primitive neuroectodermal tumor. J Clin Oncol. 2000;18(10):2187–8.
27. Wei S, Siegal GP. Round cell tumors of bone: an update on recent molecular genetic advances. Adv Anat Pathol. 2014;21(5):359–72.
28. Henderson-Jackson EB, Conley A, Bui MM. Molecular pathology of bone and soft tissue neoplasms and potential targets for novel therapy. In: Coppola D, editor. Molecular pathology and diagnostics of cancer – cancer growth and progression, vol. 16. Dordrecht: Springer; 2014.
29. Henderson-Jackson EB, Bui MM. Molecular pathology of soft-tissue neoplasms and its role in clinical practice. Cancer Control. 2015;22(2):186–92.
30. Dodd LG, Bui MM. Atlas of soft tissue and bone pathology: with histologic, cytologic, and radiologic correlations. New York: Demos Medical; 2015.
31. Elbashier SH, Nazarina AR, Looi LM. Cytokeratin immunoreactivity in Ewing sarcoma/ primitive neuroectodermal tumour. Malays J Pathol. 2013;35(2):139–45.
32. Ludwig JA. Ewing sarcoma: historical perspectives, current state-of-the-art, and opportunities for targeted therapy in the future. Curr Opin Oncol. 2008;20(4):412–8.
33. Schlauder SM, Steffensen TS, Morgan M, et al. Assessment of muscarinic and nicotinic acetylcholine receptor expression in primitive neuroectodermal tumor/ewing family of tumor and desmoplastic small round cell tumor: an immunohistochemical and Western blot study of tissue microarray and cell lines. Fetal Pediatr Pathol. 2008;27(2):83–97.
34. Bui MM, Han G, Acs G, et al. Connexin 43 is a potential prognostic biomarker for ewing sarcoma/primitive neuroectodermal tumor. Sarcoma. 2011;2011:971050.
35. Toomey EC, Schiffman JD, Lessnick SL. Recent advances in the molecular pathogenesis of Ewing's sarcoma. Oncogene. 2010;29(32):4504–16.
36. Leung CT, Brugge JS. Tumor self-seeding: bidirectional flow of tumor cells. Cell. 2009;139(7):1226–8.
37. Luo M, Clouthier SG, Deol Y, et al. Breast cancer stem cells: current advances and clinical implications. Methods Mol Biol. 2015;1293:1–49.
38. Maltoni R, Fici P, Amadori D, et al. Circulating tumor cells in early breast cancer: a connection with vascular invasion. Cancer Lett. 2015;367(1):43–8.
39. van Dalum G, Stam GJ, Scholten LF, et al. Importance of circulating tumor cells in newly diagnosed colorectal cancer. Int J Oncol. 2015;46(3):1361–8.
40. Schleiermacher G, Peter M, Oberlin O, et al. Increased risk of systemic relapses associated with bone marrow micrometastasis and circulating tumor cells in localized ewing tumor. J Clin Oncol. 2003;21(1):85–91.

41. Mallanna SK, Rizzino A. Emerging roles of microRNAs in the control of embryonic stem cells and the generation of induced pluripotent stem cells. Dev Biol. 2010;344(1):16–25.
42. Riggi N, Suva ML, De Vito C, et al. EWS-FLI-1 modulates miRNA145 and SOX2 expression to initiate mesenchymal stem cell reprogramming toward Ewing sarcoma cancer stem cells. Genes Dev. 2010;24(9):916–32.
43. Ban J, Jug G, Mestdagh P, et al. Hsa-mir-145 is the top EWS-FLI1-repressed microRNA involved in a positive feedback loop in Ewing's sarcoma. Oncogene. 2011;30(18):2173–80.
44. Franzetti GA, Laud-Duval K, Bellanger D, Stern MH, Sastre-Garau X, Delattre O. MiR-30a-5p connects EWS-FLI1 and CD99, two major therapeutic targets in Ewing tumor. Oncogene. 2013;32(33):3915–21.

Part III
Molecular & Therapeutic Advances in Neuroendocrine Tumor Pathology

Molecular Pathology of Neuroendocrine Tumor: The Era of Targeted Therapeutics

Anthony M. Magliocco

Introduction

Neuroendocrine tumors are a heterogeneous neoplasm of diverse origin arising from a multitude of organs and tissues including the gastrointestinal tract, pancreas, bronchial tissues, thymus, parathyroid, adrenal, pituitary, and calcitonin-producing cells of the thyroid gland.

The prevalence is unfortunately increasing to a current rate of over 35/100,000 [1]. Complicating this is the fact that tumors in 80 % of cases present with advanced disease and metastasis with a 5-year survival rate of less than 40 %. Consequently, there is great need for effective systemic therapy [2].

Molecular Biology

Neuroendocrine neoplasms, of both endocrine and exocrine types, share the feature that they are generally under the control of the peptide hormone somatostatin [3].

Somatostatin primarily effects its action via interaction with somatostatin receptors (SSTRs). These membrane-associated receptors function via G-coupled signaling. Somatostatin also has effects on ion channels and tyrosine kinase receptors [4].

There are five main SSTRs that all bind somatostatin but have different cellular signaling effects [5].

A.M. Magliocco, MD
Anatomic Pathology Department, Moffitt Cancer Center, Tampa, FL, USA
e-mail: anthony.magliocco@moffitt.org

A. Nasir, D. Coppola (eds.), *Neuroendocrine Tumors: Review of Pathology, Molecular and Therapeutic Advances*, DOI 10.1007/978-1-4939-3426-3_23

SSTR Biology

SSTR1 leads to MAPK pathway activation [6].

SSTR2 is most commonly expressed in GI-NETs and pancreatic NETS. SSTR2 activation results in activation of SHP1 downregulation of MAPK resulting in cell cycle suppression via Rb and p21. Its signaling is inactivated via recycling.

SSTR3 is connected with phosphotyrosine phosphatase (PTP)-dependent apoptosis, involving p53 and Bax activities. It may also have an effect on suppression of VEGF. It is downregulated via internalization and ubiquitination.

SSTR4 signaling results in upregulation of MAPK/ERK1/ERK2 pathway and subsequent cellular proliferations. SSTR4 is inactivated via internalization.

SSTR5 is connected with ion exchange channels K+/H+, voltage dependent Ca2+ and also with AMP and kainate glutamate signaling [7].

Somatostatin Analogues (SSAs)

SSTRs represent an attractive target for pharmacological targeting. Natural somatostatin has a very short half-life of only a few minutes due to rapid enzymatic digestion. Consequently more stable synthetic forms have been developed for therapeutic purposes; these include octreotide (SSTR2), lanreotide (SSTR5), pasireotide (SSTR1, SSTR2, SSTR3, SSTR5), and KE108 (SSTR1, SSTR2, SSTR3, SSTR4, SSTR5). These various SSAs have different affinities for SSTRs [8].

SSTRs Expression Patterns

SSTRs are also expressed broadly in non-endocrine cells including cells of blood vessels, stroma, and the immune system. Because of this broad distribution of SSTRs, SSAs have both direct and indirect effects on NET biology and growth [9].

Direct Effects of SSAs

The main direct effects of SSA on NETs are mediated through the action of the SSTR system and a variety of molecular signaling pathways within NET cells. These pathways and molecular mechanisms include the following:

1. Activation of p27kip1 via signaling through SHP1 and SHP2 and r-PTPeta
2. Downregulation of proliferation via suppression of PTP, cGMP, and RAS signaling

3. Triggering of apoptosis via p53 and BAX pathway activation via SSTR3 and dopamine receptor
4. Intracellular pH modification via NHE1 channel alterations
5. Induction of endogenous connexins (CX26 GJB2 and CX42) to form gap junctions

Indirect Effects of SSAs

Because SSTRs are expressed on non-NET tissues, SSAs also have indirect effects on NET growth. These indirect effects include the following molecular mechanisms:

1. Inhibition of trophic hormone release via calcium depletion. These pathways include GH, IGF1, EGF, insulin, gastrin, prolactin, VIP, serotonin, and others. This is probably mediated via transcription factor STAT5b through SSTR2 or SSTR3 activities.
2. Suppression of angiogenesis, via suppression of SSTR2 activity on neoangiogenetic endothelial cells. In addition, there may be suppression of VEGF and fibroblast growth factor via SSTR1, SSTR2, SSTR3, and SSTR5.
3. SSAs appear to possess immunomodulatory activity via triggering interferon release. In addition, there may be effects on lymphocyte proliferation and natural killer cell activities.

Interferon ALPHA

Interferon alpha appears to have a variety of inhibitory effects on NETs. These include direct effects on the neoplasms via induction of cell cycle arrest and apoptosis via a variety of signaling pathways and interferon receptors. In addition, interferon alpha has effects on angiogenesis via suppression of VEGF and the immune activity of the lymphocytes in the surrounding stroma. Unfortunately, INF-alpha has marked toxic side effects including induction of flu-like symptoms, fatigue, weight loss, and significant myelotoxicity [10, 11].

SSAs and INF-alpha have also been used in combination with synergistic results.

Carcinoid Syndrome

Carcinoid syndrome causes serious morbidity in some patients with NETs due to release of functional hormones from the neoplasm including serotonin, tachykinin, and substance P. The syndrome is characterized by flushing, diarrhea, tachycardia, abdominal pains, hypo- and hypertension, and cardiac abnormalities including heart valve fibrosis.

Carcinoid can be monitored biochemically by laboratory tests that measure chromogranin A or 5-hydroxyindoleacetic acid.

SSAs often have good effects on treating the symptoms of carcinoid syndrome by inducing stable disease or disease regression and reducing the levels of 5HIAA and chromogranin A [12].

Octreotide was approved in 1987 for the treatment of carcinoid, glucagonoma, and Verner-Morrison disease [13, 14]. Octreotide has a modified amino acid structure with a substitution of 3 amino acids resulting in an enhanced activity and stability of the molecule resulting in a 120-min half-life and an effective activity of over 12 h. The drug has low toxicity and has an effect against NET with low Ki67 proliferative indices.

Clinical Trials and SSAs

Trials such as PROMID which examined octreotide vs. placebo and CLARINET pitting lanreotide against placebo in phase II studies showed excellent signals with notable gains in progression-free survival [14–16].

Resistance to SSAs

Unfortunately, NETs often develop resistance to SSA treatment. This is via a variety of mechanisms including the following:

1. Tachyphylaxis, desensitization of the receptors
2. Development of mutated forms of the SSTR receptors (SSTR5/MD4 in pituitary adenoma)
3. Development of autoantibodies against the SSAs as SSAs are peptides and potentially immunogenic
4. Modification of other regulatory proteins such as amphiphysin IIb

Targeted Agents

Besides the SSTRs, NETs show a variety of potentially actionable molecular alterations. These include significant vascularity and overexpression of pro-angiogenic factors such as VEGF, VEGFR, and PDGF raising the possibility of using anti-angiogenic agents such as bevacizumab [17–19].

Further, several of the signaling pathways lead to mTOR activation, raising it as a potentially attractive target. This has led to the initiation of trials combining the anti-mTOR everolimus with octreotide (RADIANT 2, a phase III study) [20–22].

Sunitinib, an oral multitargeted RTK inhibitor of VEGFR, PDGFR, cKIT, RET FLT3, and others, has shown benefit in phase II and phase III trials with patients with NETs and has been approved for use by both European authorities and the FDA for treatment of metastatic unresectable PNET [23–25].

The Raf pathway has been investigated in NETs but with limited results. In melanomas and other tumors, BRAF is frequently activated via a mutational event (V600E) making BRAF an attractive and functional target. However, in NETs BRAF mutations are not observed. Some effects were noted with anti-RAF treatment using sorafenib, but the effects were most likely due to anti-angiogenic activities [26].

Following the report of EGFR expression and upregulation in some cases of NET [27], anti-EFGR therapies have also been tested in a limited number of patients.

Telotristat Etiprate (LX1606)

Telotristat etiprate is an inhibitor of tryptophan hydroxylase involved in serotonin biosynthesis and an attractive target to abrogate the effects of carcinoid syndrome [28, 29].

Chimeric Somatostatin

Evidence is emerging that there may be interactions between SSTR and D2 receptors leading to the development of a new class of chimeric molecules that target both, and these include BIM-23A758 and BIM-23A760 [30–32].

Radiotargeted Therapy

Trials are underway to evaluate the effectiveness of radiotargeted therapies using 90Y and 177Lu. Agents include 177Lu-DOTA-TYR3-octreotate [33].

Other Molecular Targets

Advances in genomic analysis technology and deep sequencing methods enable the uncovering of novel potentially actionable targetable mutations. Some targets that have emerged are of interest and include SMAD4 (targeting the TGF-beta pathway). DAXX and ATRX have also been shown to be altered [34, 35]. These genes are involved in chromatin remodeling.

Immunotherapy

Immunotherapy is rapidly emerging as a consideration in many tumor types, particularly after the spectacular results in several trials using immune checkpoint inhibitors for the treatment of advanced solid tumors including metastatic melanoma. These results are particularly encouraging given that in many instances, the checkpoint inhibitors display synergistic activity and extremely long durable responses unlike many targeted therapies. Current targets include PD-1, PD-L1, and CTLA4. These agents are currently under investigation in advanced NET [36–38].

Summary

NETs represent a diverse, heterogeneous group of neoplasms that frequently present with advanced stage and are often complicated by development of carcinoid syndrome. The mainstay of treatment is based on their proliferative activity. Tumors with high activity are subjected to cytotoxic therapy using combinations of platinum, temozolomide, and capecitabine. Biotherapy with SSAs is utilized in low- and mid-grade tumors. Interferon shows some effectiveness but has significant toxicity. Sunitinib (a multitarget TKI) and everolimus (against mTOR) have shown effect. Ongoing studies are investigating other targeted therapies and anti-angiogenic agents. Finally, immunotherapy using immune checkpoint inhibitors is under intense evaluation.

References

1. Oberg K, Knigge U, Kwekkeboom D, Perren A. Neuroendocrine gastro-entero-pancreatic tumors: ESMO Clinical Practice Guidelines for diagnosis, treatment and follow-up. Ann Oncol. 2012;23 Suppl 7:vii124–30.
2. Rubin J, Ajani J, Schirmer W, Venook AP, Bukowski R, Pommier R, Saltz L, Dandona P, Anthony L. Octreotide acetate long-acting formulation versus open-label subcutaneous octreotide acetate in malignant carcinoid syndrome. J Clin Oncol. 1999;17(2):600–6.
3. Kaltsas GA, Besser GM, Grossman AB. The diagnosis and medical management of advanced neuroendocrine tumors. Endocr Rev. 2004;25(3):458–511.
4. Oberg KE, Reubi JC, Kwekkeboom DJ, Krenning EP. Role of somatostatins in gastroenteropancreatic neuroendocrine tumor development and therapy. Gastroenterology. 2010;139(3):742–53. 753 e1.
5. Barbieri F, Pattarozzi A, Gatti M, Porcile C, Bajetto A, Ferrari A, Culler MD, Florio T. Somatostatin receptors 1, 2, and 5 cooperate in the somatostatin inhibition of C6 glioma cell proliferation in vitro via a phosphotyrosine phosphatase-eta-dependent inhibition of extracellularly regulated kinase-1/2. Endocrinology. 2008;149(9):4736–46.
6. Florio T, Yao H, Carey KD, Dillon TJ, Stork PJ. Somatostatin activation of mitogen-activated protein kinase via somatostatin receptor 1 (SSTR1). Mol Endocrinol. 1999;13(1):24–37.
7. Patel YC. Somatostatin and its receptor family. Front Neuroendocrinol. 1999;20(3):157–98.

8. Modlin IM, Pavel M, Kidd M, Gustafsson BI. Review article: somatostatin analogues in the treatment of gastroenteropancreatic neuroendocrine (carcinoid) tumours. Aliment Pharmacol Ther. 2010;31(2):169–88.
9. Sun LC, Coy DH. Somatostatin receptor-targeted anti-cancer therapy. Curr Drug Deliv. 2011;8(1):2–10.
10. Lissoni P, Barni S, Tancini G, Mainini E, Piglia F, Maestroni GJ, Lewinski A. Immunoendocrine therapy with low-dose subcutaneous interleukin-2 plus melatonin of locally advanced or metastatic endocrine tumors. Oncology. 1995;52(2):163–6.
11. Oberg K. Interferon in the management of neuroendocrine GEP-tumors: a review. Digestion. 2000;62 Suppl 1:92–7.
12. Pavel M, Kidd M, Modlin I. Systemic therapeutic options for carcinoid. Semin Oncol. 2013;40(1):84–99.
13. Basser RL, Green MD. Recent advances in carcinoids and gastrointestinal neuroendocrine tumors. Curr Opin Oncol. 1991;3(1):109–20.
14. Rinke A, Muller HH, Schade-Brittinger C, Klose KJ, Barth P, Wied M, Mayer C, Aminossadati B, Pape UF, Blaker M, Harder J, Arnold C, Gress T, Arnold R. Placebo-controlled, double-blind, prospective, randomized study on the effect of octreotide LAR in the control of tumor growth in patients with metastatic neuroendocrine midgut tumors: a report from the PROMID Study Group. J Clin Oncol. 2009;27(28):4656–63.
15. Anthony L, Freda PU. From somatostatin to octreotide LAR: evolution of a somatostatin analogue. Curr Med Res Opin. 2009;25(12):2989–99.
16. Caplin ME, Pavel M, Cwikla JB, Phan AT, Raderer M, Sedlackova E, Cadiot G, Wolin EM, Capdevila J, Wall L, Rindi G, Langley A, Martinez S, Blumberg J, Ruszniewski P. Lanreotide in metastatic enteropancreatic neuroendocrine tumors. N Engl J Med. 2014;371(3):224–33.
17. Chan JA, Stuart K, Earle CC, Clark JW, Bhargava P, Miksad R, Blaszkowsky L, Enzinger PC, Meyerhardt JA, Zheng H, Fuchs CS, Kulke MH. Prospective study of bevacizumab plus temozolomide in patients with advanced neuroendocrine tumors. J Clin Oncol. 2012;30(24):2963–8.
18. Mitry E, Walter T, Baudin E, Kurtz JE, Ruszniewski P, Dominguez-Tinajero S, Bengrine-Lefevre L, Cadiot G, Dromain C, Farace F, Rougier P, Ducreux M. Bevacizumab plus capecitabine in patients with progressive advanced well-differentiated neuroendocrine tumors of the gastro-intestinal (GI-NETs) tract (BETTER trial) – a phase II non-randomised trial. Eur J Cancer. 2014;50(18):3107–15.
19. Hobday TJ, Qin R, Reidy-Lagunes D, Moore MJ, Strosberg J, Kaubisch A, Shah M, Kindler HL, Lenz HJ, Chen H, Erlichman C. Multicenter phase II trial of temsirolimus and Bevacizumab in pancreatic neuroendocrine tumors. J Clin Oncol. 2015;33(14):1551–6.
20. Capdevila J, Sevilla I, Alonso V, Anton Aparicio L, Jimenez Fonseca P, Grande E, Reina JJ, Manzano JL, Alonso Lajara JD, Barriuso J, Castellano D, Medina J, Lopez C, Segura A, Carrera S, Crespo G, Fuster J, Munarriz J, Garcia Alfonso P. Evaluation of the efficacy and safety of lanreotide in combination with targeted therapies in patients with neuroendocrine tumours in clinical practice: a retrospective cross-sectional analysis. BMC Cancer. 2015;15:495.
21. Castellano D, Bajetta E, Panneerselvam A, Saletan S, Kocha W, O'Dorisio T, Anthony LB, Hobday T. Everolimus plus octreotide long-acting repeatable in patients with colorectal neuroendocrine tumors: a subgroup analysis of the phase III RADIANT-2 study. Oncologist. 2013;18(1):46–53.
22. Wolin EM. Long-term everolimus treatment of patients with pancreatic neuroendocrine tumors. Chemotherapy. 2014;60(3):143–50.
23. Blumenthal GM, Cortazar P, Zhang JJ, Tang S, Sridhara R, Murgo A, Justice R, Pazdur R. FDA approval summary: sunitinib for the treatment of progressive well-differentiated locally advanced or metastatic pancreatic neuroendocrine tumors. Oncologist. 2012;17(8):1108–13.
24. Reidy-Lagunes DL. Systemic therapy for advanced pancreatic neuroendocrine tumors: an update. J Natl Compr Canc Netw. 2012;10(6):777–83.

25. Peng L, Schwarz RE. Pancreatic neuroendocrine tumors: signal pathways and targeted therapies. Curr Mol Med. 2013;13(3):333–9.
26. Karhoff D, Sauer S, Schrader J, Arnold R, Fendrich V, Bartsch DK, Horsch D. Rap1/B-Raf signaling is activated in neuroendocrine tumors of the digestive tract and Raf kinase inhibition constitutes a putative therapeutic target. Neuroendocrinology. 2007;85(1):45–53.
27. Welin S, Fjallskog ML, Saras J, Eriksson B, Janson ET. Expression of tyrosine kinase receptors in malignant midgut carcinoid tumors. Neuroendocrinology. 2006;84(1):42–8.
28. Pavel M, Horsch D, Caplin M, Ramage J, Seufferlein T, Valle J, Banks P, Lapuerta P, Sands A, Zambrowicz B, Fleming D, Wiedenmann B. Telotristat etiprate for carcinoid syndrome: a single-arm, multicenter trial. J Clin Endocrinol Metab. 2015;100(4):1511–9.
29. Kulke MH, O'Dorisio T, Phan A, Bergsland E, Law L, Banks P, Freiman J, Frazier K, Jackson J, Yao JC, Kvols L, Lapuerta P, Zambrowicz B, Fleming D, Sands A. Telotristat etiprate, a novel serotonin synthesis inhibitor, in patients with carcinoid syndrome and diarrhea not adequately controlled by octreotide. Endocr Relat Cancer. 2014;21(5):705–14.
30. Kidd M, Modlin IM, Black JW, Boyce M, Culler M. A comparison of the effects of gastrin, somatostatin and dopamine receptor ligands on rat gastric enterochromaffin-like cell secretion and proliferation. Regul Pept. 2007;143(1–3):109–17.
31. Zitzmann K, Andersen S, Vlotides G, Spottl G, Zhang S, Datta R, Culler M, Goke B, Auernhammer CJ. The novel somatostatin receptor 2/dopamine type 2 receptor chimeric compound BIM-23A758 decreases the viability of human GOT1 midgut carcinoid cells. Neuroendocrinology. 2013;98(2):128–36.
32. Jaquet P, Gunz G, Saveanu A, Dufour H, Taylor J, Dong J, Kim S, Moreau JP, Enjalbert A, Culler MD. Efficacy of chimeric molecules directed towards multiple somatostatin and dopamine receptors on inhibition of GH and prolactin secretion from GH-secreting pituitary adenomas classified as partially responsive to somatostatin analog therapy. Eur J Endocrinol. 2005;153(1):135–41.
33. Hendlisz A, Flamen P, Van den Eynde M, Borbath I, Demetter P, Demolin G, Pattyn P, Pauwels S, Peeters M, Roeyen G, Van Cutsemo E, Van Hootegem P, Van Laethem JL, Verslype C, Delaunoit T. Locoregional and radioisotopic targeted treatment of neuroendocrine tumours. Acta Gastroenterol Belg. 2009;72(1):44–8.
34. Yuan F, Shi M, Ji J, Shi H, Zhou C, Yu Y, Liu B, Zhu Z, Zhang J. KRAS and DAXX/ATRX gene mutations are correlated with the clinicopathological features, advanced diseases, and poor prognosis in Chinese patients with pancreatic neuroendocrine tumors. Int J Biol Sci. 2014;10(9):957–65.
35. Reid MD, Saka B, Balci S, Goldblum AS, Adsay NV. Molecular genetics of pancreatic neoplasms and their morphologic correlates: an update on recent advances and potential diagnostic applications. Am J Clin Pathol. 2014;141(2):168–80.
36. Schultheis AM, Scheel AH, Ozretic L, George J, Thomas RK, Hagemann T, Zander T, Wolf J, Buettner R. PD-L1 expression in small cell neuroendocrine carcinomas. Eur J Cancer. 2015;51(3):421–6.
37. Alonso-Gordoa T, Capdevila J, Grande E. GEP-NETs update: biotherapy for neuroendocrine tumours. Eur J Endocrinol. 2015;172(1):R31–46.
38. Basso D, Fogar P, Falconi M, Fadi E, Sperti C, Frasson C, Greco E, Tamburrino D, Teolato S, Moz S, Bozzato D, Pelloso M, Padoan A, De Franchis G, Gnatta E, Facco M, Zambon CF, Navaglia F, Pasquali C, Basso G, Semenzato G, Pedrazzoli S, Pederzoli P, Plebani M. Pancreatic tumors and immature immunosuppressive myeloid cells in blood and spleen: role of inhibitory co-stimulatory molecules PDL1 and CTLA4. An in vivo and in vitro study. PLoS One. 2013;8(1):e54824.

Somatostatin Receptors in Human Neuroendocrine Tumors

Aejaz Nasir, Ujalla Sheikh, Jalil Muhammad, and Domenico Coppola

Peptide Receptors and NETs

Since the late twentieth century, somatostatin analogs (SSAs) have been used as a form of targeted therapies to control symptoms of hormonal hypersecretion by functional NETs. These agents are still an important treatment modality for NETs today. In recent years somatostatin receptors (SSTRs) have become a subject of active investigation as important targets for diagnosis and treatment of NETs.

Somatostatin and Somatostatin Receptors

Somatostatin (SST) is an endogenous cyclic peptide that regulates the secretion of various hormones by endocrine cells through its binding with a family of G protein-coupled transmembrane receptors, including five distinct subtypes (SSTRs 1–5) [1, 2]. SST also has a potent and broad antisecretory action, which makes it an invaluable drug target for the pharmacological management of NETs [3]. Somatostatin has a very short half-life (~3–4 min) [2], which limits its therapeutic efficacy in clinical setting. However, synthetic somatostatin analogs (SSAs) such as octreotide and lanreotide have high affinity for SSTR 2 and SSTR 5 and are without the undesirable effects of

A. Nasir, MD, MPhil, FCAP (✉)
Diagnostic and Experimental Pathology (Tailored Therapeutics), Lilly Research Laboratories, Room 2391, Building 98C/2C, Eli Lilly and Co., 893 South Delaware St., Indianapolis, IN, USA
e-mail: nasirae@lilly.com

U. Sheikh • D. Coppola, MD
Department of Anatomic Pathology, H. Lee Moffitt Cancer Center, Tampa, FL, USA

J. Muhammad
Department of Neuroscience, George Mason University, Fairfax, VA, USA

A. Nasir, D. Coppola (eds.), *Neuroendocrine Tumors: Review of Pathology, Molecular and Therapeutic Advances*, DOI 10.1007/978-1-4939-3426-3_24

somatostatin [2, 4], supporting their efficacy in clinical setting. Furthermore, the ability of SSTRs to internalize and the development of radiolabeled somatostatin analogs have further contributed to improved diagnosis and treatment of NETs [3].

SSTR Signaling and Downstream Effects

SSTRs 1, 2, 3, and 5 mediate their antiproliferative actions and SSTR 4 its pro-proliferative action through unique signaling pathways [3]. The antiproliferative effect of SSTRs is mediated by either inhibiting mitogenesis or stimulating apoptosis [5]. In fact, SSTRs 1, 2, 4, and 5 can induce G1 cell cycle growth arrest, while SSTR 3 is pro-apoptotic via the induction of p53 and BAX [6, 7].

Activation of SSTRs and Effects on NET Cells

Activation of SSTRs has a number of direct and indirect effects on NET cells [3, 8]. Direct antiproliferative effects of SSTR activation include inhibition of cell cycle and growth factor effects and induction of apoptosis (Fig. 1), which may be mediated by the PI3K/mTOR, MAPK, and Ras/ERK signaling pathways [9, 10]. Indirect effects of SSTR activation include inhibition of the release of growth factors and trophic hormones, inhibition of angiogenesis, and modulation of the immune system (Fig. 1) [3, 8].

Investigating the function of each SSTR in various human tumor types has provided insightful information on the role of signaling pathways that can suppress tumor cell proliferation, survival, and angiogenesis [3]. This has also provided the rationale for developing multi-SSTR-targeted somatostatin analogs and combination therapies with various targeted agents like inhibitors of the mammalian target of rapamycin (mTOR) and dopamine receptors [3].

Expression of SSTRs in Human NET and Normal Tissues

Somatostatin receptors (SSTRs 1, 2A and 2B, 3, 4, and 5) belong to the G protein-coupled receptor family and have shown a wide expression pattern in both normal human tissues and solid tumors [3]. Specifically, these various SSTR subtypes (SSTRs 1, 2, 3, 4, 5) have been identified in human NETs and other tumors (Table 1) and their metastases, using a variety of techniques including autoradiography [11, 12], reverse transcriptase polymerase chain reaction (rt-PCR), and immunohistochemistry (IHC) [13–15].

Although somatostatin receptor incidence and density reported in various tumors depend on the methodology used, however, the majority of NETs express SSTRs in high density (Table 1) [16]. These tumors include pituitary adenomas (in particular GH- and TSH-producing adenomas), GEP and lung NETs, pheochromocytomas, and paragangliomas (Reubi 2003). Tumors of the nervous system, such

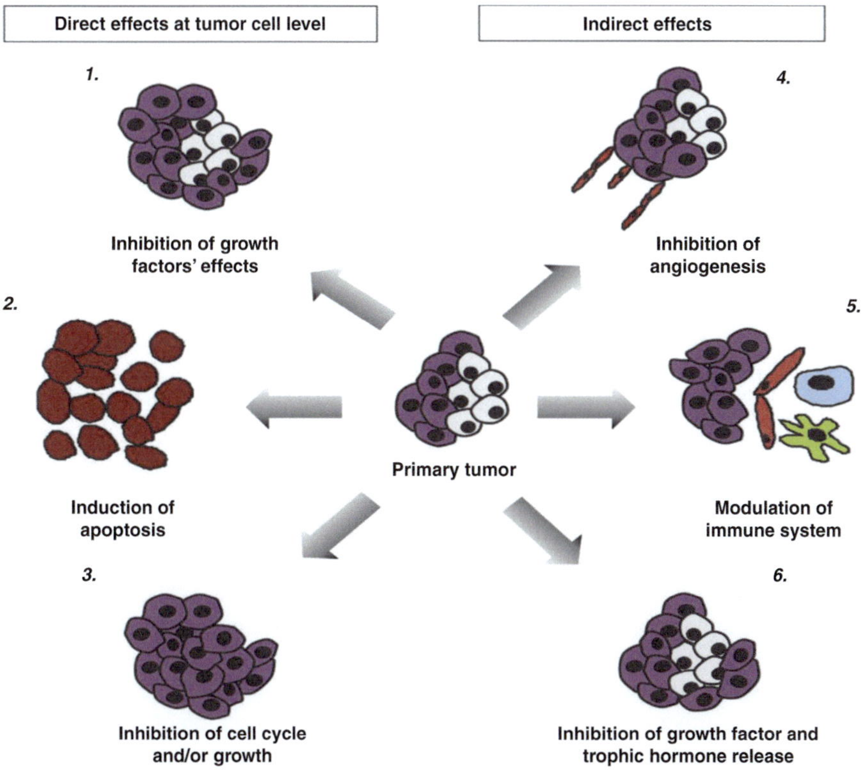

Fig. 1 Antiproliferative effect of somatostatin analogs on tumor cells. Somatostatin and its analogs may induce tumor shrinkage through direct action on the tumor cell [(*1*) inhibitory cross-talk of the SSTR signaling to the signaling induced by autocrine growth factors in the tumor cells, as well as inhibition of autocrine growth factor secretion from tumor cells; (*2*) cytostatic signaling mediated by the SSTR; (3) cytotoxic action of SSTR (e.g., by induction of apoptosis)] or indirectly by acting on components of the tumor microenvironment [(*4*) blocking of neovascularization; (*5*) inhibition of the secretion of tumor-promoting signals from immune cells; (*6*) blocking of the secretion of paracrine growth factor)]. Tumor cells are shown in fuchsia, vascular endothelial cells in red, immune cells in green and blue, and apoptotic cells in brown (Reproduced with permission from Theodoropoulou and Stalla [3])

Table 1 NETs expressing somatostatin receptors

Tumors with predominance of sst_2	Tumors with predominance of other ssts (with or without sst_2)
Pituitary adenomas (GH, TSH)	Selected GH Pituitary adenomas (sst_5; $sst_2 + sst_5$) ACTH pituitary adenomas (sst_5) Inactive pituitary adenomas (sst_3)
GEP NETs	Selected GEP NETs (insulinomas: sst_1, sst_5, with or without sst_2)
Lung NETs	Selected lung NETs
Pheochromocytomas	Medullary thyroid carcinomas
Paragangliomas	

as medulloblastomas, meningiomas, and neuroblastomas, also express somatostatin receptors at high density [16]. Furthermore, non-neural and non-NET tumors like breast, small cell lung, hepatic, renal, and gastric cancers and lymphoma also can express SSTRs with a lower incidence and/or density than NETs [16].

More recently, SSTR subtyping is being viewed as putative biomarkers of response of human NETs to somatostatin analog therapy [3]. This makes analytical and further clinical validation of SSTR subtyping methodologies an important goal for pathologists, who are engaged in supporting sub-specialty diagnostic and theranostic services in neuroendocrine pathology – at least at major referral centers.

Because of the pathobiological and clinical relevance of SSTRs, a large number of studies have investigated the expression and distribution of SSTRs in human NET tissues [13, 15, 17–19]. The distribution of SSTRs is widespread in GEP-NETs, with an overall prevalence of 50–100 % and frequent co-expression of multiple SSTRs in a given tumor [13, 15, 17–19]. Interestingly, the expression of SSTRs varies among various histological types of NETs and also among patients with the same tumor type. SSTR 2 and SSTR 5 are expressed in about 90 % and 80 % of pancreatic NET cells, respectively, making them potentially sensitive to hormone treatment [20].

In our experience, SSTR 2 was the most frequently expressed subtype in the hepatic metastases of NECs of the small intestine and pancreas, while SSTR 1 was the least commonly expressed SSTR (Fig. 2) [15]. In other studies, SSTR 2 has been shown to be absent or very low in insulinomas compared to nonfunctioning PNETs [16, 21]. Such differential expression of various SSTRs in primary and metastatic NETs/NECs further substantiates the relevance of implementation of reliable methodologies for SSTR subtyping as a potential biomarker approach to predict response to NETs/NECs to various somatostatin analog therapies.

SSTR Expression Correlates with the Pathology of Human NETs

In human NETs, the expression of SSTRs correlates with the degree of endocrine differentiation, lower histopathologic tumor grades [12], and clinical response to somatostatin analog (octreotide) therapy [22]. While the majority of well-differentiated NETs (Fig. 3) and islet cell carcinomas are SSTR-positive and respond favorably to somatostatin analog therapy, the poorly differentiated ETs are usually SSTR-negative (Figs. 4 and 5) [12] and rarely respond to somatostatin analog therapy.

Detection of SSTRs by Imaging

Overall, the most sensitive imaging modality for the detection of metastatic disease in NETs is SSTR scintigraphy (OctreoScan) [24]. This imaging technique also allows for noninvasive determination of the presence of SSTRs using radiolabeled octreotide (pentetreotide) [25]. Therefore, it is widely used for predicting the response of SSTR-positive NETs to somatostatin analogs. However, it does not identify expression of various SSTR subtypes in a given case of NET.

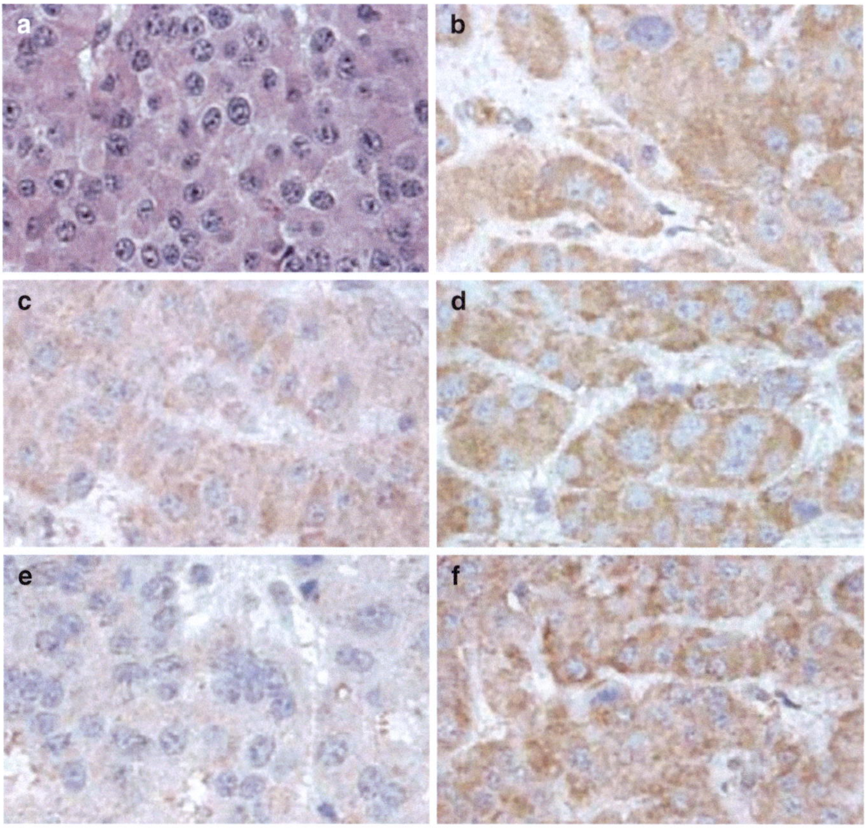

Fig. 2 (**a**) Moderately differentiated ECA of the pancreas; paraffin section from the primary pancreatic ECA (hematoxylin-eosin, ×630). (**b–f**) Paraffin sections from the primary pancreatic ECA featuring 2+, 1+, 2+, negative, and 2+ expression of SSTRs 1, 2, 3, 4, and 5, respectively (immunoperoxidase staining for SSTR subtypes 1–5, ×630) (Reproduced with permission from Nasir et al. [15])

SSTR Expression on NET Tissues and Response to Somatostatin Analogs

The expression of SSTRs on NET cells forms the basis for somatostatin analog treatment of patients with SSTR-positive NETs [26]. In malignant NETs, the presence of SSTRs has been shown to predict favorable clinical response to somatostatin analog (octreotide) therapy [22]. Therefore, SSTR subtyping is regarded as putative biomarkers of somatostatin analog response [3]. While SSTR subtyping may be useful in predicting favorable clinical response of many different types of NETs to SSA therapy, some clinical subsets of NETs may specifically benefit from SSTR subtyping on tumor tissues: These include [1] *SSTR-negative gastroenteropancreatic (GEP) NETs*, in which clinical response to somatostatin analog therapy is generally absent or suboptimal [2]; *nonfunctioning GEP-NETs*, in which role of octreotide therapy is controversial; and [3] *OctreoScan-positive GEP-NETs*, which

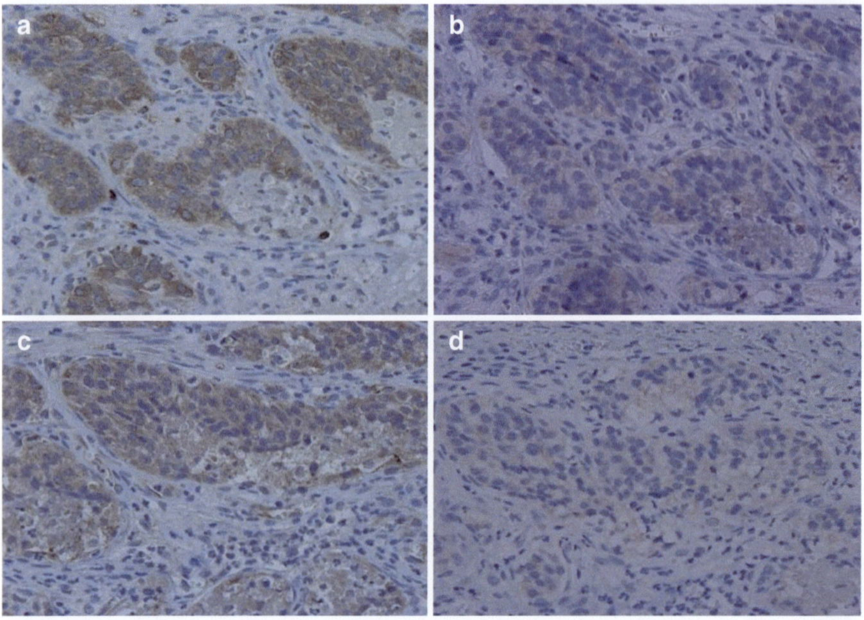

Fig. 3 Expression of SSTRs 1, 2, 3, and 5 in NET G1 (carcinoid tumor) of the appendix vermiformis. (**a**) SSTR 1, diffuse and intense positive staining identified mostly in cytoplasm of the tumor cells. (**b**) SSTR 2, weak but positive staining seen along the plasma membrane; (**c**) SSTR 3, diffuse cytoplasmic staining present; d) SSTR 5, very weak, but membranous staining seen along the plasma membrane. Original magnification ×400 (**a–d**) (Reproduced with permission from Mizutani et al. [23])

may show a variable clinical response to somatostatin analog treatment. For future studies, systematic analyses of SSTR status of NETs, based on imaging and tissue-based assays, will be an important consideration.

Clinical Usefulness of Somatostatin Analog Monotherapy and Combination

Treatment with radiolabeled somatostatin analogs is effective in the management of patients with inoperable or metastasized NETs [27]. Such therapy results in reduced hormonal overproduction and symptomatic relief in most of the NET patients, although it is seldom successful in reducing the tumor size [28]. Specifically, in patients with metastatic carcinoids, octreotide and lanreotide have shown biochemical response in 40–50 % cases, with temporary stabilization of tumor growth in more than 80 % and tumor regression in less than 10 % patients [29, 30]. More recently, co-targeting of SSTRs 1, 2, 3, and 5 (with SSA therapy) and dopamine receptor type 2 (D2DR) has been shown to yield potent therapeutic outcomes [3]. Furthermore, SSTR 2 targeting sensitizes NET cells to antitumor activity of mTOR inhibitors [3].

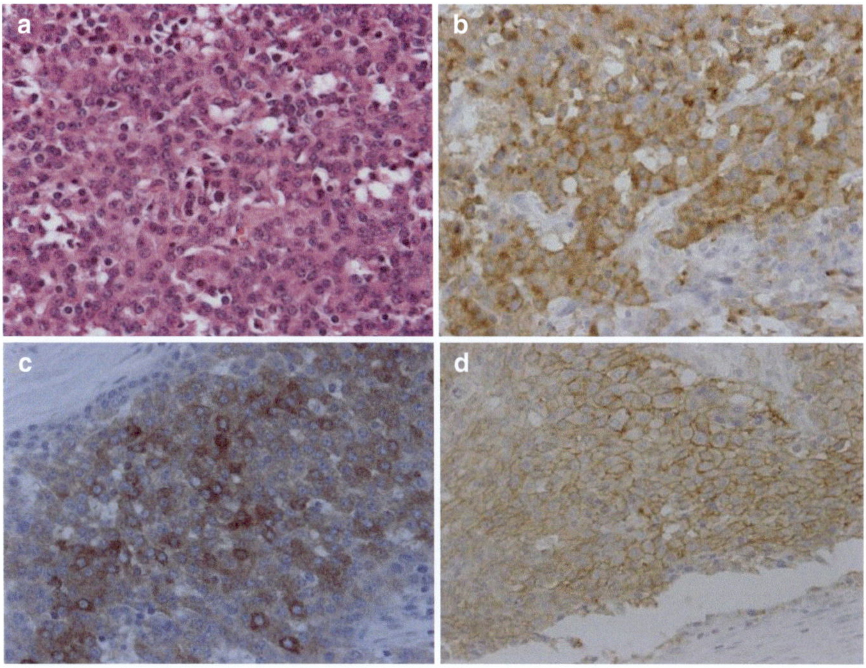

Fig. 4 Expression of SSTRs 1 and 2 in NEC G3 (neuroendocrine carcinoma) of the stomach. (**a**) H-E, rather solid growth of poorly differentiated tumor cells. (**b**) Synaptophysin: diffuse and intense cytoplasmic positive staining seen in tumor cells. (**c**) SSTR 1, diffuse cytoplasmic positivity seen in tumor cells. (**d**) SSTR 2, intense membranous staining along the plasma membrane. Original magnification ×400 (**a–d**) (Reproduced with permission from Mizutani et al. [23])

Other Peptide Receptors

With the clinical success of SSTRs in the management of NETs, patients have led to increased interest in other peptide receptors, including receptors for bombesin, cholecystokinin, and vasoactive intestinal peptide (VIP) in some types of pancreatic NETs [31–34].

Future Directions

In recent years, with the availability of newer subtype-specific ligands such as pasireotide (SOM-230) with selective affinity for various SSTR subtypes, compared to the older SSAs (like octreotide and lanreotide), it is becoming increasingly important to determine the relative expression of various SSTR subtypes in order to select the most relevant SSA(s) for optimal therapeutic effect in a given NET patient. Such a personalized approach will allow improved patient selection for SSA therapy, based on expression of various SSTRs in the patient's own GEP-NET tissues, and

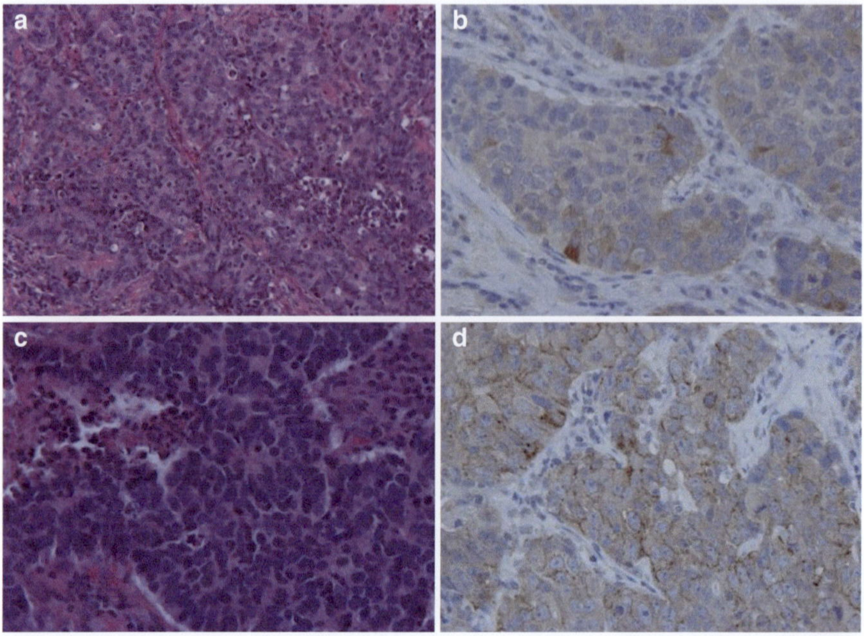

Fig. 5 Expression of SSTR 1 in two different NEC G3 (large cell neuroendocrine carcinoma; LCNEC) of lung. (**a**) H-E, rather solid growth of poorly differentiated tumor cells with incomplete peripheral nuclear palisading. (**b**) SSTR 1; in this case cytoplasmic positive staining seen. (**c**) H-E, another case of LCNEC. (**d**) Intense membranous and occasional cytoplasmic positivity identified in the tumor cells. Original magnification ×200 (**a**), ×400 (**b–d**) (Reproduced with permission from Mizutani et al. [23])

may contribute to higher clinical response rates for various SSA therapies in such patients.

Overall, lower grade NETs of the GI tract and pancreas have higher levels of various SSTRs, while PD-NECs tend to have infrequent and lower levels of SSTR expression in the tumor tissues. With the availability of newer somatostatin analogs such as pasireotide (SOM230), the determination of differential expression of various SSTR subtypes, and an assessment of heterogeneity of such expression in larger series of primary and metastatic GEP-NECs, is clinically relevant. Furthermore, SSTR-subtype expression should be correlated with the pattern of clinical response of the treated patients to somatostatin analog therapies. Based on our own experience with SSTR IHC, we believe that SSTR subtyping is feasible on formalin-fixed NET tissues. These findings merit additional SSTR-subtype analyses on larger series of patients with endocrine neoplasms. The predominance of cytoplasmic expression of various SSTR subtypes in our experience is best explained by prior Sandostatin therapy in our patients, a rational basis to explain internalization of the SSTRs.

Abbreviations

BAX	Gene promoter
ECA	Endocrine carcinoma
ERK	Extracellular regulated kinase
ET	Endocrine tumor
GEP-NET	Gastroenteropancreatic neuroendocrine tumor
G1	Growth phase 1
IHC	Immunohistochemistry
MAPK	Mitogen-activated protein kinase
mTOR	Mechanistic target of rapamycin (aka mammalian target of rapamycin)
NEC	Neuroendocrine carcinoma
NEC G3	Neuroendocrine carcinoma, grade 3
NET	Neuroendocrine tumor
NET G1	Neuroendocrine tumor, grade 1
PI3K	Phosphoinositide 3-kinase
p53	Gene promoter
rt-PCR	Reverse transcription polymerase chain reaction
SOM-230	Pasireotide (A newer somatostatin analog)
SSA	Somatostatin analog
SSTR	Somatostatin receptor
SSTR 2	Somatostatin receptor 2
SST	Somatostatin
VIP	Vasoactive intestinal peptide

References

1. Patel YC. Molecular pharmacology of somatostatin receptor subtypes. J Endocrinol Invest. 1997;20(6):348–67.
2. Lamberts SW, van der Lely AJ, de Herder WW, Hofland LJ. Octreotide. N Engl J Med. 1996;334(4):246–54.
3. Theodoropoulou M, Stalla GK. Somatostatin receptors: from signaling to clinical practice. Front Neuroendocrinol. 2013;34(3):228–52.
4. Eriksson B. New drugs in neuroendocrine tumors: rising of new therapeutic philosophies? Curr Opin Oncol. 2010;22(4):381–6.
5. Stafford ND, Condon LT, Rogers MJ, Helboe L, Crooks DA, Atkin SL. The immunohistochemical localisation of somatostatin receptors 1, 2, 3, and 5 in acoustic neuromas. J Clin Pathol. 2004;57(2):168–71.
6. Srikant CB. Human somatostatin receptor mediated antiproliferative action evokes subtype selective cytotoxic and cytostatic signaling. Yale J Biol Med. 1997;70(5–6):541–8.
7. Sharma K, Srikant CB. Induction of wild-type p53, Bax, and acidic endonuclease during somatostatin-signaled apoptosis in MCF-7 human breast cancer cells. Int J Cancer. 1998;76(2):259–66.

8. Susini C, Buscail L. Rationale for the use of somatostatin analogs as antitumor agents. Ann Oncol. 2006;17(12):1733–42.
9. Grozinsky-Glasberg S, Shimon I, Korbonits M, Grossman AB. Somatostatin analogues in the control of neuroendocrine tumours: efficacy and mechanisms. Endocr Relat Cancer. 2008;15(3):701–20.
10. Schonbrunn A. Somatostatin receptors present knowledge and future directions. Ann Oncol. 1999;10 Suppl 2:S17–21.
11. Reubi JC, Krenning E, Lamberts SW, Kvols L. Somatostatin receptors in malignant tissues. J Steroid Biochem Mol Biol. 1990;37(6):1073–7.
12. Reubi JC, Kvols L, Krenning E, Lamberts SW. In vitro and in vivo detection of somatostatin receptors in human malignant tissues. Acta Oncol. 1991;30(4):463–8.
13. Papotti M, Bongiovanni M, Volante M, Allia E, Landolfi S, Helboe L, et al. Expression of somatostatin receptor types 1–5 in 81 cases of gastrointestinal and pancreatic endocrine tumors. A correlative immunohistochemical and reverse-transcriptase polymerase chain reaction analysis. Virchows Arch. 2002;440(5):461–75.
14. Oda Y, Tanaka Y, Naruse T, Sasanabe R, Tsubamoto M, Funahashi H. Expression of somatostatin receptor and effects of somatostatin analog on pancreatic endocrine tumors. Surg Today. 2002;32(8):690–4.
15. Nasir A, Stridsberg M, Strosberg J, Su PH, Livingston S, Malik HA, et al. Somatostatin receptor profiling in hepatic metastases from small intestinal and pancreatic neuroendocrine neoplasms: immunohistochemical approach with potential clinical utility. Cancer Control. 2006;13(1):52–60.
16. Reubi JC. Peptide receptors as molecular targets for cancer diagnosis and therapy. Endocr Rev. 2003;24(4):389–427.
17. Kulaksiz H, Eissele R, Rossler D, Schulz S, Hollt V, Cetin Y, et al. Identification of somatostatin receptor subtypes 1, 2A, 3, and 5 in neuroendocrine tumours with subtype specific antibodies. Gut. 2002;50(1):52–60.
18. Fjallskog ML, Ludvigsen E, Stridsberg M, Oberg K, Eriksson B, Janson ET. Expression of somatostatin receptor subtypes 1 to 5 in tumor tissue and intratumoral vessels in malignant endocrine pancreatic tumors. Med Oncol. 2003;20(1):59–67.
19. Portela-Gomes GM, Stridsberg M, Grimelius L, Rorstad O, Janson ET. Differential expression of the five somatostatin receptor subtypes in human benign and malignant insulinomas – predominance of receptor subtype 4. Endocr Pathol. 2007;18(2):79–85.
20. Fazio N, Cinieri S, Lorizzo K, Squadroni M, Orlando L, Spada F, et al. Biological targeted therapies in patients with advanced enteropancreatic neuroendocrine carcinomas. Cancer Treat Rev. 2010;36 Suppl 3:S87–94.
21. Missiaglia E, Dalai I, Barbi S, Beghelli S, Falconi M, della Peruta M, et al. Pancreatic endocrine tumors: expression profiling evidences a role for AKT-mTOR pathway. J Clin Oncol. 2010;28(2):245–55.
22. Kvols LK, Reubi JC, Horisberger U, Moertel CG, Rubin J, Charboneau JW. The presence of somatostatin receptors in malignant neuroendocrine tumor tissue predicts responsiveness to octreotide. Yale J Biol Med. 1992;65(5):505–18; discussion 31–6.
23. Mizutani G, Nakanishi Y, Watanabe N, Honma T, Obana Y, Seki T, et al. Expression of Somatostatin Receptor (SSTR) Subtypes (SSTR-1, 2A, 3, 4 and 5) in Neuroendocrine Tumors Using Real-time RT-PCR Method and Immunohistochemistry. Acta Histochem Cytochem. 2012;45(3):167–76.
24. Oberg K, Kvols L, Caplin M, Delle Fave G, de Herder W, Rindi G, et al. Consensus report on the use of somatostatin analogs for the management of neuroendocrine tumors of the gastroenteropancreatic system. Ann Oncol. 2004;15(6):966–73.
25. McCarthy KE, Woltering EA, Anthony LB. In situ radiotherapy with 111In-pentetreotide. State of the art and perspectives. Q J Nucl Med. 2000;44(1):88–95.
26. Hofland LJ, Lamberts SW. The pathophysiological consequences of somatostatin receptor internalization and resistance. Endocr Rev. 2003;24(1):28–47.

27. Kwekkeboom DJ, Mueller-Brand J, Paganelli G, Anthony LB, Pauwels S, Kvols LK, et al. Overview of results of peptide receptor radionuclide therapy with 3 radiolabeled somatostatin analogs. J Nucl Med. 2005;46 Suppl 1:62S–6.
28. Janson ET, Oberg K. Long-term management of the carcinoid syndrome. Treatment with octreotide alone and in combination with alpha-interferon. Acta Oncol. 1993;32(2):225–9.
29. Ruszniewski P, Ducreux M, Chayvialle JA, Blumberg J, Cloarec D, Michel H, et al. Treatment of the carcinoid syndrome with the longacting somatostatin analogue lanreotide: a prospective study in 39 patients. Gut. 1996;39(2):279–83.
30. Wymenga AN, Eriksson B, Salmela PI, Jacobsen MB, Van Cutsem EJ, Fiasse RH, et al. Efficacy and safety of prolonged-release lanreotide in patients with gastrointestinal neuroendocrine tumors and hormone-related symptoms. J Clin Oncol. 1999;17(4):1111.
31. Tang C, Biemond I, Lamers CB. Expression of peptide receptors in human endocrine tumours of the pancreas. Gut. 1997;40(2):267–71.
32. Reubi JC, Waser B. Concomitant expression of several peptide receptors in neuroendocrine tumours: molecular basis for in vivo multireceptor tumour targeting. Eur J Nucl Med Mol Imaging. 2003;30(5):781–93.
33. Reubi JC, Macke HR, Krenning EP. Candidates for peptide receptor radiotherapy today and in the future. J Nucl Med. 2005;46 Suppl 1:67S–75.
34. Nakayama S, Yokote T, Kobayashi K, Hirata Y, Hiraiwa T, Komoto I, et al. VIPoma with expression of both VIP and VPAC1 receptors in a patient with WDHA syndrome. Endocrine. 2009;35(2):143–6.

Pathologic Angiogenesis in Neuroendocrine Tumors

Aejaz Nasir, Ujalla Sheikh, Jalil Muhammad, and Domenico Coppola

Introduction

Tumor angiogenesis is one of the key drivers of cancer growth and progression, involves a number of receptor tyrosine kinases (RTKs) and their ligands (Fig. 1), and represents a state of disequilibrium between pro- and antiangiogenic pathways [1]. Vascular endothelial cell growth factor (VEGF) is a potent mitogen and specific mediator of angiogenesis. The process of angiogenesis and lymphangiogenesis is mediated by three VEGF receptors (VEGFRs 1, 2, 3); VEGF signaling is predominately mediated by VEGF receptor-2 (VEGFR2 or kinase insert domain receptor [KDR]) [2, 3], which exhibits protein tyrosine kinase activity in response to its binding with the VEGF ligands [4].

Experimental Pancreatic Neuroendocrine Tumor Model and Angiogenesis

The importance of angiogenesis in the genesis of pancreatic NETs is supported by studies on the *RIP1-Tag2 mouse model* that forms well-vascularized beta-cell tumors [5, 6]. In the transgenic mouse model of PNETs, an angiogenic switch occurs in premalignant lesions, and angiogenesis persists during progression to

A. Nasir, MD, MPhil, FCAP (✉)
Diagnostic and Experimental Pathology (Tailored Therapeutics),
Lilly Research Laboratories, Room 2391, Building 98C/2C, Eli Lilly and Co.,
893 South Delaware St., Indianapolis, IN, USA
e-mail: nasirae@lilly.com

U. Sheikh • D. Coppola, MD
Department of Anatomic Pathology, H. Lee Moffitt Cancer Center, Tampa, FL, USA

J. Muhammad
Department of Neuroscience, George Mason University, Fairfax, VA, USA

A. Nasir, D. Coppola (eds.), *Neuroendocrine Tumors: Review of Pathology, Molecular and Therapeutic Advances*, DOI 10.1007/978-1-4939-3426-3_25

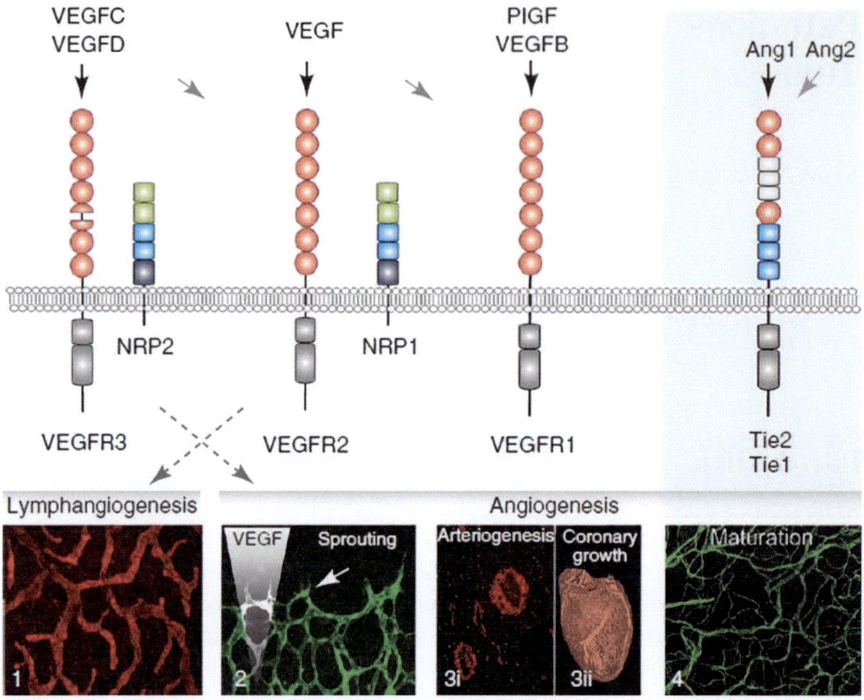

Fig. 1 VEGFs, angiopoietins, and their receptors regulate blood and lymphatic vessel formation and maturation, as part of the pathologic process of tumor angiogenesis. VEGFC and VEGFD induce lymphangiogenesis via VEGFR3, but VEGFR3 also contributes to angiogenesis (*dashed arrow*). Certain lymphangiogenic signals might also be mediated via VEGFR2 (*dashed arrow*). PlGF is involved in arteriogenesis and pathological angiogenesis, whereas VEGFB induces the growth of the coronary vessels and their branches in rat hearts. VEGFRs have an extracellular Ig homology domain (*red*), a single transmembrane region, and an intracellular tyrosine kinase domain (*gray*) interrupted by a kinase insert (Reproduced with permission from Saharinen et al. [10])

expansive solid tumors and invasive carcinomas [7]. Both vascular endothelial growth factor (VEGF)-A and its receptors, VEGFR1 and VEGFR2, are constitutively expressed in normal islets as well as in experimental PETs that develop in the RIP1-Tag2 animal model [8]. In this model VEGFA has been shown to be critical for the angiogenic switch, as well as for tumor growth [9].

While antiangiogenic (anti-VEGF/VEGFR) therapies significantly reduce pancreatic tumor growth or cause regression of established tumors in treated mice, compared with controls, and also disrupt tumor vasculature and reduce capillary density [7, 11–14], these therapies may be most efficacious when they are directed at specific stages of carcinogenesis, i.e., preventing the angiogenic switch in premalignant lesions, intervening in the rapid expansion of small tumors, or inducing the regression of large end-stage cancers [7].

Vascularity of Human NETs

Like the RIP-Tag2 animal model, human NETs are highly vascularized neoplasms that exhibit a high expression of several proangiogenic molecules, such as the principal angiogenic cytokine VEGFA [15], particularly in midgut carcinoids. VEGF may not only be required to maintain the differentiated state of the capillary vessels in these hypervascular tumors, in conjunction with the other growth factors synthesized by the NET cells, it may also have an important role in tumor growth.

VEGF and VEGF Receptors in Human Pancreatic NETs

Several studies have investigated the expression of VEGF, VEGFRs, and other markers of angiogenesis in human PNET tissues. Significant variation has been shown in the degree of (1) expression of VEGF in benign tumors [16, 17], (2) expression of VEGFC in well-differentiated NECs [18, 19], and (3) correlation between VEGF expression and tumor microvascular density (MVD) [16–19] in pancreatic NETs. In another study, expression of VEGFR2 and VEGFR3 in neoplastic cells was found to correlate with ligand expression in both primary and metastatic tumor tissue, pointing to a role for VEGFRs in regulating growth or survival of some pancreatic NETs [18].

Angiogenesis and Prognosis of Pancreatic NETs

Although in general pancreatic and other NETs are well-vascularized neoplasms, there is no consistent correlation between the expression of VEGF or the microvascular density (MVD) and the prognosis of PNET patients. Some studies have found VEGF expression to correlate with a more aggressive tumor behavior [20], while others found lower VEGF expression in malignant as compared to benign PNETs [16, 17]. These findings have recently been described as "neuroendocrine paradox" [21], to explain the possibility that intense microvascular density and VEGF expression may be typical of "well-differentiated" PNETs in recapitulating the normal pancreatic islet cell architecture. As pancreatic endocrine cells acquire more malignant phenotype as part of the neoplastic change and gain further molecular changes, their rapid growth causes hypoxia, which activates the hypoxia-inducible factors-1α (HIF-1α) pathway, leading to an increased endothelial proliferation eventually resulting in further complexity and abnormalities in the previously normal vascular architecture.

Angiopoietins (Ang-1 and Ang-2)

Angiopoietin-2 (Ang-2), a ligand of the endothelial tyrosine kinase, Tie-2, is emerging as a key regulator of vascular remodeling during tumor angiogenesis. In stable vessels, Ang-1 is produced by pericytes, Tie2 is activated in endothelial cells, and Ang-2 is stored in Weibel-Palade bodies [10]. In vessels undergoing angiogenesis in response to VEGF secreted by nearby hypoxic cells, Ang-2 is expressed predominantly in the tip cells of angiogenic sprouts, where it may regulate cell-matrix interactions by binding to integrins and connective tissue matrix. The Tie-2 receptor is expressed in the stalk cells, which become coated with pericytes and the basement membrane matrix that accumulates in between the cells in the stabilization phase of angiogenesis. Ang-1, from the perivascular cells, interacts with the Tie-2 receptor and is necessary for the stabilization of the newly formed vessels, for attenuation of angiogenesis, and for limiting the production of excess of connective tissue. In order to develop clinically relevant biomarkers for tumor angiogenesis programs, it is important to study the expression of Ang-1/Ang-2 and Tie-2 in various NET tumor tissues.

Angiopoietins and Tie-2 Receptor in Human NETs

In a recent study, several lines of scientific evidence support an important angioregulatory role for Ang-2 and its receptor (Tie2) in human GEP-NET tissues [22]: circulating Ang-2 was significantly elevated in the serum of patients with GEP-NETs compared with healthy controls; elevated serum Ang-2 levels correlated with the presence of metastatic disease; Ang-2 concentrations above the 75th percentile predicted shorter survival; increased angiopoietin-2 (Ang-2) messenger RNA (mRNA) levels were found in the endothelial cells of NET and nonneoplastic tissues [22], including the NET cells; and presence of Ang-2 in NET cells and its receptor Tie2 in NET vasculature. In orthotopic pancreatic NET xenografts, Ang-2 overexpression stimulates neo-angiogenesis (increased microvessel density) and increases lymph node metastases, indicating a functional role of Ang-2 in experimental NETs [22].

Other investigators found enhanced expression of Ang-1, Ang-2, and Tie-2 in freshly isolated tumor cells from GEP-NET both by IHC and RT-PCR and also significantly higher levels of sTie-2 and Ang-2 levels in GEP-NETs with metastases compared to those with no metastases [23]. These findings suggest involvement of the Ang/Tie-2 system in the growth and development of metastatic GEP-NETs and also in the recruitment of Tie-2C monocytes to the tumor site, where they can promote inflammation and angiogenesis [23]. In another study, serum Ang-2 (but not Ang-1) levels were significantly elevated in NET patients compared to healthy control subjects, and in NET patients with distant metastases compared to those without metastatic disease, and were associated with the volume of liver metastases and shorter time to disease progression, supporting a role for Ang-2 as a potentially useful serum marker for monitoring and prognostication in patients with NETs [24].

The induction of Ang-2 in pancreatic NETs may, therefore, represent a clinically relevant mechanism of disease progression and could constitute an adverse prognostic marker [22, 24]. Collectively, these data provide scientific rationale for Ang-2 to be a valid therapeutic target and that Ang-2 inhibition may prove to be a druggable mechanism of inhibition of angiogenesis in human NETs. In view of the Ang-2 directed experimental therapeutics already in clinical trials, it will be prudent: (1) to experimentally investigate the benefit of targeting Ang-2/Tie2 in preclinical NET models and (2) to further validate Ang-2 as a biologically relevant candidate prognostic and/or predictive marker in advanced GEP-NETs.

Platelet-Derived Growth Factor Receptors

Platelet-derived growth factor receptor (PDGFR) beta signaling is involved in autocrine growth stimulation of tumor cells, tumor angiogenesis, and regulation of tumor interstitial fluid pressure [25]. In an IHC-based analysis of 38 malignant human PNETs including eight poorly differentiated NECs, PDGFR-alpha and PDGFR-beta were frequently expressed both on tumor cells and tumor stroma [26]. Furthermore, PDGFR-beta expression was upregulated in primary pancreatic NETs and metastases compared with normal pancreatic islets and in tumor stroma compared with normal pancreatic stroma [25]. Based on an analysis of multiple tyrosine kinases in PNETs, the authors concluded that malignant PNETs that express PDGFRs and other tyrosine kinases, like c-Kit and EGFR, may be targeted by the currently available TKIs with or without chemotherapy and/or radiotherapy. However, because there is marked variation in the level of expression of these targets in individual tumors, it will be important to reliably evaluate (even quantify) these targets on available tumor tissue.

In a gene expression profiling study, PDGFR-beta was found upregulated in pancreatic NECs with metastases as compared to nonmetastatic (benign) pancreatic NETs [27]. Role of PDGFRs in PNETs has also been supported by experimental evidence from a transgenic mouse model of PNETs (RIP-Tag2), in which islet cell carcinomas develop from multifocal, hyper-proliferative nodules featuring the histological hallmarks of human carcinoma in situ. Compared to control animals, the animals treated with inhibitors of PDGFRs showed inhibition of tumor growth, regression of established pancreatic tumors, decrease in vascular density, and also disruption of tumor vasculature [7, 11, 13, 14]. Taken together these preclinical findings and frequent expression of PDGFRs in human PNETs warrants further investigation of PDGFRs as potential therapeutic targets in human PNET tissues.

Clinical Efficacy of Antiangiogenic Agents in NETs

From a clinical standpoint, therapeutic inhibition of neo-angiogenesis is a plausible treatment approach for PNETs. Several VEGF-pathway inhibitors, including the anti-VEGF monoclonal antibody, bevacizumab and the VEGF receptor (VEGFR)-targeted tyrosine kinase inhibitors (TKIs), sunitinib (targets VEGFR, PDGFR, c-KIT, Flt-3, and RET), pazopanib (targets VEGFR1, 2, and 3; PDGFRα and c-KIT), and sorafenib (targets VEGFR2, PDGFR, FGFR1, and RAF), have shown clinical activity in NETs [28–33]. After showing its activity against PNETs in preclinical models and phase 1 and 2 trials, sunitinib has shown significant improvement in progression-free survival (PFS) in PNET patients [30], resulting in its regulatory approvals.

Bevacizumab is a monoclonal antibody binding circulating VEGF with some preliminary data in patients with PNETs, as monotherapy, and also in combination with temozolomide [34], showing 86 % response rate (partial response plus stable disease), and with metronomic capecitabine and octreotide, showing partial response in 18 % and a PFS of 15 months. PNETs appear to respond better than non-pancreatic NETs [35].

Combining Antiangiogenic Agents

The signaling pathways involved in angiogenesis are heavily interlinked. For example, dual inhibition of VEGFRs and PDGFR results in a greater antiangiogenic effect in the RIP1-Tag2 model than selective inhibition of VEGFR or PDGFR alone, with substantial decreases in both endothelial cells and pericytes [36]. Therefore, a therapeutic approach combining more than one AA agents may be more efficacious than using a single antiangiogenic agent alone.

Human NETs and Resistance to Antiangiogenic Therapies

Despite remarkable scientific and clinical progress with antiangiogenic therapies, some tumors show intrinsic resistance to antiangiogenic therapies (i.e., they never respond to AA-Rxs), while others develop acquired resistance (i.e., start to progress after showing an initial clinical response). Both forms of resistance share similar molecular and cellular mechanisms (Fig. 2), mediated by several proangiogenic factors, including VEGFs, fibroblast growth factors (FGFs), angiopoietins (Ang-1/Ang-2), and ephrins, which can override the efficacy of single-agent VEGF-/VEGFR-targeted therapies [12, 37].

Upregulation of these proangiogenic factors is mediated by intra-tumor hypoxia with hypoxia-inducible factor-1alpha (HIF-1a) accumulation [39, 40], which in turn can also upregulate c-Met and promote more invasive and metastatic behavior in the

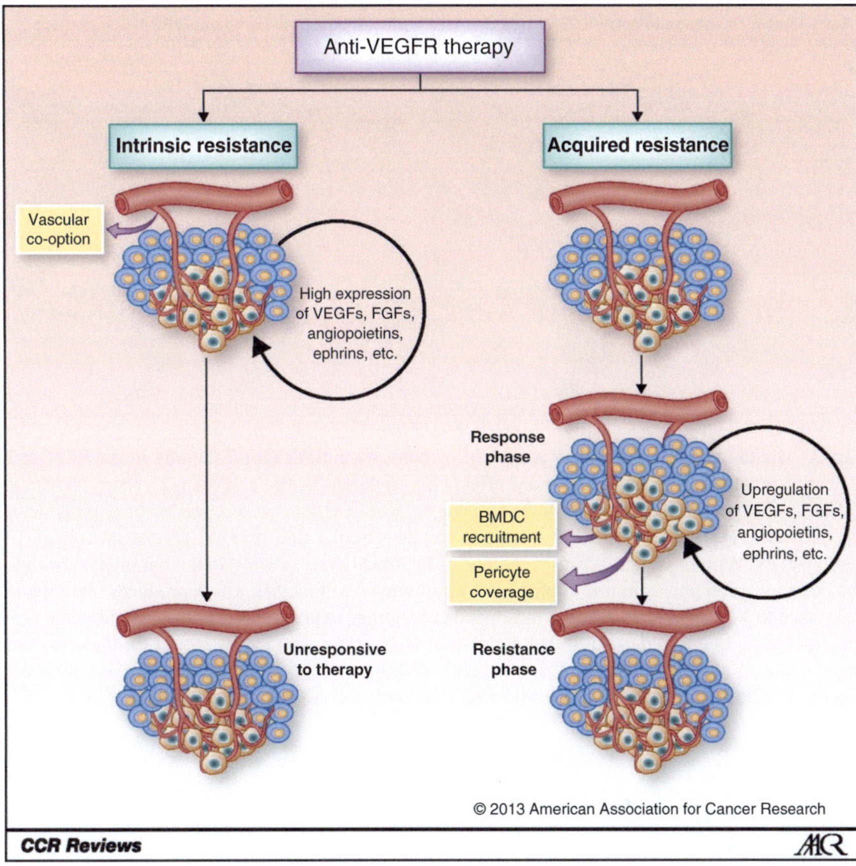

Fig. 2 Modes of resistance to antiangiogenic therapy. On the one hand, *intrinsic resistance* or refractoriness is defined as total lack of response to antiangiogenic therapy. The specific mechanisms of such resistance include the multiplicity of proangiogenic factors expressed in tumors and vascular co-option. Thus, therapy is unable to reduce or stabilize tumors and there is no benefit from antiangiogenic therapy. On the other hand, *acquired resistance* refers to the adaptive capacity present in tumors that leads them to evade the therapeutic blockade after an adequate effectiveness phase. Induced adaptive mechanisms, including overexpression of alternative proangiogenic factors, recruitment of vascular progenitor cells (*BMDCs*), and pericyte coverage, ultimately allow for revascularization despite therapy blockade, allowing tumor regrowth and disease progression. *BMDC* bone marrow-derived cell (Reproduced with permission from Oberg et al. [38])

tumor cells. This may be due to progressive selection of resistant clones of neoplastic cells that can survive in a hypoxic environment. Recent studies have shown that inhibition of c-Met can reduce the invasive and metastatic capabilities promoted by the VEGF-pathway inhibition, suggesting that simultaneous inhibition of c-Met and VEGF-targeted therapy may ultimately diminish resistance to anti-VEGF/VEGFR therapy alone [41]. Additional strategies to overcome these resistance mechanisms have been explored in animal models and also in the clinical setting [1]. These

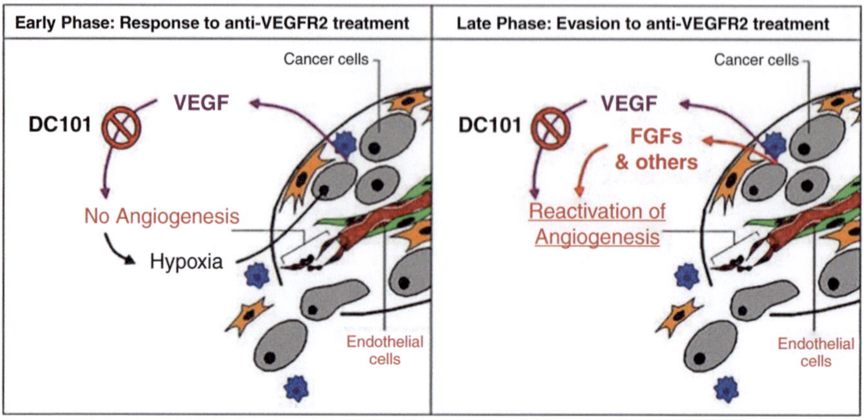

Fig. 3 Model of the early and late phases of response to anti-VEGFR2 therapy in the RIP-Tag2 islet carcinogenesis model. Differential effects are apparent in the early-stage versus late-stage anti-VEGFR2 treatment. In the initial phase (*left*), VEGF is the main regulator of angiogenesis (*purple arrows*), and the VEGFR2 blockade causes vascular and tumoral regression (objective response). Nevertheless, it also causes regions of hypoxia (*black arrows*) in the tumors that initiate the circumvention phase. In this latter phase of circumvention (*right*), which produces phenotypic resistance to VEGFR2 blockade, the tumor cells upregulate expression of other proangiogenic factors, including FGFs (*red arrows*) that are demonstrably important in this model for the observed reactivation of angiogenesis. The result is reestablishment of the tumor vasculature and progression to continuing tumor growth (Reproduced with permission from Casanovas et al. [12])

include combination of bevacizumab and HIF-1 or Sp1 inhibitors [42, 43], co-targeting of VEGF and FGF signaling pathways, which has also shown improved efficacy of VEGF inhibition in the RIP-Tag2 model of PNETs [44].

Inhibition of VEGFR2, which is the principal VEGF receptor in tumor angiogenesis, results in an initial disruption of angiogenic switch, subsequent angiogenesis, and initial tumor growth [12], but in late-stage tumors, phenotypic resistance to VEGFR2 blockade emerges, as tumors regrew during treatment after an initial period of growth suppression. This resistance to VEGFR2 blockade involves reactivation of tumor angiogenesis, independent of VEGF and is associated with hypoxia-mediated induction of other proangiogenic factors, including members of the FGF family (Fig. 3).

Counteracting such mechanisms of resistance by targeting multiple alternative proangiogenic signaling pathways may be required to achieve improved efficacy of antiangiogenic therapies [12]. In a recent study, Allen et al. (2011) suggest that co-targeting VEGF/VEGFR and FGF signaling pathways can improve efficacy and overcome adaptive resistance to VEGF inhibition in a transgenic model of PNETs [44]. In a timely commentary titled “Overcoming Antiangiogenic Resistance,” Yao and Phan (2011) discussed this important topic and illustrated the mechanisms of adaptive resistance to AA-Rxs and the various therapeutic options that can be used in clinical trials to overcome such resistance [1] (Fig. 4).

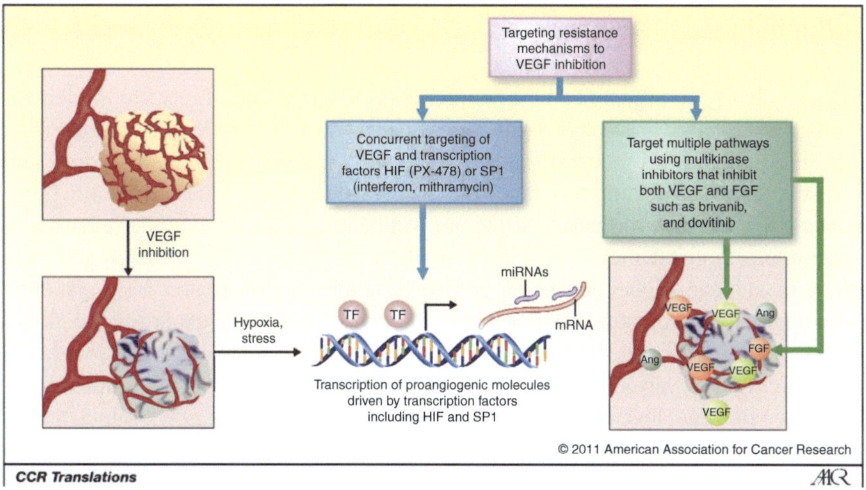

Fig. 4 Overcoming antiangiogenic resistance [1]. Successful inhibition of the VEGF signaling pathway leads to hypoxic stress, which leads to the upregulation of transcription factors. Transcription factors, such as HIF and SP1, regulate multiple proangiogenic and pro-survival pathways. Upregulated by hypoxic stress, transcription factors lead to increased expression of multiple proangiogenic molecules, including VEGF, FGF, and Ang, which may lead to the development of resistance to initial VEGF inhibition. Strategies to overcome resistance include concurrent targeting of VEGF and transcription factors or concurrent targeting of multiple angiogenic pathways, such as VEGF and FGF

Biomarkers for Antiangiogenic Therapies

Despite several regulatory approvals, based on efficacy of several antiangiogenic agents in clinical trials during last decade or so, we still do not have clinically validated biomarkers that can be used as a companion diagnostic to predict patient response or to tailor antiangiogenic therapies to individual NET patients. Systematic evaluation of members of the VEGF/VEGFR pathway will be required to identify promising candidate biomarkers that can be subjected to stringent analytical and clinical validation analyses. After initial response, evasive resistance may develop against antiangiogenic therapies resulting in more aggressive clinical course [40], due possibly to more resistant clones that can manage to survive in a hypoxic environment. Such clones may well be amenable to various combinatorial approaches, many of which are being investigated in current clinical trials. It is also important for pathologists involved in implementation of precision medicine model to be able to fully understand the biology of the underlying resistance mechanisms and to standardize reliable methodologies to evaluate and report on various resistance mechanisms that may exist in a particular case of human NET.

Conclusion

There is clearly an urgent need for neuroendocrine tumor pathologists to implement robust tissue-based assays to evaluate expression of various VEGF ligands (like VEGFA) and VEGF receptors and co-receptors and also gain insights into and investigate the therapeutic resistance mechanisms in NETs, so that systematic prognostic and predictive biomarker strategies can be implemented to guide selection of appropriate targeted therapies with or without an appropriate antiangiogenic, in order to achieve higher levels of clinical efficacy in the treated NET patients. Although many interesting studies have been carried out in the experimental model of pancreatic NETs and in human PNETs, additional and advanced studies to define the expression of various proangiogenic and antiangiogenic molecules and various resistance mechanisms in pancreatic and non-pancreatic NETs are warranted to further characterize the process of pathologic angiogenesis in these neoplasms. Such analyses will be most relevant in NETs that pursue a malignant clinical course, including those with liver and other visceral metastases.

Abbreviations

PNET	Pancreatic neuroendocrine tumor
mTOR	Mammalian target of rapamycin
VEGF	Vascular endothelial cell growth factor
VEGFR	Vascular endothelial growth factor receptor
VEGFR1	Vascular endothelial growth factor receptor 1
VEGFR2	Vascular endothelial growth factor receptor 2
VEGFR3	Vascular endothelial growth factor receptor 3
VEGFA	Vascular endothelial growth factor -A
VEGFB	Vascular endothelial growth factor -B
VEGFC	Vascular endothelial growth factor -C
VEGFD	Vascular endothelial growth factor -D
AA-Rx	Antiangiogenesis therapy
RTK	Receptor tyrosine kinase
KDR	Kinase insert domain receptor (VEGFR2)
PIGF	Placental growth factor
NET	Neuroendocrine tumor
RIP1-Tag2	Rat insulin promoter T antigen transgene
PET	Pancreatic endocrine tumor
NEC	Neuroendocrine carcinoma
MVD	Microvascular density
HIF-1α	Hypoxia-inducible factors-1α
Ang-2	Angiopoietin-2
Tie-2	Transmembrane vascular endothelial tyrosine kinase

GEP-NET	Gastro-entero-pancreatic neuroendocrine tumor
IHC	Immunohistochemistry
RT-PCR	Reverse transcriptase polymerase chain reaction
PDGFR	Platelet-derived growth factor receptor
PDGFR-beta	Platelet-derived growth factor receptor-beta
c-KIT	Tyrosine protein kinase
EGFR	Epidermal growth factor receptor
TKI	Tyrosine kinase inhibitor
RET	Rearranged during transfection (receptor)
PDGFR-alpha	Platelet-derived growth factor receptor-alpha
FGFR1	Fibroblast growth factor receptor 1
PFS	Progression-free survival
NET	Neuroendocrine tumor
AA	Antiangiogenesis
FGF	Fibroblast growth factor
BMDC	Bone marrow-derived cell
c-Met	The mesenchymal epithelial transition
HIF	Hypoxia-inducible factor
RAF	Rapidly accelerated fibrosarcoma (protein kinase family)

References

1. Yao JC, Phan A. Overcoming antiangiogenic resistance. Clin Cancer Res. 2011;17(16):5217–9.
2. Ferrara N, Gerber HP, LeCouter J. The biology of VEGF and its receptors. Nat Med. 2003;9(6):669–76.
3. Hoeben A, Landuyt B, Highley MS, Wildiers H, Van Oosterom AT, De Bruijn EA. Vascular endothelial growth factor and angiogenesis. Pharmacol Rev. 2004;56(4):549–80.
4. Yang XH, Man XY, Cai SQ, Yao YG, Bu ZY, Zheng M. Expression of VEGFR-2 on HaCaT cells is regulated by VEGF and plays an active role in mediating VEGF induced effects. Biochem Biophys Res Commun. 2006;349(1):31–8.
5. Hanahan D. Heritable formation of pancreatic beta-cell tumours in transgenic mice expressing recombinant insulin/simian virus 40 oncogenes. Nature. 1985;315(6015):115–22.
6. Folkman J, Watson K, Ingber D, Hanahan D. Induction of angiogenesis during the transition from hyperplasia to neoplasia. Nature. 1989;339(6219):58–61.
7. Bergers G, Javaherian K, Lo KM, Folkman J, Hanahan D. Effects of angiogenesis inhibitors on multistage carcinogenesis in mice. Science. 1999;284(5415):808–12.
8. Christofori G, Naik P, Hanahan D. Vascular endothelial growth factor and its receptors, flt-1 and flk-1, are expressed in normal pancreatic islets and throughout islet cell tumorigenesis. Mol Endocrinol. 1995;9(12):1760–70.
9. Inoue M, Hager JH, Ferrara N, Gerber HP, Hanahan D. VEGF-A has a critical, nonredundant role in angiogenic switching and pancreatic beta cell carcinogenesis. Cancer Cell. 2002;1(2):193–202.
10. Saharinen P, Eklund L, Pulkki K, Bono P, Alitalo K. VEGF and angiopoietin signaling in tumor angiogenesis and metastasis. Trends Mol Med. 2011;17(7):347–62.
11. Parangi S, O'Reilly M, Christofori G, Holmgren L, Grosfeld J, Folkman J, et al. Antiangiogenic therapy of transgenic mice impairs de novo tumor growth. Proc Natl Acad Sci U S A. 1996;93(5):2002–7.

12. Casanovas O, Hicklin DJ, Bergers G, Hanahan D. Drug resistance by evasion of antiangiogenic targeting of VEGF signaling in late-stage pancreatic islet tumors. Cancer Cell. 2005;8(4):299–309.
13. Pietras K, Hanahan D. A multitargeted, metronomic, and maximum-tolerated dose "chemo-switch" regimen is antiangiogenic, producing objective responses and survival benefit in a mouse model of cancer. J Clin Oncol. 2005;23(5):939–52.
14. Mancuso MR, Davis R, Norberg SM, O'Brien S, Sennino B, Nakahara T, et al. Rapid vascular regrowth in tumors after reversal of VEGF inhibition. J Clin Invest. 2006;116(10):2610–21.
15. Terris B, Scoazec JY, Rubbia L, Bregeaud L, Pepper MS, Ruszniewski P, et al. Expression of vascular endothelial growth factor in digestive neuroendocrine tumours. Histopathology. 1998;32(2):133–8.
16. Marion-Audibert AM, Barel C, Gouysse G, Dumortier J, Pilleul F, Pourreyron C, et al. Low microvessel density is an unfavorable histoprognostic factor in pancreatic endocrine tumors. Gastroenterology. 2003;125(4):1094–104.
17. Couvelard A, O'Toole D, Turley H, Leek R, Sauvanet A, Degott C, et al. Microvascular density and hypoxia-inducible factor pathway in pancreatic endocrine tumours: negative correlation of microvascular density and VEGF expression with tumour progression. Br J Cancer. 2005;92(1):94–101.
18. Hansel DE, Rahman A, Hermans J, de Krijger RR, Ashfaq R, Yeo CJ, et al. Liver metastases arising from well-differentiated pancreatic endocrine neoplasms demonstrate increased VEGF-C expression. Mod Pathol. 2003;16(7):652–9.
19. Rubbia-Brandt L, Terris B, Giostra E, Dousset B, Morel P, Pepper MS. Lymphatic vessel density and vascular endothelial growth factor-C expression correlate with malignant behavior in human pancreatic endocrine tumors. Clin Cancer Res. 2004;10(20):6919–28.
20. Zhang J, Jia Z, Li Q, Wang L, Rashid A, Zhu Z, et al. Elevated expression of vascular endothelial growth factor correlates with increased angiogenesis and decreased progression-free survival among patients with low-grade neuroendocrine tumors. Cancer. 2007;109(8):1478–86.
21. Scoazec JY. Angiogenesis in neuroendocrine tumors: therapeutic applications. Neuroendocrinology. 2013;97(1):45–56.
22. Detjen KM, Rieke S, Deters A, Schulz P, Rexin A, Vollmer S, et al. Angiopoietin-2 promotes disease progression of neuroendocrine tumors. Clin Cancer Res. 2010;16(2):420–9.
23. Figueroa-Vega N, Diaz A, Adrados M, Alvarez-Escola C, Paniagua A, Aragones J, et al. The association of the angiopoietin/Tie-2 system with the development of metastasis and leukocyte migration in neuroendocrine tumors. Endocr Relat Cancer. 2010;17(4):897–908.
24. Srirajaskanthan R, Dancey G, Hackshaw A, Luong T, Caplin ME, Meyer T. Circulating angiopoietin-2 is elevated in patients with neuroendocrine tumours and correlates with disease burden and prognosis. Endocr Relat Cancer. 2009;16(3):967–76.
25. Fjallskog ML, Hessman O, Eriksson B, Janson ET. Upregulated expression of PDGF receptor beta in endocrine pancreatic tumors and metastases compared to normal endocrine pancreas. Acta Oncol. 2007;46(6):741–6.
26. Fjallskog ML, Lejonklou MH, Oberg KE, Eriksson BK, Janson ET. Expression of molecular targets for tyrosine kinase receptor antagonists in malignant endocrine pancreatic tumors. Clin Cancer Res. 2003;9(4):1469–73.
27. Couvelard A, Hu J, Steers G, O'Toole D, Sauvanet A, Belghiti J, et al. Identification of potential therapeutic targets by gene-expression profiling in pancreatic endocrine tumors. Gastroenterology. 2006;131(5):1597–610.
28. Mendel DB, Laird AD, Xin X, Louie SG, Christensen JG, Li G, et al. In vivo antitumor activity of SU11248, a novel tyrosine kinase inhibitor targeting vascular endothelial growth factor and platelet-derived growth factor receptors: determination of a pharmacokinetic/pharmacodynamic relationship. Clin Cancer Res. 2003;9(1):327–37.
29. Kulke MH, Lenz HJ, Meropol NJ, Posey J, Ryan DP, Picus J, et al. Activity of sunitinib in patients with advanced neuroendocrine tumors. J Clin Oncol. 2008;26(20):3403–10.
30. Raymond E, Dahan L, Raoul JL, Bang YJ, Borbath I, Lombard-Bohas C, et al. Sunitinib malate for the treatment of pancreatic neuroendocrine tumors. N Engl J Med. 2011;364(6):501–13.

31. Ahn HK, Choi JY, Kim KM, Kim H, Choi SH, Park SH, et al. Phase II study of pazopanib monotherapy in metastatic gastroenteropancreatic neuroendocrine tumours. Br J Cancer. 2013;109(6):1414–9.
32. Chan JA, Mayer RJ, Jackson N, Malinowski P, Regan E, Kulke MH. Phase I study of sorafenib in combination with everolimus (RAD001) in patients with advanced neuroendocrine tumors. Cancer Chemother Pharmacol. 2013;71(5):1241–6.
33. Castellano D, Capdevila J, Sastre J, Alonso V, Llanos M, Garcia-Carbonero R, et al. Sorafenib and bevacizumab combination targeted therapy in advanced neuroendocrine tumour: a phase II study of Spanish Neuroendocrine Tumour Group (GETNE0801). Eur J Cancer. 2013;49(18):3780–7.
34. Chan JA, Stuart K, Earle CC, Clark JW, Bhargava P, Miksad R, et al. Prospective study of bevacizumab plus temozolomide in patients with advanced neuroendocrine tumors. J Clin Oncol. 2012;30(24):2963–8.
35. Berruti A, Fazio N, Ferrero A, Brizzi MP, Volante M, Nobili E, et al. Bevacizumab plus octreotide and metronomic capecitabine in patients with metastatic well-to-moderately differentiated neuroendocrine tumors: the XELBEVOCT study. BMC Cancer. 2014;14:184.
36. Yao VJ, Sennino B, Davis RB, et al. Combined anti- VEGFR and anti-PDGFR actions of sunitinib on blood vessels in preclinical tumor models. 18th EORTIC-NCI-AACR Symposium on Molecular Targets and Cancer Therapeutics, Prague; 2006.
37. Bergers G, Hanahan D. Modes of resistance to anti-angiogenic therapy. Nat Rev Cancer. 2008;8(8):592–603.
38. Oberg K, Casanovas O, Castano JP, Chung D, Delle Fave G, Denefle P, et al. Molecular pathogenesis of neuroendocrine tumors: implications for current and future therapeutic approaches. Clin Cancer Res. 2013;19(11):2842–9.
39. Carmeliet P. Angiogenesis in life, disease and medicine. Nature. 2005;438(7070):932–6.
40. Paez-Ribes M, Allen E, Hudock J, Takeda T, Okuyama H, Vinals F, et al. Antiangiogenic therapy elicits malignant progression of tumors to increased local invasion and distant metastasis. Cancer Cell. 2009;15(3):220–31.
41. Sennino B, Ishiguro-Oonuma T, Wei Y, Naylor RM, Williamson CW, Bhagwandin V, et al. Suppression of tumor invasion and metastasis by concurrent inhibition of c-Met and VEGF signaling in pancreatic neuroendocrine tumors. Cancer Discov. 2012;2(3):270–87.
42. Jia Z, Zhang J, Wei D, Wang L, Yuan P, Le X, et al. Molecular basis of the synergistic antiangiogenic activity of bevacizumab and mithramycin A. Cancer Res. 2007;67(10):4878–85.
43. Rapisarda A, Hollingshead M, Uranchimeg B, Bonomi CA, Borgel SD, Carter JP, et al. Increased antitumor activity of bevacizumab in combination with hypoxia inducible factor-1 inhibition. Mol Cancer Ther. 2009;8(7):1867–77.
44. Allen E, Walters IB, Hanahan D. Brivanib, a dual FGF/VEGF inhibitor, is active both first and second line against mouse pancreatic neuroendocrine tumors developing adaptive/evasive resistance to VEGF inhibition. Clin Cancer Res. 2011;17(16):5299–310.

Molecular Targets in Human Neuroendocrine Tumors

Ujalla Sheikh, Jalil Muhammad, Domenico Coppola, and Aejaz Nasir

Introduction

Recent data demonstrate that the incidence of gastroenteropancreatic neuroendocrine tumors (GEP-NETs) has increased exponentially (overall ~500 %) over the last three decades, thus refuting the erroneous concept of their rarity [1, 2], due in part to improved diagnostic services and greater public awareness. Diagnosis of these neoplasms is usually delayed since there is no biochemical screening test and symptoms are protean and overlooked. Although grouped as a neoplastic entity (NETs), each lesion is derived from distinct cell precursors, produces specific bioactive products, exhibits distinct chromosomal abnormalities and somatic mutation events, and has uniquely dissimilar clinical presentations. GEP-NETs demonstrate very different survival rates reflecting the intrinsic differences in malignant potential and variations in proliferative regulation [1]. Specifically for PNETs, the clinical course depends primarily on the type of primary tumor, the tumor size, and histological grade [3]. Functional tumors may present at an early stage due to hormonal symptoms arising from secretion of various hormones or amines by the tumor [3]. The vast majority of PNETs, however, are nonfunctional, tend to remain clinically silent and may result in larger tumor size at presentation, compared to their functional counterparts. About two-thirds of patients with pancreatic NETs have distant metastases at diagnosis [2].

U. Sheikh • D. Coppola, MD
Department of Anatomic Pathology, H. Lee Moffitt Cancer Center, Tampa, FL, USA

J. Muhammad
Department of Neuroscience, George Mason University, Fairfax, VA, USA

A. Nasir, MD, MPhil, FCAP (✉)
Diagnostic and Experimental Pathology (Tailored Therapeutics), Lilly Research Laboratories, Eli Lilly and Co., Room 2391, Building 98C/2C, 893 South Delaware St., Indianapolis, IN, USA
e-mail: nasirae@lilly.com

A. Nasir, D. Coppola (eds.), *Neuroendocrine Tumors: Review of Pathology, Molecular and Therapeutic Advances*, DOI 10.1007/978-1-4939-3426-3_26

In recent years, there has been a dramatic increase in the number of molecularly targeted agents to treat cancer as a result of improved understanding of the complex pathobiologic processes and molecular pathways that are involved in the development, growth and progression of cancer, including NETs. Here we would like to review some of the key molecular targets that have been investigated as potential therapeutic targets in pancreatic NETs in recent years and review some of the emerging data, which may be of relevance to the diagnostic pathologists who are actively engaged in multidisciplinary care of patients with GEP/pancreatic neuroendocrine tumors. The molecular targets that have been under active clinical and scientific investigation in recent years [4] include peptide hormone receptors and receptor tyrosine kinases, including those that have a well-defined role in pathologic angiogenesis in PNETs and intracellular molecular targets like the mammalian target of rapamycin (mTOR).

Peptide Receptors and NETs

For many years somatostatin analogs (SSAs) have been used as a form of targeted therapies to control symptoms of hormonal hypersecretion by functional NETs. These agents are still an important treatment modality for NETs. In recent years somatostatin receptors (SSTRs) have been under active investigation as important targets for diagnosis and treatment of NETs.

Somatostatin and Somatostatin Receptors (SSTRs)

Somatostatin is an endogenous cyclic peptide that regulates the secretion of growth hormone, insulin, glucagon, and gastrin by the respective endocrine cells [5], through a family of G protein-coupled transmembrane receptors, including five distinct subtypes (SSTRs 1–5) [6, 7]. Somatostatin has a very short half-life (~3–4 min) [7], limiting its therapeutic efficacy in clinical setting. However, synthetic somatostatin analogs (SSAs) such as octreotide and lanreotide have high affinity for SSTR2 and SSTR5 and are without the undesirable effects of somatostatin [7, 8], supporting their clinical usefulness.

Activation of SSTRs has a number of direct and indirect effects on NET cells [9]. Direct antiproliferative effects of SSTR activation include inhibition of cell cycle and growth factor effects and induction of apoptosis, which may be mediated by the PI3K/mTOR, MAPK, and Ras/ERK signaling pathways [10, 11]. Indirect effects of SSTR activation include inhibition of the release of growth factors and trophic hormones, inhibition of angiogenesis, and modulation of the immune system [9].

Because of clinical and biologic relevance of SSTRs, a number of studies have investigated the expression and distribution of SSTRs in archival human NET tissues [12–14]. The distribution of SSTRs is widespread in GEP-NETs, with an overall prevalence of 50–100 % and frequent co-expression of multiple SSTRs in a given tumor. The expression of SSTRs varies among various histological types of

NETs and also among patients with the same tumor type. SSTR2 and SSTR5 are expressed in about 90 % and 80 % of pancreatic NET cells, respectively, making them potentially sensitive to hormone treatment [15]. Somatostatin receptor 2 (SSTR2) was absent or very low in insulinomas compared with nonfunctioning PNETs; differential expression of various SSTRs in PNETs makes evaluation of SSTRs relevant as markers of response to somatostatin analogs [16].

Other Peptide Receptors

With the clinical success of SSTRs in the management of NETs, patients have led to increased interest in other peptide receptors, including receptors for bombesin, cholecystokinin, and vasoactive intestinal peptide (VIP) in some types of pancreatic NETs [17–19].

Epidermal Growth Factor Receptor (EGFR)

Epidermal growth factor family of receptors (EGFR, ErbB) consists of four structurally related receptor tyrosine kinases (RTKs), including HER1 (aka EGFR, ErbB1), HER2 (ErbB2), HER3 (ErbB3), and HER4 (ErbB4). Eleven growth factor ligands can activate EGFR family of receptors, including EGF and TGF-alpha. EGFR (ErbB-1) is one of the regulator of the PI3K/Akt and the MAPKs pathways, which are important in regulating a number of cell functions, including cell growth, proliferation, differentiation, motility, and survival. EGFR activation pathways have been well characterized using tumor cell lines and are known to involve EGFR activation through autophosphorylation [20]. EGFR activation results in phosphorylation/upregulation of downstream signaling molecules, such as ERK1/2 (extracellular regulated kinase 1 and 2) and PKB/Akt (protein kinase B), which leads to enhanced tumor cell survival and proliferation [20]. Regulation of EGFR activity can be disrupted by several mechanisms: increased production of ligands; overexpression of EGFR; impaired downregulation of EGFR; cross-talk between EGFR and other EGFR family members, TKIs, and receptors; and activation of mutations in EGFR.

EGFR in NET Cell Lines

In a mutational survey of 36 kinase genes, including RTKs (EGFR, c-Kit, HER2, PDGFR-alpha), 6 genes from the Akt/mTOR pathway (AKT2, PIK3CA, RPS6K1, STK11, PDPK1, FRAP1-mTOR), and 25 genes that are frequently mutated in cancer, revealed alterations in targetable kinases in neuroendocrine cancer cell lines. PNET cell lines QGP1, CM, and BON harbored mutations in FGFR3, FLT1/VEGFR1, and PIK3CA, respectively, rendering these models useful for preclinical studies involving pathway-specific therapies [21].

In a recent study the effect of transactivation of EGFR by EGF, TGF-alpha, and various GI hormones to stimulate the growth of human foregut carcinoid (BON), the somatostatinoma (QGP-1), and the rat islet tumor (Rin-14B) cell lines showed an increased Tyr(1068) EGFR phosphorylation [22]. Furthermore, the stimulated phosphorylation of EGFR was dependent on Src kinases, PKCs, MMPs, and reactive oxygen species. These findings suggest that disruption of EGFR signaling cascade by EGFR inhibition alone or combined with other receptor antagonists may be a novel therapeutic approach for treatment of foregut NETs and PETs [22].

Cell Lines with Mutations in Other Tyrosine Kinase Genes

PNET cell lines QGP1, CM, and BON have been shown to harbor mutations in FGFR3, FLT1/VEGFR1, and PIK3CA genes, respectively [21]. These findings may have relevance to design preclinical studies with respective targeted therapies.

EGFR in Human NETs/PNETs

Several immunohistochemical studies have reported EGFR expression in human pancreatic NETs [23], with the proportion of samples expressing EGFR ranging from 18 to 65 %, including variation in the intensity of EGFR staining. The observed variation among studies may reflect differences in the patient populations or antibodies used [24] and need careful evaluation of this important therapeutic target in larger cohorts of pancreatic and non-pancreatic NETs.

Differential Expression of EGFR in Human GI and Pancreatic NETs

In an IHC-based analysis of 140 human PNETs, EGFR was immunopositive in 18 (13 %), HER2 in 3 (2 %), KIT in 16 (11 %), and PDGFR-alpha in 135 (96 %) [21]. These RTKs were expressed in PNET cells with variable frequency and/or in the surrounding tumor endothelium (Fig. 1).

Of the 130 PNETs evaluated as a tissue microarray (TMA) by FISH, 2 (1.5 %) cases had HER2 gene amplification [21]. All of these PNETs were disomic, monosomic (Fig. 2), or polysomic-trisomic, but there was no EGFR gene amplification [21].

An IHC, Western blot, and qPCR-based analysis of EGFR and P-EGFR expression in GI carcinoids and PETs showed a higher percentage of primary and metastatic GI carcinoids expressed EGFR and P-EGFR compared to PNETs. However, PNET patients with activated EGFR had worse prognosis [24]. These findings implicate the EGFR and P-EGFR signal transduction pathway in the pathogenesis of these tumors and suggest that targeted therapy directed against the EGFR tyrosine kinase domain may be a useful therapeutic approach in patients with unresectable metastatic GI carcinoids and PNETs [24].

In another IHC-based investigation of human PNETs, 96 % of tumor samples were *positive* for EGFR expression, 63 % for activated EGFR, 76 % for activated

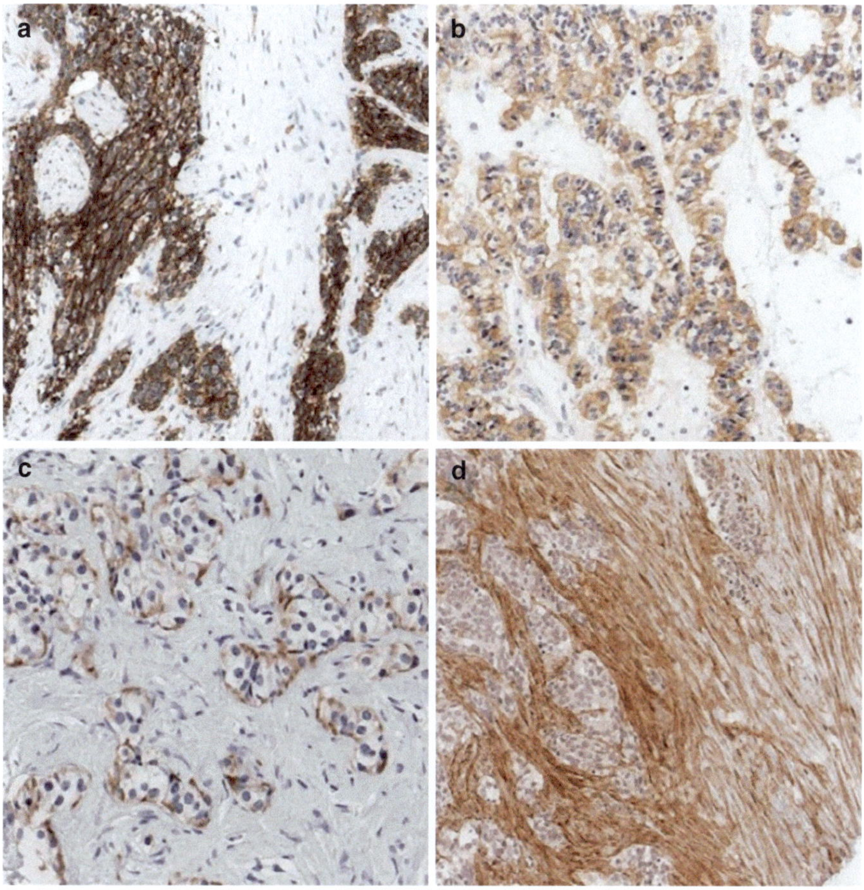

Fig. 1 Immunohistochemical staining for receptor tyrosine kinases in pancreatic endocrine tumors. Shown are positive staining for KIT (**a**), EGFR (**b**), and HER2 (**c**) in tumor cells; positive staining in tumor cells and in the stroma is shown for PDGFR-alpha (**d**). Original magnification, ×20 (Reproduced with permission from Corbo et al. [21])

Akt, and 96 % for activated ERK1/2 [20]. Furthermore, the histological score for the activation of Akt and ERK1/2 correlated with the histological score for activated EGFR. Based on these findings, the investigators suggested that therapeutic inhibition of EGFR with or without concomitant inhibition of Akt and ERK1/2 may provide newer therapeutic options for NET patients [20].

EGFR as a Prognostic Factor in Pancreatic NETs

Co-expression of transforming growth factor-alpha (TGF-alpha) and its receptor epidermal growth factor receptor (EGFR) is known to be associated with aggressive biologic behavior and adverse clinical outcome in a variety of tumors, including pancreatic adenocarcinomas [25]. Although expression of EGFR has been disputed as a

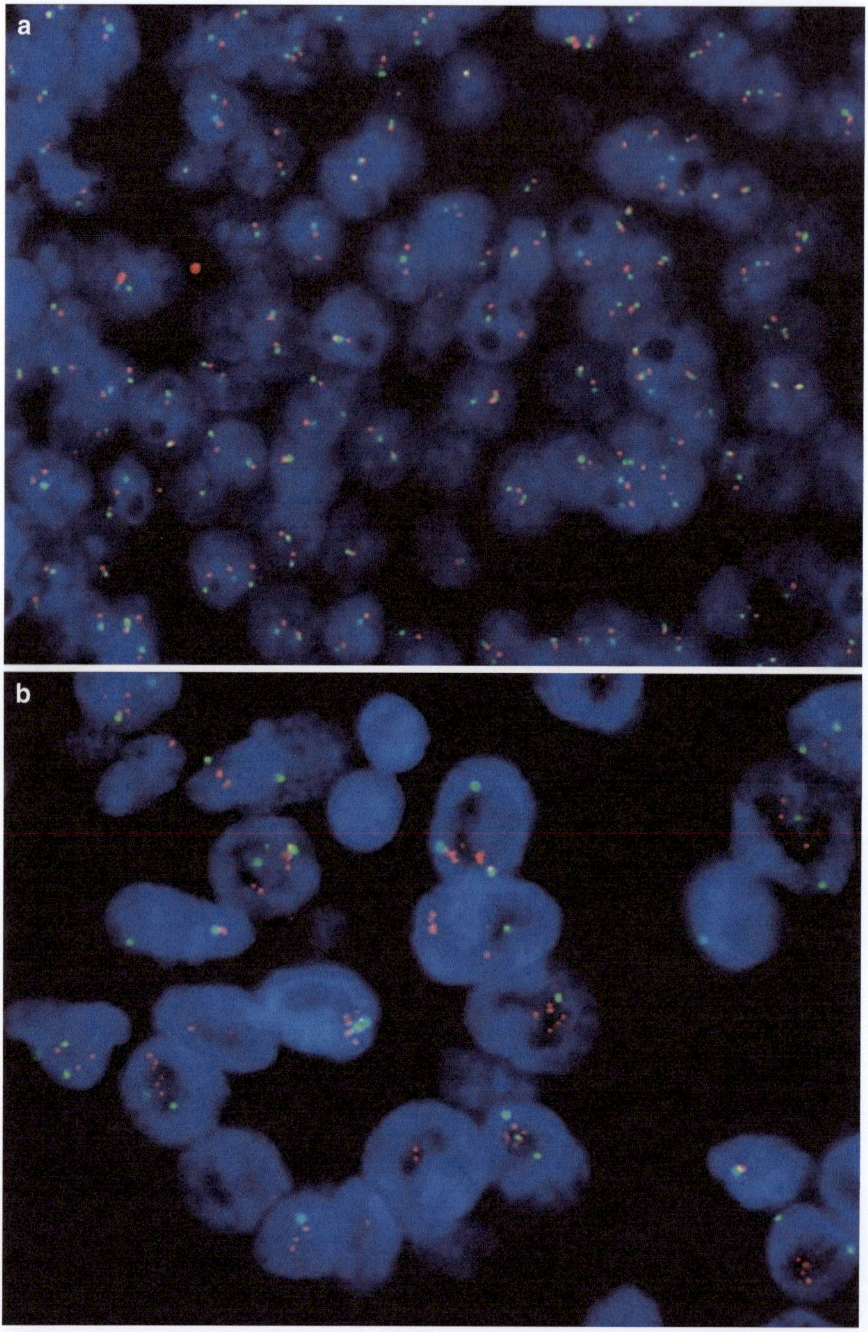

Fig. 2 Fluorescent in situ hybridization (FISH) analysis for EGFR and HER2 in pancreatic endocrine tumor. FISH analysis showing monosomy for EGFR (**a**) and gene amplification for HER2 (**b**). Originalmagnification,·100. EGFR and HER2 signal red, centromeric probes signal green (Reproduced with permission from Corbo et al. [21])

marker of malignancy in NETs [25, 26], a recent study showed significant correlation between EGFR expression and grade of malignancy in pancreatic NETs with low levels of expression in benign tumors and those of uncertain behavior to high levels of expression in well and poorly differentiated tumors [27]. Furthermore, patients with pancreatic NET expressing activated EGFR have been found to have significantly worse prognosis than those whose tumors did not express activated EGFR [24].

Collectively, findings in the above studies suggest that EGFR may provide useful information both as a prognostic marker in GEP-NETs. Furthermore, targeted therapy against the tyrosine kinase domain of EGFR may be a clinically relevant approach for patients with GI and pancreatic NETs.

Stem Cell Factor Receptor (SCFR aka c-Kit, Tyrosine Protein Kinase, CD117)

c-Kit is a protein that in humans is encoded by the gene, KIT. KIT is expressed on the surface of hematopoietic stem cells and other cell types. Receptor is activated by binding with its ligand, stem cell factor (SCF, or KIT-ligand). A number of studies have evaluated expression of c-Kit in human pancreatic NET tissue samples [28–31]. The proportion of c-Kit positive samples varied over a wide range between these studies and within one study varied substantially with the type of antibody used to detect c-Kit [29]. Inconsistencies between studies may, therefore, be related to technique or antibodies used rather than c-Kit levels. It is, therefore, important to define the most optimal approach to assess the KIT status of a given PNET and to determine if c-Kit expression by NETs can be translated into therapeutic benefit with agents like imatinib mesylate [29]. More recently, in a multivariate analysis of several prognostic factors, only WHO criteria and c-Kit expression were identified as independent markers of unfavorable prognosis in pancreatic NETs [32]. Furthermore, based on IHC expression of KIT and CK19 expression, PNETs were grouped into three prognostic categories: low risk (KIT−/CK19−), intermediate risk (KIT−/CK19+), and high risk (KIT+/CK19+), with significantly different patient survival, metastases, and recurrence of PETs among the three groups.

Sarcoma Kinase (Src)

The Src family of kinases (SFK) is a family of non-receptor tyrosine kinases involved in the transduction of signals from the cell membrane to different targets involved in cell cycle, cell adhesion, and cell motility. SFK activity has been shown to regulate adhesion, spreading, and migration of pancreatic NET cells in vitro [33]. Similarly, SFKs were found to be overexpressed in human PNETs [34] and are also involved in the transactivation of EGFR [22]. Inhibition of Src activity decreases adherence, spreading, and migration of pancreatic NET cells in vitro [33]. Furthermore, SFKs regulate mTOR activity during adhesion and simultaneous inhibition of SFKs and mTOR reduces proliferation of PNET cells without inducing PI3K/Akt activity [33].

Intracellular and Downstream Targets

Intracellular molecules mediating signal transduction downstream of RTKs form the basis of additional therapeutic approaches against pancreatic NETs. One of these targets is mTOR – a serine/threonine kinase, which regulates cell growth, metabolism, and apoptosis.

mTOR Pathway

mTOR is one of the most important target among a large number of extracellular and intracellular signaling molecules. Being a key regulator of several different cell functions, mTOR activation is tightly controlled by several positive and feedback regulatory loops [35]. Furthermore, mTOR forms two distinct protein complexes (mTORC1, mTORC2) (Fig. 3), which can be activated in different ways and exert different but related functions [37]. Mutations in the mTOR pathway genes have been reported in 15 % of PNETs [38]. Among these, the most important regulatory genes include phosphatase and tensin homolog (PTEN) [39], the tuberous sclerosis complex 2 gene (TSC2) [40, 41], and neurofibromatosis type 1 (NF1) [42, 43]. Loss-of-function mutations in TSC1 and TSC2, tumor suppressor genes that inhibit mTOR, occur in tuberous sclerosis – a hereditary cancer syndrome associated with the development of PNETs [44]. PTEN regulates the activity of mTOR through the Akt pathway and, along with TSC2, is downregulated in approximately 75 % of the primary PNETs, supporting a role for the PI3K/Akt/mTOR pathway in the development of pancreatic NETs. Also, low expression of these molecules was associated with shorter disease-free and overall survival in primary PNETs [16].

Clinical Success with mTOR Inhibitors and Future Clinical Opportunities

The mTOR inhibitor everolimus, which specifically inhibits mTORC1 and also mTORC2 (on prolonged exposure to drug), showed activity in a phase II study, followed by randomized, placebo-controlled phase III trials in patients with advanced PNETs and extra-pancreatic carcinoids. Based on significant increase in PFS in patients, receiving everolimus (vs. placebo) led to its approval [45]. One of the major clinical challenge is posed by the concomitant activation of the PI3K and MAPK pathways [46–48], which may interfere with the activity of mTOR inhibitors and may need alternative therapeutic approaches, like using mTOR inhibitors with or without SSTR analogs or as dual PI3K/mTOR inhibitors in advanced NETs

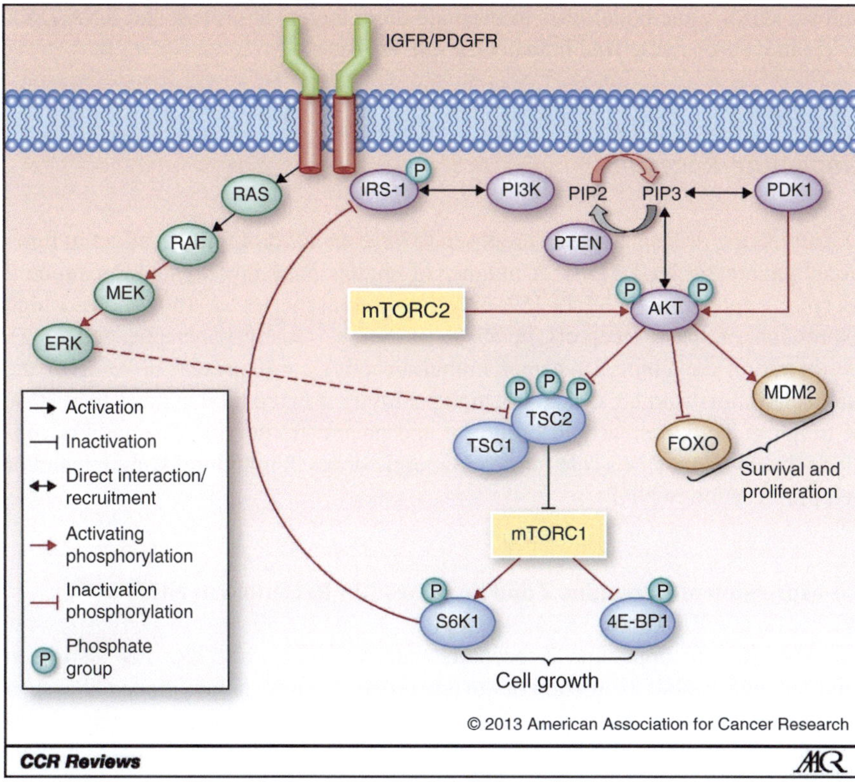

Fig. 3 Schematic representation of the mTOR pathway and associated regulatory circuitries. mTOR exists as two different complexes (mTORC1 and mTORC2) that are activated through different signaling cascades. Here the activation of mTORC1 by receptor tyrosine kinases–triggered signaling is depicted. Positive and feedback regulatory loops are also described. *PIP2* phosphatidylinositol (4,5)-bisphosphate, *ERK* extracellular signal-regulated kinase, *IGFR* insulin-like growth factor receptor, *MEK* MAP-ERK kinase, *PDGFR* platelet-derived growth factor receptor, *PI3K* phosphoinositide 3-kinase, *PIP2* phosphatidylinositol (4,5)-bisphosphate, *PIP3* phosphatidylinositol (3,4,5)-trisphosphate (Reproduced with permission from Oberg et al. [36])

(pancreatic and extra-pancreatic) [49, 50]. The rationale for combination of mTOR inhibition with SSTR analogs is to inhibit the IGF1R/PI3K/Akt axis (Bousquet, 2006 #167).

Other Potentially "Druggable" Targets

Several other potential therapeutic targets have been identified in human pancreatic NETs, including IGF-1, B-Raf [51], COX-2 [52], MTA-1 [53], CDK4 [54], claudin 3 and 7 [55], MAGE1 [56], and activated Akt [57]. Clearly there is need to develop and standardize methodologies to evaluate these targets at protein and RNA/DNA levels in well-characterized human GEP-NET tissues.

Dopamine Receptors

Dopaminergic drugs have been proposed to have an antiproliferative effect in functional pancreatic NETs [58]. A number of studies have investigated dopamine 2 receptor expression in NETs [59–62]. Grossrubatscher et al. [60] showed high expression of these receptors in 85 % of NETs (mostly pancreatic and lung). Furthermore, dopamine 2 receptor immunoreactivity was present in 93 % of the islet cell tumors studied. Generally, high positivity was reported in more than 70 % of tumor cells, particularly in bronchial and pancreatic tumors. The authors conclude that there may be a role for dopaminergic drugs in inhibiting secretion and/or cell proliferation in NETs.

Co-expression of Dopamine 2 and Somatostatin Receptors in NETs

Co-expression of dopamine 2 receptors with SSTR2 and SSTR5 has also been reported, with higher expression of the dopamine receptors in low-grade rather than high-grade NET [63]. Kidd et al. [64] report variable expression of dopamine 2 and somatostatin receptors depending on cell type and tissue of origin. In future studies, it will be valuable to develop methodologies that can reliable quantify both of these two receptors in archival human NET tissues.

Abbreviations

Akt	Protein kinase B
AKT2	kt/mTOR pathway gene
ALDH+	Aldehyde dehydrogenase positive
ATM	Protein kinase
BON	Pancreatic neuroendocrine tumors cell line
c-Kit	Stem cell growth factor receptor
CK19	Cytokeratin 19
CM	Pancreatic neuroendocrine tumors cell line
CSC	Cancer stem cells
EGF	Epidermal growth factor
EGFR	Epidermal growth factor receptor
ErbB-1	Epidermal growth factor receptor
ERK	Extracellular-regulated kinase
ERK1	Extracellular-regulated kinase 1

ERK2	Extracellular-regulated kinase 2
FGFR3	Fibroblast growth factor receptor 3
FLT1	EGFR gene
FRAP1-mTOR	Akt/mTOR pathway gene
GEP-NET	Gastroenteropancreatic neuroendocrine tumor
GI	Gastrointestinal
HER	Human epidermal growth factor receptor
HER2	Human epidermal growth factor receptor 2
HER3	Human epidermal growth factor receptor 3
IHC	Immunohistochemistry/immunohistochemical
KIT	c-Kit encoding gene
MAPK	Mitogen-activated protein kinase
MMP	Matrix metalloproteinases
mTOR	Mammalian target of rapamycin
mTOR	Mammalian target of rapamycin
NET	Neuroendocrine tumor
NF1	Neurofibromatosis type 1
PDGFR-alpha	Platelet-derived growth factor receptor-alpha
PDPK1	Akt/mTOR pathway gene
P-EGFR	Phosphorylated EGFR
PIK3CA	Akt/mTOR pathway gene
PI3K	Phosphoinositide-3-kinase
PKB	Protein kinase B
PMET	Phosphorylated MET
PNET	Primitive neuroendocrine tumor
PTEN	Phosphatase and tensin homolog
QGP-1	Pancreatic neuroendocrine tumors cell line
qPCR	Quantitative polymerase chain reaction
Rin-14B	Pancreatic delta cell line
RPS6K1	Akt/mTOR pathway gene
RTK	Receptor tyrosine kinase
SCF	Stem cell factor
SFK	Sarcoma family of kinases
siRNA	Small interfering RNA
Src	Sarcoma
SSA	Somatostatin analog
SSTR	Somatostatin receptors
SSTR2	Somatostatin receptor 2
SSTR5	Somatostatin receptor 5
STK11	Akt/mTOR pathway gene
TGFα	Transforming growth factor-alpha
TSC1	Tuberous sclerosis complex 1 gene
TSC2	Tuberous sclerosis complex 2 gene
VEGFR1	VEGF receptor
VIP	Vasoactive intestinal peptide

References

1. Schimmack S, Svejda B, Lawrence B, Kidd M, Modlin IM. The diversity and commonalities of gastroenteropancreatic neuroendocrine tumors. Langenbecks Arch Surg. 2011;396(3):273–98.
2. Yao JC, Hassan M, Phan A, Dagohoy C, Leary C, Mares JE, et al. One hundred years after "carcinoid": epidemiology of and prognostic factors for neuroendocrine tumors in 35,825 cases in the United States. J Clin Oncol. 2008;26(18):3063–72.
3. Wiedenmann B, Pavel M, Kos-Kudla B. From targets to treatments: a review of molecular targets in pancreatic neuroendocrine tumors. Neuroendocrinology. 2011;94(3):177–90.
4. Metz DC, Jensen RT. Gastrointestinal neuroendocrine tumors: pancreatic endocrine tumors. Gastroenterology. 2008;135(5):1469–92.
5. Kumar U, Grant M. Somatostatin and somatostatin receptors. Results Probl Cell Differ. 2010;50:137–84.
6. Patel YC. Molecular pharmacology of somatostatin receptor subtypes. J Endocrinol Invest. 1997;20(6):348–67.
7. Lamberts SW, van der Lely AJ, de Herder WW, Hofland LJ. Octreotide. N Engl J Med. 1996;334(4):246–54.
8. Eriksson B. New drugs in neuroendocrine tumors: rising of new therapeutic philosophies? Curr Opin Oncol. 2010;22(4):381–6.
9. Susini C, Buscail L. Rationale for the use of somatostatin analogs as antitumor agents. Ann Oncol. 2006;17(12):1733–42.
10. Grozinsky-Glasberg S, Shimon I, Korbonits M, Grossman AB. Somatostatin analogues in the control of neuroendocrine tumours: efficacy and mechanisms. Endocr Relat Cancer. 2008;15(3):701–20.
11. Schonbrunn A. Somatostatin receptors present knowledge and future directions. Ann Oncol. 1999;10 Suppl 2:S17–21.
12. Kulaksiz H, Eissele R, Rossler D, Schulz S, Hollt V, Cetin Y, et al. Identification of somatostatin receptor subtypes 1, 2A, 3, and 5 in neuroendocrine tumours with subtype specific antibodies. Gut. 2002;50(1):52–60.
13. Papotti M, Bongiovanni M, Volante M, Allia E, Landolfi S, Helboe L, et al. Expression of somatostatin receptor types 1–5 in 81 cases of gastrointestinal and pancreatic endocrine tumors. A correlative immunohistochemical and reverse-transcriptase polymerase chain reaction analysis. Virchows Arch. 2002;440(5):461–75.
14. Fjallskog ML, Ludvigsen E, Stridsberg M, Oberg K, Eriksson B, Janson ET. Expression of somatostatin receptor subtypes 1 to 5 in tumor tissue and intratumoral vessels in malignant endocrine pancreatic tumors. Med Oncol. 2003;20(1):59–67.
15. Fazio N, Cinieri S, Lorizzo K, Squadroni M, Orlando L, Spada F, et al. Biological targeted therapies in patients with advanced enteropancreatic neuroendocrine carcinomas. Cancer Treat Rev. 2010;36 Suppl 3:S87–94.
16. Missiaglia E, Dalai I, Barbi S, Beghelli S, Falconi M, della Peruta M, et al. Pancreatic endocrine tumors: expression profiling evidences a role for AKT-mTOR pathway. J Clin Oncol. 2010;28(2):245–55.
17. Tang C, Biemond I, Lamers CB. Expression of peptide receptors in human endocrine tumours of the pancreas. Gut. 1997;40(2):267–71.
18. Reubi JC, Waser B, Gugger M, Friess H, Kleeff J, Kayed H, et al. Distribution of CCK1 and CCK2 receptors in normal and diseased human pancreatic tissue. Gastroenterology. 2003;125(1):98–106.
19. Reubi JC, Waser B. Concomitant expression of several peptide receptors in neuroendocrine tumours: molecular basis for in vivo multireceptor tumour targeting. Eur J Nucl Med Mol Imaging. 2003;30(5):781–93.
20. Shah T, Hochhauser D, Frow R, Quaglia A, Dhillon AP, Caplin ME. Epidermal growth factor receptor expression and activation in neuroendocrine tumours. J Neuroendocrinol. 2006;18(5):355–60.

21. Corbo V, Beghelli S, Bersani S, Antonello D, Talamini G, Brunelli M, et al. Pancreatic endocrine tumours: mutational and immunohistochemical survey of protein kinases reveals alterations in targetable kinases in cancer cell lines and rare primaries. Ann Oncol. 2012;23(1):127–34.
22. Di Florio A, Sancho V, Moreno P, Delle Fave G, Jensen RT. Gastrointestinal hormones stimulate growth of Foregut Neuroendocrine Tumors by transactivating the EGF receptor. Biochim Biophys Acta. 2013;1833(3):573–82.
23. Wulbrand U, Wied M, Zofel P, Goke B, Arnold R, Fehmann H. Growth factor receptor expression in human gastroenteropancreatic neuroendocrine tumours. Eur J Clin Invest. 1998;28(12):1038–49.
24. Papouchado B, Erickson LA, Rohlinger AL, Hobday TJ, Erlichman C, Ames MM, et al. Epidermal growth factor receptor and activated epidermal growth factor receptor expression in gastrointestinal carcinoids and pancreatic endocrine carcinomas. Mod Pathol. 2005;18(10):1329–35.
25. Srivastava A, Alexander J, Lomakin I, Dayal Y. Immunohistochemical expression of transforming growth factor alpha and epidermal growth factor receptor in pancreatic endocrine tumors. Hum Pathol. 2001;32(11):1184–9.
26. Srirajaskanthan R, Shah T, Watkins J, Marelli L, Khan K, Caplin ME. Expression of the HER-1-4 family of receptor tyrosine kinases in neuroendocrine tumours. Oncol Rep. 2010;23(4):909–15.
27. Bergmann F, Breinig M, Hopfner M, Rieker RJ, Fischer L, Kohler C, et al. Expression pattern and functional relevance of epidermal growth factor receptor and cyclooxygenase-2: novel chemotherapeutic targets in pancreatic endocrine tumors? Am J Gastroenterol. 2009;104(1):171–81.
28. Fjallskog ML, Lejonklou MH, Oberg KE, Eriksson BK, Janson ET. Expression of molecular targets for tyrosine kinase receptor antagonists in malignant endocrine pancreatic tumors. Clin Cancer Res. 2003;9(4):1469–73.
29. Kostoula V, Khan K, Savage K, Stubbs M, Quaglia A, Dhillon AP, et al. Expression of c-kit (CD117) in neuroendocrine tumours – a target for therapy? Oncol Rep. 2005;13(4):643–7.
30. Lankat-Buttgereit B, Horsch D, Barth P, Arnold R, Blocker S, Goke R. Effects of the tyrosine kinase inhibitor imatinib on neuroendocrine tumor cell growth. Digestion. 2005;71(3):131–40.
31. Ferrari L, Della Torre S, Collini P, Martinetti A, Procopio G, De Dosso S, et al. Kit protein (CD117) and proliferation index (Ki-67) evaluation in well and poorly differentiated neuroendocrine tumors. Tumori. 2006;92(6):531–5.
32. Zhang L, Smyrk TC, Oliveira AM, Lohse CM, Zhang S, Johnson MR, et al. KIT is an independent prognostic marker for pancreatic endocrine tumors: a finding derived from analysis of islet cell differentiation markers. Am J Surg Pathol. 2009;33(10):1562–9.
33. Di Florio A, Capurso G, Milione M, Panzuto F, Geremia R, Delle Fave G, et al. Src family kinase activity regulates adhesion, spreading and migration of pancreatic endocrine tumour cells. Endocr Relat Cancer. 2007;14(1):111–24.
34. Capurso G, Di Florio A, Sette C, Delle Fave G. Signalling pathways passing Src in pancreatic endocrine tumours: relevance for possible combined targeted therapies. Neuroendocrinology. 2013;97(1):67–73.
35. Efeyan A, Sabatini DM. mTOR and cancer: many loops in one pathway. Curr Opin Cell Biol. 2010;22(2):169–76.
36. Oberg K, Casanovas O, Castano JP, Chung D, Delle Fave G, Denefle P, et al. Molecular pathogenesis of neuroendocrine tumors: implications for current and future therapeutic approaches. Clin Cancer Res. 2013;19(11):2842–9.
37. Laplante M, Sabatini DM. mTOR signaling in growth control and disease. Cell. 2012;149(2):274–93.
38. Jiao Y, Shi C, Edil BH, de Wilde RF, Klimstra DS, Maitra A, et al. DAXX/ATRX, MEN1, and mTOR pathway genes are frequently altered in pancreatic neuroendocrine tumors. Science. 2011;331(6021):1199–203.
39. Wang L, Ignat A, Axiotis CA. Differential expression of the PTEN tumor suppressor protein in fetal and adult neuroendocrine tissues and tumors: progressive loss of PTEN expression in

poorly differentiated neuroendocrine neoplasms. Appl Immunohistochem Mol Morphol. 2002;10(2):139–46.
40. Francalanci P, Diomedi-Camassei F, Purificato C, Santorelli FM, Giannotti A, Dominici C, et al. Malignant pancreatic endocrine tumor in a child with tuberous sclerosis. Am J Surg Pathol. 2003;27(10):1386–9.
41. Merritt 2nd JL, Davis DM, Pittelkow MR, Babovic-Vuksanovic D. Extensive acrochordons and pancreatic islet-cell tumors in tuberous sclerosis associated with TSC2 mutations. Am J Med Genet A. 2006;140(15):1669–72.
42. Johannessen CM, Reczek EE, James MF, Brems H, Legius E, Cichowski K. The NF1 tumor suppressor critically regulates TSC2 and mTOR. Proc Natl Acad Sci U S A. 2005;102(24):8573–8.
43. Perren A, Wiesli P, Schmid S, Montani M, Schmitt A, Schmid C, et al. Pancreatic endocrine tumors are a rare manifestation of the neurofibromatosis type 1 phenotype: molecular analysis of a malignant insulinoma in a NF-1 patient. Am J Surg Pathol. 2006;30(8):1047–51.
44. Yao JC. Neuroendocrine tumors. Molecular targeted therapy for carcinoid and islet-cell carcinoma. Best Pract Res Clin Endocrinol Metab. 2007;21(1):163–72.
45. Capdevila J, Salazar R, Halperin I, Abad A, Yao JC. Innovations therapy: mammalian target of rapamycin (mTOR) inhibitors for the treatment of neuroendocrine tumors. Cancer Metastasis Rev. 2011;30 Suppl 1:27–34.
46. Zhang H, Bajraszewski N, Wu E, Wang H, Moseman AP, Dabora SL, et al. PDGFRs are critical for PI3K/Akt activation and negatively regulated by mTOR. J Clin Invest. 2007;117(3):730–8.
47. Carracedo A, Ma L, Teruya-Feldstein J, Rojo F, Salmena L, Alimonti A, et al. Inhibition of mTORC1 leads to MAPK pathway activation through a PI3K-dependent feedback loop in human cancer. J Clin Invest. 2008;118(9):3065–74.
48. Sarbassov DD, Guertin DA, Ali SM, Sabatini DM. Phosphorylation and regulation of Akt/PKB by the rictor-mTOR complex. Science. 2005;307(5712):1098–101.
49. Pavel ME, Hainsworth JD, Baudin E, Peeters M, Horsch D, Winkler RE, et al. Everolimus plus octreotide long-acting repeatable for the treatment of advanced neuroendocrine tumours associated with carcinoid syndrome (RADIANT-2): a randomised, placebo-controlled, phase 3 study. Lancet. 2011;378(9808):2005–12.
50. Guertin DA, Sabatini DM. The pharmacology of mTOR inhibition. Sci Signal. 2009;2(67):e24.
51. Karhoff D, Sauer S, Schrader J, Arnold R, Fendrich V, Bartsch DK, et al. Rap1/B-Raf signaling is activated in neuroendocrine tumors of the digestive tract and Raf kinase inhibition constitutes a putative therapeutic target. Neuroendocrinology. 2007;85(1):45–53.
52. Ohike N, Morohoshi T. Immunohistochemical analysis of cyclooxygenase (COX)-2 expression in pancreatic endocrine tumors: association with tumor progression and proliferation. Pathol Int. 2001;51(10):770–7.
53. Hofer MD, Chang MC, Hirko KA, Rubin MA, Nose V. Immunohistochemical and clinicopathological correlation of the metastasis-associated gene 1 (MTA1) expression in benign and malignant pancreatic endocrine tumors. Mod Pathol. 2009;22(7):933–9.
54. Lindberg D, Hessman O, Akerstrom G, Westin G. Cyclin-dependent kinase 4 (CDK4) expression in pancreatic endocrine tumors. Neuroendocrinology. 2007;86(2):112–8.
55. Borka K, Kaliszky P, Szabo E, Lotz G, Kupcsulik P, Schaff Z, et al. Claudin expression in pancreatic endocrine tumors as compared with ductal adenocarcinomas. Virchows Arch. 2007;450(5):549–57.
56. Hansel DE, House MG, Ashfaq R, Rahman A, Yeo CJ, Maitra A. MAGE1 is expressed by a subset of pancreatic endocrine neoplasms and associated lymph node and liver metastases. Int J Gastrointest Cancer. 2003;33(2–3):141–7.
57. Ghayouri M, Boulware D, Nasir A, Strosberg J, Kvols L, Coppola D. Activation of the serine/threonine protein kinase Akt in enteropancreatic neuroendocrine tumors. Anticancer Res. 2010;30(12):5063–7.
58. Pathak RD, Tran TH, Burshell AL. A case of dopamine agonists inhibiting pancreatic polypeptide secretion from an islet cell tumor. J Clin Endocrinol Metab. 2004;89(2):581–4.

59. Lemmer K, Ahnert-Hilger G, Hopfner M, Hoegerle S, Faiss S, Grabowski P, et al. Expression of dopamine receptors and transporter in neuroendocrine gastrointestinal tumor cells. Life Sci. 2002;71(6):667–78.
60. Grossrubatscher E, Veronese S, Ciaramella PD, Pugliese R, Boniardi M, De Carlis L, et al. High expression of dopamine receptor subtype 2 in a large series of neuroendocrine tumors. Cancer Biol Ther. 2008;7(12):1970–8.
61. Pivonello R, Ferone D, de Herder WW, Faggiano A, Bodei L, de Krijger RR, et al. Dopamine receptor expression and function in corticotroph ectopic tumors. J Clin Endocrinol Metab. 2007;92(1):65–9.
62. Srirajaskanthan R, Watkins J, Marelli L, Khan K, Caplin ME. Expression of somatostatin and dopamine 2 receptors in neuroendocrine tumours and the potential role for new biotherapies. Neuroendocrinology. 2009;89(3):308–14.
63. Srirajaskanthan R, Dancey G, Hackshaw A, Luong T, Caplin ME, Meyer T. Circulating angiopoietin-2 is elevated in patients with neuroendocrine tumours and correlates with disease burden and prognosis. Endocr Relat Cancer. 2009;16(3):967–76.
64. Kidd M, Drozdov I, Joseph R, Pfragner R, Culler M, Modlin I. Differential cytotoxicity of novel somatostatin and dopamine chimeric compounds on bronchopulmonary and small intestinal neuroendocrine tumor cell lines. Cancer. 2008;113(4):690–700.

Recent Advances in Molecular Pathology of Neuroendocrine Neoplasms

Aejaz Nasir, Ujalla Sheikh, Kevin G Neill, Kun Jiang, Jalil Muhammad, and Domenico Coppola

Although grouped as a neoplastic entity (NETs), each neoplasm is derived from distinct cell precursors, produces specific bioactive products, exhibits distinct chromosomal abnormalities and somatic mutation events, and has uniquely dissimilar clinical presentations [1]. In recent clinical trials, VEGF pathway inhibitor sunitinib and the mTOR inhibitor everolimus have shown efficacy in patients with advanced pancreatic NETs [2]. The efficacy of these targeted therapies in NETs suggests that the molecular characterization of NETs may provide an avenue to predict which patients may benefit most from the treatment and how to overcome potential drug resistance [2].

In recent years, a wide range of molecular approaches are being used both for characterization of NETs and also for discovery and validation of novel candidate biomarkers in NETs. Some of these molecular approaches elaborate on the genesis, growth, and progression of these neoplasms, others serve as prognostic markers, and still others have the potential to be used as biomarkers that can predict response or resistance of NETs to various targeted and other emerging therapies, as reviewed in the following sections.

A. Nasir, MD, MPhil, FCAP (✉)
Diagnostic and Experimental Pathology (Tailored Therapeutics), Lilly Research Laboratories, Eli Lilly and Co., Room 2391, Building 98C/2C, 893 South Delaware St., Indianapolis, IN, USA
e-mail: nasirae@lilly.com

U. Sheikh • K.G. Neill, MD • K. Jiang, MD • D. Coppola, MD
Department of Anatomic Pathology, H. Lee Moffitt Cancer Center, Tampa, FL, USA

J. Muhammad
Department of Neuroscience, George Mason University, Fairfax, VA, USA

A. Nasir, D. Coppola (eds.), *Neuroendocrine Tumors: Review of Pathology, Molecular and Therapeutic Advances*, DOI 10.1007/978-1-4939-3426-3_27

The Mammalian Target of Rapamycin (mTOR)

The mammalian target of rapamycin (mTOR) is an intracellular serine/threonine kinase that functions as a transduction factor to which a wide variety of physiological and pathologic extra and intracellular signals converge [3]. mTOR is involved in the regulation of cell metabolism, survival, proliferation, and motility, through the regulation of protein translation. Multiple somatic mutations in the mTOR pathway have been identified in pancreatic NETs [4, 5].

Specifically, PTEN was found mutated in 7 %, TSC2 in 8.8 %, and PIK3CA in only 1.4 % [6]. Expression levels of PTEN and TSC2 have also recently been linked to outcome in pancreatic NETs [7]. In other studies, PTEN was mutated or lost in about 10–29 % of sporadic PNETs [8, 9]. The expression of PTEN in PNETs has been positively correlated with longer survival especially when correlated with low expression of p-mTOR [8]. Furthermore, positive p-mTOR expression and PTEN loss may have a synergic effect on tumorigenesis and proliferation of PNETs.

The expression and activity of mTOR have been proved to be higher in PNET tissue than in normal pancreatic islet cells. Expression of mTOR or of its activated downstream target p4EBP1 has also been associated with a higher proliferative index and shorter survival in patients with NETs. The expression of mTOR, p-mTOR, and S6K is significantly related to tumor aggressiveness in the form of higher mitotic count, tumor size, staging, vascular invasion, and metastasis [10]. Also, low levels of 4EBP1 or high levels of eIF4E are thought to confer resistance to rapamycin analogs [11]. Therefore, mTOR and its effectors might be biomarkers of aggressive disease, but are not mutated in PNETs, and most molecular changes occur upstream in the PI3K/Akt/mTOR pathway.

Taken together, the above data suggest that targeted therapy based on mTOR/PTEN signaling pathway and its associated molecular mechanisms may play a role in the medical management of PNETS. However, since biomarkers to select individual patients who would respond to treatment with mTOR inhibitors are still lacking, future analytical and clinical validation studies and evaluation of the clinical utility of the various members of the mTOR pathway in human NETs will be an important molecular advance in the near future. Independent validation of the above findings in prospective studies will further facilitate the development of more personalized approaches to treatment of NET patients.

EGFR Family of Receptors as Biomarkers

Epidermal growth factor receptor (EGFR) is expressed in many cancers and is associated with poor prognosis [12]. Furthermore, co-expression of transforming growth factor alpha (TGF-alpha) and its receptor, EGFR, is also associated with aggressive biologic behavior and adverse clinical outcome in a variety of tumors, including pancreatic adenocarcinomas [13]. Although in NETs, the expression of EGFR has been disputed as a marker of malignancy [13, 14], a recent study showed significant correlation between EGFR expression and grade of malignancy in pancreatic NETs with low levels of expression in benign tumors and those of uncertain behavior but high levels of expression in well- and poorly differentiated tumors [15]. Furthermore, patients with pancreatic NETs expressing activated EGFR had significantly worse prognosis than those whose tumors did not express activated EGFR [16]. In another recent study, only rare primary PNETs revealed HER2 amplification and mutations in KIT and ATM genes [5]. On independent validation using IHC staining of 140 human PNETs, EGFR was immunopositive in 18 (13 %), HER2 in 3 (2 %), KIT in 16 (11 %), and PDGFR-alpha in 135 (96 %) [5]. Therefore, a number of studies have shown EGFR expression as a marker of adverse clinical outcome in PNETs.

c-KIT

In a multivariate analysis of several prognostic factors, only WHO criteria and c-kit expression were identified as independent markers of unfavorable prognosis in pancreatic NETs [17]. Furthermore, based on IHC expression of KIT and CK19, three prognostic groups of PNETs were identified: low risk (KIT−/CK19−), intermediate risk (KIT−/CK19+), and high risk (KIT+/CK19+), with significantly different patient survival, metastases, and recurrence of PETs among the three groups [17].

MGMT

Emerging data suggest that high methylguanine-methyltransferase (MGMT) expression is associated with therapeutic resistance to temozolomide [18, 19]. The sensitivity of tumor cells to alkylating agents, including temozolomide, has been associated with low MGMT levels, which through its ability to restore DNA to its normal form can prevent chemotherapy-induced cell death [20]. MGMT deficiency seems to be more common in pancreatic NETs than in carcinoid tumors, potentially explaining the greater sensitivity of pancreatic NETs to treatment with the alkylating agents streptozocin and temozolomide and raising the possibility of using MGMT expression as a predictive marker in future studies of these tumors [18]. If confirmed in future prospective studies, low MGMT expression could help select patients for such treatments. Therefore, *quantification of tumor MGMT expression levels is warranted in future studies of alkylating agents in NETs* [19].

Chromogranin A (CgA)

Chromogranin A (CgA) is a 49-kDa protein, found in the neurosecretory vesicles of NET cells, and is commonly detected in the plasma of patients with endocrine neoplasms [21, 22]. Elevated plasma CgA levels have been associated with poor overall prognosis in patients with NETs [22]. Early decreases in CgA levels have been associated with favorable treatment outcome in some studies [23, 24]. Both plasma CgA and 24-h urinary 5HIAA levels have been evaluated in prior NET studies as surrogate markers of response. Serial measurements of plasma CgA need to be incorporated into prospective clinical trials. Also, further validation of CgA as a prognostic and potentially predictive biomarker study is warranted [19].

In the past decade, knowledge regarding molecular pathology of sporadic pancreatic neuroendocrine tumors (PNETs) has increased substantially, thanks to microarray studies and novel mutational analysis methods [25]. Over the same period of time, a number of targeted agents have been tested in clinical trials in this tumor type. For some of these agents, there is a strong biological rationale. Among them, the mammalian target of rapamycin (mTOR) inhibitor (everolimus) and the antiangiogenic agent sunitinib are approved for the treatment of PNETs. However, there is lack of knowledge regarding biomarkers able to predict their efficacy and about mechanisms of resistance to these targeted agents [26]. It has also been ascertained that the most common mutations in sporadic PNETs are of the multiple endocrine neoplasia type 1 (MEN1) gene and of the genes ATRX and DAXX. Currently, the clinical significance and potential for treatment of these mutations are uncertain. In this chapter, we will review the main molecular changes occurring in GEP-NETs and emphasize as to how they may be linked to various treatment options.

MENIN

MENIN is a nuclear protein, encoded by the MEN1 gene, which regulates gene transcription by coordinating chromatin remodeling. It is involved in the negative modulation of cell cycle inhibitors, such as p27KIPI and p18INK4c, of transcription factors such as SMAD3 and JUND, and interacts with the DNA repair machinery [27]. MENIN is considered a tumor suppressor, although its exact role is not completely clear and its action is often controversial. In fact, MENIN works as an inhibitor of proliferation, maintaining the promoter activity of CDKN2C (p18) and CDKN1B (p27) through H3K4 methylation, thus regulating the expression of cell cycle progression inhibitors [27, 28]. Nevertheless, under physiological or pathological conditions, such as obesity or pregnancy, MENIN stimulates pancreatic endocrine cell proliferation controlling G1 to S progression [27, 29].

While the role of MENIN has been extensively investigated in patients with MEN1 syndrome, mutations of the MEN1 gene have also been found in about 25–44 % of sporadic PNETs [6, 30], suggesting a role in the pathogenesis of these tumors. Interestingly, MEN1 mutations have been associated with prolonged survival in patients with metastatic disease [6]. Although mutations of MEN1 are the most frequent alterations in sporadic PNETs, this does not represent a target for treatment yet, although there have been successful attempts of gene therapy to replace the MEN1 gene in PNET models. However, the relation between MENIN and other "druggable" pathways is gaining increasing interest. MENIN is able to suppress Akt activity reducing its translocation from the cytoplasm to the cell membrane during stimulation with growth factors, therefore reducing Akt-induced proliferation and anti-apoptosis activity [31]. On the other hand, MENIN expression is modulated by PI3K/Akt activity, which leads to phosphorylation of the transcription factor Foxo1, which in turn negatively regulates the expression of MENIN, enhancing proliferation [27, 32].

MENIN has also a role in preventing the RAS-driven activation of the mitogen-activated protein kinase (MAPK) pathway, leaving the RASSFA inhibitory pathway intact. The removal of this mechanism of MAPK pathway blockage could explain why the loss of MENIN causes proliferation in PNETs [33]. However, targeting the RAF or MAPK pathway alone does not seem to be a promising strategy in PNETs. Recently, a novel link between MENIN and the Hedgehog (Hh) signaling pathway has been suggested by Gurung et al. [34]. Furthermore, Fendrich et al. showed how cyclopamine, a Hedgehog inhibitor, decreased tumor cell proliferation, reduced tumor volume, and significantly prolonged median survival in the transgenic mouse model of PNET [35]. The orally available smoothened antagonist LDE225 is therefore under investigation for PNETs. Finally, a valuable target therapy for MENIN could possibly arrive with RNA antagonist (s)-based strategies, as suggested by Luzi et al., but further studies are needed to explore this field [36].

About 15–20 % of NETs are part of inherited genetic syndromes, including multiple endocrine neoplasia type 1 and type 2 (MEN1 and MEN2), von Hippel-Lindau syndrome (vHL), neurofibromatosis type 1 (NF1), and tuberous sclerosis complex (TSC). The genes involved in pancreatic NETs (PNETs) are quite different and fewer than those involved in ductal adenocarcinomas of the pancreas [37]. The genes commonly mutated in PNETs include MEN1 (44 %), DAXX and ATRX (43 %; associated with better prognosis), and those coding for members of the mTOR pathway (15 %) [6, 38–40]. Immunohistochemical assays for DAXX and ATRX proteins demonstrate positive nuclear labeling for DAXX in large cell NEC and absence of nuclear staining for DAXX in a well-differentiated NET (Fig. 1). Similarly, nuclear positivity for ATRX protein has been shown in small cell NEC with absence of nuclear staining for ATRX protein in a well-differentiated NET (Fig. 1). Somatic mutations in DAXX and ATRX appear to be late events in PNETs, since they were absent in microadenomas [4]. On exomic sequence analysis of sporadic pancreatic NETs, an average of 16 nonsynonymous mutations per PNET is far fewer than in ductal adenocarcinoma [6].

The VHL/HIF pathway is also important in PNET pathogenesis [42]. Pancreatic neuroendocrine microadenomas are present in more than 70 % of patients with von Hippel-Lindau syndrome. Sporadic PNETs rarely harbor somatic VHL gene mutation, but promoter hyper-methylation and deletion of VHL occur in up to 25 % sporadic PNETs and are associated with an adverse prognosis [43].

In contrast to pancreatic adenocarcinoma, activation of classical oncogene-mediated pathways does not seem a common event in PNETs [1]. Little is known in respect of pancreatic neuroendocrine oncogenesis and the molecular basis of the progression of sporadic NETs [44]. Mutations in main driver genes like k-Ras, P53,

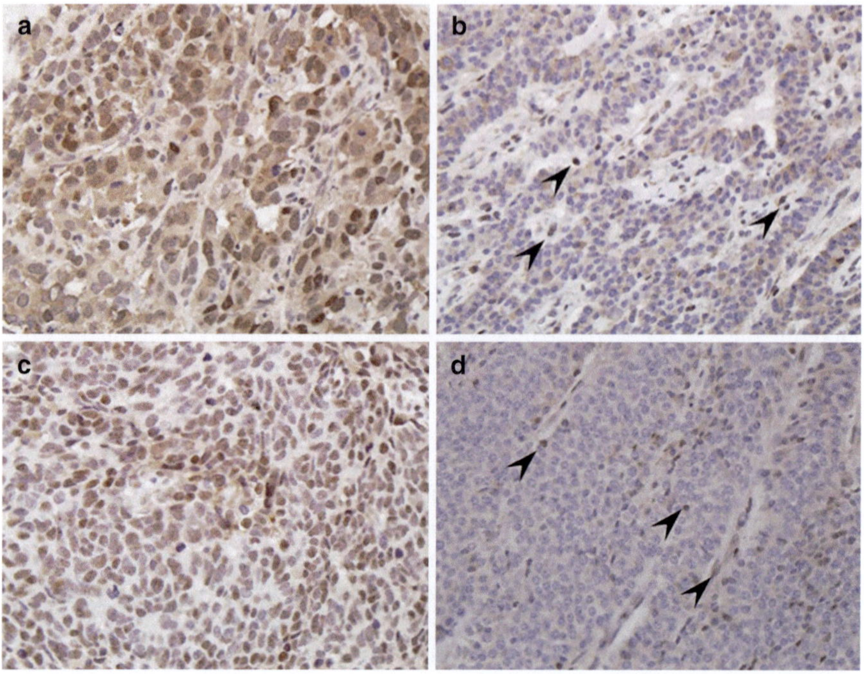

Fig. 1 Immunohistochemical labeling patterns for DAXX and ATRX. (**a**) Example of positive nuclear labeling for DAXX in a large cell NEC. (**b**) Loss of nuclear labeling of DAXX in a well-differentiated neuroendocrine tumor. Endothelial cells and lymphocytes within the stroma are positive (indicated by *arrowheads*). (**c**) Positive nuclear labeling for ATRX in a small cell NEC. (**d**) Loss of nuclear labeling of ATRX in a well-differentiated neuroendocrine tumor. Similar to that for DAXX shown in (**b**), endothelial cells and lymphocytes within the stroma are positive (original magnifications ×200) (Reproduced from Yachida et al. [41] with kind permission by Lippincott Williams & Wilkins)

myc, FOS, Jun, src, and Rb have not been specifically implicated [45, 46]. However, copy number alterations in proteins that regulate some of these pathways, MDM2 and P53, have been observed [47].

MDM2 and p53

The tumor suppressor p53 plays a critical role in maintaining genomic stability and tumor prevention [48]. The p53 pathway is tightly regulated by a number of proteins, including the critical negative regulators MDM2, MDM4, and WIP1 [48]. Extra gene copies of MDM2 (22 %), MDM4 (30 %), and WIP1 (51 %) have been reported in PNETs, which may lead to an attenuated p53 function [47]. Thus, development of MDM2 inhibitors and related molecules can restore p53 tumor suppressor function and may provide tangible therapeutic options for PNETs [2].

Molecular Changes in CTCs in NETs

CTCs are associated with progressive NETs and could be used as a prognostic marker. In a prospective study of 120 patients with metastatic NETs, presence of CTCs conferred poorer overall survival, with an HR of 14 [49]. Furthermore, a reduction of CTCs 3–5 weeks after treatment predicted response to therapy in addition to better survival compared with those patients in whom CTCs were increased [50]. Therefore, patients on ineffective or potentially toxic therapies can have their treatment changed appropriately and their management tailored according to CTC changes [2].

CTCs have been reported in blood samples from a number of patients with metastatic NETs, including pancreas, midgut, and bronchial NETs [49] but without any correlation between CTC counts and Ki-67 or CgA levels. In patients with lung cancer treated with anti-EGF receptor (EGFR) therapy, a resistance-associated EGFR mutation has been reported in CTCs [51]. Therefore, molecular characterization of CTCs could potentially assist in understanding NET metastasis and resistance to therapy in addition to their use as biomarkers [2].

Transcription Factors in NETs (PAX8, TTF-1, and CDX2)

PAX8 is a transcription factor expressed in normal adult pancreatic islet cells and is also in primary and metastatic well-differentiated PNETs [52]. Loss of PAX8 may have prognostic significance since PAX8-negative PNETs tend to be larger and are associated with malignant behavior and increased incidence of liver metastases [52].

Tissue-specific transcription factors, such as TTF1 and CDX2, will be increasingly utilized to support origin of an occult primary NETs when one is faced with a metastatic neuroendocrine carcinoma (NEC) of unknown primary.

Cyclin-Dependent Kinases and Rb

Cyclin-dependent protein kinases 4 (CDK4) and 6 are involved in phosphorylation of the retinoblastoma (Rb) tumor suppressor gene leading to inactivation [53]. CDK4/CDK6 amplification and expression have been shown in PNETs as well as its activator, cyclin D [54]. Loss of Rb protein via RB1 gene mutation is also frequently observed in poorly differentiated and high-grade NETs (Figs. 2 and 3) [41]. Furthermore, growth of the human PNET cell line QGP1 can be inhibited in a xenograft mouse model by the CDK4/CDK6-specific inhibitor PD 0332991, which reactivates the Rb pathway [55]. Therefore, gene amplification and overexpression of CDK4 and CDK6 suggest that a subset of patients with PNETs may respond favorably to CDK4/CDK6 inhibitors that are currently entering clinical trials [2].

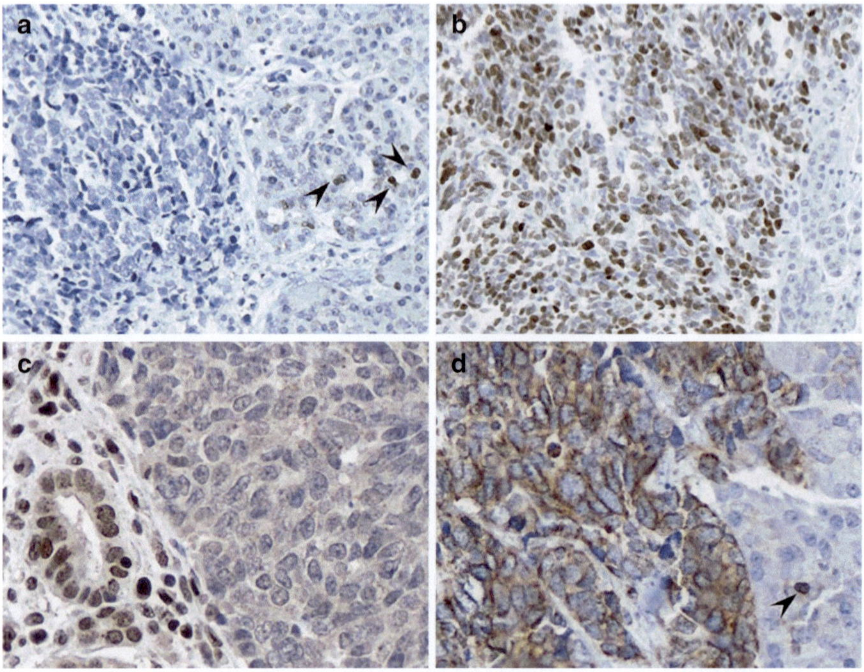

Fig. 2 Immunohistochemical labeling for p53, Rb, and Bcl-2 in small cell neuroendocrine carcinomas. (**a**) Example of loss of nuclear labeling for p53. Scattered reactive acinar cells with positive nuclear labeling are present in the adjacent normal tissue (*arrowheads*). Sequencing analysis for TP53 in this patient revealed a nonsense mutation (p.E307X). (**b**) Example of diffusely positive nuclear labeling for p53. (**c**) Example of loss of nuclear labeling for retinoblastoma (Rb) protein. Adjacent nonneoplastic cells show positive nuclear labeling (*left side*). (**d**) Diffuse cytoplasmic positivity for Bcl-2 protein. Note the reactive lymphocyte regarded as an internal positive control for this protein (*arrowhead*) (original magnifications ×200) (Reproduced from Yachida et al. [41] with kind permission by Lippincott Williams & Wilkins)

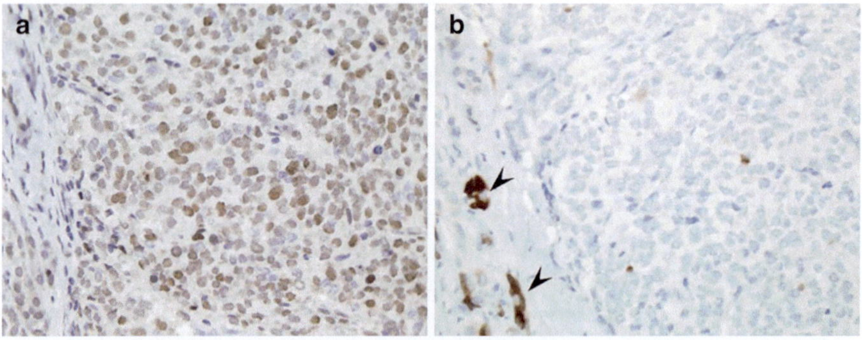

Fig. 3 Immunohistochemical labeling for Rb and p16 in a large cell NEC. (**a**) Positive nuclear immunolabeling for Rb. (**b**) Loss of p16 labeling in a serial section of the same large cell NEC. Reactive acinar cells (*arrowheads*) serve as positive internal controls for labeling (original magnifications ×200) (Reproduced from Yachida et al. [41] with kind permission by Lippincott Williams & Wilkins)

Chromosomal Abnormalities

Characteristic allelic imbalances have been observed in sporadic carcinoid and pancreatic NETs [19]. Comparative genomic hybridization (CGH) studies have identified a number of chromosomal alterations in PNETs, among which chromosomal losses are somewhat more frequent than gains, while amplifications are uncommon [56, 57]. In PNETs, the most common chromosomal losses occur on 6, 11, X, and Y, while most common gains include Chr 9, 12, and 17 [1]. Loss of chromosome 18, for example, seems to be a frequent and characteristic feature of small intestinal NETs [1, 58–60], while chromosomes 17 and 19 exhibit the most common gains [1]. It is obvious that pancreatic and small intestinal NETs express significantly different patterns of chromosomal rearrangements; however, the precise implications of the alterations are as still unknown.

Exomic sequence analysis of small intestinal NETs (SI-NETs) showed a much lower rate of somatic single nucleotide variants (SNVs) with an average of 0.1 per 106 nucleotides, suggesting their mutational quiescence [61]. Another study in SI-NETs identified recurrent somatic mutations and deletions in *CDKN1B* [62]. Furthermore, several recurrent somatic copy number alterations (CNAs) were discovered in cancer-related pathways, including PI3K/Akt/mTOR, tumor growth factor (alterations in *SMAD* genes), and *SRC*. Independent large-scale validation of these genetic findings is warranted to confirm these preliminary data, to examine novel epigenetic alterations, and to further determine their value as prognostic or predictive biomarkers in NETs.

Initial proof of concept novel molecular diagnostic studies using comparative genomic hybridization (CGH) and single nucleotide polymorphism (SNP) analyses have shown distinct patterns of allelic alternations in pancreatic and ileal NETs. Most frequent allelic imbalances in WD-NETs were losses of chromosome 18 in 10 tumors (34 %), chromosome 21 or 21q in six (21 %), chromosome 13 or 13q in five (17 %), and chromosome 16 or 16q in four (14 %) tumors and amplification of chromosome 20 or 20p in seven (24 %) tumors. Chromosomal aberrations were significantly less common in WD-NETs from lung and gastrointestinal tract compared to PETs [60]. Also, the observed genetic alterations differed significantly with the anatomical subsite of the NET: allelic loss of chromosome 18 was present in 69 % of ileal carcinoids, 13 % of non-ileal carcinoids, and 6 % of pancreatic NETs [63].

Epigenetic Mechanisms in NETs

Epigenetic mechanisms are an essential component of normal development and gene expression patterns in mammals [2]. Mutations in epigenetic regulators have the potential to lead to misregulation of gene expression that contributes to tumorigenesis, and it has been suggested that epigenetic rather than genetic changes may play a key role in NETs [64]. The long-standing observation that menin mutations are associated with NETs supports a role for epigenetic regulation of menin in the pathogenesis of NETs [2].

Discovery and Validation of Novel Molecular Biomarkers in PNETs

Gene Expression Profiling

In addition to clinic-pathologic criteria, the discovery of novel molecular markers of metastases may allow development of newer objective criteria to determine patient prognosis and may improve our understanding of the biology of clinical progression in PETs [65]. In recent years, we [66–70] and others [71–77] have carried out gene expression profiling analyses in PNETs. To identify candidate progression genes in PNETs, we used Affymetrix 2.0 gene chip on fresh-frozen metastatic primary PECAs (MP PECAs) that already had metastasized to the liver at the time of resection of the pancreatic primary and a set of frozen non-MP PETs that remained free of clinically detectable metastases until the last patient follow-up. All of the pancreatic endocrine primaries used in this experiment were nonfunctional. Using rigorous thresholds for *P*-values and fold changes in the differentially expressed genes, including gene function/class and pathway analysis, we selected our leading "candidate progression genes" that were differentially expressed between the two sets of pancreatic primaries (metastatic and nonmetastatic). Among these, CD24 antigen, insulin receptor, TMPRSS6, SERPINA1, SMURF1, RNF43, and AKR1C2 were notably upregulated, whereas RUNX1T1, protocadherin 9, RASSF5, RERG, ST14, glucagon, and PDGFRL were notably downregulated [66–68, 78, 79].

From our "candidate progression gene list," we validated under-expression of several leading candidate progression genes including RUNX1T1 and overexpression of TMPRSS6, SERPINA1, and others on an independent test set of archival PECAs (with liver metastases) using quantitative real-time polymerase chain reaction [70]. We then went on to further validate several of our novel genes, including RUNX1T1 and palladin as progression genes at the protein level using immunohistochemistry on independent test sets of metastatic and non-MP pancreatic endocrine neoplasms [65, 70]. Because IHC expression of RUNX1T1 protein showed a striking difference between the two sets of primaries (metastatic and nonmetastatic), we used ROC curve analysis to further elucidate the relationship between sensitivity and specificity of RUNX1T1 as a prognostic test to predict the presence of liver metastases. Using a cutoff of RUNX1T1 score of four or less in the primary tumor tissue as a predictor of liver metastases, we found low RUNX1T1 expression to have a sensitivity of 85 % and specificity of 96 %.

Based on these data, decreased IHC expression of RUNX1T1 protein in the primary PNET tissue appears to be a surrogate end point for prediction of risk of liver metastases in patients with surgically resected primary PETs [70]. Under-expression of this novel prognostic marker may identify patients with resected primary PETs who are at high risk for metastatic recurrence and may be candidates for closer follow-up for early detection of metastatic disease. Furthermore, RUNX1T1 protein expression in the primary tumor tissue emerges as a stronger predictor of liver metastases as compared with the other conventional pathological criteria, such as tumor size, grade, and Ki-67 index. A genome-wide screen to detect somatic mutations of genes in colorectal cancer also identified RUNX1T1 as 1 of the 189 new candidate cancer genes, related to TGF-alpha signaling [80]. Another leading gene that was validated as progression gene in PNETs was palladin [65, 69] which was a known metastasis-associated gene with a defined role in cell motility and cell-cell interactions [81, 82]. It is possible that palladin protein may be contributing to liver metastases in case on PNETs by intensifying the invasive properties of the tumor cells.

Using a liquid chromatography-mass spectrometry (LC-MS)-based proteomic approach to identify proteins that can be used as biomarkers for malignant (metastatic) vs. benign (nonmetastatic) insulinomas, 16 (out of 3000) proteins were found differentially expressed between the two insulinoma subsets [83]. IHC validation on tissue microarrays containing 62 insulinomas revealed ALDH1A1, VDAC1, and TPD52 to fulfill the requirements for biologic markers that can be used beyond ENETS and WHO criteria for prognostic stratification of resected insulinomas [83]. Based on these data, additional investigations using proteomic biomarker discovery approach and further validation of these and other promising protein biomarkers in other types of PNETs and non-pancreatic NETs are warranted.

Conclusion

With increasing recognition of the differences in biology and clinical behavior among various NETs, advances in molecular pathology of NETs will facilitate development, validation, and qualification of robust prognostic and predictive biomarkers that can play important roles in pathologic classification, prognostication, and optimal management of NETs. The rigorous analysis of molecular aberrations and clinical outcomes in annotated bio-specimens would represent a useful and feasible first step in defining clinically relevant molecular subgroups of pancreatic and non-pancreatic NETs. A more in-depth understanding of the molecular abnormalities in NETs will be increasingly relevant as additional molecularly targeted therapies are developed. Although large-scale, prospective studies enrolling patients with specific molecular NET subtypes may not be entirely feasible at this point, useful information regarding the activity of specific drugs in molecular subtypes can be gained from retrospective/exploratory analyses of relevant human cancer tissues and annotated clinical data either from clinical trials or through academic-industry collaborations. This will create more and more opportunities for diagnostic pathologists in the academia and community to build and advance molecular pathology expertise using the gold standard and newer molecular methodologies, as part of the implementation of personalized NET oncology model in the twenty-first century.

Abbreviations

4EBP1	Eukaryotic translational initiation factor 4E-binding protein 1
AKR1C2	Candidate progression aldo-keto reductase family 1, member C2 gene
Akt	Protein kinase B
ALDH1A1	Aldehyde dehydrogenase 1 family member A1 gene
ATM	Ataxia Telangiectasia Mutated gene
ATRX	Alpha thalassemia/mental retardation syndrome X-linked gene
CAN	Copy number alterations
CDKN1B	Cyclin-dependent kinase inhibitor 1B gene
CDKN2C	Cyclin-dependent kinase inhibitor 2C gene
CDX2	Caudal type homeobox 2 gene (a transcription factor)
CGH	Comparative genomic hybridization
CK19	Cytokeratin 19
c-Kit	Stem cell growth factor receptor
DAXX	Death-domain associated protein
EGFR	Epidermal growth factor receptor
eIF4E	Eukaryotic translation initiation factor 4E gene
Foxo1	Forkhead box O1 gene
GEP	Gastroenteropancreatic
HER2	Human epidermal growth factor receptor 2
HIF	Hypoxia-inducible factor
IHC	Immunohistochemical
JUND	Jun D proto-oncogene
KIT	c-Kit encoding gene
LC-MS	Liquid chromatography-mass spectrometry
LDE225	Signaling pathway inhibitor
MAPK	Mitogen-activated protein kinase
MEN1	Multiple endocrine neoplasia type 1 gene
MEN2	Multiple endocrine neoplasia type 2 gene
MENIN	Protein encoded by MEN1 gene
MGMT	Methylguanine-methyltransferase
MP	Metastatic primary
mTOR	Mechanistic target of rapamycin
NET	Neuroendocrine tumor
p18INK4c	Cell cycle inhibitor
p27KIPI	Cell cycle inhibitor
p4EBP1	Phosphorylated 4EBP1
PDGFR-alpha	Platelet-derived growth factor receptor alpha
PDGFRL	Platelet derived growth factor receptor like gene candidate progression gene
PECA	Pancreatic endocrine carcinoma
PET	Pancreatic endocrine tumor
PI3K	Phosphoinositide 3-kinase

PIK3CA	Akt/mTOR pathway gene
p-mTOR	Phosphorylated mechanistic target of rapamycin
PNET	Primitive neuroendocrine tumor
PTEN	Phosphatase and tensin homolog
RASSF5	Candidate progression gene
RERG	Candidate progression gene
RNF43	Candidate progression gene
ROC	Receiver operating characteristic
RUNX1T1	Candidate progression gene
S6K	Ribosomal protein S6 kinase
SERPINA1	Candidate progression gene
SI-NET	Small intestinal neuroendocrine tumors
SMAD	Homologs of both the *Drosophila* protein, mothers against decapentaplegic (MAD) and the *Caenorhabditis elegans* protein SMA
SMAD3	Transcription factor
SMURF1	Candidate progression gene
SNP	Single nucleotide polymorphism
SNV	Single nucleotide variants
SRC	SRC proto-oncogene, non-receptor tyrosine kinase
ST14	Candidate progression gene
TGF	Transforming growth factor
TGF-alpha	Transforming growth factor alpha
TMPRSS6	Candidate progression gene
TPD52	Tumor protein D52
TSC	Tuberous sclerosis complex
TSC2	Tuberous sclerosis complex 2 gene
TTF1	Transcription termination factor, RNA polymerase I
VDAC1	Voltage dependent anion channel 1 gene
vHL	von Hippel-Lindau syndrome
WD-NET	Well-differentiated neuroendocrine tumors
WHO	World Health Organization

References

1. Schimmack S, Svejda B, Lawrence B, Kidd M, Modlin IM. The diversity and commonalities of gastroenteropancreatic neuroendocrine tumors. Langenbecks Arch Surg. 2011;396(3): 273–98.
2. Oberg K, Casanovas O, Castano JP, Chung D, Delle Fave G, Denefle P, et al. Molecular pathogenesis of neuroendocrine tumors: implications for current and future therapeutic approaches. Clin Cancer Res. 2013;19(11):2842–9.
3. Capurso G, Archibugi L, Delle Fave G. Molecular pathogenesis and targeted therapy of sporadic pancreatic neuroendocrine tumors. J Hepatobiliary Pancreat Sci. 2015;22(8):594–601.
4. de Wilde RF, Edil BH, Hruban RH, Maitra A. Well-differentiated pancreatic neuroendocrine tumors: from genetics to therapy. Nat Rev Gastroenterol Hepatol. 2012;9(4):199–208.

5. Corbo V, Beghelli S, Bersani S, Antonello D, Talamini G, Brunelli M, et al. Pancreatic endocrine tumours: mutational and immunohistochemical survey of protein kinases reveals alterations in targetable kinases in cancer cell lines and rare primaries. Ann Oncol. 2012;23(1):127–34.
6. Jiao Y, Shi C, Edil BH, de Wilde RF, Klimstra DS, Maitra A, et al. DAXX/ATRX, MEN1, and mTOR pathway genes are frequently altered in pancreatic neuroendocrine tumors. Science. 2011;331(6021):1199–203.
7. Missiaglia E, Dalai I, Barbi S, Beghelli S, Falconi M, della Peruta M, et al. Pancreatic endocrine tumors: expression profiling evidences a role for AKT-mTOR pathway. J Clin Oncol. 2010;28(2):245–55.
8. Han X, Ji Y, Zhao J, Xu X, Lou W. Expression of PTEN and mTOR in pancreatic neuroendocrine tumors. Tumour Biol. 2013;34(5):2871–9.
9. Perren A, Komminoth P, Saremaslani P, Matter C, Feurer S, Lees JA, et al. Mutation and expression analyses reveal differential subcellular compartmentalization of PTEN in endocrine pancreatic tumors compared to normal islet cells. Am J Pathol. 2000;157(4):1097–103.
10. Komori Y, Yada K, Ohta M, Uchida H, Iwashita Y, Fukuzawa K, et al. Mammalian target of rapamycin signaling activation patterns in pancreatic neuroendocrine tumors. J Hepatobiliary Pancreat Sci. 2014;21(4):288–95.
11. Carew JS, Kelly KR, Nawrocki ST. Mechanisms of mTOR inhibitor resistance in cancer therapy. Target Oncol. 2011;6(1):17–27.
12. Shah T, Hochhauser D, Frow R, Quaglia A, Dhillon AP, Caplin ME. Epidermal growth factor receptor expression and activation in neuroendocrine tumours. J Neuroendocrinol. 2006;18(5):355–60.
13. Srivastava A, Alexander J, Lomakin I, Dayal Y. Immunohistochemical expression of transforming growth factor alpha and epidermal growth factor receptor in pancreatic endocrine tumors. Hum Pathol. 2001;32(11):1184–9.
14. Srirajaskanthan R, Shah T, Watkins J, Marelli L, Khan K, Caplin ME. Expression of the HER-1-4 family of receptor tyrosine kinases in neuroendocrine tumours. Oncol Rep. 2010;23(4):909–15.
15. Bergmann F, Breinig M, Hopfner M, Rieker RJ, Fischer L, Kohler C, et al. Expression pattern and functional relevance of epidermal growth factor receptor and cyclooxygenase-2: novel chemotherapeutic targets in pancreatic endocrine tumors? Am J Gastroenterol. 2009;104(1):171–81.
16. Papouchado B, Erickson LA, Rohlinger AL, Hobday TJ, Erlichman C, Ames MM, et al. Epidermal growth factor receptor and activated epidermal growth factor receptor expression in gastrointestinal carcinoids and pancreatic endocrine carcinomas. Mod Pathol. 2005;18(10):1329–35.
17. Zhang L, Smyrk TC, Oliveira AM, Lohse CM, Zhang S, Johnson MR, et al. KIT is an independent prognostic marker for pancreatic endocrine tumors: a finding derived from analysis of islet cell differentiation markers. Am J Surg Pathol. 2009;33(10):1562–9.
18. Kulke MH, Hornick JL, Frauenhoffer C, Hooshmand S, Ryan DP, Enzinger PC, et al. O6-methylguanine DNA methyltransferase deficiency and response to temozolomide-based therapy in patients with neuroendocrine tumors. Clin Cancer Res. 2009;15(1):338–45.
19. Kulke MH, Siu LL, Tepper JE, Fisher G, Jaffe D, Haller DG, et al. Future directions in the treatment of neuroendocrine tumors: consensus report of the National Cancer Institute Neuroendocrine Tumor clinical trials planning meeting. J Clin Oncol. 2011;29(7):934–43.
20. Gerson SL. Clinical relevance of MGMT in the treatment of cancer. J Clin Oncol. 2002;20(9):2388–99.
21. Eriksson B, Oberg K, Stridsberg M. Tumor markers in neuroendocrine tumors. Digestion. 2000;62 Suppl 1:33–8.
22. Janson ET, Holmberg L, Stridsberg M, Eriksson B, Theodorsson E, Wilander E, et al. Carcinoid tumors: analysis of prognostic factors and survival in 301 patients from a referral center. Ann Oncol. 1997;8(7):685–90.
23. Kouvaraki MA, Ajani JA, Hoff P, Wolff R, Evans DB, Lozano R, et al. Fluorouracil, doxorubicin, and streptozocin in the treatment of patients with locally advanced and metastatic pancreatic endocrine carcinomas. J Clin Oncol. 2004;22(23):4762–71.

24. Yao JC, Lombard-Bohas C, Baudin E, Kvols LK, Rougier P, Ruszniewski P, et al. Daily oral everolimus activity in patients with metastatic pancreatic neuroendocrine tumors after failure of cytotoxic chemotherapy: a phase II trial. J Clin Oncol. 2010;28(1):69–76.
25. Capurso G, Festa S, Valente R, Piciucchi M, Panzuto F, Jensen RT, et al. Molecular pathology and genetics of pancreatic endocrine tumours. J Mol Endocrinol. 2012;49(1):R37–50.
26. Jensen RT, Delle Fave G. Promising advances in the treatment of malignant pancreatic endocrine tumors. N Engl J Med. 2011;364(6):564–5.
27. Karnik SK, Hughes CM, Gu X, Rozenblatt-Rosen O, McLean GW, Xiong Y, et al. Menin regulates pancreatic islet growth by promoting histone methylation and expression of genes encoding p27Kip1 and p18INK4c. Proc Natl Acad Sci U S A. 2005;102(41):14659–64.
28. Balogh K, Racz K, Patocs A, Hunyady L. Menin and its interacting proteins: elucidation of menin function. Trends Endocrinol Metab. 2006;17(9):357–64.
29. Yang Y, Gurung B, Wu T, Wang H, Stoffers DA, Hua X. Reversal of preexisting hyperglycemia in diabetic mice by acute deletion of the Men1 gene. Proc Natl Acad Sci U S A. 2010;107(47):20358–63.
30. Corbo V, Dalai I, Scardoni M, Barbi S, Beghelli S, Bersani S, et al. MEN1 in pancreatic endocrine tumors: analysis of gene and protein status in 169 sporadic neoplasms reveals alterations in the vast majority of cases. Endocr Relat Cancer. 2010;17(3):771–83.
31. Wang Y, Ozawa A, Zaman S, Prasad NB, Chandrasekharappa SC, Agarwal SK, et al. The tumor suppressor protein menin inhibits AKT activation by regulating its cellular localization. Cancer Res. 2011;71(2):371–82.
32. Zhang H, Li W, Wang Q, Wang X, Li F, Zhang C, et al. Glucose-mediated repression of menin promotes pancreatic beta-cell proliferation. Endocrinology. 2012;153(2):602–11.
33. Chamberlain CE, Scheel DW, McGlynn K, Kim H, Miyatsuka T, Wang J, et al. Menin determines K-RAS proliferative outputs in endocrine cells. J Clin Invest. 2014; 124(9):4093–101.
34. Gurung B, Feng Z, Iwamoto DV, Thiel A, Jin G, Fan CM, et al. Menin epigenetically represses Hedgehog signaling in MEN1 tumor syndrome. Cancer Res. 2013;73(8):2650–8.
35. Fendrich V, Rehm J, Waldmann J, Buchholz M, Christofori G, Lauth M, et al. Hedgehog inhibition with cyclopamine represses tumor growth and prolongs survival in a transgenic mouse model of islet cell tumors. Ann Surg. 2011;253(3):546–52.
36. Luzi E, Marini F, Giusti F, Galli G, Cavalli L, Brandi ML. The negative feedback-loop between the oncomir Mir-24-1 and menin modulates the Men1 tumorigenesis by mimicking the "Knudson's second hit". PLoS One. 2012;7(6):e39767.
37. Rishi A, Goggins M, Wood LD, Hruban RH. Pathological and molecular evaluation of pancreatic neoplasms. Semin Oncol. 2015;42(1):28–39.
38. Chiang HC, O'Dorisio TM, Huang SC, Maton PN, Gardner JD, Jensen RT. Multiple hormone elevations in Zollinger-Ellison syndrome. Prospective study of clinical significance and of the development of a second symptomatic pancreatic endocrine tumor syndrome. Gastroenterology. 1990;99(6):1565–75.
39. Jonkers YM, Ramaekers FC, Speel EJ. Molecular alterations during insulinoma tumorigenesis. Biochim Biophys Acta. 2007;1775(2):313–32.
40. Hessman O, Lindberg D, Einarsson A, Lillhager P, Carling T, Grimelius L, et al. Genetic alterations on 3p, 11q13, and 18q in nonfamilial and MEN 1-associated pancreatic endocrine tumors. Genes Chromosomes Cancer. 1999;26(3):258–64.
41. Yachida S, Vakiani E, White CM, Zhong Y, Saunders T, Morgan R, et al. Small cell and large cell neuroendocrine carcinomas of the pancreas are genetically similar and distinct from well-differentiated pancreatic neuroendocrine tumors. Am J Surg Pathol. 2012;36(2):173–84.
42. Speisky D, Duces A, Bieche I, Rebours V, Hammel P, Sauvanet A, et al. Molecular profiling of pancreatic neuroendocrine tumors in sporadic and Von Hippel-Lindau patients. Clin Cancer Res. 2012;18(10):2838–49.
43. Schmitt AM, Schmid S, Rudolph T, Anlauf M, Prinz C, Kloppel G, et al. VHL inactivation is an important pathway for the development of malignant sporadic pancreatic endocrine tumors. Endocr Relat Cancer. 2009;16(4):1219–27.

44. Oberg K, Eriksson B. Endocrine tumours of the pancreas. Best Pract Res Clin Gastroenterol. 2005;19(5):753–81.
45. Rindi G, Candusso ME, Solcia E. Molecular aspects of the endocrine tumours of the pancreas and the gastrointestinal tract. Ital J Gastroenterol Hepatol. 1999;31 Suppl 2:S135–8.
46. Yoshimoto K, Iwahana H, Fukuda A, Sano T, Katsuragi K, Kinoshita M, et al. ras mutations in endocrine tumors: mutation detection by polymerase chain reaction-single strand conformation polymorphism. Jpn J Cancer Res. 1992;83(10):1057–62.
47. Hu W, Feng Z, Modica I, Klimstra DS, Song L, Allen PJ, et al. Gene amplifications in well-differentiated pancreatic neuroendocrine tumors inactivate the p53 pathway. Genes Cancer. 2010;1(4):360–8.
48. Levine AJ, Hu W, Feng Z. The P53 pathway: what questions remain to be explored? Cell Death Differ. 2006;13(6):1027–36.
49. Khan MS, Tsigani T, Rashid M, Rabouhans JS, Yu D, Luong TV, et al. Circulating tumor cells and EpCAM expression in neuroendocrine tumors. Clin Cancer Res. 2011;17(2):337–45.
50. Khan MS, Kirkwood A, Tsigani T, Garcia-Hernandez J, Hartley JA, Caplin ME, et al. Circulating tumor cells as prognostic markers in neuroendocrine tumors. J Clin Oncol. 2013;31(3):365–72.
51. Maheswaran S, Sequist LV, Nagrath S, Ulkus L, Brannigan B, Collura CV, et al. Detection of mutations in EGFR in circulating lung-cancer cells. N Engl J Med. 2008;359(4):366–77.
52. Long KB, Srivastava A, Hirsch MS, Hornick JL. PAX8 expression in well-differentiated pancreatic endocrine tumors: correlation with clinicopathologic features and comparison with gastrointestinal and pulmonary carcinoid tumors. Am J Surg Pathol. 2010;34(5):723–9.
53. Molenaar JJ, Ebus ME, Koster J, van Sluis P, van Noesel CJ, Versteeg R, et al. Cyclin D1 and CDK4 activity contribute to the undifferentiated phenotype in neuroblastoma. Cancer Res. 2008;68(8):2599–609.
54. Tang LH, Contractor T, Clausen R, Klimstra DS, Du YC, Allen PJ, et al. Attenuation of the retinoblastoma pathway in pancreatic neuroendocrine tumors due to increased cdk4/cdk6. Clin Cancer Res. 2012;18(17):4612–20.
55. Tang LH, Gonen M, Hedvat C, Modlin IM, Klimstra DS. Objective quantification of the Ki67 proliferative index in neuroendocrine tumors of the gastroenteropancreatic system: a comparison of digital image analysis with manual methods. Am J Surg Pathol. 2012;36(12):1761–70.
56. Speel EJ, Richter J, Moch H, Egenter C, Saremaslani P, Rutimann K, et al. Genetic differences in endocrine pancreatic tumor subtypes detected by comparative genomic hybridization. Am J Pathol. 1999;155(6):1787–94.
57. Speel EJ, Scheidweiler AF, Zhao J, Matter C, Saremaslani P, Roth J, et al. Genetic evidence for early divergence of small functioning and nonfunctioning endocrine pancreatic tumors: gain of 9Q34 is an early event in insulinomas. Cancer Res. 2001;61(13):5186–92.
58. Kim JW, Woo OH, Cho KR, Seo BK, Yong HS, Kim A, et al. Primary large cell neuroendocrine carcinoma of the breast: radiologic and pathologic findings. J Korean Med Sci. 2008;23(6):1118–20.
59. Kulke MH, Freed E, Chiang DY, Philips J, Zahrieh D, Glickman JN, et al. High-resolution analysis of genetic alterations in small bowel carcinoid tumors reveals areas of recurrent amplification and loss. Genes Chromosomes Cancer. 2008;47(7):591–603.
60. Kim do H, Nagano Y, Choi IS, White JA, Yao JC, Rashid A. Allelic alterations in well-differentiated neuroendocrine tumors (carcinoid tumors) identified by genome-wide single nucleotide polymorphism analysis and comparison with pancreatic endocrine tumors. Genes Chromosomes Cancer. 2008;47(1):84–92.
61. Banck MS, Kanwar R, Kulkarni AA, Boora GK, Metge F, Kipp BR, et al. The genomic landscape of small intestine neuroendocrine tumors. J Clin Invest. 2013;123(6):2502–8.
62. Francis JM, Kiezun A, Ramos AH, Serra S, Pedamallu CS, Qian ZR, et al. Somatic mutation of CDKN1B in small intestine neuroendocrine tumors. Nat Genet. 2013;45(12):1483–6.
63. Wang GG, Yao JC, Worah S, White JA, Luna R, Wu TT, et al. Comparison of genetic alterations in neuroendocrine tumors: frequent loss of chromosome 18 in ileal carcinoid tumors. Mod Pathol. 2005;18(8):1079–87.

64. Elsasser SJ, Allis CD, Lewis PW. Cancer. New epigenetic drivers of cancers. Science. 2011;331(6021):1145–6.
65. Henderson-Jackson EB, Helm J, Strosberg J, Nasir NA, Yeatman TJ, Kvols LK, et al. Palladin is a marker of liver metastasis in primary pancreatic endocrine carcinomas. Anticancer Res. 2011;31(9):2957–62.
66. Nasir A, McCarthy SM, Nasir NA, Chen DT, Agarwal D, Skaf J, et al. Discovery and validation of a novel set of putative progression markers in well differentiated primary pancreatic endocrine carcinomas. North American Neuroendocrine Tumor Society (NANETS), Neuroendocrine Tumor Symposium. Charlotte; 2009.
67. Nasir A, Henderson-Jackson EB, Helm J, Strosberg J, Nasir NA, Cheema A, et al. RUNX1T1 and Palladin outperform pathologic criteria of malignancy in predicting liver metastases in primary pancreatic endocrine carcinoma. North American Neuroendocrine Tumor Society (NANETS), NeuroEndocrine Tumor Symposium. Charlotte; 2009.
68. Nasir A, Helm J, Turner LM, Henderson-Jackson EB, Strosberg J, Nasir NA, et al. RUNX1T1: a novel predictor of liver metastasis in primary pancreatic endocrine neoplasms. North American Neuroendocrine Tumor Society (NANETS), Neuroendocrine Tumor Symposium. Charlotte; 2009.
69. Nasir A, Henderson-Jackson EB, Helm J, Strosberg J, Nasir NA, Coppola D, et al. Palladin is a reliable marker of liver metastasis in primary pancreatic endocrine neoplasms. North American Neuroendocrine Tumor Society (NANETS), Neuroendocrine Tumor Symposium. Charlotte; 2009.
70. Nasir A, Helm J, Turner L, Chen DT, Strosberg J, Hafez N, et al. RUNX1T1: a novel predictor of liver metastasis in primary pancreatic endocrine neoplasms. Pancreas. 2011;40(4):627–33.
71. Maitra A, Hansel DE, Argani P, Ashfaq R, Rahman A, Naji A, et al. Global expression analysis of well-differentiated pancreatic endocrine neoplasms using oligonucleotide microarrays. Clin Cancer Res. 2003;9(16 Pt 1):5988–95.
72. Bloomston M, Durkin A, Yang I, Rojiani M, Rosemurgy AS, Enkmann S, et al. Identification of molecular markers specific for pancreatic neuroendocrine tumors by genetic profiling of core biopsies. Ann Surg Oncol. 2004;11(4):413–9.
73. Capurso G, Lattimore S, Crnogorac-Jurcevic T, Panzuto F, Milione M, Bhakta V, et al. Gene expression profiles of progressive pancreatic endocrine tumours and their liver metastases reveal potential novel markers and therapeutic targets. Endocr Relat Cancer. 2006;13(2):541–58.
74. Dilley WG, Kalyanaraman S, Verma S, Cobb JP, Laramie JM, Lairmore TC. Global gene expression in neuroendocrine tumors from patients with the MEN1 syndrome. Mol Cancer. 2005;4(1):9.
75. Couvelard A, Hu J, Steers G, O'Toole D, Sauvanet A, Belghiti J, et al. Identification of potential therapeutic targets by gene-expression profiling in pancreatic endocrine tumors. Gastroenterology. 2006;131(5):1597–610.
76. Duerr EM, Mizukami Y, Ng A, Xavier RJ, Kikuchi H, Deshpande V, et al. Defining molecular classifications and targets in gastroenteropancreatic neuroendocrine tumors through DNA microarray analysis. Endocr Relat Cancer. 2008;15(1):243–56.
77. Shida T, Furuya M, Kishimoto T, Nikaido T, Tanizawa T, Koda K, et al. The expression of NeuroD and mASH1 in the gastroenteropancreatic neuroendocrine tumors. Mod Pathol. 2008;21(11):1363–70.
78. McCarthy SM, Nasir NA, Chen DT, Agarwal D, Skaf J, Gruidle M, et al. Discovery and validation of a novel set of putative progression markers in sporadic well differentiated primary pancreatic endocrine carcinomas. AACR Annual Meeting. San Diego; 2008.
79. Hafez N, Coppola D, Helm J, Turner L, Nasir N, Hakem A, et al. p21 upregulation not p53 predicts liver metastases in primary pancreatic endocrine carcinomas. Granada: European Neuroendocrine Tumor Society (ENETS); 2009.
80. Sjoblom T, Jones S, Wood LD, Parsons DW, Lin J, Barber TD, et al. The consensus coding sequences of human breast and colorectal cancers. Science. 2006;314(5797):268–74.

81. Parast MM, Otey CA. Characterization of palladin, a novel protein localized to stress fibers and cell adhesions. J Cell Biol. 2000;150(3):643–56.
82. Rachlin AS, Otey CA. Identification of palladin isoforms and characterization of an isoform-specific interaction between Lasp-1 and palladin. J Cell Sci. 2006;119(Pt 6):995–1004.
83. Alkatout I, Friemel J, Sitek B, Anlauf M, Eisenach PA, Stuhler K, et al. Novel prognostic markers revealed by a proteomic approach separating benign from malignant insulinomas. Mod Pathol. 2015;28(1):69–79.

Targeted Therapies for Neuroendocrine Neoplasms

Heloisa Prado Soares and Jonathan Strosberg

Introduction

Neuroendocrine tumors (NETs) are neoplasms that arise in the diffuse neuroendocrine system and are characterized by the ability to synthesize, store, and secrete a variety of neuroamines and peptides [11]. They commonly originate in the gastrointestinal tract and bronchopulmonary system. NETs comprise a spectrum of diseases ranging from well-differentiated, low-grade tumors to poorly differentiated, high-grade carcinomas. Significant progress in the understanding of their molecular biology has been made in recent years. While most targeted therapies in this field have been developed empirically, knowledge of genomic landscape [2, 16] and signaling pathways has led to better understanding of their mechanisms of action. In this chapter, we describe the current available targeted therapies for neuroendocrine tumors as well as drugs in development.

H.P. Soares, MD, PhD (✉)
Department of Gastrointestinal Oncology, H. Lee Moffitt Cancer Center and Research Institute, FOB 2nd Floor, 12902 Magnolia Ave, Tampa, FL 33612, USA

Oncologic Sciences, University of South Florida, Tampa, FL USA
e-mail: Heloisa.Soares@moffitt.org

J. Strosberg, MD
Department of Gastrointestinal Oncology, H. Lee Moffitt Cancer Center and Research Institute, FOB 2nd Floor, 12902 Magnolia Ave, Tampa, FL 33612, USA

Oncologic Sciences, University of South Florida, Tampa, FL USA

Neuroendocrine Program, Department of Gastrointestinal Oncology, H. Lee Moffitt Cancer Center and Research Institute, Tampa, FL USA
e-mail: Strosberg@moffitt.org

A. Nasir, D. Coppola (eds.), *Neuroendocrine Tumors: Review of Pathology, Molecular and Therapeutic Advances*, DOI 10.1007/978-1-4939-3426-3_28

Somatostatin Receptor Pathway

Somatostatin Analogs

Somatostatin was initially identified as an inhibitor of growth hormone and was subsequently found to perform numerous other inhibitory functions within the diffuse endocrine system including suppression of other hormones such as gastrin, cholecystokinin, and serotonin. The human hormone somatostatin has two bioactive forms consisting of 14 and 28 amino acids [31]. It interacts with somatostatin receptors which belong to a family of G-protein coupled receptors [23]. The vast majority of differentiated NETs (over 80 %) express somatostatin receptors on their cell surface, thereby representing an attractive target for medical therapy. Five types of somatostatin receptors (SST1, SST2, SST3, SST4, and SST5) have been identified in NET cells [8]. Octreotide and lanreotide are both somatostatin analogs (SSA) that share similar somatostatin receptor affinity profiles, binding avidly to SST2 and moderately to SST5 [25]. Both drugs have been used to treat hormonal symptoms associated with NETs for decades.

The first clinical trial of octreotide evaluated the drug in 25 patients with malignant carcinoid syndrome [20]. This study showed significant improvement of flushing and diarrhea as well as major 5-HIAA reductions in urine in roughly 80 % of patients, leading to the approval of octreotide by the Food and Drug Administration (FDA) for management of the carcinoid syndrome. A subsequent crossover trial comparing octreotide versus lanreotide in 33 patients with carcinoid syndrome demonstrated similar symptom control and biochemical responses between the two analogs [26]. Additional trials have also demonstrated that both SSAs can palliate hormonal syndromes associated with functioning pancreatic NETs, particularly VIPomas and glucagonomas [24].

In recent years, high-level evidence has emerged that SSAs can significantly inhibit growth of well-differentiated gastroenteropancreatic neuroendocrine tumors (GEP-NETs) [36]. The antiproliferative effect of SSAs can be divided into two categories: "direct" and "indirect". The direct effect involves interaction between SSAs and somatostatin receptors on tumor cells. Although the precise signaling transduction pathways are not fully understood, the initial steps appear to involve activation of phosphotyrosine phosphatases (PTPs) and modulation of the MAP-kinase pathway [30]. The indirect antiproliferative effect is mediated through suppression of circulating growth factors such as vascular-endothelial growth factor (VEGF) and insulin-like growth factor (IGF) [41].

The PROMID study [32] was a randomized phase III trial that compared octreotide LAR 30 mg versus placebo in 85 patients with advanced carcinoid tumors originating in the midgut. Time to tumor progression (TTP) increased from 6 months in the placebo arm to 14.3 months in the octreotide LAR arm ($p = 0.000072$). A subgroup analysis showed that patients with low tumor burden (<10 % hepatic involvement) and resected primary tumors benefitted most significantly from treatment with octreotide LAR. There was no significant difference in the adverse effects profiles of both arms. The results were seen with caution as some felt that the early termination of the study after an interim analysis could have overestimated the benefit of octreotide LAR. However, the CLARINET study [3] confirmed the antiproliferative effects of SSAs. This randomized phase III study compared depot-lanreotide 120 mg to placebo in 204 patients with hormonally nonfunctioning GEP-NETs. A 53 % improvement in progression free survival (PFS) was seen with lanreotide (hazard ratio 0.47, 95 % CI: 0.30–0.73; $p=0.0002$), meeting the trial's primary endpoint. The most common adverse effects associated with lanreotide were diarrhea, abdominal pain, and cholelithiasis. While both octreotide and lanreotide inhibit tumor growth in a clinically and statistically significant fashion, objective responses with both somatostatin analogs are exceptionally rare.

Pasireotide is a newer SSA that was developed with a particularly strong binding affinity to SST5, SST1, and SST3. It is still unclear whether this enhanced binding affinity results in improved clinical outcomes. While a phase II study of pasireotide in patients with refractory carcinoid syndrome demonstrated symptom improvement in 27 % of patients [21], a randomized phase III trial comparing pasireotide to octreotide LAR 40 mg in patients with poor symptom control showed no difference in palliation of flushing and diarrhea [42]. A phase II clinical trial of pasireotide in a heterogeneous population of treatment-naïve NET patients demonstrated a median PFS of 11 months [6]. Pasireotide is associated with a high rate of hyperglycemia due to binding of SST5. Its future development in NETs is uncertain.

Peptide Receptor Radionuclide Therapy

The use of radiolabeled somatostatin analogs is another promising option to target NETs that express high levels of somatostatin receptors. In addition to being used for diagnostic purposes, they can be used to deliver therapeutic radiation directly to tumor cells. Radiolabeled somatostatin analogs consist of three parts: a cyclic octapeptide, a chelator, and a radionuclide. Several variants of such conjugates have been developed, with indium-111 (^{111}In), yttrium-90 (^{90}Y), and lutetium-177 (^{177}Lu) being the most comprehensively evaluated [22].

The initial studies of Peptide Receptor Radionuclide Therapy (PRPT) used ^{111}In, but the characteristics of ^{111}In as a radionuclide were not optimal for the management of NETs. Currently, the most commonly used isotopes are ^{90}Y and ^{177}Lu, but no randomized trials have been performed comparing those two radionuclides. The reported radiographic response rates range from 4 to 47 %, with much of the heterogeneity in response rates likely relating to primary tumor site as well as line of therapy [22, 40]. Overall, PRRT is well tolerated, seems to significantly slow progression, and is associated with relatively few serious adverse events. Rates of renal insufficiency are low when prophylactic amino acids are infused. Long-term bone marrow toxicity, including myelodysplastic syndrome and acute leukemia, appears to occur in roughly 1 % of treated patients. Despite its common use in Europe in a quasi-investigational basis, PRRT has not been approved for use in the USA. The

NETTER-1 study is the first phase III multicentric, randomized, controlled, parallel-group study, comparing ^{177}Lu-DOTATATE with Octreotide LAR. In this study, treatment with PRRT plus best supportive care (30 mg Octreotide LAR) is compared to treatment with high dose (60 mg) Octreotide LAR in patients with inoperable and progressive somatostatin receptor positive midgut carcinoid tumors (ClinicalTrials.gov Identifier: NCT01578239). Results of the NETTER-1 will hopefully shed further light on the role of PRRT in the management of NETs.

mTOR Pathway

The mammalian target of rapamycin (mTOR) is a serine/threonine kinase that is currently the focus of intense interest because it integrates signals from growth factors, G protein-coupled receptor (GPCR) agonists, nutrients (amino acids and glucose), cellular energy levels (AMP/ATP ratio), and stress conditions to determine whether a cell proceeds to grow and divide [43]. Therefore it is a key module in the regulation of metabolism, migration, survival, autophagy, and growth [33].

Germline mutations of *TSC2*, an endogenous inhibitor of mTOR, are a risk factor for the development of pancreatic NETs. Somatic mutations in mTOR pathway genes, including *PTEN*, *PIK3CA*, and *TSC2* occur in roughly 15 % of pancreatic NETs [16]. Other alterations in mTOR pathway genes, including amplifications of *AKT1/2*, are observed in nearly one-third of small bowel carcinoid tumors [2].

Several inhibitors of mTOR have been developed and evaluated for the treatment of NETS, including the so-called rapalogs, temsirolimus and everolimus.

Everolimus

The oral mTOR inhibitor everolimus has been studied extensively in GEP-NETs. A phase II study, known as the RADIANT-1 trial, of 160 patients with pancreatic NETs investigated everolimus monotherapy ($N=115$) or everolimus plus octreotide ($N=45$) [46]. Response rates and median PFS were 9 % and 9.7 months with monotherapy versus 4 % and 16.7 months with combination therapy. A subsequent phase III study (RADIANT-2 trial) randomly assigned 429 patients with hormonally functional carcinoid tumors to treatment with everolimus 10 mg plus octreotide versus placebo plus octreotide. On central radiographic review, median PFS increased from 11.3 months on the placebo arm to 16.4 months on the everolimus arm (HR 0.77; $p=0.026$) [27]. While clinically significant, the primary endpoint fell short of its prespecified statistical significance threshold of $p<0.0246$. A potential explanation for the lack of statistical significance was the discrepancy between central versus local radiographic review. There was no trend towards improvement in overall survival in the everolimus arm, possibly due to the high rate of crossover to everolimus in the placebo arm.

Another phase III study (RADIANT-3 trial) randomly assigned 410 patients with low- and intermediate-grade pancreatic NETs to treatment with everolimus 10 mg versus placebo [48]. Concurrent SSA therapy was allowed. Despite an objective response rate of only 5 % in the everolimus arm, the study demonstrated a clinically and statistically significant improvement in PFS. Median PFS increased from 4.6 months on the placebo arm to 11 months on the everolimus arm (HR 0.35, $p<0.001$). Median overall survival was not reached and no statistically significant survival difference between the groups was observed; however, updated survival data has demonstrated a trend towards improvement with everolimus. Everolimus has since been approved by the FDA for treatment of patients with advanced pancreatic NETs.

To possibly expand the role of everolimus in NETs, the RADIANT-4 trial was designed to enroll patients with hormonally nonfunctioning carcinoid tumors. In this phase III study, 285 adults with histologically confirmed well-differentiated advanced NET of GI or lung origin, with no history of symptoms related to carcinoid syndrome were randomized to receive everolimus versus placebo with no crossover upon progression. Results are expected to be presented soon (ClinicalTrials.gov Identifier: NCT01524783). Also, multiple trials are ongoing to examine the use of everolimus in combination with various other agents. Examples of combinatory therapies under investigation include everolimus in addition to pasireotide, bevacizumab, erlotinib, cixutumumab, vatalanib, and several cytotoxic agents.

In general, side effects of everolimus include aphthous oral ulcers, rash, diarrhea, hyperglycemia, and cytopenias. Pneumonitis is a relatively rare but potentially serious toxicity that can be managed with dose reductions or interruptions and glucocorticoid therapy in symptomatic patients. Everolimus is an immunosuppressive drug, and atypical infections such as tuberculosis or aspergillosis are occasionally observed. While most toxicities are mild, chronic side effects may adversely impact patients' quality of life.

Temsirolimus

A phase II trial of temsirolimus in 37 patients with advanced NETs showed limited objective response as monotherapy [9]. Given the relatively modest activity of single-agent mTOR inhibitors in NETs, there is interest in developing novel combinatory treatment strategies. Hobday et al. [14] published results from a multicenter trial of temsirolimus and bevacizumab in 56 patients with progressive pancreatic NETs. Response rate (RR) was 41 % (23 of 56 patients) and median PFS was 13.2 months (95 % CI, 11.2–16.6). Median overall survival was 34 months (95 % CI, 27.1 to not reached). The most common grade 3 to 4 adverse events attributed to therapy were hypertension (21 %), fatigue (16 %), lymphopenia (14 %), and hyperglycemia (14 %). This study suggested that the combination of temsirolimus and bevacizumab had substantial activity and reasonable tolerability.

VEGF Pathway

Neuroendocrine tumors are highly vascular and frequently express the vascular-endothelial growth factor (VEGF) ligand and receptor (VEGFR) [34, 38, 47]. Increased levels of circulating VEGF have been associated with tumor progression. Consequently, inhibition of the VEGF pathway has been identified as a therapeutic strategy. The VEGF pathway can be targeted by circulating VEGF inhibitors such as bevacizumab or with the use of multitargeted tyrosine kinase inhibitors against VEGFR, including sunitinib, pazopanib, and sorafenib.

Bevacizumab

Bevacizumab is a humanized monoclonal antibody that binds to circulating VEGF-A. In a randomized phase II trial, 44 patients with metastatic carcinoid tumors were randomly assigned to treatment with bevacizumab or pegylated interferon (PEG-IFN) for 18 weeks, followed by both agents in combination [47]. At the week 18 time point, the rate of PFS was 95 % on the bevacizumab arm versus 68 % on the PEG-IFN arm. On functional CT scans performed at baseline and on day 2 of therapy, bevacizumab treatment caused average reductions in tumor blood flow of 49 %. Despite this promising phase II data, a randomized phase III trial sponsored by the Southwest Oncology Group (SWOG) failed to show a significant difference in PFS comparing bevacizumab to IFN-alpha in carcinoid tumor patients with high risk prognostic features. In this study of 427 patients, median PFS was 16.6 months in the bevacizumab arm and 15.4 months with the IFN arm ($p=0.55$) [44].

Combinations of bevacizumab and other agents are also under investigation, with several phase II trials reporting promising data. In one study, the combination of bevacizumab plus temozolomide was shown to be effective in patients with advanced NET, particularly in the subgroup of pancreatic NETs [5]. In a small phase II study of 31 evaluable patients, a combined regimen of bevacizumab plus capecitabine and oxaliplatin resulted in PR in 23 % and SD in 71 % [19]. Of particular note, 6 of 7 patients with pancreatic NET had PR. Overall, the 1-year PFS with this treatment combination was 52 % and median PFS was 13.7 months. The combination of bevacizumab and FOLFOX (oxaliplatin, 5-fluorouracil, and leucovorin) has also been evaluated in a small study of patients with NET [39]. Two of 6 patients with pancreatic NET had PR compared with 1 of 5 patients with small-bowel (carcinoid) NET, whereas SD was observed in the majority of patients regardless of primary site. A bevacizumab/everolimus combination has also demonstrated promising early results. In a small, randomized run-in study of 39 patients with low- to intermediate-grade NET, 26 % experienced PR and 67 % had SD [45].

A randomized phase II study of everolimus plus bevacizumab versus everolimus monotherapy demonstrated improvement response rates in the combination group (31 % versus 12 %) and PFS (16.7 months versus 14.0 months; $p=0.12$) [17].

Sunitinib

Sunitinib is a tyrosine kinase inhibitor (TKI) that targets VEGFR1, -2, and -3, as well as platelet-derived growth factor receptor (PDGFR). This drug showed promising results in a subgroup of patients with pancreatic NETs in a phase II trial [18]. Therefore, a multinational randomized phase III trial comparing sunitinib 37.5 mg/day versus placebo in 171 patients with low- and intermediate-grade pancreatic NETs was conducted. There was a statistically significant improvement in median PFS from 5.5 months on the placebo arm to 11.1 months on the sunitinib arm ($p<0.001$) [29]. A trend towards improvement in overall survival was also noted but was not statistically significant. The objective response rate associated with sunitinib was 9.3 %. Side effects of sunitinib included nausea, diarrhea, fatigue, cytopenias, palmar-plantar erythrodysesthesia, and hypertension. Based on the results of this study, sunitinib is FDA approved for treatment of pancreatic NETs.

Sorafenib

Sorafenib is a small-molecule TKI that inhibits both intracellular and cell surface kinases (BRAF, CRAF, KIT, FLT-3, RET, VEGFR1, VEGFR2, VEGFR3, and PDGFRβ) [10]. This drug, which was initially approved by the FDA in the USA for the treatment of renal cell carcinoma, has shown modest activity as single agent for the treatment of metastatic NETs [15]. The combination of sorafenib with bevacizumab was also tested [4]. Although it showed some clinical activity in patients with advanced NETs, the combination was associated with an unfavorable safety profile [4].

Other Inhibitors of VEGFR

Other VEGFR targeting TKIs, including pazopanib and axitinib, are being investigated in clinical trials of GEP-NET patients. A phase II study that included 70 patients with advanced pancreatic NETs and carcinoid tumors evaluated the efficacy of pazopanib with octreotide LAR. No responses were seen in patients with carcinoid tumors and 21 % of pancreatic NETs patients achieved an objective response [28]. Another phase II trial showed clinical activity of pazopanib as a single agent in advanced NETs regardless of previous treatments [12]. Currently, a randomized phase II study is investigating pazopanib versus placebo in patients with advanced, progressive carcinoid tumors.

Additional Pathways

Epidermal growth factor receptor (EGFR), a transmembrane tyrosine kinase receptor, is activated when a ligand (EGF or related factors) binds to its extracellular domain. Activation of EGFR leads to downstream activation of three major signaling pathways including the Ras/Raf/MEK/ERK and the PI3K-Akt pathways [1]. Despite showing activity in NET cell lines [35], the use of EGFR inhibitors (gefitinib) did not result in significant clinical activity [13]. Preclinical data suggest that concomitant inhibition of two nonredundant amplified pathways (mTOR and EGFR) could reverse potential drug resistance and lead to tumor growth inhibition. Therefore, the efficacy of erlotinib, another EGFR inhibitor, is currently being assessed in a phase II study to evaluate the safety and efficacy of everolimus plus erlotinib in patients with well- to moderately-differentiated neuroendocrine tumors (ClinicalTrials.gov Identifier: NCT00843531).

It has been showed that IGF-1 receptor (IGF-1R) is overexpressed in NETs making it another attractive target for therapy. Preclinical data suggest multiple roles for the IGF-1R in NETs, including mediation of resistance to mTOR inhibitors. Cixutumumab, a monoclonal antibody (MAB) against IGF-1R, was tested in combination with everolimus and octreotide in patients with well-differentiated NET, but results have been disappointing [7]. Ganitumab, another human MAB against IGF-1R, was tested in metastatic low- and intermediate-grade carcinoids or pNETs. Although well tolerated, treatment with single-agent ganitumab failed to result in significant tumor responses among patients with metastatic well-differentiated carcinoid or pancreatic NET [37]. Histone deacetylase inhibitors, proteasome inhibitors, and c-Kit and PDGFR inhibitors have been also tested.

Conclusions

Somatostatin analogs continue to represent the primary first-line treatment for most well-differentiated metastatic NETs due to their antisecretory and antiproliferative activity combined with a tolerable side effect profile. In recent years, new targeted therapies, including mTOR inhibitors and VEGF inhibitors, have been approved for treatment of pancreatic NETs. Their scope may also expand to treatment of advanced carcinoid tumors based on results of recent clinical trials, including the RADIANT-4 study. Radiolabeled somatostatin analogs may also be approved for somatostatin-receptor-expressing tumors' pending results of the NETTER study. Appropriate selection and sequencing of therapies will be the focus of future trials.

References

1. Arteaga CL, Engelman JA. ERBB receptors: from oncogene discovery to basic science to mechanism-based cancer therapeutics. Cancer Cell. 2014;25(3):282–303. doi:10.1016/j.ccr.2014.02.025.
2. Banck MS, Kanwar R, Kulkarni AA, Boora GK, Metge F, Kipp BR, Zhang L, Thorland EC, Minn KT, Tentu R, Eckloff BW, Wieben ED, Wu Y, Cunningham JM, Nagorney DM, Gilbert JA, Ames MM, Beutler AS. The genomic landscape of small intestine neuroendocrine tumors. J Clin Invest. 2013;123(6):2502–8. doi:10.1172/JCI67963. 67963 [pii].
3. Caplin M. Phase III trial results favour lanreotide therapy. In: Patients with gastroenteropancreatic neuro-endocrine tumours. Amsterdam: European Society of Medical Oncology (ESMO); 2013.
4. Castellano D, Capdevila J, Sastre J, Alonso V, Llanos M, Garcia-Carbonero R, Manzano Mozo JL, Sevilla I, Duran I, Salazar R. Sorafenib and bevacizumab combination targeted therapy in advanced neuroendocrine tumour: a phase II study of Spanish Neuroendocrine Tumour Group (GETNE0801). Eur J Cancer. 2013;49(18):3780–7. doi:10.1016/j.ejca.2013.06.042.
5. Chan JA, Stuart K, Earle CC, Clark JW, Bhargava P, Miksad R, Blaszkowsky L, Enzinger PC, Meyerhardt JA, Zheng H, Fuchs CS, Kulke MH. Prospective study of bevacizumab plus temozolomide in patients with advanced neuroendocrine tumors. J Clin Oncol Off J Am Soc Clin Oncol. 2012;30(24):2963–8. doi:JCO.2011.40.3147 [pii] 10.1200/JCO.2011.40.3147.
6. Cives M, Kunz PL, Morse B, Coppola D, Schell MJ, Campos T, Nguyen PT, Nandoskar P, Khandelwal V, Strosberg JR. Phase II clinical trial of pasireotide long-acting repeatable in patients with metastatic neuroendocrine tumors. Endocr Relat Cancer. 2015;22(1):1–9. doi:10.1530/ERC-14-0360.
7. Dasari A, Phan A, Gupta S, Rashid A, Yeung SC, Hess K, Chen H, Tarco E, Chen H, Wei C, Anh-Do K, Halperin D, Meric-Bernstam F, Yao J. Phase I study of the anti-IGF1R antibody cixutumumab with everolimus and octreotide in advanced well-differentiated neuroendocrine tumors. Endocr Relat Cancer. 2015;22(3):431–41. doi:10.1530/ERC-15-0002.
8. de Herder WW, Hofland LJ, van der Lely AJ, Lamberts SW. Somatostatin receptors in gastroentero-pancreatic neuroendocrine tumours. Endocr Relat Cancer. 2003;10(4):451–8.
9. Duran I, Kortmansky J, Singh D, Hirte H, Kocha W, Goss G, Le L, Oza A, Nicklee T, Ho J, Birle D, Pond GR, Arboine D, Dancey J, Aviel-Ronen S, Tsao MS, Hedley D, Siu LL. A phase II clinical and pharmacodynamic study of temsirolimus in advanced neuroendocrine carcinomas. Br J Cancer. 2006;95(9):1148–54. doi:6603419 [pii] 10.1038/sj.bjc.6603419.
10. Eads JR, Meropol NJ. A new era for the systemic therapy of neuroendocrine tumors. Oncologist. 2012;17(3):326–38. doi:10.1634/theoncologist.2011-0356.
11. Feyrter F. Über diffuse endocrine epitheliale Organe. Leipzig: Barth; 1938.
12. Grande E, Capdevila J, Castellano D, Teule A, Duran I, Fuster J, Sevilla I, Escudero P, Sastre J, Garcia-Donas J, Casanovas O, Earl J, Ortega L, Apellaniz-Ruiz M, Rodriguez-Antona C, Alonso-Gordoa T, Diez JJ, Carrato A, Garcia-Carbonero R. Pazopanib in pretreated advanced neuroendocrine tumors: a phase II, open-label trial of the Spanish Task Force Group for Neuroendocrine Tumors (GETNE) dagger. Ann Oncol Off J Eur Soc Med Oncol. 2015. doi:10.1093/annonc/mdv252.
13. Hobday TJ, Holen K, Donehower R, Camoriano J, Kim G, Picus J, Philip P, Lloyd R, Mahoney M, Erlichman E. A phase II trial of gefitinib in patients (pts) with progressive metastatic neuroendocrine

tumors (NET): a phase II consortium (P2C) study. J Clin Oncol Off J Am Soc Clin Oncol. 2006;24(18):Suppl 4043.
14. Hobday TJ, Qin R, Reidy-Lagunes D, Moore MJ, Strosberg J, Kaubisch A, Shah M, Kindler HL, Lenz HJ, Chen H, Erlichman C. Multicenter phase II trial of temsirolimus and bevacizumab in pancreatic neuroendocrine tumors. J Clin Oncol Off J Am Soc Clin Oncol. 2015;33(14):1551–6. doi:10.1200/JCO.2014.56.2082.
15. Hobday TJ, Rubin J, Holen K, Picus J, Donehower R, Marschke R, Maples W, Lloyd R, Mahoney M, Erlichman C. MC044h, a phase II trial of sorafenib in patients (pts) with metastatic neuroendocrine tumors (NET): a phase II consortium (P2C) study. J Clin Oncol Off J Am Soc Clin Oncol. 2007;25(18):Suppl 4504.
16. Jiao Y, Shi C, Edil BH, de Wilde RF, Klimstra DS, Maitra A, Schulick RD, Tang LH, Wolfgang CL, Choti MA, Velculescu VE, Diaz Jr LA, Vogelstein B, Kinzler KW, Hruban RH, Papadopoulos N. DAXX/ATRX, MEN1, and mTOR pathway genes are frequently altered in pancreatic neuroendocrine tumors. Science. 2011;331(6021):1199–203. doi:science.1200609 [pii] 10.1126/science.1200609.
17. Kulke M, Niedzwiecki D, Foster N, Briant Fruth B, Kunz P, Kennecke H, Wolin E, Venook A. Randomized phase II study of everolimus (E) versus everolimus plus bevacizumab (E+B) in patients (Pts) with locally advanced or metastatic pancreatic neuroendocrine tumors (pNET), CALGB 80701 (Alliance). J Clin Oncol Off J Am Soc Clin Oncol. 2015;33:Suppl; abstr 4005.
18. Kulke MH, Lenz HJ, Meropol NJ, Posey J, Ryan DP, Picus J, Bergsland E, Stuart K, Tye L, Huang X, Li JZ, Baum CM, Fuchs CS. Activity of sunitinib in patients with advanced neuroendocrine tumors. J Clin Oncol Off J Am Soc Clin Oncol. 2008;26(20):3403–10. doi:26/20/3403 [pii] 10.1200/JCO.2007.15.9020.
19. Kunz PL, Kuo T, Zhan JM, Kaiser HL, Norton JA, Visser BC, Longacre TA, Ford M, Balise RR, Fisher GA. A phase II study of capecitabine, oxaliplatin, and bevacizumab for metastatic or unresectable neuroendocrine tumors. J Clin Oncol. 2010;28:15s Suppl; abstr 4104.
20. Kvols LK, Moertel CG, O'Connell MJ, Schutt AJ, Rubin J, Hahn RG. Treatment of the malignant carcinoid syndrome. Evaluation of a long-acting somatostatin analogue. N Engl J Med. 1986;315(11):663–6.
21. Kvols LK, Oberg KE, O'Dorisio TM, Mohideen P, de Herder WW, Arnold R, Hu K, Zhang Y, Hughes G, Anthony L, Wiedenmann B. Pasireotide (SOM230) shows efficacy and tolerability in the treatment of patients with advanced neuroendocrine tumors refractory or resistant to octreotide LAR: results from a phase II study. Endocr Relat Cancer. 2012;19(5):657–66. doi:10.1530/ERC-11-0367.
22. Kwekkeboom DJ, de Herder WW, Krenning EP. Somatostatin receptor-targeted radionuclide therapy in patients with gastroenteropancreatic neuroendocrine tumors. Endocrinol Metab Clin North Am. 2011;40(1):173–85, ix. doi:10.1016/j.ecl.2010.12.003.
23. Lamberts SW, van der Lely AJ, de Herder WW, Hofland LJ. Octreotide. N Engl J Med. 1996;334(4):246–54.
24. Maton PN. Use of octreotide acetate for control of symptoms in patients with islet cell tumors. World J Surg. 1993;17(4):504–10.
25. Maurer R, Reubi JC. Somatostatin receptors. JAMA. 1985;253(18):2741.
26. O'Toole D, Ducreux M, Bommelaer G, Wemeau JL, Bouche O, Catus F, Blumberg J, Ruszniewski P. Treatment of carcinoid syndrome: a prospective crossover evaluation of lanreotide versus octreotide in terms of efficacy, patient acceptability, and tolerance. Cancer. 2000;88(4):770–6.10.1002/(SICI)1097-0142(20000215)88:4<770::AID-CNCR6>3.0.CO;2-0 [pii].
27. Pavel ME, Hainsworth JD, Baudin E, Peeters M, Horsch D, Winkler RE, Klimovsky J, Lebwohl D, Jehl V, Wolin EM, Oberg K, Van Cutsem E, Yao JC. Everolimus plus octreotide long-acting repeatable for the treatment of advanced neuroendocrine tumours associated with carcinoid syndrome (RADIANT-2): a randomised, placebo-controlled, phase 3 study. Lancet. 2011;378(9808):2005–12. doi:S0140-6736(11)61742-X [pii] 10.1016/S0140-6736(11)61742-X.

28. Phan AT, Halperin DM, Chan JA, Fogelman DR, Hess KR, Malinowski P, Regan E, Ng CS, Yao JC, Kulke MH. Pazopanib and depot octreotide in advanced, well-differentiated neuroendocrine tumours: a multicentre, single-group, phase 2 study. Lancet Oncol. 2015;16(6):695–703. doi:10.1016/S1470-2045(15)70136-1.
29. Raymond E, Dahan L, Raoul JL, Bang YJ, Borbath I, Lombard-Bohas C, Valle J, Metrakos P, Smith D, Vinik A, Chen JS, Horsch D, Hammel P, Wiedenmann B, Van Cutsem E, Patyna S, Lu DR, Blanckmeister C, Chao R, Ruszniewski P. Sunitinib malate for the treatment of pancreatic neuroendocrine tumors. N Engl J Med. 2011;364(6):501–13. doi:10.1056/NEJMoa1003825.
30. Reardon DB, Dent P, Wood SL, Kong T, Sturgill TW. Activation in vitro of somatostatin receptor subtypes 2, 3, or 4 stimulates protein tyrosine phosphatase activity in membranes from transfected Ras-transformed NIH 3T3 cells: coexpression with catalytically inactive SHP-2 blocks responsiveness. Mol Endocrinol. 1997;11(8):1062–9.
31. Reichlin S. Somatostatin. N Engl J Med. 1983;309(24):1495–501.
32. Rinke A, Muller HH, Schade-Brittinger C, Klose KJ, Barth P, Wied M, Mayer C, Aminossadati B, Pape UF, Blaker M, Harder J, Arnold C, Gress T, Arnold R. Placebo-controlled, double-blind, prospective, randomized study on the effect of octreotide LAR in the control of tumor growth in patients with metastatic neuroendocrine midgut tumors: a report from the PROMID Study Group. J Clin Oncol Off J Am Soc Clin Oncol. 2009;27(28):4656–63.
33. Shimobayashi M, Hall MN. Making new contacts: the mTOR network in metabolism and signalling crosstalk. Nat Rev Mol Cell Biol. 2014;15(3):155–62. doi:10.1038/nrm3757.
34. Silva SR, Bowen KA, Rychahou PG, Jackson LN, Weiss HL, Lee EY, Townsend Jr CM, Evers BM. VEGFR-2 expression in carcinoid cancer cells and its role in tumor growth and metastasis. Int J Cancer. 2011;128(5):1045–56. doi:10.1002/ijc.25441.
35. Stilling GA, Zhang H, Ruebel KH, Leontovich AA, Jin L, Tanizaki Y, Zhang S, Erickson LA, Hobday T, Lloyd RV. Characterization of the functional and growth properties of cell lines established from ileal and rectal carcinoid tumors. Endocr Pathol. 2007;18(4):223–32. doi:10.1007/s12022-007-9001-3.
36. Strosberg J, Kvols L. Antiproliferative effect of somatostatin analogs in gastroenteropancreatic neuroendocrine tumors. World J Gastroenterol. 2010;16(24):2963–70.
37. Strosberg JR, Chan JA, Ryan DP, Meyerhardt JA, Fuchs CS, Abrams T, Regan E, Brady R, Weber J, Campos T, Kvols LK, Kulke MH. A multi-institutional, phase II open-label study of ganitumab (AMG 479) in advanced carcinoid and pancreatic neuroendocrine tumors. Endocr Relat Cancer. 2013;20(3):383–90. doi:10.1530/ERC-12-0390.
38. Terris B, Scoazec JY, Rubbia L, Bregeaud L, Pepper MS, Ruszniewski P, Belghiti J, Flejou J, Degott C. Expression of vascular endothelial growth factor in digestive neuroendocrine tumours. Histopathology. 1998;32(2):133–8.
39. Venook AP, Ko AH, Tempero MA, Uy J, Weber T, Korn M, EK B. Phase II trial of FOLFOX plus bevacizumab in advanced, progressive neuroendocrine tumors. J Clin Oncol. 2008;26: 15_Suppl 15545, 26(15):Suppl 15545.
40. Vinjamuri S, Gilbert TM, Banks M, McKane G, Maltby P, Poston G, Weissman H, Palmer DH, Vora J, Pritchard DM, Cuthbertson DJ. Peptide receptor radionuclide therapy with (90) Y-DOTATATE/(90)Y-DOTATOC in patients with progressive metastatic neuroendocrine tumours: assessment of response, survival and toxicity. Br J Cancer. 2013;108(7):1440–8. doi:10.1038/bjc.2013.103.
41. Weckbecker G, Lewis I, Albert R, Schmid HA, Hoyer D, Bruns C. Opportunities in somatostatin research: biological, chemical and therapeutic aspects. Nat Rev Drug Discov. 2003;2(12):999–1017.
42. Wolin E, Jarzab B, Eriksson B, Walter T, Toumpanakis C, Morse M, Tomassetti P, Weber M, Fogelman D, Ramage J, Poon D, Huang J, Hudson M, Zhi X, Pasieka JL, Mahamat A, Swahn F, Newell-Price J, Mansoor W, Oberg K. A multicenter, randomized, blinded, phase III study of pasireotide LAR versus octreotide LAR in patients with metastatic neuroendocrine tumors with disease-related symptoms inadequately controlled by somatostatin analogs. J Clin Oncol Off J Am Soc Clin Oncol. 2013;(31):Suppl;abstr 4031.

43. Wullschleger S, Loewith R, Hall MN. TOR signaling in growth and metabolism. Cell. 2006;124(3):471–84.
44. Yao J, Guthrie K, Moran C, Strosberg J, Kulke M, Chan J, LoConte N, McWilliams R, Wolin E, Mattar B, McDonough S, Chen H, Blanke C, Hochster H. SWOG S0518: phase III prospective randomized comparison of depot octreotide plus interferon alpha-2b versus depot octreotide plus bevacizumab (NSC #704865) in advanced, poor prognosis carcinoid patients (NCT00569127). J Clin Oncol Off J Am Soc Clin Oncol. 2015;33:Suppl;abstr 4004.
45. Yao J, Phan A, Fogelman D, Ng C, Jacobs C, Dagohoy C, Leary C, Hess K. Randomized run-in study of bevacizumab and everolimus in low- to intermediate-grade neuroendocrine tumors (LGNETs) using perfusion CT as functional biomarker. J Clin Oncol Off J Am Soc Clin Oncol. 2010;28(15):Suppl 4002.
46. Yao JC, Lombard-Bohas C, Baudin E, Kvols LK, Rougier P, Ruszniewski P, Hoosen S, St Peter J, Haas T, Lebwohl D, Van Cutsem E, Kulke MH, Hobday TJ, O'Dorisio TM, Shah MH, Cadiot G, Luppi G, Posey JA, Wiedenmann B. Daily oral everolimus activity in patients with metastatic pancreatic neuroendocrine tumors after failure of cytotoxic chemotherapy: a phase II trial. J Clin Oncol Off J Am Soc Clin Oncol. 2010;28(1):69–76. doi:JCO.2009.24.2669 [pii] 10.1200/JCO.2009.24.2669.
47. Yao JC, Phan A, Hoff PM, Chen HX, Charnsangavej C, Yeung SC, Hess K, Ng C, Abbruzzese JL, Ajani JA. Targeting vascular endothelial growth factor in advanced carcinoid tumor: a random assignment phase II study of depot octreotide with bevacizumab and pegylated interferon alpha-2b. J Clin Oncol Off J Am Soc Clin Oncol. 2008;26(8):1316–23.
48. Yao JC, Shah MH, Ito T, Bohas CL, Wolin EM, Van Cutsem E, Hobday TJ, Okusaka T, Capdevila J, de Vries EG, Tomassetti P, Pavel ME, Hoosen S, Haas T, Lincy J, Lebwohl D, Oberg K. Everolimus for advanced pancreatic neuroendocrine tumors. N Engl J Med. 2011;364(6):514–23. doi:10.1056/NEJMoa1009290.

Future Prospects in Neuroendocrine Tumor Pathology

Aejaz Nasir and Domenico Coppola

Because of the lower incidence of neuroendocrine neoplasms, limited experience at most institutions in diagnosing and treating such patients, and lack of uniformly agreed diagnostic and treatment guidelines, the science of Neuroendocrine Tumor Pathology has gradually matured to its current state in recent years. With the unprecedented progress in molecular discoveries, rapid advancements in modern technology, and prioritization of personalized approaches in the diagnosis and treatment of human cancer, the years ahead are among the most exciting time in this field, during which we are going to see not only more uniform diagnostic standards in this field but also some of the most remarkable achievements in targeted therapeutic approaches for patients with these unusual malignancies.

Heterogeneity of these uncommon neoplasms, lack of internationally agreed nomenclature and classification schemes, rather unique association between tumor histology, grades and clinical course, diversity of histologic hallmarks, levels of differentiation, anatomic sites of origin, and hormone secretion are some of the key factors that make diagnosis and treatment of these neoplasms particularly challenging for general pathologists and clinicians. Even in the developed world, uniform practice of higher standards of pathologic diagnosis and treatment is mostly limited to the major tertiary care referral centers (centers of excellence), where large multidisciplinary teams work in a well-coordinated manner to offer these patients the highest standards of clinical care. At H. Lee Moffitt Cancer Center, Neuroendocrine Tumor Pathology has been part of a large multidisciplinary team effort for many years led by

A. Nasir, MD, MPhil, FCAP (✉)
Diagnostic & Experimental Pathology (Tailored Therapeutics),
Lilly Research laboratories, Eli Lilly & Co.,
893 South Delaware St., Indianapolis, IN, USA
e-mail: nasirae@lilly.com

D. Coppola, MD
Department of Anatomic Pathology,
H. Lee Moffitt Cancer Center, Tampa, FL, USA

A. Nasir, D. Coppola (eds.), *Neuroendocrine Tumors: Review of Pathology, Molecular and Therapeutic Advances*, DOI 10.1007/978-1-4939-3426-3_29

a world leader and oncologist, Professor Larry Kvols. His pioneer work and close collaborations with many of the other world leaders from Mayo Clinic, Yale University, Dana-Farber Cancer Institute, Memorial Sloan-Kettering and MD Anderson Cancer Centers, Universities of Berlin and Uppsala, and other global centers of excellence have moved this field to its current level of scientific and clinical advancement.

Such remarkable progress is now evident in the form comprehensive diagnostic and clinical guidelines that have been put forward by the North American and European Neuroendocrine Tumor Societies (NANETS, ENETS), World Health Organization, and other agencies in recent years. These important developments will serve as a landmark in future advancement of the field of Neuroendocrine Oncology and will set the new directions for higher standards and uniformity in diagnostic services and clinical care of these patients across the globe. In addition, in the years to follow, we will be able to pool scientific and clinical data sets together to identify newer and more valuable insights to drive the field toward more advanced implementation of personalized oncology in order to maximize benefit to these patients.

Some of the key areas in which we, the pathologists who are actively engaged with our clinical oncology colleagues in multidisciplinary care of neuroendocrine tumor patients, will see significant progress will be as follows:

More Unified Classification, Grading, and Reporting Schemes for NETs

In the past, variations in classification systems have interfered with clinical trial design, epidemiologic studies, and patient care. More recently, WHO has published revised histologic classifications of neuroendocrine neoplasms of the GI system [1] and lung [2] with clinical, histopathologic, and molecular genetic features. It is hoped that with the availability of such advanced references, pathologists will be more consistent in their experience with these otherwise not-so-common malignancies.

While low-grade NETs follow a relatively indolent course, high-grade NETs (NECs) are highly aggressive malignancies. It is important for diagnostic pathologists to adopt consistent means of assessment of NET cell proliferation index, based on the number of mitoses per 10 HPFs or the percentage of Ki67-positive tumor cells. Furthermore, since management of high-grade NECs is different from that of low- and intermediate-grade NETs, diagnostic pathologists need to implement a unified NET pathology reporting system, including an accurate and reproducible assessment of histologic grade. Although several systems of NET nomenclature, grading, and staging have been proposed, none has achieved universal acceptance. To help define the underlying common features of these classification systems and to identify the minimal pathology data that should be reported to ensure consistent clinical management and reproducibility of data from clinical trials, a multidisciplinary team of physicians interested in NETs was successful in putting forward a consensus statement on minimal data to be included in the NET pathology reports [3]. Agreement was reached about the importance of tumor grading, the staging landmarks, the prognostic factors assessable by routine histology, the potential for tumors to metastasize, and the current status of advanced immunohistochemical and molecular testing for treatment-related biomarkers. The lack of utility of a variety of immunohistochemical stains and pathologic findings was also agreed upon. A consensus could not be reached on many areas, including the extent of disease assessment, terminology, routine immunohistochemical staining for general neuroendocrine markers, use of Ki67 staining to assess proliferation, and the relationship of tumor grade to degree of differentiation. Although experts could not agree on a specific classification system, agreement was reached on the fundamental pathology data that should be reported [3]. In order to achieve standardization in pathologic assessment and reporting of NETs, we are in support of implementation of such a unified NET pathology reporting system. Of course, any such reporting guidelines will need to be modifiable, based on the local institutional pathology and clinical oncology expertise in the NET specialty centers, where large populations of NET patients are diagnosed and managed in multidisciplinary setting. Such a unified NET pathology reporting approach will not only encourage more uniform reporting among pathologists in various parts of the world, it will also provide neuroendocrine oncologists with the required pathology-related data elements that can be utilized in their clinical patient management decisions.

Newer Schemes for NET Staging

Another important advance in recent years is the addition of NET staging to the *seventh* edition of the AJCC Cancer Staging Handbook [4]. The TNM staging for NETs of the GI tract and pancreas was proposed in line with the respective adenocarcinomas. Several studies [5–8] have evaluated the prognostic validity of these new NET staging systems with mixed results. There is, therefore, an obvious need for uniform application and evaluation of clinical utility of these staging systems in NET patient management in the era of personalized oncology.

Future Applications of Immunohistochemistry in NET Pathology

With the current and future progress in precision medicine, as we move forward more with the personalized diagnostic approaches and treatment options for NET patients, in diagnostic NET pathology practice, neuroendocrine markers, tissue-specific transcription factors (TTF1, CDX2), and other immunohistochemical markers will need to be used more effectively by incorporating their use in the overall patient management plan. This will create more valuable contributions by pathologists in recognizing neuroendocrine differentiation in human cancer tissues, to identify sites of occult primary NETs in case of metastatic neuroendocrine carcinomas (NEC) with unknown primaries, and to validate and assess newer molecular biomarkers of prognostic or therapeutic relevance, which will make substantial contributions to advance the field of personalized oncology for NET patients.

Molecular Characterization of NETs

About 15–20 % of NETs are part of *inherited genetic syndromes* (MEN1, MEN2, vHL, NF1 and TSC). Sporadic P*NETs* show frequent mutations in *MEN1*, *DAXX/ATRX*, and mTOR pathway genes [9]. While recurrent somatic mutations and deletions in *CDKN1B gene were found in small intestinal NETs* [10], in other analyses, small intestinal NETs were found to be mutationally quiescent [11]. In addition, several recurrent somatic copy number alterations (CNAs) have been discovered in cancer-related pathways, including PI3K/Akt/mTOR, tumor growth factors (SMAD genes), and SRC. *Independent large-scale validation of these preliminary findings is warranted* to further determine their value as prognostic or predictive biomarkers in NETs.

Molecular Diagnostics for NETs

With increasing recognition of the differences in biology and clinical course of pancreatic, thoracic, and gastrointestinal NETs, advanced imaging and molecular diagnostics will play progressively important roles in the classification of NETs. Initial proof-of-concept studies using comparative genomic hybridization (CGH) and single-nucleotide polymorphism (SNP) analyses have shown distinct patterns of allelic alternations in pancreatic and ileal NETs. More frequent allelic imbalances in WD-NETs were losses of chromosomes 18, 21 or 21q, 13 or 13q, and 16 or 16q and amplification of chromosome 20 or 20p; chromosomal aberrations were much less common in WD-NETs from lung and GI tract compared to PETs [12]. Also, the observed genetic alterations differed significantly with the anatomical subsite of the NET: allelic loss of chromosome 18 was far more frequent in ileal carcinoids compared to non-ileal carcinoids and PNETs [13].

Origin of NETs and Management Decisions

Although traditionally NETs have been classified based on embryologic origin (foregut, midgut, hindgut), anatomic location (lung, pancreas, GI tract), and their secreted products (insulin, glucagon, gastrin, vasoactive intestinal peptide [VIP], somatostatin [SST]), the *anatomic site of origin (pancreatic vs. non-pancreatic) is now being recognized as a key determinant of therapeutic decisions because of important differences in NET biology and clinical course at these sites.* Some NETs actively secrete hormones resulting in well-recognized clinical syndromes and are called functional, e.g., insulinomas, VIPomas, etc. *To be of value in patient management, pathologists need to work up NET cases to be able to render both histopathologic and clinical classification in each case.*

Prospects for Treatment of NET Patients

With current refinements in our understanding of diverse biology and clinical course of NETs/NECs, it is becoming obvious that NETs need to be separated into pancreatic and non-pancreatic NETs for the purposes of enrollment in clinical trials and treatment in the clinic. Until recently, there were only a few therapeutic options for oncologic control of low- and intermediate-grade NETs. The PROMID study showed that octreotide long-acting repeatable (octreotide-LAR) formulation can delay tumor growth in midgut NETs. Some recent phase III studies have shown improved progression-free survival with everolimus and sunitinib in patients with pancreatic NETs, validating the PI3K/Akt/mTOR pathway and angiogenesis as important "druggable" therapeutic targets. Other targeted approaches are under active investigation and will bring forward additional targeted therapeutic options for NET patients in the coming years.

Personalized Therapies for NET Patients: Future is Here....

NETs are heterogeneous in their biologic behavior and aggressiveness. This characteristic, along with the recent emergence of multiple active therapies, has led to considerable interest in predictive and prognostic biomarkers that may allow us to tailor therapies for specific subpopulations of NET patients. In addition to the known prognostic value of tumor grade, recent studies have also confirmed the prognostic value of plasma levels of CGA and neuron-specific enolase (NSE). In a multinational study with central radiology review, patients with baseline-elevated CGA or NSE had significantly shorter PFS and overall survival [14]. Also, early CGA or NSE response was linked to favorable therapeutic benefit [14, 15]. If these findings are validated in subsequent studies, biomarkers could be used to select patients for therapy versus active surveillance among newly diagnosed patients with significant tumor burden and to guide frequency of monitoring among patients on active therapy.

Emerging data suggest that high methylguanine-methyltransferase (MGMT) expression is associated with therapeutic resistance to temozolomide [16, 17]. If confirmed in future prospective studies, low MGMT expression could help select patients for treatment. Predictive biomarkers of therapeutic benefits for mTOR and VEGF inhibitors remain to be identified and validated. Multiple somatic mutations in the mTOR pathway, however, have been identified [9]. Expression levels of PTEN and TSC2 have also recently been linked to outcome [18]. These findings suggest that future studies evaluating the mTOR pathway may reveal predictive markers of benefit. Confirmation of the above findings in prospective studies will facilitate more personalized approaches to treatment of NETs.

In conclusion, the future of Neuroendocrine Tumor Pathology is brighter than ever before. With uniform implementation of recent pathologic typing, grading, and staging guidelines along with radiologic and targeted therapeutic advances as part of a well-integrated multidisciplinary model of clinical oncology, pathologists can become major contributors to the twenty-first-century management of neuroendocrine tumor patients.

Abbreviations

AJCC	American Joint Committee on Cancer Staging
Akt	v-akt murine thymoma viral oncogene homolog 1
ATRX	Alpha thalassemia/mental retardation syndrome X-linked gene
CNA	Copy number alteration
CDKN1B	A gene that encodes for the cyclin-dependent kinase inhibitor, p27KIP1
CDX2	Caudal type homeobox 2
CGA	Chromogranin A
CGH	Comparative genomic hybridization
DAXX	Death-domain associated protein
ENETS	The European Neuroendocrine Tumor Society
GI system	Gastrointestinal system
HPF	High power field (40X)
MEN	Multiple endocrine neoplasia
MGMT	Methylguanine-methyltransferase
mTOR	Mammalian Target of Rapamycin
NANETS	The North American Neuroendocrine Tumor Society
NEC	Neuroendocrine carcinoma
NET	Neuroendocrine tumor
NSE	Neuron-specific enolase
PFS	Progression-free survival
PI3K	PI3kinase
PNET	Pancreatic neuroendocrine tumor
PTEN	phosphatase and tensin homolog
SNP	Single- nucleotide polymorphism
SST	Somatostatin
TNM	Tumor, nodes, metastases (staging criteria)
TSC2	Tuberous sclerosis 2
TTF1	Thyroid transcription factor 1
VEGF	Vascular endothelial growth factor
VIP	Vasoctive intestinal peptide
WHO	World Health Organization

References

1. Bosman FT, Carneiro F, Hruban RH, Theise ND, Editors. WHO Classification of Tumors of the Digestive System. 4th ed. Lyon: IARC; 2010.
2. Kleihues P, Sobin L, editors. Tumors of the lung, pleura, thymus and heart. Lyon: IARC Press; 2004.
3. Klimstra DS, Modlin IR, Adsay NV, Chetty R, Deshpande V, Gonen M, et al. Pathology reporting of neuroendocrine tumors: application of the Delphic consensus process to the development of a minimum pathology data set. Am J Surg Pathol. 2010;34(3):300–13.
4. Sobin LH, Gospodarowicz MK, Wittekind C, Eds. AJCC Cancer Staging Handbook. 7th ed. New York: Springer; 2011.
5. Ellison TA, Wolfgang CL, Shi C, Cameron JL, Murakami P, Mun LJ, et al. A single institution's 26-year experience with nonfunctional pancreatic neuroendocrine tumors: a validation of current staging systems and a new prognostic nomogram. Ann Surg. 2014;259(2):204–12.
6. Strosberg JR, Cheema A, Weber J, Han G, Coppola D, Kvols LK. Prognostic validity of a novel American Joint Committee on Cancer Staging Classification for pancreatic neuroendocrine tumors. J Clin Oncol. 2011;29(22):3044–9.
7. Strosberg JR, Weber JM, Feldman M, Coppola D, Meredith K, Kvols LK. Prognostic validity of the American Joint Committee on Cancer staging classification for midgut neuroendocrine tumors. J Clin Oncol. 2013;31(4):420–5.
8. Qadan M, Ma Y, Visser BC, Kunz PL, Fisher GA, Norton JA, et al. Reassessment of the current American Joint Committee on Cancer staging system for pancreatic neuroendocrine tumors. J Am Coll Surg. 2014;218(2):188–95.
9. Jiao Y, Shi C, Edil BH, de Wilde RF, Klimstra DS, Maitra A, et al. DAXX/ATRX, MEN1, and mTOR pathway genes are frequently altered in pancreatic neuroendocrine tumors. Science. 2011;331(6021):1199–203.
10. Francis JM, Kiezun A, Ramos AH, Serra S, Pedamallu CS, Qian ZR, et al. Somatic mutation of CDKN1B in small intestine neuroendocrine tumors. Nat Genet. 2013;45(12):1483–6.
11. Banck MS, Kanwar R, Kulkarni AA, Boora GK, Metge F, Kipp BR, et al. The genomic landscape of small intestine neuroendocrine tumors. J Clin Invest. 2013;123(6):2502–8.
12. Kim do H, Nagano Y, Choi IS, White JA, Yao JC, Rashid A. Allelic alterations in well-differentiated neuroendocrine tumors (carcinoid tumors) identified by genome-wide single nucleotide polymorphism analysis and comparison with pancreatic endocrine tumors. Genes Chromosomes Cancer. 2008;47(1):84–92.
13. Wang GG, Yao JC, Worah S, White JA, Luna R, Wu TT, et al. Comparison of genetic alterations in neuroendocrine tumors: frequent loss of chromosome 18 in ileal carcinoid tumors. Mod Pathol. 2005;18(8):1079–87.
14. Yao JC, Pavel M, Phan AT, Kulke MH, Hoosen S, St Peter J, et al. Chromogranin A and neuron-specific enolase as prognostic markers in patients with advanced pNET treated with everolimus. J Clin Endocrinol Metab. 2011;96(12):3741–9.
15. Kouvaraki MA, Ajani JA, Hoff P, Wolff R, Evans DB, Lozano R, et al. Fluorouracil, doxorubicin, and streptozocin in the treatment of patients with locally advanced and metastatic pancreatic endocrine carcinomas. J Clin Oncol. 2004;22(23):4762–71.
16. Kulke MH, Hornick JL, Frauenhoffer C, Hooshmand S, Ryan DP, Enzinger PC, et al. O6-methylguanine DNA methyltransferase deficiency and response to temozolomide-based therapy in patients with neuroendocrine tumors. Clin Cancer Res. 2009;15(1):338–45.
17. Kulke MH, Bendell J, Kvols L, Picus J, Pommier R, Yao J. Evolving diagnostic and treatment strategies for pancreatic neuroendocrine tumors. J Hematol Oncol. 2011;4:29.
18. Missiaglia E, Dalai I, Barbi S, Beghelli S, Falconi M, della Peruta M, et al. Pancreatic endocrine tumors: expression profiling evidences a role for AKT-mTOR pathway. J Clin Oncol. 2010;28(2):245–55.

Index

A
Achaete-scute homolog 1 (ASH1), 64
Achlorhydria, 10, 225–227
Acinar adenocarcinoma, 370
Acromegaly, 81
Adamantinoma Ewing sarcoma, 421
Adenocarcinoma
  gastric, 224, 226, 227, 229
  NETs *vs.,* 31–33
  neuroendocrine markers, 32
  with paneth cell-like NE
    differentiation, 369
Adrenal Gland Scaled Score, 14
AJCC. *See* American Joint Committee on
    Cancer (AJCC)
Akt/mTOR pathways, 469
Aldo-keto reductase family one member C3
    (AKR1C3), 280
Alpha thalassemia/mental retardation
    syndrome X-linked (ATRX),
    255, 485, 487
Alveolar rhabdomyosarcoma, 423
American Joint Committee on Cancer (AJCC)
  guidelines, 404
  NETs classification, 22, 24–26
Angiogenesis, 207
  experimental pancreatic neuroendocrine
    tumor model and, 452
  and NET, 452–453
  and prognosis, 454
Angiogenic switch, 452–453, 459
Angiopoietins
  Ang-1 and Ang-2, 455
  Tie-2 receptor, 455–456
Antiangiogenic agents
  combining, 457
  resistance to, 457–460
Antiangiogenic therapies
  biomarkers, 460
AntiEGFR therapies, 435
Anti-VEGF monoclonal antibody, 457
Anti-VEGF/VEGFR therapies, 453
Apoptosis, 433, 440
Appendiceal carcinoids in children
  clinical features, 292–293
  demographics, 292
  prognosis, 293
  treatment, 293
Appendiceal NETs
  in children (*see* Appendiceal carcinoids in
    children)
  clinical presentation, 287
  diagnosis, 287
  epidemiology, 286–287
  mixed adenoneuroendocrine carcinomas
    (MANECs), 293–294
  molecular pathology, 290
  pathogenesis, 286
  pathologic findings
    EC Cell NETs, 287–288
    L Cell NETs, 288
    tubular carcinoid, 288–290
  primary neuroendocrine carcinomas
    (NECs), 294–295
  prognosis and postoperative monitoring,
    290–291
  treatment, 292
APUDoma. *See* Merkel cell
    carcinoma (MCC)
ASH1, 64

A. Nasir, D. Coppola (eds.), *Neuroendocrine Tumors: Review of Pathology, Molecular and Therapeutic Advances*, DOI 10.1007/978-1-4939-3426-3

Ataxia telangiectasia mutated (ATM) gene, 207, 231
Atrophic gastritis
  associated, 225
  carcinoid–adenocarcinoma lesions, 226
  chronic, 215, 216, 224–227, 232
  prevalence, 225
ATRX, 255, 485, 487
Atypical carcinoid (AC), 141, 152, 156–158
Atypical central neurocytomas (WHO Grade II), 90
Atypical Ewing sarcoma, 421
Atypical pituitary adenoma, 84, 87
Autoimmune chronic atrophic gastritis (A-CAG)-associated gastric NETs, 224
Autoradiography, 442
Azzopardi phenomenon, 160, 392

B
BCL-2, 167, 205
Bevacizumab, 457, 458, 504–505
BIM-23A758, 435
BIM-23A760, 435
BIN-1, 93
Biomarkers
  for antiangiogenic therapies, 460
  EGFR family of receptors, 484
  Ewing sarcoma/primitive neuroectodermal tumor (ES/PNET), 424
  putative, 442, 445
  SI-NENs, 280–282
Bladder cancer
  carcinoid, 353–354
  large cell neuroendocrine carcinoma (LCNEC), 356–357
  paraganglioma, 358–360
  small cell carcinoma (SCC), 354–356
  telomerase reverse transcriptase (TERT) promoter mutations, 360
Bombesin, 446, 468
Bone malignancy in children. *See* Ewing sarcoma/primitive neuroectodermal tumor (ES/PNET)
Bone marrow (BM), 424, 458, 501
BRAF, 435, 505
Breast neuroendocrine carcinoma
  clinical features and prognosis, 185–190
  histopathology
    invasive breast carcinoma with neuroendocrine differentiation (NEBC), 179–184
    neuroendocrine carcinoma, poorly differentiated (NEC-PD), 177–179
    neuroendocrine tumor, well differentiated (NET-WD), 177
  immunohistochemistry and differential diagnosis, 191–192
  molecular and genetic features, 192–193
  treatment, 193
Bronchial and thymic neuroendocrine NETs, 13–14
Bronchial carcinoid tumor, 152–156
Bronchial tumorlets, 14

C
Calcitonin, 117, 364, 431
CAM 5.2, 63
Cancer
  clinically aggressive, 59
  colorectal, 58
  high-grade, 66
Carcinoembryonic antigen (CEA), 63, 119–120
Carcinoid
  cytologic variability, 365, 366
  diagnostic criteria, 365
  monitoring, 434
  proliferation marker Ki67, 367
  prostatic adenocarcinoma, 365
  PSA, 365, 367
  synaptophysin, 365, 366
  syndrome, 433–434
Carcinoid tumor, 9, 152–156, 176, 270, 374
Carcinoma
  large cell carcinoma (LCC), 56–57
  large cell neuroendocrine cell carcinoma (LCNEC), 138, 141, 143
  mixed adenoneuroendocrine carcinoma (MANEC), 57
  neuroendocrine (*see* Neuroendocrine carcinoma (NEC))
  small cell carcinoma (SCC), 56
  small cell neuroendocrine cell carcinoma (SCNEC), 138, 141
C-cell(s)
  characteristics, 127
  proliferations, 127–129
C-cell hyperplasia (CCH), 15, 114, 127
CCND1 gene and cyclin D1 expression, 83–84
CD56, 62–63
CDX2, 35, 63, 489
Cell block preparations, 117, 118
Central neurocytoma (CN)
  atypical central neurocytomas (WHO Grade II), 90

chromosomal abnormalities, 92
clinical features, 11
differential diagnosis, 89–90
genetic and oncogenesis pathways
insulin-like growth factor 2, 93
neuregulin (NRG), 94
N-MYC and BIN-1, 93
platelet-derived growth factor (PDGF), 94
PTEN, 93
histogenesis
multipotential central neurocytoma cells, 91
neural cell of origin, 91
neural stem cells, 91–92
intraventricular tumor, 88
Cervical NET, 378–379
CGH. *See* Comparative genomic hybridization (CGH)
Children's Oncology Group (COG) risk categories, 344–345
Chimeric somatostatin, 435
Cholecystokinin, 446, 468
Chromogranin A (CgA), 62, 324–325, 485–486
Chromosomal abnormalities, 92, 231, 489–491, 491
Chromosomal instability (CIN), 311
Chronic atrophic gastritis, 215, 216, 224–227, 232
Chronic lymphocytic leukemia/small lymphocytic lymphoma (CLL/SLL), 394, 399
Circulating tumor cell (CTC), 424
c-Kit, 469, 471–473, 484–485
Classic Ewing sarcoma, 421
Classification systems
anterior pituitary, 15–16
differentiation, 6
distal colon and rectum (hindgut), 13
grading, 7–8
inherited conditions, 6
jejunum, ileum, appendix and cecum (midgut NETs), 12–13
lung and thymus (thorax, foregut), 13–14
neuroendocrine neoplasm
anatomic distribution, 5–6
embryologic classification, 5
WHO, 22
neuroendocrine tumors (NETs)
AJCC system, 24–26
ENETS system, 23
functional, 5
markers, 4
TNM, 22
UICC system, 24
pancreas, 9–12
pheochromocytoma, paraganglioma and medullary thyroid cancer, 14–15
pituitary adenomas, functional classification, 16–17
pituitary tumors
radiologic classification, 17
WHO classification, 17
stomach, 8–9
Clear cell sarcoma, 423
Cleared out chromatin, 392, 396
c-Met, 458
CN. *See* Central neurocytoma (CN)
Collagen IV IHC stain, 129
Colon
carcinoembryonic antigen (CEA) AND, 63
carcinoma cell line HT29, 63
PD-NEC, 58–59
small cell neuroendocrine carcinoma, 56
Colorectal cancer (CRC)
chromosomal instability (CIN), 311
CpG island methylator phenotype (CIMP), 312
hereditary, 310
MSI, 311
sporadic, 310
Colorectal LCCs, 65
Colorectal NETs, 12, 310
Colorectal neuroendocrine tumor
etiology and associated conditions, 307
genetic mechanisms
insulin-like peptide 5 (INSL5), 313–314
methylation, 312–313
mutations, 312
Notch1, 313
Wnt pathway/PROX1 protein, 313
histopathology
large-cell NEC, 309
MANEC, 310
neuroendocrine carcinomas (NECs), 308
NOTCH 1 gene pathway and its interaction, 307–308
small-cell NEC, 309
molecular pathways
chromosomal instability (CIN), 311
colorectal neuroendocrine tumors, 310
CpG island methylator phenotype (CIMP), 312
MSI, 311
Colorectal SCCs, 65
Companion diagnostic, 460

Comparative genomic hybridization (CGH), 47, 424, 489, 491
Congenital hypoventilation syndrome, 342
Copy number alterations (CNAs), 488, 491
CpG island methylator phenotype (CIMP), 312
Cushing's disease, 81
CXCL14 and NKX2–NKX3, 276
Cyclin-dependent kinases and Rb, 489
Cyclin D1 expression, 83–84
Cyfra 21–1, 169
Cystic teratoma, 375, 376
Cytokeratin, 32, 63
Cytokeratin fragments (CKfr), 281

D
DAXX (death-domain-associated protein), 48, 255, 485, 487
Degenerative nuclear atypia, 30
Deletions in CDKN1B, 489
Desmoplastic round cell tumor (DRCT), 423
Desmoplastic small round cell tumor, 423
Differential diagnosis
  breast neuroendocrine carcinoma, 191–192
  central neurocytoma (CN), 89–90
  Ewing sarcoma (ES), 423
  fine-needle aspiration (FNA) cytology, 117–118
  mediastinum, NETs, 141–142
  medullary thyroid carcinoma (MTC), 129–130
  Merkel cell carcinoma pathology, 395
  NETs
    adenocarcinomas *vs.,* 31–33
    Ki-67 antibody, 30
    metastatic, 35
    MIB-1, 30
    neoplasms *vs.,* 33–34
    neuroendocrine carcinoma (NEC), 31
    neuroendocrine neoplasms from various malignancies, 37
    nonepithelial neoplasms *vs.,* 35
    paragangliomas *vs.,* 34
    primary tumors originated in liver *vs.,* 33
    prostate cancer *vs.,* 35–36
    solid pseudopapillary neoplasm (SPN) *vs.,* 34
    tumor proliferation index, 30
  thymic NETs, 141–142

Diffuse idiopathic pulmonary NE cell hyperplasia (DIPNECH), 151
Dopamine receptors, 475
Dopamine receptor type 2 (D2DR), 446
Ductal carcinoma in situ (DCIS), 181
Duodenal SI-NENs, 272

E
E-cadherin-catenin, 169
EC Cell NETs, 287–288
Elective lymphadenectomy, 405
Endocrine carcinoma (ECA), 443
Endocrine differentiation within adenocarcinoma, 364–365
Endocrine tumor (ET). *See* Neuroendocrine tumors (NET)
Endometrium NET, 379–381
Endoscopic mucosal resection (EMR), 226
Endoscopic submucosal dissection (ESD), 226
Endothelial cells, Tie2 activation, 455
Enterochromaffin-like cell carcinoids (ECL cell NETs), 216
Enterochromaffin-like (ECL) cells
  hyperplasia, 228, 232
  NETs, 218
  serotonin-producing NETs, 218
EpCAM expression, SI-NENs, 277–278
Epidermal growth factor receptor (EGFR)
  as biomarkers, 484
  cell lines with mutations, 469
  differential expression, 470–471
  human NETs/PNETs, 456, 469–470
  in NET cell lines, 469, 506
  peptide receptors and NETs, 468–469
  prognostic factor in pancreatic NETs, 471
  sarcoma kinase (Src), 473
  SCFR, 471–473
Epigenetic mechanisms in NETs, 491
Epithelial neuroendocrine cells (ENC), 286
Esophageal neuroendocrine
  classification, 202
  diagnosis, 208
  gastrointestinal neuroendocrine lesions, 200
  gross, 203
  histologic features, 203
  management approach, 209
  molecular pathways
    angiogenesis, 207

ataxia telangiectasia mutated (ATM) gene, 207
Bcl-2, 205
Fox Chase Cancer Center (FCCC), 204
gastrointestinal and pancreatic neuroendocrine, 204
GEP-NEN gene co-expression network, 204, 205
heparanase, 206
instability in neuroendocrine tumorigenesis, 204–205
KIT and PDGFRA, 208
location-specific phenomena, 203
mammalian target of rapamycin (mTOR), 207
MEN gene inactivation, 203
NETs genomics, 203–204
p53 and Rb, 206–207
somatostatin receptor signaling, 208
neuroendocrine neoplasms, 200–202
treatment, 209
Esophagus, PD-NEC, 57
ES/PNET. *See* Ewing sarcoma/primitive neuroectodermal tumor (ES/PNET)
Esthesioneuroblastoma (ENB), 423
Estrogen receptors (ERs), 181
European Neuroendocrine Tumour Society (ENETS), 7–9, 22, 23, 216, 273
Everolimus, 502–503
Ewing sarcoma (ES)
chromosomal rearrangement and genes fusion, 420
differential diagnosis, 423
ES/PNET *vs.*, 422
fusion genes of, 420
immunophenotype, 421
management, 424
Merkel cell carcinoma pathology, 395
microscopic appearance, 421
neuroectodermal differentiation in, 422
pathogenesis, 420
subtypes, 421
Ewing sarcoma/primitive neuroectodermal tumor (ES/PNET)
biomarkers, 424
defined, 420
differential diagnosis, 423
differentiation, 422
immunophenotype, 421–422
management, 424
microscopic appearance, 421
pathogenesis, 420
EWSR1 gene, 420
Exomic sequence analysis, 487, 489
Extracellular regulated kinase (ERK), 441
Extraskeletal myxoid chondrosarcoma, 423

F

Fallopian tube NET, 378
Familial/hereditary NETs, 47
Familial medullary thyroid cancer, 115, 120
Familial paraganglioma, hereditary pheochromocytoma, 327, 329
FCCC. *See* Fox Chase Cancer Center (FCCC)
Female genital tract
endometrium, 379–381
fallopian tube, 378
ovaries
carcinoid tumors, 374
cystic teratoma, 375, 376
insular carcinoids, 374, 375
metastatic carcinoid, 375, 377
mucinous carcinoids, 374–375
small cell carcinoma of hypercalcemic type (SSC-H), 377
small cell carcinoma of the ovary-pulmonary type (SSC-P), 377–378
strumal and mucinous carcinoids, 374
uterine cervix, 378–379
vagina and vulva, 381
Fibroblast growth factors (FGFs), 458
Fine needle aspiration cytology (FNAC)
breast carcinomas, 181
calcitonin measurement, 117
cell block preparations, 117, 118
cellular specimen, 117
differential diagnosis, 117–118
mucosa-associated lymphoid tissue (MALT) lymphoma, 119
multinucleation, 117, 118
oncocytic features, 117, 118
paragangliomas, 119
plasmacytoma, 119
sensitivity, 117
undifferentiated thyroid carcinoma, 119
FLI-1 gene, 421
FLI-1 protein expression, 421
FNAC. *See* Fine needle aspiration cytology (FNAC)
Follicular adenomas, 129–130
Foregut neuroendocrine tumors, 200, 203, 209
Fox Chase Cancer Center (FCCC), 204

Fragile histidine triad gene (FHIT), 166, 168
Functional PNETs (FPNETs), 10
Fusion oncogenes, 420

G

Ganglioneuroblastoma, 334, 336, 337, 342
Ganglioneuroma, 334, 339, 340, 342
Gastric adenocarcinoma, 224, 226, 227, 229
Gastric inhibitory polypeptide receptor (GIPR), 280
Gastric MANECs, 222
Gastric neuroendocrine carcinomas, 220, 223, 224
Gastric neuroendocrine tumors (G-NETs)
  diagnostic approach
    biochemical investigations, 216
    endoscopy, 215
    gastric biopsies, 215–216
    imaging, 216
  epidemiology, 214
  etiology and pathogenesis, 215
  histologic grading, 222, 224
  histopathologic classification
    categories, 217
    ECL cell NETs, 218
    ECL cell serotonin-producing NETs, 218
    ENETS, 216
    enterochromaffin-like cell carcinoids (ECL cell NETs), 216
    gastric MANECs, 222
    gastric neuroendocrine carcinomas, 220, 223, 224
    gastrin-producing NETs (gastrinomas), 218, 221, 222
    gross, 217
    microscopic, 218–220
    subtypes, 217
  molecular advances, 230–231
  multidisciplinary approach, 231–232
  prognosis, 224
  proton pump inhibitors and, 232
  type I, 225–227
  type II, 227–228
  type III, 228–230
  type IV, 230
Gastrinoma, 10, 227–228, 246–247
Gastrin-producing NETs (gastrinomas), 218, 221, 222
Gastro-entero-pancreatic
  clinical considerations, 67–68
  diagnostic challenges for pathologists, 67
  epidemiology, 54–55
  histopathologic classification schemes, 55
  molecular pathology, 55
  PD-NECs
    clinical features of, 61
    immunohistochemistry role in, 61–65
    prognosis, 66
    response to therapy in, 66–67
    site-specific, 57–60
  poorly differentiated neuroendocrine carcinomas, 56–57
  site-specific PD-NECs, 57–60
Gastroenteropancreatic-neuroendocrine neoplasms (GEP-NEN), 306
Gastroenteropancreatic neuroendocrine tumor (GEP-NET), 6, 7, 214, 222, 442, 467
Gastroenteropancreatic (GEP) tumor, 445
Gastrointestinal (GI) epithelium, 306
Gastrointestinal neuroendocrine neoplasms (GI-NENs), 200
Gastrointestinal PD-NECs, 65
Gastrointestinal tract, NET, 40. *See also* Gastro-entero-pancreatic
GCC. *See* Goblet cell carcinoids (GCC)
GCDFP-15. *See* Gross cystic disease fluid protein 15 (GCDFP-15)
G1 cell cycle growth, 440
G-coupled signaling, 431
Gene expression
  profiling, 151, 491–492
  signatures, 231
Gene promoter (BAX), 440
Genetic(s)
  abnormalities, G-NETs, 231
  in colorectal neuroendocrine carcinomas
    insulin-like peptide 5 (INSL5), 313–314
    methylation, 312–313
    mutations, 312
    Notch1, 313
    Wnt pathway/PROX1 protein, 313
  small intestine neuroendocrine neoplasms (SI-NENs), 273–276
  testing
    hereditary pheochromocytoma, 329–330
Genetic and oncogenesis pathways, CN
  insulin-like growth factor 2, 93
  neuregulin (NRG), 94
  N-MYC and BIN-1, 93
  platelet-derived growth factor (PDGF), 94
  PTEN, 93

Genetic profiling, SI-NENs, 273–276
GEP-NEN gene co-expression network, 204, 205
Germline screening, hereditary pheochromocytoma, 330
Glucagonoma, 10, 246
G-NETs. *See* Gastric neuroendocrine tumors (G-NETs)
Goblet cell carcinoids (GCC)
  adenocarcinoid, 295
  clinical presentation, 296
  demographics, 296
  diagnosis, 299
  electron microscopy, 298
  histopathologic findings
    gross, 296–297
    microscopic, 297
  imaging, 299
  immunohistochemistry
    differentiation markers, 298
    Ki67 index, 298
    neuroendocrine markers, 297
  metastatic spread, 299–300
  molecular pathology, 298–299
  pathogenesis, 296
  prognosis, 300
  special stains, 297
  treatment, 300
  tumors, 12–13
G-protein-coupled receptor, 279, 442
Grading, 7–8, 222, 224
Gross cystic disease fluid protein 15 (GCDFP-15), 192
Gross total surgical resection (GTR), 94
GSP, pituitary adenomas, 82–83
G3 well differentiated neuroendocrine carcinoma, 68

H
Helicobactor pylori, 216, 225, 226, 229
Hematoxylin and Eosin (H&E) stains, 127
Heparanase, 206
Hepatocellular carcinoma (HCC) and NETs, 33
HER2 (ErbB2), 468, 484
Her-2 oncoprotein, 181
Heterogeneity, 447
HIF-1α, 454, 458
High-grade
  large-cell neuroendocrine carcinomas, 68
  neuroendocrine carcinomas, 13
  PD-NECs and NETs, 68
Hindgut
  carcinoids, 12
  NENs, 5
Hirschsprung disease, 342
Hormonal active tumors, 81
Hormonal hypersecretion, 440
Human chorionic gonadotropin (hCG), 191
Human hormone somatostatin, 500
Hürthle cell tumors, 130
Hyalinizing trabecular tumors, 129
Hypergastrinemia, 225–227, 227–228
Hyperparathyroidism, 115, 120
Hyper-proliferative nodules, 456
Hypokalemia, 10
Hypomethylation and promoter methylation, 275–276
Hypoxia-inducible factors-1α (HIF-1α) pathway, 454, 458

I
Ileal NETs (INETs), 272
Image-defined risk factors (IDRF), 343
Immunohistochemistry (IHC). *See also* Marker
  angiopoietins and Tie-2 receptor, 455, 457
  CgA immunoreactivity, 68
  EGFR, differential expression, 470
  Ewing sarcoma (ES), 421, 423
  markers, 56
  MLH1 protein loss, 66
  in PD-NEC, 61–65
  SSTRs expression, 442
Immunomodulatory activity, 433
Immunophenotypical profile
  epithelial differentiation and neuroendocrine tumors, 42
  epithelial *vs.* site-specific immunohistochemical markers, 44
  immunohistochemistry
    role, 46
    secretory proteins and receptors, 43
  neuroendocrine differentiation, 42–43
  neuroendocrine neoplasms
    immunohistochemistry and grade, 44–46
    location, 44
Inappropriate miRNA expression patterns, 87
Incidental-type I G-NETs, 214
Index
  Ki-67, 61
  labeling, 60
  mitotic and Ki-67, 67
  proliferative, 68

Inherited genetic syndromes, 487
Instability in neuroendocrine tumorigenesis, 204–205
Insular carcinoids, 374, 375
Insulin-like growth factor (IGF), 93, 500
Insulin-like peptide 5 (INSL5), 313–314
Insulinoma, 10, 245, 492
Interferon alpha, 433
Internalization, SSTRs, 447
International Agency for Research on Cancer (IARC), 270
International Association for the Study of Lung Cancer (IASLC), 14
International Neuroblastoma Risk Group (INRG) Staging System, 342–344
International Neuroblastoma Staging System (INSS), 342–343
Intestine. *See also* Small intestine neuroendocrine neoplasms (SI-NENs)
  MANECs, 58
  NECs, 54
Intracranial neoplasms, 81
Intrahepatic cholangiocarcinoma, 33–34
Intraventricular tumor, 88
Invasive breast carcinoma with neuroendocrine differentiation (NEBC), 179–184
131-Iodine-labeled metaiodobenzylguanidine (131I-MIBG), 330
ISL1, 65
Islet cell
  carcinogenesis model, 456
  carcinomas, 443–444

J
Jejunoileal SI-NENs, 272–273
Jun-D- activated transcription, 47

K
Karyotyping, 424
Ki-67 index
  CTCs in NETs, 488
  gastric NETs, 218, 220, 222
  goblet cell carcinoids (GCC), 298
  labeling index, 8
  Pancreas NETs, 252–254
  in PD-NEC, 61, 65, 67
  pituitary adenomas, 88, 90, 98
Kinase insert domain receptor (KDR), 452
KIT (c-Kit encoding gene)
  and ATM genes, 484
  and PDGFRA, 208
Kulchitsky cells and bronchioles, 150

L
Lanreotide, 440, 446, 447
Large cell carcinoma (LCC), 56–57
Large cell lung cancer (LCLC)
  CDX-2, 161–162
  clinical symptoms and treatment, 164–165
  genetic markers, 161
  immunohistochemical identification, 161
  necrosis, 162–164
  SCLC, morphological similarities, 164
Large-cell NEC, 309
Large cell neuroendocrine cell carcinoma (LCNEC), 138, 141, 143, 356–357, 370, 446
Large-scale validation of genetic findings, 491
L Cell NETs, 288
LCLC. *See* Large cell lung cancer (LCLC)
LCNEC. *See* Large cell neuroendocrine cell carcinoma (LCNEC)
Leiomyosarcoma, 130
Liquid chromatography-mass spectrometry (LC-MS), 492
Liver metastases, 488
Loss of heterozygosity (LOH) analysis, 81
177Lu-DOTA-TYR3-octreotate, 435
Lung neuroendocrine tumors
  historical aspects, 150
  intervention and chemoprevention, 169–170
  Kulchitsky cells and bronchioles, 150
  molecular pathways in
    chromosomal changes, 165–166
    proliferation markers, 168–169
    tumor suppressor genes, 166–168
  oat cell carcinoma, 150
  pathogenesis, 150–151
  precursor lesions, 151
  SSTRs expression, 442
  terminology and classification
    atypical carcinoid, 152, 156–158
    carcinoid tumor, 152–158
    large cell lung cancer (LCLC), 161–165
    small cell lung cancer (SCLC), 158–161
Lymphangiogenesis, 452, 453
Lymphatic invasion, 124

Lymphoblastic lymphoma (LBL), 423
Lymphovascular invasion (LVI), 391, 393

M
Malignant neoplasms, 423
Mammaglobin, 192
Mammalian target of rapamycin (mTOR), 207, 483–484
MANEC. *See* Mixed adenoneuroendocrine carcinoma (MANEC)
MAPK pathway activation, 432, 441
Marker
  neuroendocrine and other IHC
    achaete-scute homolog 1 (ASH1), 64
    CAM 5.2, 63
    carcinoembryonic antigen (CEA), 63
    CD56, 62–63
    CDX2, 63
    chromogranin A (CgA), 62
    neuron-specific enolase (NSE), 62
    P53, 64
    synaptophysin, 62
    thyroid transcription factor (TTF)-1, 64
  organ-specific IHC, 64–65
  prognostic, 66
MCC. *See* Merkel cell carcinoma (MCC)
MCPyV. *See* Merkel cell polyomavirus (MCPyV)
MDM2 and p53, 488
Mechanistic target of rapamycin (mTOR), 441
Mediastinum, NETs
  classification, 141
  diagnostic radiology, 139
  differential diagnosis, 141–142
  epidemiology, 138
  gross features, 140
  immunohistochemical stains, 141
  location, 138–139
  management and follow-up, 143
  microscopic features, 140–141
  molecular pathology, 142
  prognosis, 143
  response evaluation, 143
  symptoms, 139
  terminology, 138
  tumorigenesis, 139
Medullary thyroid carcinoma (MTC)
  clinical presentation, 116
  differential diagnosis, 129–130
  histopathology findings
    C-cells, 127–129
    sporadic tumors, 121, 124, 127
  inherited forms, 114–115
  presurgical diagnosis and initial evaluation
    fine-needle aspiration (FNA) cytology, 117–119
    preoperative imaging studies, 120–122, 123–126
    RET germline mutations, 120, 121
    serum calcitonin and CEA, 119–120
  prognostic factors, 131–132
  sporadic, 115
  thyroid C cells, 14–15
  treatment, 130–131
Melatonin, 95, 96, 103
Memorial Sloan-Kettering criteria, 252
MEN1, 84
MEN2A, 114–115
MEN2B, 114–115
MEN1 gene, 482
MEN gene inactivation, 203
MENIN, 486–488
MEN2 syndromes, 114
Merkel cell carcinoma (MCC), 381
  clinical presentation, 390
  epidemiological and clinical features, 389–391
  immunohistochemical aspects
    CD56, 400
    CK7 positivity, 397
    Ewing sarcoma/primitive neuroectodermal tumor (PNET), 400
    imatinib, 398
    neuron-specific enolase (NSE), 396
    nuclear signal, 397, 402
    paranuclear dot-like accentuation, 396
    p63 expression, 397, 398
    Rb protein expression, 398
    small cell lung carcinoma (SCLC), 399
    small metastatic deposits, 396, 401
    staining patterns, 399, 402
    thyroid transcription factor 1 (TTF-1), 399
  light microscopic findings (*see* Merkel cell carcinoma pathology)
  lymph nodes, 389
  molecular aspects and pathogenesis, 403–404
  multicentric presentations, 390
  pericolic adipose tissue, 391
  prognostic factors, staging and management, 404–406
  ultrastructural features, 401–403

Merkel cell carcinoma pathology
Azzopardi phenomenon, 392
chronic lymphocytic leukemia/small lymphocytic lymphoma (CLL/SLL), 394, 399
"cleared out" chromatin, 392, 396
differential diagnosis, 395
Ewing sarcoma, 395
growth patterns, 391–392, 395
lymphovascular invasion (LVI), 391, 393
small cell pattern, 392, 394
small round blue cell" (SRBC) proliferation, 391
squamous cell carcinoma, 393, 397, 398
sun-damaged skin, 393
tumor borders, 391–392
Merkel cell polyomavirus (MCPyV), 403–404
Mesenchymal chondrosarcoma (MCS), 423
Metalloproteinases (MMP), 169
Metastasis, NET and malignant paraganglioma, 34, 35
Metastatic carcinoid, 186, 375, 377
Metastatic GI carcinoid, 189
Metastatic neuroendocrine carcinoma (NEC), 489
Metastatic tumor, 34, 118, 375
Methylation, 66, 82, 142, 312–313
Methylguanine-methyltransferase (MGMT), 481, 485
MIB-1, 88, 90
Micro-MTC, 124
MicroRNAs (miRNAs), 87, 424
Microsatellite instability (MSI), 311, 379
Microsatellites, 166
Microvascular density (MVD), 454
Midgut NENs, 5
Mitogen-activated protein kinase (MAPK), 432, 441
Mitosis-karyorrhexis index (MKI) score, 344
Mixed adenoneuroendocrine carcinoma (MANEC)
adenocarcinoma ex goblet cell carcinoid, 293, 294
colon and rectum, 310
diffuse infiltrative growth pattern, 293
exocrine and endocrine carcinoma, 293
gastric carcinomas, 217, 222
mucosal epithelium, 293
neuroendocrine tumor *vs.* adenocarcinoma, 32–33
Mixed carcinoid tumors, 354
Molecular biomarkers
discovery and validation, 491–493
in PNETs, gene expression profiling, 491–492
Molecular changes in CTCs in NETs, 488
Molecular genetics
abnormalities, 48–49
genotype-phenotype correlations, 47
GI NETs, 47–48
hereditary disorders and, 47
immunohistochemistry, 49
Jun-D- activated transcription, 47
microRNA expression patterns, 49
mTOR (mammalian target of rapamycin) pathway mutation, 48
multiple endocrine neoplasia (MEN) types, 46–47
nuclear transcriptional machinery in tumor cells, 46–47
pancreatic NETs, 48
Molecular mechanisms, 432, 433, 484
Molecular pathology of neuroendocrine neoplasms
chromogranin A (CgA), 485–486
chromosomal abnormalities, 489–491
c-Kit, 484–485
cyclin-dependent kinases and Rb, 489
EGFR family of receptors as biomarkers, 484
epigenetic mechanisms in NETs, 491
mammalian target of rapamycin (mTOR), 483–484
MDM2 and p53, 488
MENIN, 486–488
MGMT, 485
molecular biomarkers in PNETs, 491–492
molecular changes in CTCs in NETs, 488
transcription factors in NETs, 489
Molecular pathway
in colorectal neuroendocrine carcinomas
chromosomal instability (CIN), 311
colorectal neuroendocrine tumors, 310
CpG island methylator phenotype (CIMP), 312
MSI, 311
esophageal neuroendocrine
angiogenesis, 207
ataxia telangiectasia mutated (ATM) gene, 207
Bcl-2, 205
Fox Chase Cancer Center (FCCC), 204
gastrointestinal and pancreatic neuroendocrine, 204
GEP-NEN gene co-expression network, 204, 205
heparanase, 206
instability in neuroendocrine tumorigenesis, 204–205

KIT and PDGFRA, 208
location-specific phenomena, 203
mammalian target of rapamycin (mTOR), 207
MEN gene inactivation, 203
NETs genomics, 203–204
p53 and Rb, 206–207
somatostatin receptor signaling, 208
small intestine neuroendocrine neoplasms (SI-NENs), 273
Molecular targets in human NETs, 465–476
Molecular testing, Ewing sarcoma (ES), 421
MTC. *See* Medullary thyroid carcinoma (MTC)
mTOR activation, 434
mTOR inhibitor, 475
mTOR pathway
everolimus, 502–503
genes, 255, 502
in human NETs, 484
in pancreatic NETs, 483
temsirolimus, 503–504
Mucinous carcinoids, 374–375
Mucinous carcinoma, 181, 183
Mucosa-associated lymphoid tissue (MALT) lymphoma, 119
Multinucleation, 117, 118
Multiple endocrine neoplasia type 1 (MEN1), 46–47, 230, 243, 487
Multiple endocrine neoplasia type 2 (MEN2), 46–47, 327–328
syndromes, 114, 487
Multipotential central neurocytoma cells, 91
Muscarinic acetylcholine receptor, 424
Mutations, 312
MYC-associated factor X (MAX), 329
MYC protein, 167

N

National Comprehensive Cancer Network (NCCN), 291
Neo-angiogenesis, 455, 457
Nesidioblastosis
adult type, 258
in children, 258
clinical criteria, 258
clinical diagnostic criteria, 260–261
definition, 257–258, 257–262
diffuse type, 258
histopathology, 261–262
pathogenesis and molecular biology, 258–260
treatment, 262
varieties, 258
NET. *See* Neuroendocrine tumors (NET)
Neural cell of origin, 91
Neural stem cells, 91–92
Neuregulin (NRG), 94
Neuroblastic tumors
epidemiological and clinical features, 331–332
immunohistochemistry, 337–339
light microscopic findings
classification schemes, 332
differentiation features, 332
ganglioneuroblastoma, 334, 336, 337
ganglioneuroma, 334, 339, 340
neuroblastomas, 332–336
poorly differentiated neuroblastoma, 337
molecular pathogenesis and testing, 341–342
prognostic factors, staging, and management, 342–345
ultrastructure, 339–341
Neuroblastoma (NB), 332–336, 423
Neuroendocrine carcinoma (NEC)
colon and rectum, 308
esophageal (*see* Esophageal neuroendocrine)
poorly differentiated
clinical features of, 61
immunohistochemistry role in, 61–65
large cell carcinoma (LCC), 56–57
mixed adenoneuroendocrine carcinoma (MANEC), 57
prognosis, 66
response to therapy in, 66–67
site-specific, 57–60
small cell carcinoma (SCC), 56
poorly differentiated (NEC-PD), 177–179
SI-NENs (*see* small intestine neuroendocrine neoplasms (SI-NENs))
SSTRs expression, 442
Neuroendocrine differentiation, 191–194, 421
Neuroendocrine ductal carcinoma in situ (NE-DCIS), 181
Neuroendocrine markers
adenocarcinoma, 32
goblet cell carcinoids (GCC), 297
hepatocellular lesions and, 33
immunoexpression, 218
immunohistochemical examination, 40–41
immunohistochemical negativity, 45
immunoreactivity, 43
NETs stain, 44
primary liver endothelial neoplasms, 33

Neuroendocrine neoplasm (NEN)
anatomic distribution, 5–6
of brain
CN (*see* Central neurocytoma (CN))
pineal region tumors, 95–104
pituitary (*see* Pituitary adenomas)
EGFR, 506
embryologic classification, 5
inhibitors of VEGFR, 505–506
Ki-67 proliferation index, 31
malignancies and, 36–37
mimickers and, 36
mTOR pathway, 502
everolimus, 502–503
temsirolimus, 503–504
SI-NENs (*see* small intestine neuroendocrine neoplasms (SI-NENs))
somatostatin analogs, 506–507
somatostatin receptor pathway
peptide receptor radionuclide therapy, 501–502
somatostatin analogs, 500–501
of stomach (*see* Gastric neuroendocrine tumors (G-NETs))
VEGF pathway
bevacizumab, 504–505
sorafenib, 505
sunitinib, 505
WHO classification, 22
Neuroendocrine tumor
molecular pathology (*see* Targeted therapies)
pathology
classification, grading, and reporting schemes, 513–514
immunohistochemistry in NET pathology, 514
management decisions, 515
molecular characterization of NETs, 514
molecular diagnostics of NETs, 515
NET staging, 514
personalized therapies, 516
treatment of NET patients, 515–516
Neuroendocrine tumors (NET)
and angiogenesis, 452–454
angiopoietins (Ang-1 and Ang-2), 455–456
antiangiogenic agents, 457–460
biomarkers for antiangiogenic therapies, 460
characteristics, 40
chimeric somatostatin, 435
classification systems (*see* Staging, NETs)
clinical syndromes, 11
defined, 431
differential diagnosis
adenocarcinomas *vs.,* 31–33
Ki-67 antibody, 30
metastatic, 35
MIB-1, 30
neoplasms *vs.,* 33–34
neuroendocrine carcinoma (NEC), 31
neuroendocrine neoplasms from various malignancies, 37
nonepithelial neoplasms *vs.,* 35
paragangliomas *vs.,* 34
primary tumors originated in liver *vs.,* 33
prostate cancer *vs.,* 35–36
solid pseudopapillary neoplasm (SPN) *vs.,* 34
tumor proliferation index, 30
in female (*see* Female genital tract)
functional, 5, 11
gastric neoplasms, 8–9
gastroenteropancreatic, 9
immunotherapy, 436
in lung (*see* Lung neuroendocrine tumors)
markers, 4
molecular biology, 431
molecular genetics of, 46–49
molecular targets, 435
PDGFR, 456
prognosis, 454
radiotargeted therapy, 435
somatostatin analogues (SSAs)
clinical trials, 434
resistence to, 434
somatostatin receptors, 442
SSTR biology
carcinoid syndrome, 433–434
direct effects of SSAs, 432–433
indirect effects of SSAs, 433
interferon alpha, 433
staging system (*see* TNM)
stomach and pancreas, 8–9
targeted agents, 434–435
telotristat etiprate, 435
vascularity of human, 454
VEGF and VEGF receptors, 454
Neuroendocrine tumor, well differentiated (NET-WD), 177
Neuroepithelial bodies (NEBs), 150

Neurofibromatosis, 242–243
Neurofibromatosis type 1 (NF-1), 47, 487
G-NETs, 230
hereditary pheochromocytoma, 327–328
Neurofilament (NF), 91, 98
Neurokinin A, 281
Neuron-specific enolase (NSE), 62, 270
Nicotinic acetylcholine receptor, 424
NKX2.2 gene, 421
Nm23, 85
N-MYC, 93
Nonepithelial neoplasms *vs.* NETs, 35
Nonfunctional PNETs (NFPNETs), 10–12
Non-lesional gastric biopsies, 226
North American Neuroendocrine Tumor Society (NANETS) guidelines, 23, 291
NOTCH 1 gene pathway and its interaction, 307–308, 313
Novel biomarker, 491–492
NSE. *See* Neuron-specific enolase (NSE)

O
OctreoScan, 444
Octreotide, 434, 440, 443, 445, 446, 447
Oncogenes
CCND1 gene and cyclin D1 expression, 83–84
GSP, 82–83
pituitary tumor-transforming gene (PTTG), 83
ras, 83

P
P53 (Gene promotor), 64, 84, 206–207, 440
Palladin, 256–257, 488
Palliative radiation therapy, 131
Pancreatic endocrine primaries, 488
Pancreatic endocrine tumors (PET), 481
Pancreatic neuroendocrine tumor (PNETs)
ancillary studies
Ki-67, 252–254
PHH3, 254
angiogenesis and prognosis, 454
classification, 243–244
clinical, 242–244
cystic degeneration, 244
cytogenetic abnormalities, 256
functional
gastrinoma, 246–247
glucagonoma, 246
insulinomas, 245
pancreatic polypeptide-secreting tumor (PPoma), 248
polyfunctional pancreatic endocrine tumor, 248
somatostatin-secreting pancreatic neuroendocrine tumor, 247–248
vasoactive intestinal peptide-secreting tumor (VIPoma), 247
genes associated with familial syndromes, 255–256
imaging, 244
microRNA, 257
molecular alterations, 255, 256
mutants, 48
nesidioblastosis, adult type, 257–262
nonfunctional, 253
octreotide scintigraphy, 244
palladin and RUNX1T1, 256–257
pathological classification, 9–12
pathology
cytopathology, 251–252
gross, 248
histopathology, 249–251
Pancreatic PD-NECs, 65
Pancreatic polypeptide-secreting tumor (PPoma), 248
Pancreatobiliary, NET, 40
Pancreatobiliary-related markers, 32
Papillary tumor of the pineal region (PTPR), 95
Paraganglioma
cystoscopy, 358
diffuse reactivity for synaptophysin, 358, 359
eosinophilic granular cytoplasm, 358
in FNA cytology and intraoperative cytology, 119
infiltrating into muscularis propria, 358, 359
NETs *vs.*, 34
organoid (nesting) pattern, 130
prostate, 369
therapy, 360
zellballen pattern, 358
Pasireotide (SOM-230), 447
P16/CDKN2A, 85
PDGFR-alpha, 469, 484
Peptic ulcers, 227–228
Peptide receptor radionuclide therapy (PRRT), 230, 501–502

Peptide receptors and NETs
EGFR
cell lines with mutations, 469
composition, 468
differential expression, 470–471
human NETs/PNETs, 469–470
in NET cell lines, 469
prognostic factor in pancreatic NETs, 471
sarcoma kinase (Src), 473
SCFR, 471–473
intracellular and downstream targets
dopamine 2 and somatostatin receptors in NETs, 476
dopamine receptors, 475
druggable targets, 475
mTOR inhibitors, 475
mTOR pathway, 473–475
SSTR
activation and effects on NET cells, 440–441, 468
detection by imaging, 444
expression correlates with pathology of human NETs, 443–444
expression on NET tissues, 444–445
in human NET and normal tissues, 442–443
signaling and downstream effects, 440
somatostatin analog monotherapy, 445–446
Pericytes, 455, 457
Periodic acid–Schiff–diastase (PAS-D) special stain, 32
Peripheral blood (PB), 424
Pheochromocytoma
in adrenal gland, 318
epidemiological and clinical features, 318
immunohistochemistry, 324–326
light microscopic findings
behavior, 320–323
biopsy, 320, 324
characteristics, 318, 319
ganglion cells, 320
nests of tumor, 318, 319
pathologic features, 323
molecular pathogenesis and testing, 327–330
neuroendocrine tumors, 14
penetrance, 115
prognostic factors, staging, and management, 330–331
RET germline mutation, 120
somatostatin receptor, 442
ultrastructure, 326–327
Pheochromocytoma of the Adrenal Gland Scaled Score (PASS), 331
PHH3, 254
Phosphatase and tensin homolog (PTEN), 483
Phosphoinositide 3-kinase (PI3K), 441
Phosphotyrosine phosphatases (PTPs), 500
PI3K/Akt/mTOR pathway, 276, 277, 484, 491
PIK3CA, 483
Pineal cyst, 95
Pineal parenchymal tumor of intermediate differentiation (PPTID), 95–98, 100–103
Pineal region tumors
clinical features of, 96
electron microscopic study, 101
genetics, 102–103
immunohistochemistry, 98–101
neuroimaging study, 96
pathology, 96–98
pineoblastoma, MRI characteristics, 97
prognosis, 103–104
Pineocytoma, 95–98
Pineocytomatous rosettes, 98
$P16^{INK4A}$, 167
Pituitary adenomas
classification, 16
clinical manifestation, 15–16
diagnostic and clinical management, 87–88
epigenetics, 81–82
functional classification of, 16–17
hormonal active tumors, 81
intracranial neoplasms, 81
oncogenes
CCND1 gene and cyclin D1 expression, 83–84
GSP, 82–83
pituitary tumor-transforming gene (PTTG), 83
ras, 83
pathology diagnosis, 82
radiologic classification, 17
tumor suppressor genes (TSG)
inappropriate miRNA expression patterns, 87
loci, 81
MEN1, 84
microRNA, 87
nm23, 85
p53, 84
p16/CDKN2A, 85
pituitary tumor-associated methylome, 86–87
p27/Kip1, 85–86
putative TSG loci, 86

retinoblastoma susceptibility gene (Rb), 84
WHO classification, 17
Pituitary tumor-associated methylome, 86–87
Pituitary tumor-transforming gene (PTTG), 83
P27/Kip1, 85–86, 432
Plasma chromogranin A (CgA), 244–245
Plasmacytoma, 119
Platelet-derived growth factor (PDGF), 94
Platelet-derived growth factor receptor (PDGFR), 456
Pleomorphism, 30
p-mTOR, 483, 484
PNET pathogenesis, 488
Polyfunctional pancreatic endocrine tumor, 248
Poorly differentiated invasive ductal carcinoma, 186–188
Poorly differentiated neuroblastoma, 337
Poorly differentiated neuroendocrine carcinoma
clinical features of, 61
gastric NETs, 214, 232
immunohistochemistry role in, 61–65
large cell carcinoma (LCC), 56–57
mixed adenoneuroendocrine carcinoma (MANEC), 57
prognosis, 66
response to therapy in, 66–67
site-specific, 57–60
small cell carcinoma (SCC), 56
Poorly differentiated synovial sarcomas (PDSS), 423
Postoperative levothyroxine, 131
PPoma. *See* Pancreatic polypeptide-secreting tumor (PPoma)
P16 promoter methylation, 276
PPTID. *See* Pineal parenchymal tumor of intermediate differentiation (PPTID)
1p/19q co-deletion, 92
Primary breast small cell carcinoma, 191
Primary NETs, 489
Primary neuroendocrine carcinoma of skin, 388. *See also* Merkel cell carcinoma (MCC)
Primary neuroendocrine carcinomas (NECs), 294–295
Primary small cell carcinoma, 381
Primary tumor, 405, 441, 467, 492
Primitive neuroectodermal tumor (PNET). *See also* Ewing sarcoma (ES)
composition, 420–421
differentiation, 421
Proangiogenic, human NETs, 454, 457–461
Progesterone receptors (PRs), 181
Prognosis, 66, 103–104, 143, 224, 290–291, 293, 300, 454, 484
Progression-free survival (PFS), 458
Progression genes, 488
Proliferation markers, 168–169
PROMID study, 434, 500
Prophylactic total thyroidectomy, 131
Prostate cancer
acinar adenocarcinoma, 370
adenocarcinoma with paneth cell-like NE differentiation, 369
carcinoid tumor, 365–367
endocrine differentiation within adenocarcinoma, 364–365
large-cell neuroendocrine carcinoma (LCNEC), 370
molecular features, 370–371
NETs *vs.*, 35–36
paraganglioma, 369
small cell carcinoma, 367–368
Proton pump inhibitors and G-NETs, 232
Pseudo-dysplastic foci, 30
PTEN, 93
PTPR. *See* Papillary tumor of the pineal region (PTPR)
Pure carcinoid tumors, 354
Putative TSG loci, 86

Q

qPCR, 471

R

Radiolabeled somatostatin analogs, 445
Radiotargeted therapy, 435
Raf pathway, 435
RAS genes, 83, 167
RASSF1A, 275–276
Receptor tyrosine kinases (RTKs), 452
Rectal NETs, 13
Rectum, PD-NEC, 58–59
Resistance
to temozolomide, 485
to VEGFR2 blockade, 459
RET germline mutations, 120, 121
Retinal S-antigen, 98, 101
Retinoblastoma gene, 166–167
Retinoblastoma susceptibility gene (Rb), 84
Retinoic acid, 169
Reverse-transcriptase polymerase chain reaction (rt-PCR), 442, 455, 457

Rhabdomyosarcoma (RMS), 423
Rhodopsin, 98
RIP1-Tag2 mouse model, 452–453
ROC curve analysis, 488
RUNX1T1, 256–257, 488

S

"Salt-pepper-like" chromatin pattern, 40
Sarcoma kinase (Src), 473
SCC. *See* Small cell carcinoma (SCC)
SCLC. *See* Small cell lung cancer (SCLC)
Sclerosing Ewing sarcoma, 421
SCNEC. *See* Small cell neuroendocrine cell carcinoma (SCNEC)
Sensitivity of RUNX1T1, 488
Sentinel lymph node biopsy (SLNB), 405
Serotonin, 95, 98, 433
Serum calcitonin and CEA, 119–120
Serum pancreatic polypeptide levels, PanNETs, 245
Signaling pathways, 441, 457, 459, 460
SI-NENs. *See* Small intestine neuroendocrine neoplasms (SI-NENs)
Single nucleotide polymorphism (SNP), 424
Single nucleotide variants (SNVs), 489
S6K, 484
SMAD genes, 491
Small cell carcinoma (SCC)
  mixed carcinoid tumors, 354
  nuclear molding and salt and pepper chromatin, 354, 355
  organoid and nested pattern, 354, 355
  PDNEC subtypes, 56
  prognosis, 354
  prostate cancer, 367–368
  pure carcinoid tumors, 354
  survival rate, 356
  urinary bladder cancer, 354–356
Small cell carcinoma of hypercalcemic type (SSC-H), 377
Small cell carcinoma of ovary-pulmonary type (SSC-P), 377–378
Small Cell Carcinoma of the Breast (SCCB), 177–179
Small cell lung cancer (SCLC)
  Azzopardi phenomenon, 160
  clinical symptoms and treatment, 160–161
  Ki-67 proliferative marker, 160
  low magnification, 159
Small-cell NEC, 309
Small cell neuroendocrine carcinoma of esophagus, 202
Small cell neuroendocrine cell carcinoma (SCNEC), 138, 141
Small cell pattern, MCC, 392, 394
Small intestine neuroendocrine neoplasms (SI-NENs)
  biomarkers, 280–282
  cancer-related pathways
    aldo-keto reductase family one member C3 (AKR1C3), 280
    EpCAM expression, 277–278
    gastric inhibitory polypeptide receptor (GIPR), 280
    G-protein-coupled receptors, 279
    PI3K/Akt/mTOR pathway, 276, 277
    receptor and membrane proteins changes, 278–279
    somatostatin receptor (SSTR), 280
    SRC oncogene pathway, 279
    TGF-β pathway, 276
    VEGF-R and IGF-R, 277
  diagnosis
    duodenal, 272
    jejunoileal, 272–273
  genetic profiling, 273–276
  gross features, 271
  microscopic features, 271–272
  molecular features, 273
  pathognomonic carcinoid syndrome, 271
  prognosis, 282
  treatment, 282
Small round blue cell (SRBC) proliferation, 391
Solid papillary carcinomas (SPC), 181, 184
Solid pseudopapillary neoplasm (SPN) *vs.* NETs, 34
Somatic mutations, 483
Somatostatin (SST), 431, 440, 441
Somatostatin analogs (SSAs)
  antiproliferative effect, 441
  clinical trials, 434
  direct effects of, 432–434
  monotherapy, 445–446
  octreotide therapy, 443, 445
  resistence to, 434
  targeted therapies, 467, 500–501, 506–507
  type I G-NETs, 226–227
Somatostatin and somatostatin receptors (SSTRs)
  activation and effects on NET cells, 440–441, 468
  detection by imaging, 444
  expression correlates with pathology of human NETs, 443–444
  expression on NET tissues, 444–445

in human NET and normal tissues, 442–443
scintigraphy, 444
signaling and downstream effects, 440
SI-NENs, 280
somatostatin analog monotherapy, 445–446
targeted therapies, 467
Somatostatinoma, 10–11, 247–248
Somatostatin receptor pathway
peptide receptor radionuclide therapy, 501–502
somatostatin analogs, 500–501
Somatostatin receptor signaling, 208
Somatostatin-secreting pancreatic neuroendocrine tumor, 247–248
Sorafenib, 505
Specificity of RUNX1T1, 488
S-100, pheochromocytoma, 324, 326
Spindle cell Ewing sarcoma, 421
Spindle cell tumors, 130
Sporadic gastric NETs, 228–230
Sporadic MTC, 15, 115
Sporadic tumors, 121, 124, 127
Squamous cell carcinoma, 393, 397, 398
SRC oncogene pathway, SI-NENs, 279
SSAs. *See* Somatostatin analogs (SSAs)
SSTR1, 432
SSTR2, 432
SSTR3, 432
SSTR4, 432
SSTRs. *See* Somatostatin and somatostatin receptors (SSTRs)
Staging, NETs
AJCC system for classification, 24–26
blood/lymphatic system, 23
ENETS system for classification, 23
TNM systems, 22
UICC system for classification, 24
WHO 2000 classification system, 22
Stomach, gastric PD-NEC, 57, 67
Strumal and mucinous carcinoids, 374
Subepithelial neuroendocrine cells (SNC), 286
Substance P, 433
Sunitinib, 435, 505
Surveillance, Epidemiology and End Results (SEER) program, 22
Synaptophysin, 62, 324–325

T

Tachykinin, 433
Targeted therapies
chimeric somatostatin, 435
clinical trials and SSAs, 434
immunotherapy, 436
molecular biology, 431
for neuroendocrine neoplasms
EGFR, 506
inhibitors of VEGFR, 505–506
mTOR pathway
mTOR pathway: everolimus, 502–503
mTOR pathway: temsirolimus, 503–504
somatostatin analogs, 506–507
somatostatin receptor pathway
somatostatin receptor pathway: peptide receptor radionuclide therapy, 501–502
somatostatin receptor pathway: somatostatin analogs, 500–501
VEGF pathway
VEGF pathway: bevacizumab, 504–505
VEGF pathway: sorafenib, 505
VEGF pathway: sunitinib, 505
radiotargeted therapy, 435
somatostatin analogues (SSAs), 432
SSTRs expression patterns
biology, 432
carcinoid syndrome, 433–434
direct effects, 432–433
indirect effects, 433
interferon ALPHA, 433
targeted agents, 434–435
telotristat etiprate (LX1606), 435
Tau protein, 98
Telomerase reverse transcriptase (TERT) promoter mutations, 360
Telotristat etiprate (LX1606), 435
Temsirolimus, 503–504
TGF-β pathway, SI-NENs, 276
Thymic NETs
classification, 141
diagnostic radiology, 139
differential diagnosis, 141–142
epidemiology, 138
gross features, 140
immunohistochemical stains, 141
location, 138–139
management and follow-up, 143
microscopic features, 140–141
molecular pathology, 142
prognosis, 143
response evaluation, 143
symptoms, 139
terminology, 138
tumorigenesis, 139

Thyroidectomy, 130–131
Thyroid transcription factor 1 (TTF-1), 64, 191
Tie-2 receptor, 455–456
Time to tumor progression (TTP), 500
Tissue microarrays, 492
TNM staging system
AJCC system, 22
appendiceal NEN, 26
gastric NENs, 25
gastroenteropancreatic (GEP) NETs, 23
NETs classification, 22
pancreatic NENs, 25
Transcription factors, 460, 489
Transforming growth factor alpha (TGF-alpha), 484
TTF-1, 489
Tuberous sclerosis, 47
Tuberous sclerosis complex (TSC), 242–243, 487
Tuberous sclerosis complex 2 gene (TSC2), 483
Tubular carcinoid, 12, 288–290
Tumor
angiogenesis, 452
atypical carcinoid (AC), 141
large cell neuroendocrine cell carcinoma (LCNEC), 138, 141, 143
mediastinum (*see* Mediastinum, NETs)
small cell neuroendocrine cell carcinoma (SCNEC), 138, 141
suppressor genes, 166–168
thymic (*see* Thymic NETs)
typical carcinoid (TC), 141
Tumor suppressor genes (TSG)
inappropriate miRNA expression patterns, 87
loci, 81
MEN1, 84
microRNA, 87
nm23, 85
p53, 84
p16/CDKN2A, 85
pituitary tumor-associated methylome, 86–87
p27/Kip1, 85–86
putative TSG loci, 86
retinoblastoma susceptibility gene (Rb), 84
Typical carcinoid (TC), 141
Tyrosine kinase inhibitors (TKIs), 458

U
Undifferentiated thyroid carcinoma, 119
Union for International Cancer Control (UICC), 24
Urine 5-HIAA, serological and laboratory markers, 32
Uterine cervix NET, 378–379

V
Vascular-endothelial growth factor (VEGF), 453, 454, 500
Vascularity of human, 454
Vascular remodeling, 455
Vasoactive Intestinal Peptide (VIP), 446, 468
Vasoactive intestinal peptide-secreting tumor (VIPoma), 10, 247
VEGF-C, 453, 454
VEGF-pathway
bevacizumab, 504–505
inhibition, 458–459
sorafenib, 505
VEGFR, 460
VEGFR1, 453, 457
VEGFR2, 459
VEGFR3, 453, 454
VEGFR2 blockade, 459
VEGF receptor (VEGFR), 277, 458, 460
Verner-Morrison Syndrome, 10
Vesicular monoamine transporter 2 (VMAT2), 218
VIPoma. *See* Vasoactive intestinal peptide-secreting tumor (VIPoma)
von Hippel-Lindau (vHL) syndrome
hereditary pheochromocytoma, 327–328
NET patients, 47, 487
PanNETs, 242–243, 249
von Recklinghausen's disease, 47

W
Watery Diarrhea, 10
WDHA Syndrome, 10
Weibel-Palade bodies, 455
WHO
digestive and pancreatic NETs, 4–5
gastroenteropancreatic NETs, 22

GEP-NENs, grading nomenclature, 8
GEP-NETs, 7
lung and thymus, 14
NET grading criteria, 8
neuroendocrine tumor classification, 9
pituitary tumors, 15
pulmonary and thymic tumors, 8
tumor classification, 177
WIF1, 275
Wilms' tumor (WT), 423
Wnt pathway/PROX1 protein, 313

X
X-chromosomal inactivation analysis, 81

Z
Zollinger-Ellison syndrome (ZES), 9, 10, 216, 227–228

MIX
Papier aus verantwortungsvollen Quellen
Paper from responsible sources
FSC® C105338
FSC
www.fsc.org

If you have any concerns about our products,
you can contact us on
ProductSafety@springernature.com

In case Publisher is established outside the EU,
the EU authorized representative is:
Springer Nature Customer Service Center GmbH
Europaplatz 3, 69115 Heidelberg, Germany

Printed by Libri Plureos GmbH
in Hamburg, Germany